Medicinal Plants, Trees and Herbs

Volume 2 and Volume 3 are available through Starrisingpublishers.com

Volume 2 contains I-Z listings

Volume 3 Contains full color images of plants, trees and herbs.

Library of Congress Cataloging-in-Publication Data:

Grieve, Sophia

Medicinal Plants, Trees and Herbs (Volume 1 A-H)/ Sophia Grieve

ISBN-10: 1-893774-75-9

ISBN-13: 978-1-893774-75-9

Printed in the United States of America

Book Design by Star Rising Publishers

First Edition: April 2012

10 9 8 7 6 5 4 3 2 1

Medicinal Plants, Trees and Herbs

The Medicinal, Culinary, Cosmetic and Economic Properties,
Cultivation and History of Herbs, Plants & Trees
with Their Scientific Uses

Volume 1 (A-F)

Sophia Grieve

Contents

INTRODUCTION

BOTANY and medicine came down the ages hand in hand until the seventeenth century; then both arts became scientific, their ways parted, and no new herbals were compiled. The botanical books ignored the medicinal properties of plants and the medical books contained no plant lore.

The essence of a herbal was the combination of traditional plant lore, the medicinal properties of the herbs, and their botanical classification. From the time of Dioscorides down to Parkinson in 1629 this herbal tradition was unbroken. Culpeper's popular herbal was discredited with scientific people because it was astrological.

The death of the herbal was one of the reasons why, with a few exceptions, the only plants which have retained their place in the Allopaths' pharmacopoeias are poisonous ones like Aconite, Belladonna, Henbane and the Opium Poppy.

Dandelion, Gentian and Valerian for some reason have survived and the Homeopaths use many more, but such useful plants as Agrimony, Slippery Elm, Horehound, Bistort, Poplar, Bur Marigold, Wood Betony, Wood Sanicle, Wild Carrot, Raspberry leaves, and the Sarsaparillas are now only used by Herbalists.

All serious Herbalists have long realized that a new Herbal is badly needed - a herbal which must include the traditional lore and properties of plants, and the modern use of properly standardized extracts and tinctures which were unknown in the days of Gerard and Parkinson, and even in the days of Culpeper, and which have been made possible by the development of modern chemistry.

The interest for the amateur can only be an historical one, because the herbal tinctures and extracts are too potent to be prescribed or experimented with by the unskilled or the inexperienced; in fact, it is as dangerous for amateurs to doctor themselves indiscriminately with herbs, as is would be for them to administer drugs in their alkaloid form.

A knowledge of herbs is as necessary as a knowledge of Pathology, if herbal treatment for all but the simplest ailments is to be successful.

Each herb has its own indications for use, and successful prescribing depends upon the correspondence between these indications and the patient's symptoms. Then, and only then, will the result be altogether successful.

Most of the modern scientific work on the right use of herbs we owe to Hahnemann and his successors.

That famous head master, Edward Thring, first taught me botany when I was a baby, in the School House garden and Uppingham fields. I still remember the pride I felt when he strapped the black japanned tin lined with green to my tiny back, and though at the time I was only four and much too young to enjoy searching in the heat for rare plants like Ladies' Tresses and Green Hellebore, the names of the plants, like the dates of the English kings, were impressed upon my mind so vividly that it has been impossible for me ever to forget them.

After Edward Thring's death, his daughter Sarah carried on my lessons, and I have never lost touch with the subject.

At one time there was an idea of my entering the medical profession, but I was put off by my first lesson in dissection.

I have always experimented in the innocent alchemy of scent blending and cooking, but it was not until I had written my first book on herbs that the idea came to me to found the Society of Herbalists, and since 1926 I have done nothing else but research work in herbal medicine.

Just before I opened Culpeper House, a list of Sophia Grieve's monographs on herbs came to me through the post. I made her acquaintance, and after examining the pamphlets, thought they might be the nucleus of the much-needed modern herbal.

I took the monographs and the suggestion to Mr.

Cape, who agreed to publish them if I would collate and edit them and see that the American herbs were also included.

Sophia Grieve's original pamphlets only included the English herbs, many of which she grew in her Buckinghamshire garden

During the War, when there was a shortage of medicinal plants because they could no longer be imported from abroad, Sophia Grieve made practical use of her knowledge and trained pupils in the work of drying and preparing herbs for the chemists' market.

She did a great deal to revive the herb industry in England.

The arrangement and the editing of the vast quantity of material which Sophia Grieve had accumulated has been a task of some difficulty. I have arranged the plants alphabetically under their most familiar names, hoping to interest flower-lovers as well as doctors, and in this way they are as easily found as the words in a dictionary. The country names are in the index.

This is not the orthodox arrangement either from the Herbalist's, or the Homeopath's, or the Allopath's, point of view.

Herbalists talk about Jalap and Black Haw, but to the uninitiated Bindweed and Guelder Rose are far more familiar, and it is under these names that they will be found in this herbal.

In homeopathy the Anemone and the Forget-me-not are known as Pulsatilla and Myosotis, and chemists accustomed to the Latin names may be shocked to find Taraxacum under Dandelion, Podophyllum under Mandrake, and Calendula under Marigold.

The very names of the plants are so interesting; the names are often derived from their original use in medicine, and the traditional use has been derived from some peculiarity of the plant based on the doctrine of signatures, its shape, growth, colour, scent or taste, or habitat.

For instance, the flower of the Scullcap, one of the best cures for insomnia, has a strong resemblance to the shape of the human skull. The Yellow Cedar has a curious sinister appearance and is used to cure fungoid growths. The little blue flower of the Eyebright with its yellow centre suggests the human eye, and is so useful for tired eyes that the French have called it 'casse lunettes.'

The flowers of many of the herbs which purify the blood are red in colour, e.g. the Scarlet Pimpernel, the Burdock, the Red Clover.

The medicinal value of Nettles is indicated by their sting; they are used internally to stimulate the circulation.

When a plant has a particularly unpleasant smell like the stinking Arrach, it usually points to a particular use - the stinking Arrach is used for foul ulcers.

The bark of the Willow cures rheumatism brought on by damp, and the tree grows in wet places.

Most of the flowers used for jaundice are yellow, like the Dandelion, Agrimony, Celandine, Hawkweed and Marigold.

Viper's Buglass is considered an antidote to snakebite, and its seed is not unlike the reptile's head.

Lungwort, because of its spotted leaves, was used for diseased lungs.

The classical names often embody the tradition which goes back to legendary times. For instance, Bellis Perennis chronicles the wound-healing properties of the Daisy. Tussilago Farfara is the botanical name for the Coltsfoot, which is used to cure coughs and colds, and Valerian is derived from the Latin word Valere.

Surely it makes a garden more romantic and wonderful to know that Wallflowers, Irises, Lupins, Delphiniums, Columbines, Dahlias and Chrysanthemums, every flower in the garden from the first Snowdrop to the Christmas Rose, are not only there for man's pleasure but have their compassionate use in his pain.

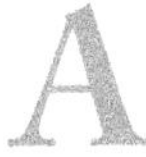

ABSCESS ROOT

Botanical: Polemonium reptans
Family: N.O. Polemoniaceae
Synonyms: American Greek Valerian. Blue Bells. False Jacob's Ladder. Sweatroot.
Habitat: United States.

Description

This plant grows from New York to Wisconsin, in woods, damp grounds, and along shady river-banks. It has creeping roots, by which it multiplies very quickly. The stems are 9 to 10 inches high, much branched, bearing pinnate leaves with six or seven pairs of leaflets. The nodding, blue flowers are in loose, terminal bunches.

The slender rootstock, when dried and used as the drug, is 1 to 2 inches long and 1/8 inch in diameter, with the bases of numerous stems on the upper surface, and tufts of pale, slender, smooth, wiry, brittle roots on the underside. The rootstock has a slightly bitter and acrid taste.

Medicinal Action and Uses

Astringent, alterative, diaphoretic, expectorant. The drug has been recommended for use in febrile and inflammatory eases, all scrofulous diseases, in bowel complaints requiring an astringent, for the bites of venomous snakes and insects, for bronchitis and laryngitis and whenever an alterative is required. It is reported to have cured consumption; an infusion of the root in wine glassful doses is useful in coughs, colds and all lung complaints, producing copious perspiration.

The tincture of the root is made of whisky.

Dosage

1 to 2 fluid ounces, two or three times a day.

ACACIAS

Family: N.O. Leguminosae

Acacias (nat. order, Leguminosae) are composed of handsome trees and shrubby bushes scattered over the warmer regions of the globe. The flowers are arranged in rounded or elongated clusters, the leaves generally compoundly pinnate, i.e. divided into leaflets up to the mid-rib and each leaflet similarly cut into narrow segments.

In several of the Australian species the leaflets are suppressed and the leaf stalks, vertically flattened serve the purpose of leaves. Some species afford valuable timber: the black wood of Australia, which is used for furniture because it takes such a high polish, is the wood of the . melanoxylon. The bark of another Australian species, known as Wattles, is rich in tannin and forms a valuable article of export. The pods of other species are employed in Egypt and Nubia for their tannin. The pods of the A. Concuine are used by Indian women in the same way as the soapnut for washing the head; and the leaves of the same tree are employed in cookery for their acidity.

Certain tribes on the Amazon use the seeds of another species, the Acacia Niopo, for snuff combined with lime and cocculus. Various species of acacia yield gum; but the best gum arabic used in medicine is an exudation from the A. Senegal. This species grows abundantly in East and West tropical Africa, forming forests in Senegambia north of the River Senegal. Most of the gum acacia collected in Upper Egypt and the Sudan is produced by the A. verek, and is known locally as Hachah.

ACACIA BARK

Botanical: Acacia decurrens, Acacia arabica
Family: N.O. Leguminosae
Synonym: Wattle Bark

Acacia Bark, known as Wattle Bark, is obtained from the chief of the Australian Wattles, A. decurrens (Willd.), the Black Wattle, and, more recently, A. arabica has been similarly used in East Africa for its astringency.

The bark is collected from wild or cultivated trees, seven years old or more, and must be allowed to mature for a year before being used medicinally.

Description

The bark of A. decurrens is usually in curved pieces, externally greyish brown, darkening with age, often with irregular longitudinal ridges and sometimes transverse cracks. Inner surface longitudinally striated, fracture irregular and coarsely fibrous. It has a slight tan-like odor and astringent taste.

The bark of A. arabica is hard and woody, rusty brown and tending to divide into several layers. The outer surface of older pieces is covered with thick blackish periderm, rugged and fissured. The inner surface is red, longitudinally striated and fibrous. Taste, astringent and mucilaginous.

Constituents

Acacia Bark contains from 24 to 42 per cent. of tannin and also gallic acid.

Its powerful astringency causes it to be extensively employed in tanning.

Medicinal Action and Uses

Medicinally it is employed as a substitute for Oak Bark. It has special use in diarrhea, mainly in the form of a decoction, the British Pharmacopoeia preparation being 6 parts in 100 administered in doses of 1/2 to 2 fluid ounces. The decoction also is used as an astringent gargle, lotion, or injection.

A liquid extract is prepared from the bark of A. arabica, administered in India for its astringent properties in doses of 1/2 to 1 fluid drachm, but the use of both gum and bark for industrial purposes is much larger than their use in medicine. The bark, under the name of Babul, is used in Scinde for tanning, and also for dyeing various shades of brown.

ACACIA (FALSE)

Botanical: Robinia pseudacacia
Family: N.O. Leguminosae
Synonym: Locust Tree

In common language, the term Acacia is often applied to species of the genus Robinia which also belongs to the family Leguminosae, though to a different section.

R. pseudacacia, the False Acacia or Locust Tree, one of the most valuable timber trees of the American forest, where it grows to a very large size, was one of the first trees introduced into England from America, and is cultivated as an ornamental tree in the milder parts of Britain, forming a large tree, with beautiful pea-like blossoms.

The timber is supposed to unite the qualities of strength and durability to a degree unknown in any other kind of tree, being very hard and close-grained. It has been extensively used for ship-building, being superior for the purpose to American Oak, and is largely used in the construction of the wooden pins called trenails, used to fasten the planks to the ribs or timber of ships. Instead of decaying, it acquires an extraordinary degree of hardness with time. It is also suitable for posts and fencing and other purposes where durability in contact with the ground is essential, and is used for axle-trees and other mechanical purposes, though not for general purposes of construction.

The roots and inner bark have a sweetish, but somewhat offensive and nauseating taste, and have been found poisonous to foraging animals.

Medicinal Action and Uses

The inner bark contains a poisonous proteid substance, Robin, which possesses strong emetic and purgative properties. It is capable of coagulating the casein of milk and of clotting the red corpuscles of certain animals.

Tonic, emetic and purgative properties have been ascribed to the root and bark, but the locust tree is rarely, if ever, prescribed as a therapeutic agent.

Occasional cases of poisoning are on record in which boys have chewed the bark and swallowed the juice: the principal symptoms being dryness of the throat, burning pain in the abdomen, dilatation of the pupils, vertigo and muscular twitches; excessive quantities causing also weak and irregular heart action.

Though the leaves of Robinia have also been stated to produce poisonous effects careful examination has failed to detect the presence of any soluble proteid or of alkaloids, and by some the leaves have been recorded as even affording wholesome food for cattle.

The flowers contain a glucoside, Robinin, which, on being boiled with acids, is resolved into sugar and quercetin

ACACIA (GUM)

Botanical: Acacia nilotica (LINN.)
Family: N.O. Leguminosae
Part Used: Gummy Exudation from stem.

ACACIA NILOTICA (LINN.) All the gum-yielding Acacias exhibit the same habit and general appearance, differing only in technical characters. They are spiny shrubs or small trees, preferring sandy or sterile regions, with the climate dry during the greater part of the year.

The gum harvest from the various species lasts about five weeks. About the middle of November, after the rainy season, it exudes spontaneously from the trunk and principal branches, but the flow is generally stimulated by incisions in the bark, a thin strip, 2 to 3 feet in length and 1 to 3 inches wide being torn off. In about fifteen days it thickens in the furrow down which it runs, hardening on exposure to the air, usually in the form of round or oval tears, about the size of a pigeon's egg, but sometimes in vermicular forms, white or red, according to whether the species is a white or red gum tree.

About the middle of December, the Moors commence the harvesting. The masses of gum are collected, either while adhering to the bark, or after it falls to the ground, the entire product, often of various species, thus collected, is packed in baskets and very large sacks of tanned leather and brought on camels and bullocks to the centres of accumulation and then to the points of export, chiefly Suakin, Alexandria, or - in Senegambia - St. Louis. It is then known as 'Acacia sorts," the term being equivalent to 'unassorted Acacia." The unsorted gums show the widest variation as to size of fragments, whiteness, clearness, freedom from adhering matter, etc. It is next sorted or 'picked' in accordance with these differences.

There are many kinds of Acacia Gum in commerce:

KORDOFAN GUM, collected in Upper Egypt and the Sudan, in Kordofan, Dafur and Arabia, and exported from Alexandria, is considered the best and is the kind generally used in pharmacy. It consists of small, irregular pieces, commonly whitish, or slightly tinged with yellow, and is freer from impurities than most other commercial varieties. But those known in commerce as 'Turkey sorts' and 'Trieste picked," which are brought from the Sudan by way of Suakin, are equally suitable for medicinal use.

SENEGAL GUM, of two varieties, produced by two different trees, one yielding a white, the other a red gum, is usually in roundish or oval unbroken pieces of various sizes, larger than those of Turkey Gum, less brittle and pulverizable, less fissured and often occurs in long, cylindrical or curved pieces.

The term 'Gum Senegal' is not, strictly speaking, synonymous with Gum Acacia, though it is commonly so used. Gum Acacia is the name originally pertaining to Sudan, Kordofan or Egyptian (hashabi) Gum, which possesses properties rendering it superior and always preferred to any other known to commerce. During the political and military disturbances in Egypt between 1880 and 1890, this gum became so nearly unobtainable that occasional packages only were seen in the market. Among the many substitutes then offered, the best was Gum Senegal, which was adopted as the official equivalent of Gum Acacia. In this way, it came about that the names were regarded as synonymous. In 1890, the original Acacia again came into the market and eventually became as abundant as ever, but it is no longer possible to entirely separate the two names. Most of the characteristically distinct grades of Acacia Gum are now referred to particular species of the genus Acacia. Most works state that both the Kordofan and Senegal Gums are products of A. Senegal (Willd.), the range of which is thus given as Senegambia in West Africa, the Upper Nile region in Eastern Africa, with more or less of the intervening central region.

A. glaucophylla (Staud.) and A. Abyssinica (Hochst.) are said to yield an equally good gum, but little of it is believed to reach the market.

Mogadore Gum, from A. gummifera (Willd), a tall tree found in Morocco and in the Isle of Bourbon, occurs in rather large pieces, closely resembling Kordofan Gum in appearance.

Indian Gum, the product of A. arabica, the Gum Arabic tree of India. The gum of this and other Indian species of Acacia is there used as a substitute for the official Gum Acacia, to which it is, however, inferior. Indian Gum is sweeter in taste than that of the other varieties, and usually contains portions of a different kind of gum.

Cape Gum is also imported. It is of a pale yellow color and is considered of inferior quality.

AUSTRAILIAN GUM, imported from South Australia, is in elongated or globular pieces, rough and even wrinkled on the surface and of a violet tint, which distinguishes it from other varieties. It is not entirely soluble in water, to which it imparts less viscidity than ordinary Gum Acacia. It frequently contains tannin.

Gum Acacia for medicinal purposes should be in roundish 'tears' of various sizes, colorless or pale yellow, or broken into angular fragments with a glass-like, sometimes iridescent fracture, often opaque from numerous fissures, but transparent and nearly colorless in thin pieces; taste insipid, mucilaginous; nearly inodorous. It should be almost entirely soluble in water, forming a viscid neutral solution, or mucilage, which, when evaporated, yields the gum unchanged. It is insoluble in alcohol and ether, but soluble in diluted alcohol in proportion to the amount of water present. It should be slowly but completely soluble in two parts of water: this solution shows an acid reaction with litmuspaper. The powdered gum is not coloured blue (indicating absence of starch) or red (indicating absence of dextrin) by the iodine test solution. It should not yield more than 4 per cent of ash.

Adulteration

Adulteration in the crude state is confined almost wholly to the addition of similar and inferior gums, the detection of which requires only familiarity with the genuine article.

In the ground condition it is adulterated oftenest with starch and dextrins, tests for which are given in the official description. Tannin is present in inferior gums and can be detected by the bluish-black coloration produced on adding ferric chloride. Gums of a yellow or brown color usually contain tannin, and these, together with such as are incompletely soluble in water and which yield ropy or glairy solutions, should not be used for medicinal purposes.

Chemical Constituents

Gum Acacia consists principally of Arabin, a compound of Arabic acid with calcium, varying amounts of the magnesium and potassium salts of the same acid being present. It is believed, also, that small amounts of other salts of these bases occur. (Arabic acid can be obtained by precipitating with alcohol from a solution of Acacia acidulated with hydrochloric acid.) The gum also contains 12 to 17 per cent of moisture and a trace of sugar, and yields 2.7 to 4 per cent of ash, consisting almost entirely of calcium, magnesium and potassium carbonates.

Medicinal Action and Uses

Gum Acacia is a demulcent and serves by the viscidity of its solution to cover and sheathe inflamed surfaces.

It is usually administered in the form of a mucilage - Mucilago Acaciae, British Pharmacopoeia and United States Pharmacopoeia made from small pieces of Gum Acacia dissolved in water and strained (1 in 8.75).

Dose

in syrup, 1 to 4 drachms of the gum. Mucilage of Acacia is a nearly transparent, colorless or scarcely yellowish, viscid liquid, having a faint, rather agreeable odor and an insipid taste. It is employed as a soothing agent in inflammatory conditions of the respiratory, digestive and urinary tract, and is useful in diarrhea and dysentery. It exerts a soothing influence upon all the surfaces with which it comes in contact. It may be diluted and flavoured to suit the taste. In low stages of typhoid fever, this mucilage, sweetened, is greatly recommended. The ordinary dose of the mucilage is from 1 to 4 fluid drachms.

In dispensing, Mucilage of Acacia is used for suspending insoluble powders in mixtures, for emulsifying oils and other liquids which are not miscible with water, and as an ingredient of many cough linctures. The British Pharmacopoeia directs it to be used as an excipient in the preparation of troches. Compound Mucilage of Acacia - Pill-coating Acacia - is made from Gum Acacia, 1 in 10, with tragacanth, chloroform and water, and is used for moistening pills previous to coating.

Gum Acacia is an ingredient of the official Pilula Ferri, Pulvis Amygdalae compositus, Pulvis Tragacanthae compositus, all the official Trochisci, and various syrups, pastes and pastilles or jujubes.

Acacia Mixture, Mistura Acaciae of the British Pharmacopoeia Codex, is made from Gum Acacia (6 in 100) with syrup and diluted orange-flower water, employed as a demulcent in cough syrups and linctures.

Dose

1 to 4 fluid drachms. Syrup of Acacia, British Pharmacopoeia Codex, used chiefly as a demulcent in cough mixtures, is freshly prepared as required, from 1 part of Gum Acacia Mucilage and 3 of syrup, the dose, 1 to 4 fluid drachms.

The United States Pharmacopoeia Syrup of Acacia, though regarded as a useful demulcent, is chiefly employed as an agent for suspending powders in mixtures.

The French Pharmacopoeia has a Syrup of Acacia and a potion gommeuse made from powdered Acacia, syrup and orange-flower water.

As a dry excipient, powdered Acacia is employed, mixed in small proportion with powdered Marsh Mallow root, or powdered Liquorice root. A variation of this is a mixture of Acacia, 50 parts; Liquorice root, 34 parts; Sugar, 16 parts, all in fine powder. Another compound Acacia Powder used sparingly as an absorbent pill excipient, is made of equal parts of Gum Acacia and Tragacanth.

Gum Acacia is highly nutritious. During the time of the gum harvest, the Moors of the desert are said to live almost entirely on it, and it has been proved that 6 oz. is sufficient to support an adult for twenty-four hours. It is related that the Bushman Hottentots have been known in times of scarcity to support themselves on it for days together. In many cases of disease, it is considered that a solution of Gum Arabic may for a time constitute the exclusive drink and food of the patient.

ACONITE

POISON
Steadman Shorter's Medical Dictionary, Poisons & Antidotes: Aconite
Botanical: Aconitum napellus (LINN.)
Family: N.O. Ranunculaciae
Synonyms: Monkshood. Blue Rocket. Friar's Cap. Auld Wife's Huid.
Part Used: The whole plant.

Habitat

Lower mountain slopes of North portion of Eastern Hemisphere. From Himalayas through Europe to Great Britain.

Aconite is now found wild in a few parts of England, mainly in the western counties and also in South Wales, but can hardly be considered truly indigenous. It was very early introduced into England, being mentioned in all the English vocabularies of plants from the tenth century downwards, and in Early English medical recipes.

Description

The plant is a hardy perennial, with a fleshy, spindle-shaped root, palecoloured when young, but subsequently acquiring a dark brown skin. The stem is about 3 feet high, with dark green, glossy leaves, deeply divided in palmate manner and flowers in erect clusters of a dark blue color. The shape of the flower is specially designed to attract and utilize bee visitors, especially the humble bee. The sepals are purple - purple being specially attractive to bees - and are fancifully shaped, one of them being in the form of a hood. The petals are only represented by the two very curious nectaries within the hood, somewhat in the form of a hammer; the stamens are numerous and lie depressed in a bunch at the mouth of the flower. They are pendulous at first, but rise in succession and place their anthers forward in such a way that a bee visiting the flower for nectar is dusted with the pollen, which he then carries to the next flower he visits and thereby fertilizes the undeveloped fruits, which are in a tuft in the centre of the stamens, each carpel containing a single seed.

In the Anglo-Saxon vocabularies it is called thung, which seems to have been a general name for any very poisonous plant. It was then called Aconite (the English form of its Greek and Latin name), later Wolf's Bane, the direct translation of the Greek Iycotonum, derived from the idea that arrows tipped with the juice, or baits anointed with it, would kill wolves - the species mentioned by Dioscorides seems to have been Aconitum lycotonum. In the Middle Ages it became Monkshood and Helmet-flower, from the curious shape of the upper sepal overtopping the rest of the flower. This was the ordinary name in Shakespeare's days.

The generic name is said to have been derived from , a dart, because it was used by barbarous races to poison their arrows, or from akone, cliffy or rocky, because the species grow in rocky glens. Theophrastus, like Pliny, derived the name from Aconae, the supposed place of its origin. The specific name, Napellus, signifies a little turnip, in allusion to the shape of the roots.

Cultivation

The chief collecting centres for foreign Aconite root have been the Swiss Alps, Salzburg, North Tyrol and Vorarlberg. Much was also formerly collected in Germany. Supplies from Spain and Japan are imported, so that the demand for English Aconite is somewhat restricted. The official Aconite is directed by the British Pharmacopeia to be derived only from plants cultivated in England, and a certain amount of home-grown Aconite has been regularly produced by the principal drug-farms, though good crops are grown with some difficulty in England, and cultivation of Aconite has not paid very well in recent years.

Aconite prefers a soil slightly retentive of moisture, such as a moist loam, and flourishes best in shade. It would probably grow luxuriantly in a moist, open wood, and would yield returns with little further trouble than weeding, digging up and drying.

In preparing beds for growing Aconite, the soil should be well dug and pulverized by early winter frosts - the digging in of rotten leaves or stable manure is advantageous.

It can be raised from seed, sown 1/2 inch deep in a cold frame in March, or in a warm position outside in April, but great care must be exercised that the right kind is obtained, as there are many varieties of Aconite- about twenty-four have been distinguished - and they have not all the same active medicinal properties. It takes two or three years to flower from seed.

Propagation is usually by division of roots in the autumn. The underground portion of the plants are dug up after the stem has died down, and the smaller of the 'daughter' roots that have developed at the side of the old roots are selected for replanting in December or January to form new stock, the young roots being planted about a foot apart each way. The young shoots appear above ground in February. Although the plants are perennial, each distinct root lasts only one year, the plant being continued by 'daughter' roots.

This official Aconite is also the species generally cultivated in gardens, though nearly all the species are worth growing as ornamental garden flowers, the best perhaps being A. Napellus, both white and blue,

A. paniculatum, A. Japonicum and A. autumnale. All grow well in shade and under trees. Gerard grew four species in his garden: A. lyocotonum, A. variegatum, A. Napellus and A. Pyrenaicum.

Part Used

Collection and Drying. The leaves, stem, flowering tops and root: the leaves and tops fresh, the root dried. The leaves and flowering tops are of less importance, they are employed for preparing Extract of Aconitum, and for this purpose are cut when the flowers are just breaking into blossom and the leaves are in their best condition, which is in June.

The roots should be collected in the autumn, after the stem dies down, but before the bud that is to produce the next year's stem has begun to develop. As this bud grows and forms a flowering stem, in the spring, some of the lateral buds develop into short shoots, each of which produces a long, slender, descending root, crowned with a bud. These roots rapidly thicken, filled with reserve material produced by the parent plant, the root of which dies as the 'daughter' roots increase in size. Towards the autumn, the parent plant dies down and the daughter roots which have then reached their maximum development are now full of starch. If allowed to remain in the soil, the buds that crown the daughter roots begin to grow, in the late winter, and this growth exhausts the strength of the root, and the proportion of both starch and alkaloid it contains is lessened.

On account of the extremely poisonous properties of the root, it is considered desirable that the root should be grown and collected under the same conditions, so that uniformity in the drug is maintained. The British Pharmacopeia specifies, therefore, that the roots should be collected in the autumn from plants cultivated in Britain and should consist of the dried, full-grown 'daughter' roots: much of the Aconite root that used to come in large quantities from Germany was the exhausted parent root of the wild-flowering plants.

When the roots are dug up, they are sorted over, the smallest laid aside for replanting and the plumper ones reserved for drying. They are first well washed in cold water and trimmed of all rootlets, and then dried, either entire, or longitudinally sliced to hasten drying.

Drying may at first be done in the open air, spread thinly, the roots not touching. Or they may be spread on clean floors or on shelves in a warm place for about ten days, turning frequently. When somewhat shrunken, they must be finished more quickly by artificial heat in a drying room or shed near a stove or gas fire, care being taken that the heated air can escape at the top of the room. Drying in an even temperature will probably take about a fortnight or more. It is not complete till the roots are dry to the core and brittle, snapping when bent.

Dried Aconite root at its upper extremity, when crowned with an undeveloped bud, enclosed by scaly leaves, is about 3/4 inch in diameter, tapering quickly downwards. It is dark brown in color and marked with the scars of rootlets. The surface is usually longitudinally wrinkled, especially if it has been dried entire. The root breaks with a short fracture and should be whitish and starchy within. A transverse section shows a thick bark, separated from the inner portion by a well-marked darker line, which often assumes a stellate appearance. Aconite root as found in commerce is, however, often yellowish or brownish internally with the stellate markings not clearly shown, probably from having been collected too early. It should be lifted in the autumn of the second year.

Aconite root is liable to attack by insects, and after being well dried should be kept in securely closed vessels.

Chemical Constituents

Aconite root contains from 0.3 to 1 per cent alkaloidal matter, consisting of Aconitine - crystalline, acrid and highly toxic - with the alkaloids Benzaconine (Picraconitine) and Aconine.

Aconitine, the only crystallizable alkaloid, is present to the extent of not more than 0.2 per cent, but to it is due the characteristic activity of the root. Aconite acid, starch, etc., are also present. On incineration, the root yields about 3 per cent ash.

The Aconitines are a group of highly toxic alkaloids derived from various species of Aconite, and whilst possessing many properties in common are chemically distinguishable according to the source from which they are obtained. The Aconitines are divided into two groups: (1) the Aconitines proper, including Aconitine, Japaconitine and Indaconitine, and (2) the Pseudaconitines - Pseudaconitine and Bikhaconitine.

This disparity between Aconites is a very important matter for investigation, though perhaps not so serious from a pharmaceutical point of view as might at first appear, since in the roots of several different species the alkaloid is found to possess similar physiological action; but this action varies in degree and the amount of alkaloid may be found to vary considerably. It is considered that the only reliable method of standardizing the potency of any of the Aconite preparations is by a physiological method: the lethal dose for the guinea-pig being considered to be the most convenient and satisfactory standard. Tinctures vary enormously as to strength, some proving seven times as powerful as others.

The Aconite which contains the best alkaloid, A. Napellus, is the old-fashioned, familiar garden variety, which may be easily recognized by its very much cut-up leaves, which are wide in the shoulder of the leaf - that part nearest the stem - and also by the purplish-blue flowers, which have the 'helmet' closely fitting over the rest of the flower, not standing up as a tall hood. All varieties of Aconite are useful, but this kind with the close set in helmet to the flower is the most valuable.

The Aconite derived from German root of A. Napellus appears to possess somewhat different properties to that prepared from English roots. The German roots may be recognized by the remains of the stem which crown the root. They are also generally less starchy, darker externally and more shrivelled than the English root and considered to be less active, probably because they are generally the exhausted parent roots.

Medicinal Action and Uses

Anodyne, diuretic and diaphoretic. The value of Aconite as a medicine has been more fully realized in modern times, and it now rank as one of our most useful drugs. It is much used in homeopathy. On account of its very poisonous nature, all medicines obtained from it come, however, under Table 1 of the poison schedule: Aconite is a deadly poison.

Both tincture and liniment of Aconite are in general use, and Aconite is also used in ointment and sometimes given as hypodermic injection. Preparations of Aconitc are employed for outward application locally to the skin to diminish the pain of neuralgia, lumbago and rheumatism.

The official tincture taken internelly diminishes the rate and force of the pulse in the early stages of fevers and slight local inflammations, such as feverish cold, larnyngitis, first stages of pneumonia and erysipelas; it relieves the pain of neuralgia, pleurisy and aneurism. In cardiac failure or to prevent same it has been used with success, in acute tonsilitis children have been well treated by a dose of 1 to 2 minims for a child 5 to 10 years old; the dose for adults is 2 to 5 minims, three times a day.

Note

The tincture of Aconite of the British Pharmacopoeia 1914 is nearly double the strength of that in the old Pharmacopoeia of 1898.

Externally the linament as such or mixed with chloroform or belladonna liniment is useful in neuralgia or rheumatism.

Poisoning from, and Antidotes

The symptons of poisoning are tingling and numbness of tongue and mouth and a sensation of ants crawling over the body, nausea and vomiting with epigastric pain, laboured breathing, pulse irregular and weak, skin cold and clammy, features bloodless, giddiness, staggering, mind remains clear. A stomach tube or emetic should be used at once, 20 minims of Tincture of Digitalis given if available, stimulants should be given and if not retained diluted brandy injected per rectum, artificial respiration and friction, patient to be kept lying down.

All the species contain an active poison Aconitine, one of the most formidable poisons which have yet been discovered: it exists in all parts of the plant, but especially in the root. The smallest portion of either root or leaves, when first put into the mouth, occasions burning and tingling, and a sense of numbness immediately follows its continuance. One-fiftieth grain of Aconitine will kill a sparrow in a few seconds; one-tenth grain a rabbit in five minutes. It is more powerful than prussic acid and acts with tremendous rapidity. One hundredth grain will act locally, so as to produce a well-marked sensation in any part of the body for a whole day. So acrid is the poison, that the juice applied to a wounded finger affects the whole system, not only causing pains in the limbs, but a sense of suffocation and syncope.

Some species of Aconite were well known to the ancients as deadly poisons. It was said to be the invention of Hecate from the foam of Cerberus, and it was a species of Aconite that entered into the poison which the old men of the island of Ceos were condemned to drink when they became infirm and no longer of use to the State. Aconite is also supposed to have been the poison that formed the cup which Medea prepared for Theseus.

Various species of Aconite possess the same narcotic properties as A. Napellus, but none of them equal in energy the A. ferox of the East Indies, the root of which is used there as an energetic poison under the name of Bikh or Nabee. Aconite poisoning of wells by A. ferox has been carried out by native Indians to stop the progress of an army. They also use it for poisoning spears, darts and arrows, and for destroying tigers.

All children should be warned against Aconite in gardens. It is wiser not to grow Aconite among kitchen herbs of any sort. The root has occasionally been mistaken for horse-radish, with fatal results - it is, however, shorter, darker and more fibrous - and the leaves have produced similar fatal results. In Ireland a poor woman once sprinkled powdered Aconite root over a dish of greens, and one man was killed and another seriously affected by it.

In 1524 and 1526 it is recorded that two criminals, to whom the root was given as an experiment, quickly died.

The older herbalists described it as venomous and deadly. Gerard says: 'There hath beene little heretofore set down concerning the virtues of the Aconite, but much might be saide of the hurts that have come thereby." It was supposed to be an antidote against other poisons. Gerard tells us that its power was 'So forcible that the herb only thrown before the scorpion or any other venomous beast, causeth them to be without force or strength to hurt, insomuch that they cannot moove or stirre untill the herbe be taken away." Ben Jonson, in his tragedy Sejanus, says:

'I have heard that Aconite
Being timely taken hath a healing might
Against the scorpion's stroke."

Linnaeus reports Aconite to be fatal to cattle and goats when they eat it fresh, but when dried it does no harm to horses, a peculiarity in common with the buttercups, to which the Aconites are related. Field-mice are well aware of its evil nature, and in hard times, when they will attack almost any plant that offers them food, they leave this severely alone.

OTHER VARIETIES

Japanese Aconite - syn. Aconitum Chinense - is regularly imported in considerable quantities. It used formerly to be ascribed to A. Fischer (Reichb.), but is now considered to be derived from A. uncinatum, var. Faponicum (Regel.) and possibly also from A. volubile (Pallas). It has conical or top-shaped, gradually tapering tuberous roots, 1 to 2 inches long, 1/3 to 1 inch in thickness at the top, externally covered with a brown, closely adhering skin internally white. Dried roots do not contain much alkaloid, if steeped when fresh in a mixture of common salt, vinegar and water. The poisonous alkaloid present is called Japaconitine, to distinguish it from the official Aconitine and the Pseudaconitine of A. laciniatum. Japaconitine is similar in constituents and properties with the Aconitine of A. Napellus.

Indian Aconite root or Nepal Aconite consists of

the root of A. laciniatum (Staph.). It is also called Bikh or Bish, and is collected in Nepal. It is much larger than the English variety, being a conical, not suddenly tapering root, 2 to 4 inches long and an inch or more at the top, of a lighter brown than the official variety, the rootlet scars much fewer than the official root. Internally it is hard and almost resinous, the taste intensely acrid and is much shriveiled longitudinally. This root yields a very active alkaloid, Pseudoaconitine, which is allied to Aconitine and resembles it in many of its properties; it is about twice as active as Aconitine. Indian Aconite root was formerly attributed to A. ferox (Wall). Their large size and less tapering character sufficiently distinguish these from the official drug.

Other varieties of Aconite are A. chasmanthum (Staph.), known in India as Mohri, which contains Indaconitine, and A. spicatum, another Indian species containing Bikhaconitine, resembling Pseudaconitine.

Russian Aconite, A. orientale, grows abundantly in the Crimea and Bessarabia. It has a small, compact, greyish-black root with a transverse section similar to that of A. Napellus. Its taste is hot and acrid. When treated by a process which gave 0.0526 per cent of crystalline Aconitine from a sample of powdered root of A. Napellus, the dried root of A. orientale yielded 2.207 per cent of total alkaloids, which were, however, amorphous. The total alkaloid has not yet been investigated further.

A. heterophyllum (Wall), Atis root, is a plant growing in the Western temperate Himalayas. This species does not contain Aconitine and is said to be non-poisonous. Its chief constituent is an intensely bitter alkaloid - Atisine - possessing tonic and antiperiodic principles. A. palmatum, of Indian origin, yields a similar alkaloid, Palmatisine.

The province of Szechwen in West China grows large quantities of medicinal plants, among them A. Wilsoni, which is worth about 4s. per cwt., of which 55,000 lb. a year can be produced in this province; A. Fischeri, about four times the price, of which rather less are yearly available, and A. Hemsleyan, about the same price as the latter, of which about 27,000 lb. are available in an average year.

Other Species

The Anthora, or Wholesome Aconite described by Culpepper, is a small plant about a foot high, with pale, divided green leaves, and yellow flowers - a native of the Alps. Its stem is erect, firm, angular and hairy; the leaves alternate and much cut into. The flowers are large, hooded with fragrant scent, growing on top of the branches in spikes of a pale yellow color, smaller than the ordinary Monkshood and succeeded by five horn-like, pointed pods, or achenes, containing five angular seeds. It flowers in July and the seeds ripen at the end of August. The root is tuberous.

Culpepper tells us that the herb was used in his time, but not often. It was reputed to be very serviceable against vegetable poisons and 'a decoction of the root is a good lotion to wash the parts bitten by venomous creatures." . . . 'The leaves, if rubbed on the skin will irritate and cause soreness and the pollen is also dangerous if blown in the eyes ."

As a matter of fact, this species of Aconite by no means deserves its reputation of harmlessness, for it is only poisonous in a less degree than the rest of the same genus, and the theory that it is a remedy against poison, particularly that of the other Aconites, is now an exploded one.

Parkinson, speaking of the Yellow Monkshood, calls it:

'The "counter-poison monkeshood" - the roots of which are effectual, not only against the poison of the poisonful Helmet Flower and all others of that kind, but also against the poison of all venomous beasts, the plague or pestilence and other infectious diseases, which raise spots, pockes, or markes in the outward skin, by expelling the poison from within and defending the heart as a most sovereign cordial."

The so-called Winter Aconite, Aeranthis hyemalis, is not a true Aconite, though closely allied, being also a member of the Buttercup family, whose blossoms it more nearly resembles.

ADDER'S TONGUE (AMERICAN)

Botanical: Erythronium Americanum (KER-GAWL)
Family: N.O. Liliaceae
Synonyms: Serpent's Tongue. Dog's Tooth Violet. Yellow Snowdrop.
Parts Used: Leaves, bulbs.

Habitat

Eastern United States of America, from New Brunswick to Florida, and westwards to Ontario and Arkansas.

The American Dog's Tooth Violet or Adder's Tongue, Erythronium Americanum (Ker Gawl), is a very beautiful early spring flower of the Eastern United States of America, belonging to the Lily family. It grows in damp, open woodlands from New Brunswick to Florida and westwards to Ontario and Arkansas.

Description

The plant, which is quite smooth, grows from a small, slender, ovoid, fawn-coloured corm, 1/3 to 1 inch long which is quite deeply buried in the soil and is of solid, firm consistence and white and starchy internally.

The stem is slender, a few inches high, and bears near the ground, on footstalks 2 to 3 inches long, a pair of oblong, dark-green, purplish-blotched leaves, the blades about 2 1/2 inches long and 1 inch wide, minutely wrinkled, with parallel, longitudinal veins. The stem terminates in a handsome, large, pendulous, lily-like flower, an inch across, with the perianth divisions strongly recurved, bright yellow in color, often tinged with purple and finely dotted within at the base, and with six stamens. It flowers in the latter part of April and early in May.

Medicinal Action and Uses

The constituents of the plant have not yet been analysed. The fresh leaves and corm, and to a lesser degree the rest of the plant, are emetic.

The fresh leaves having emollient and anti-scrofulous properties are mostly used in the form of a stimulating poultice, applied to swellings, tumors and scrofulous ulcers.

The infusion is taken internally in wine glassful doses. It is reputed of use in dropsy, hiccough and vomiting.

The recent bulbs have been used as a substitute for colchicum. They are emetic in doses of 25 to 30 grains.

ADRUE

Botanical: Cyperus articulatus (LINN.)
Family: N.O. Cyperaceae

Part Used

The drug Adrue is the tuberous rhizome of the Guinea Rush (Cyperus articulatus Linn.), a tall sedge, common in Jamaica, and on the banks of the Nile.

Description

The blackish-red, somewhat top-shaped tubers are 3/4 to 1 inch long, 1/2 to 3/4 inch in diameter, sometimes in a series of two or three, connected by an underground stem 1/8 inch in diameter and 1 to 2 inches long. Internally, the tubers are pale in color, a transverse section showing a central column with darker points indicating vascular bundles. The dried tubers often bear the bristly remains of former leaves on their upper ends. The drug has a bitterish, aromatic taste, recalling that of Lavender. The odor of the fresh tubers has been likened to that of the Sweet Sedge, Calamus aromaticus.

Medicinal Action and Uses

Carminative, sedative, very useful in vomiting of pregnancy.

The aromatic properties of the drug cause a feeling of warmth to be diffused throughout the whole system and it acts as a sedative in dyspeptic disorders.

Preparations

A fluid extract is made from the tubers. Dose, 10 to 30 minims.

AGAR-AGAR

Botanical: Gelidium amansii (KUTZ)
Family: N.O. Algae
Synonyms: Japanese Isinglass.
Part Used: The mucilage dried, after boiling the seaweed.
Habitat: Japan, best variety; Ceylon and Macassar.

Description

A seaweed gathered on the East Indian coast and sent to China, it is derived from the various species of Sphaerococcus Euchema and Gelidium. It is brownish-white in color with thorny projections on its branches; the best variety, known as Japanese Isinglass, contains large quantities of mucilage. The seaweed after collection is spread out on the shore until bleached, and then dried; it is afterwards boiled in water and the mucilaginous solution strained, the filtrate being allowed to harden, and then it is dried in the sun. The time for collection of the Algae is summer and autumn when the bleaching and drying can take place, but the final preparation of Agar-Agar is carried out in winter from November to February. The Japanese variety is derived from several kinds of Algae and comes into European commerce in two forms: (1) In transparent pieces 2 feet long, the thickness of a straw, prepared in Singapore by treating it in hot water. (2) In yellowish white masses about 1 inch wide and 1 foot long. The latter is the form considered the more suitable for the culture of bacteria.

Constituents

Agar-Agar contains glose, which is a powerful gelatinizing agent. It is precipitated from solution by alcohol. Glose is a carbohydrate. Acetic, hydrochloric and oxalic acids prevent gelatinization of Agar-Agar.

Medicinal Action and Uses

Agar-Agar is widely used as a treatment for constipation, but is usually employed with Cascara when atony of the intestinal muscles is present. It does not increase peristaltic action. Its therapeutic value depends on the ability of the dry Agar to absorb and retain moisture. Its action is mechanical and analogous to that of the cellulose of vegetable foods, aiding the regularity of the bowel movements. It is sometimes used as an adulterant of jams and jellies.

Dosage and Preparations

It is usually administered in small shreds mixed with fruit, milk or any convenient vehicle. It is not wise to give it in powder, as this gives rise to irritation in some cases. 1/2 to 1 ounce may be taken at a time. 1 ounce to a pint of boiling water makes a suitable jelly for invalids and may be flavoured with lemon.

Other Species

Ceylon Agar-Agar, or Agal Agal, which is the native name of Gracillaria lichenoides, is largely used in the East for making soups and jellies. Gigartina speciosa, a variety found on the Swan River, was erroneously supposed to have formed the edible swallow's nest, but it has been ascertained that this delicacy comes from a peculiar secretion in the birds themselves. Macassar Agar-Agar comes from the straits between Borneo and Celebes and consists of impure Euchema Spinolum incrusted with salt.

AGRIMONY

Botanical: Agrimonia Eupatoria (LINN.)
Family: N.O. Rosaceae
Synonyms: Common Agrimony. Church Steeples. Cockeburr. Sticklewort. Philanthropos.
Part Used: The herb.

Habitat

The plant is found abundantly throughout England, on hedge-banks and the sides of fields, in dry thickets and on all waste places. In Scotland it is much more local and does not penetrate very far northward.

Agrimony has an old reputation as a popular, domestic medicinal herb, being a simple well known to all country-folk. It belongs to the Rose order of plants, and its slender spikes of yellow flowers, which are in bloom from June to early September, and the singularly beautiful form of its much-cut-into leaves, make it one of the most graceful of our smaller herbs.

Description

From the long, black and somewhat woody perennial root, the erect cylindrical and slightly rough stem rises 1 or 2 feet, sometimes more, mostly unbranched, or very slightly branched in large specimens. The leaves are numerous and very rich in outline, those near the ground are often 7 or 8 inches long, while the upper ones are generally only about 3 inches in length. They are pinnate in form, i.e. divided up to the mid-rib into pairs of leaflets. The graduation in the size and richness of the leaves is noticeable: all are very similar in general character, but the upper leaves have far fewer leaflets than the lower, and such leaflets as there are, are less cut into segments and have altogether a simpler outline. The leaflets vary very considerably in size, as besides the six or eight large lateral leaflets and the terminal one, the mid-rib is fringed with several others that are very much smaller than these and ranged in the intervals between them. The main leaflets increase in size towards the apex of the leaf, where they are 1 to 1 1/2 inches long. They are oblong-oval in shape, toothed, downy above and more densely so beneath.

The flowers, though small, are numerous, arranged closely on slender, terminal spikes, which lengthen much when the blossoms have withered and the seed-vessels are maturing. At the base of each flower, which is placed stalkless on the long spike, is a small bract, cleft into three acute segments. The flowers, about 3/8 inch across, have five conspicuous and spreading petals, which are egg-shaped in form and somewhat narrow in proportion to their length, slightly notched at the end and of a bright yellow color. The stamens are five to twelve in number. The flowers face boldly outwards and upwards towards the light, but after they have withered, the calyx points downwards. It becomes rather woody, thickly covered at the end with a mass of small bristly hairs, that spread and develop into a burr-like form. Its sides are furrowed and nearly straight, about 1/5 inch long, and the mouth, about as wide, is surmounted by an enlarged ring armed with spines, of which the outer ones are shorter and spreading, and the inner ones longer and erect.

The whole plant is deep green and covered with soft hairs, and has a slightly aromatic scent; even the small root is sweet scented, especially in spring. The spikes of flowers emit a most refreshing and spicy odor like that of apricots. The leaves when dry retain most of their fragrant odor, as well as the flowers, and Agrimony was once much sought after as a substitute or addition to tea, adding a peculiar delicacy and aroma to its flavor. Agrimony is one of the plants from the dried leaves of which in some country districts is brewed what is called 'a spring drink," or 'diet drink," a compound made by the infusion of several herbs and drunk in spring time as a purifier of the blood. In France, where herbal teas or tisanes are more employed than here, it is stated that Agrimony tea, for its fragrancy, as well as for its virtues, is often drunk as a beverage at table.

The plant is subject to a considerable amount of variation, some specimens being far larger than others, much more clothed with hairs and with other minor differences. It has, therefore, by some botanists, been divided into two species, but the division is now scarcely maintained. The larger variety, having also a greater fragrance, was named Agrimonia odorata.

The long flower-spikes of Agrimony have caused the name of 'Church Steeples' to be given the plant in some parts of the country. It also bears the title of 'Cockeburr," 'Sticklewort' or 'Stickwort," because its seed-vessels cling by the hooked ends of their stiff hairs to any person or animal coming into contact with the plant. It was, Gerard informs us, at one time called Philanthropos, according to some old writers, on account of its beneficent and valuable properties, others saying that the name arose from the circumstance of the seeds clinging to the garments of passers-by, as if desirous of accompanying them, and Gerard inclines to this latter interpretation of the name.

The whole plant yields a yellow dye: when gathered in September, the color given is pale, much like that called nankeen; later in the year the dye is of a darker hue and will dye wool of a deep yellow. As it gives a good dye at all times and is a common plant, easily cultivated, it seems to deserve the notice of dyers.

Sheep and goats will eat this plant, but cattle, horses and swine leave it untouched.

History

The name Agrimony is from Argemone, a word given by the Greeks to plants which were healing to the eyes, the name Eupatoria refers to Mithridates Eupator, a king who was a renowned concoctor of herbal remedies. The magic power of Agrimony is mentioned in an old English medical manuscript:

'If it be leyd under mann's heed,
He shal sleepyn as he were deed;
He shal never drede ne wakyn
Till fro under his heed it be takyn."

Agrimony was one of the most famous vulnerary herbs. The Anglo-Saxons, who called it Garclive, taught that it would heal wounds, snake bites, warts, etc. In the time of Chaucer, when we find its name appearing in the form of Egrimoyne, it was used with Mugwort and vinegar for 'a bad back' and 'alle woundes': and one of these old writers recommends it to be taken with a mixture of pounded frogs and human blood, as a remedy for all internal hemorrhages. It formed an ingredient of the famous arquebusade water as prepared against wounds inflicted by an arquebus, or hand-gun, and was mentioned by Philip de Comines, in his account of the battle of Morat in 1476. In France, the eau de arquebusade is still applied for sprains and bruises, being carefully made from many aromatic herbs. It was at one time included in the London Materia Medica as a vulnerary herb, but modern official medicine does not recognize its virtues, though it is still fully appreciated in herbal practice as a mild astringent and tonic, useful in coughs, diarrhea and relaxed bowels. By pouring a pint of boiling water on a handful of the dried herb - stem, leaves and flowers - an excellent gargle may be made for a relaxed throat, and a teacupful of the same infusion is recommended, taken cold three or four times in the day for looseness in the bowels, also for passive losses of blood. It may be given either in infusion or decoction.

Constituents

Agrimony contains a particular volatile oil, which may be obtained from the plant by distillation and also a bitter principle. It yields in addition 5 per cent of tannin, so that its use in cottage medicine for gargles and as an astringent applicant to indolent ulcers and wounds is well justified. Owing to this presence of tannin, its use has been recommended in dressing leather.

Medicinal Action and Uses

Astringent tonic, diuretic. Agrimony has had a great reputation for curing jaundice and other liver complaints. Gerard believed in its efficacy. He says: 'A decoction of the leaves is good for them that have naughty livers': and he tells us also that Pliny called it a 'herb of princely authoritie." Dioscorides stated that it was not only 'a remedy for them that have bad livers," but also 'for such as are bitten with serpents." Dr. Hill, who from 1751 to 1771 published several works on Herbal medicine, recommends 'an infusion of 6 oz. of the crown of the root in a quart of boiling water, sweetened with honey and half a pint drank three times a day," as an effectual remedy for jaundice. It gives tone to the system and promotes assimilation of food.

Agrimony is also considered a very useful agent in skin eruptions and diseases of the blood, pimples, blotches, etc. A strong decoction of the root and leaves, sweetened with honey or sugar, has been taken successfully to cure scrofulous sores, being administered two or three times a day, in doses of a wine glassful, persistently for several months. The same decoction is also often employed in rural districts as an application to ulcers.

Preparation

Fluid extract dose, 10 to 60 drops.

In North America, it is said to be used in fevers with great success, by the Indians and Canadians.

In former days, it was sometimes given as a vermifuge, though that use; of it is obsolete.

In the Middle Ages, it was said to have magic powers, if laid under a man's head inducing heavy sleep till removed, but no narcotic properties are ascribed to it.

Green (Universal Herbal, 1832) tells us that 'its root appears to possess the properties of Peruvian bark in a very considerable degree, without manifesting any of its inconvenient qualities, and if taken in pretty large doses, either in decoction or powder, seldom fails to cure the ague."

Culpepper (1652) recommends it, in addition to the uses already enumerated, for gout, 'either used outwardly in an oil or ointment, or inwardly, in an electuary or syrup, or concreted juice." He praises its use externally, stating how sores may be cured 'by bathing and fomenting them with a decoction of this plant," and that it heals 'all inward wounds, bruises, hurts and other distempers." He continues: 'The decoction of the herb, made with wine and drunk, is good against the biting and stinging of serpents . . . it also helpeth the colic, cleanseth the breath and relieves the cough. A draught of the decoction taken warm before the fit first relieves and in time removes the tertian and quartian ague." It 'draweth forth thorns, splinters of wood, or any such thing in the flesh. It helpeth to strengthen members that are out of joint."

There are several other plants, not actually related botanically to the Common Agrimony, that were given the same name by the older herbalists because of their similar properties. These are the COMMON HEMP AGRIMONY, Eupatorium Cannabinum (Linn.) called by Gerard the Common Dutch Agrimony, and by Salmon, in his English Herbal (1710), Eupatorium Aquaticum mas, the Water Agrimony- also the plant now called the Trifid Bur-Marigold, Bidens tripartita (Linn.), but by older herbalists named the Water Hemp, Bastard Hemp and Bastard Agrimony. The name Bastard Agrimony has also been given to a species of true Agrimony, Agrimonium Agrimonoides, a native of Italy, growing in moist woods and among bushes.

AGRIMONY (HEMP)

Botanical: Eupatorium cannabinum (LINN.)
Family: N.O. Compositae
Synonyms: Holy Rope. St. John's Herb.
Part Used: Herb.

The Hemp Agrimony, Eupatorium Cannabinum, belongs to the great Composite order of plants. It is a very handsome, tall-growing perennial, common on the banks of rivers, sides of ditches, at the base of cliffs on the seashore, and in other damp places in most parts of Britain, and throughout Europe.

Description

The root-stock is woody and from it rises the erect round stems, growing from 2 to 5 feet high with short branches springing from the axils of the leaves, which are placed on it in pairs. The stems are reddish in color, covered with downy hair and are woody below. They have a pleasant aromatic smell when cut.

The root-leaves are on long stalks, but the stem-leaves have only very short root-stalks. They are divided to their base into three, more rarely five, lance-shaped toothed lobes, the middle lobe much larger than the others, the general form of the leaf being similar to that of the Hemp (hence both the English name and the Latin specific name, deriven from cannabis, hemp). In small plants the leaves are sometimes undivided. They have a bitter taste, and their pungent smell is reminiscent of an umbelliferous rather than of a composite plant. All the leaves bear distinct, short hairs, and are sparingly sprinkled with small inconspicuous, resinous dots.

The plant blooms in late summer and autumn, the flower heads being arranged in crowded masses of a dull lilac color at the top of the stem or branches. Each little composite head consists of about five or six florets. The corolla has five short teeth; though generally light purple or reddish lilac, it sometimes may be nearly white; it is covered with scattered resinous points. The anthers of the stamens are brown, and the very long style is white. The crown of hairs, or pappus, on the angled fruit is of a dirty white color.

We sometimes find the plant called 'St. John's

Herb," and on account of the hempen-shaped leaves, it was also formerly called, in some districts, 'Holy Rope," being thus named after the rope with which the Saviour was bound.

Constituents

The leaves contain a volatile oil, which acts on the kidneys, and likewise some tannin and a bitter chemical principle which will cut short the chill of intermittent fever.

Medicinal Action and Uses

Alternative and febrifuge. Though now little used medicinally, herbalists recognize its cathartic, diuretic and anti-scorbutic properties, and consider it a good remedy for purifying the blood, either used by itself, or in combination with other herbs. A homeopathic tincture is prepared, given in frequent small well-diluted doses with water, for influenza, or for a similar feverish chill, and a tea made with boiling water poured on the dry leaves will give prompt relief if taken hot at the onset of a bilious catarrh or of influenza.

In Holland it was used by the peasants for jaundice with swollen feet, and given as an alternative or purifier of the blood in the spring and against scurvy. The leaves have been used in infusion as a tonic, and in the fen districts where it prevails, such medicines are very necessary. Country people used to lay the leaves on bread, considering that they thus prevented it from becoming mouldy.

Preparation

Fluid extract, 10 to 60 drops.

According to Withering, an infusion of a handful of the fresh herb acts as a strong purgative and emetic. Boerhaave, the famous Dutch physician (1668-1738), recommends an infusion of the plant for fomenting ulcers and putrid sores, and Tournefort (Materia Medica, 1708) affirmed that the fresh-gathered root, boiled in ale, purges briskly, but without producing any bad effects, and stated that there were many instances of its having cured dropsy.

It had also the reputation of being a good wound herb, whether bruised or made into an ointment with lard.

Goats are said to be the only animals that will eat this plant.

AGRIMONY (WATER)

Botanical: Bidens tripartita (LINN.)
Family: N.O. Compositae
Synonym: Bur Marigold.
Part Used: Whole plant.

The Water Agrimony, now called the Bur Marigold is an annual flowering in late summer and autumn, abounding in wet places, such as the margins of ponds and ditches, and common in England, but rather less so in Scotland.

Description

The root is tapering, with many fibres attached to it. The erect stem grows about 2 feet high, sometimes more, and is wiry and nearly smooth, angular, solid and marked with small brown spots, so as to almost give it the dark purple appearance described by Culpepper. It is very leafy and the upper portion branches freely from the axils of the leaves, which are placed opposite one another and are of a dark green color 2 to 3 inches in length. All except the uppermost are narrowed into winged foot-stalks at the bases, which are united together across the stem. They are smooth and sharp-pointed, with coarsely toothed margins, and are divided into three segments (hence the specific name of the plant), occasionally into five, the centre lobe much larger and also often deeply three-cleft. The uppermost leaves are sometimes found undivided.

The composite flowers are in terminal heads, brownish-yellow in color and somewhat drooping, usually without ray florets the disk florets being perfectly regular. The heads are surrounded by a leafy involucre, the outer leaflets of which, about eight in number, pointed and spreading, extend much behind the flower-head. The fruits have four ribs, which terminate in long, spiky projections, or awns, two of which, as well as the ribs, are armed with reflexed prickles, causing them to cling to any rough substance they touch, such as the coat of an animal, thus helping in the dissemination of the seeds. From these burr-like fruits, the plant has been given the name it now universally bears. These burrs, when the plant has been growing on the borders of a fish-pond, have been known to destroy gold fish by adhering to their gills. The flower-heads smell rather like rosin or cedar when burnt.

Medicinal Action and Uses

This plant was formerly valued for its diuretic and astringent properties, and was employed in fevers, gravel, stone and bladder and kidney troubles generally, and was considered also a good stypic and an excellent remedy for ruptured blood-vessels and bleeding of every description, of benefit to consumptive patients.

Culpepper tells us that it was called Hepatorium 'because it strengthens the liver':

'it healeth and drieth, cutteth and cleanseth thick and tough humours of the breast and for this I hold it inferior to few herbs that grow . . . it helpeth the dropsy and yellow jaundice; it opens the obstruction of the liver, mollifies the hardness of the spleen, being applied outwardly. . . it is an excellent remedy for the third day ague; . . . it kills worms and cleanseth the body of sharp humours which are the cause of itch and scab; the herb being burnt, the smoke thereof drives away flies, wasps, etc. It strengthens the lungs exceedingly. Country people give it to their cattle when they are troubled with cough or are broken-winded."

It has sometimes been employed on the Continent as a yellow dye, but the color yielded is very indifferent. The yarn or thread must be first steeped in alum water, then dried and steeped in a decoction of the plant and afterwards boiled in the decoction.

A nearly-allied species, Bidens bipinnata (Linn.), popularly called Spanish Needles, is a native of North America, where the roots and seeds have been used as emmenagogues and in laryngeal and bronchial diseases.

MARIGOLD (NODDING). Another species of Bidens, called B. cernua, popularly known as the Nodding Marigold. The flowers are somewhat larger than B. tripartita,and have a much more decided droop, hence the name 'Nodding." The leaves are not made up of three leaflets but are of lanceolate form, deeply serrated. It is found by streams and ditches, and flowers during the later summer and autumn.

ALDER, BLACK AMERICAN

Botanical: Prinos verticillatus (LINN.)
Family: N.O. Aquiloliaceae
Synonyms: Ilex Verticillata. Black Alder Winterberry. Deciduous Winterberry. Virginian Winterberry. P. Gronovii. P. Confertus. Fever Bush. Apalachine a feuilles de Prunier.
Parts Used: The fresh bark and fruit.
Habitat: The United States, from western Florida northwards.

Description

This shrub is the most ornamental of the American deciduous hollies. It grows from 6 to 1O feet in height, with thin, oval or lanceolate leaves, white flowers and bright scarlet berries the size of a large pea, causing it to be very conspicuous in the autumn, when the surrounding vegetation is leafless.

The bark is found in thin fragments, the outer surface brownish, with whitish patches and black dots and lines, the cork layer easily separating from the pale-greenish or yellowish white inner tissue. The fracture is short, the odor almost imperceptible, and the taste bitter and slightly astringent.

It was widely used by the aborigines of North America for its astringent properties.

Constituents

The bark contains about 4-8 per cent tannin, two resins, the one soluble and the other insoluble in alcohol, albumen, gum, sugar, and a bitter principle and a yellow coloring matter not yet isolated. There is no berberine.

The fresh bark and fruit are gathered before the

first autumnal frost.

Medicinal Action and Uses

Cathartic, antiseptic, tonic, and astringent bitter. The decoction of the bark is prepared by boiling 2 ounces of bark in 3 pints of water down to 2 pints, this being given internally in diarrhea and malarial disorders, and externally in indolent sores and chronic skin disease. The berries should not be used as a substitute for the bark. In intermittent fever it can be used like Peruvian Bark, and is valuable in jaundice, gangrenous affections, dropsy, and when the body is devitalized by discharges. The bark is well known as an ingredient in several alternative syrups.

The berries are cathartic, and with Cedar apples form a mild anthelmintic for children.

An observed case, after eating twenty-five berries, had a sensation of nausea, not interfering with appetite, vomiting of bile without retching, painless and profuse evacuation of the bowels, followed by a second evacuation in half an hour, and as a result, a feeling of great lightness and well-being, with appetite and digestion better than usual.

For dyspepsia, 2 drachms of the powdered bark, and 1 drachm of powdered Golden Seal infused in a pint of boiling water, taken, when cold, in the course of one day in wine-glassful doses, will be found very helpful.

Dosage

Of the decoction, 2 to 3 fluid ounces. Of the powdered bark, 1/2 to 1 drachm.

ALDER, COMMON

Botanical: Alnus Glutinosa (GAERTN.)
Family: N.O. Betulaceae
Synonym: Betula Alnus.
Parts Used: The bark and the leaves.
Habitat: Europe south of the Arctic Circle, including Britain, Western Asia, North Africa.

History

The English Alder is a moderately-sized tree or large shrub of dark color, usually growing in moist woods or pastures or by streams. The leaves are broadly ovate, stalked, and usually smooth. The catkins are formed in the autumn, the fruiting ones having scales rather like a tiny-fir-cone; the flowers appear in early spring, before the leaves are fully out. The woody, nearly globular female catkins are the so-called 'berries." The trees are often grown in coppices, which afford winter shade for stock on mountain grazings without appearing to injure the grass beneath, and can be cut down for poles every nine or ten years.

The wood is much used. When young it is brittle and very easily worked. When more mature it is tinted and veined; in the Highlands of Scotland it is used for making handsome chairs, and is known as Scottish mahogany. It has the quality of long endurance under water, and so is valuable for pumps, troughs, sluices, and particularly for piles, for which purpose it is said to have been used in sixteenth-century Venice and widely in France and Holland. The roots and knots furnish good material for cabinet-makers, and for the clogs of Lancashire mill-towns and the south of Scotland the demand exceeds the supply, and birch has to be used instead. It is also used for cart and spinning wheels, bowls, spoons, wooden heels, herring-barrel staves, etc. On the Continent it is largely used for cigar-boxes, for which its reddish, cedar-like wood is well adapted. After lying in bogs the wood has the color but not the hardness of ebony. The branches make good charcoal, which is valuable for making gunpowder.

The bark is used by dyers, tanners, leather dressers, and for fishermen's nets.

Dyeing

The bark is used as a foundation for blacks, with the addition of copperas. Alone, it dyes woollens a reddish color (Aldine Red). The Laplanders chew it, and dye leathern garments with their saliva. An ounce dried and powdered, boiled in three-quarters of a pint of water with an equal amount of logwood, with solution of copper, tin, and bismuth, 6 grains of each, and 2 drops of iron vitriol, will dye a deep boue de Paris.

Both bark and young shoots dye yellow, and with a little copper as a yellowish-grey, useful in the half-tints and shadows of flesh in tapestry. The shoots cut in March will dye cinnamon, and if dried and powdered a tawny shade. The fresh wood yields a pinkish-fawn dye, and the catkins a green.

The leaves have been used in tanning leather. They are clammy, and if spread in a room are said to catch fleas on their glutinous surface.

Constituents

The bark and young shoots contain from 16 to 20 per cent of tannic acid, but so much coloring matter that they are not very useful for tanning. This tannin differs from that of galls and oak-bark, and does not yield glucose when acted upon by sulphuric acid, which, it is stated, resolves it into almine red and sugar.

Medicinal Action and Uses

Tonic and astringent. A decoction of the bark is useful to bathe swellings and inflammations, especially of the throat, and has been known to cure ague.

Peasants on the Alps are reported to be frequently cured of rheumatism by being covered with bags full of the heated leaves.

Horses, cows, sheep and goats are said to eat it, but swine refuse it. Some state that it is bad for horses, as it turns their tongues black.

ALDER, TAG

Botanical: Alnus serrulata (WILLD.)
Family: N.O. Betulaceae
Synonyms: Alnus rubra (obsolete). Smooth Alder. Red Alder.
Parts Used: Bark. Cones.
Habitat: United States and Europe.

Description

A well-known shrub, growing in clumps and forming thickets on the borders of ponds or rivers, or in swamps. It bears flowers of a reddish-green color in March and April. The bark is blackish grey, with small, corky warts, the inner surface being orange-brown, striated. The taste is astringent and somewhat bitter. It is almost odourless.

The name Alnus rubra should no longer be applied to Alnus serrulata, though some authorities retain it. That is the correct name of the Oregon Alder.

Medicinal Action and Uses

Alterative, tonic, astringent, emetic. A decoction or extract is useful in scrofula, secondary syphilis and several forms of cutaneous disease. The inner bark of the root is emetic, and a decoction of the cones is said to be astringent, and useful in haematuria and other hemorrhages.

When diarrhea, indigestion and dyspepsia are caused by debility of the stomach, it will be found helpful, and also in intermittent fevers.

It is said that an excellent ophthalmic powder can be made as follows: bore a hole from 1/2 to 1 inch in diameter, lengthwise, through a stout piece of limb of Tag Alder. Fill the opening with finely-powdered salt, and close it at each end. Put into hot ashes, and allow it to remain until the Tag is almost charred (three to four days), then split it open, take out the salt, powder, and keep it in a vial. To use it, blow some of the powder upon the eye, through a quill.

Dosage

Of fluid extract, 1/2 to 1 drachm. Infusion of 1 OZ. of bark in 1 pint of boiling water - in wine glassful doses. Almim, 4 to 10 grains.

ALKANETS

Botanical: Alkanna tinctoria (TAUSCH.), Lithosfermum tinctorium (VAH L.)
Family: N.O. Boraginaceae
Synonyms: Anchusa. Dyer's Bugloss. Spanish Bugloss. Orchanet.
Part Used: Root.

The name Anchusa is derived from the Greek anchousa=paint, from the use of the root as a dye.

The species are hispid or pubescent herbs, with oblong, entire leaves, and bracteated racemes, rolled up before the flowers expand. The corolla is rather small, between funnel and salver-shaped; usually purplish-blue, but in some species yellow or whitish; the calyx enlarges in fruit. The root, which is often very large in proportion to the size of the plant, yields in many of the species a red dye from the rind.

Alkanet (A. tinctoria) is cultivated in Central and Southern Europe for its dye, which is readily extracted by oils and spirit of wine. It is employed in pharmacy to give a red color to salves, etc., and in staining wood in imitation of rosewood, or mahogany. This is done by rubbing it with oil in which the Alkanet root has been soaked. About 8 to 10 tons were annually imported from France and Germany. The plant is sometimes also cultivated in Britan, but by far the greater portion of the Alkanet used here is imported either from the Levant or from the neighborhood of Montpellier, in France.

Though Alkanet imparts a fine deep red color to oily substances and to spirit of wine, it tinges water with a dull brownish hue. Wax tinged with Alkanet, and applied to the surface of warm marble, stains it flesh-color and sinks deep into the stone. It is also used in coloring spurious 'port-wine," for which purpose it is perfectly harmless.

Our British species, the Common Alkanet (A. officinalis), is a soft, hairy plant with an angular stem, narrow, lanceolate leaves; and forked, one-sided cymes of violet flowers; calyx longer than the funnel-shaped corolla. It is an occasional escape from gardens. It is a biennial, and flowers from June to July.

The Evergreen Alkanet (A. sempervireus) is also found in Great Britain. This is a stout bristly plant, with deep green, ovate leaves, and long-stalked axillary, crowded clusters of rather large flowers, which are of an intense azure blue and have a short tube to the corolla. It is not generally considered a native, but it is not an uncommon hedgeplant in Devonshire. It is a perennial and flowers from May to August.

Parkinson says that the French ladies of his day coloured their faces with an ointment containing anchusa and the color did not last long.

Medicinal Action and Uses

Culpepper says:

'It is an herb under the dominion of Venus, and indeed one of her darlings, though somewhat hard to come by. It helps old ulcers, hot inflammations, burnings by common fire and St. Anthony's fire . . . for these uses your best way is to make it into an ointment also if you make a vinegar of it, as you make a vinegar of roses, it helps the morphy and leprosy . . . it helps the yellow jaundice, spleen, and gravel in the kidneys. Dioscorides saith, it helps such as are bitten by venomous beasts, whether it be taken inwardly or applied to the wound, nay, he saith further, if any that hath newly eaten it do but spit into the mouth of a serpent, the serpent instantly dies.... It also kills worms. Its decoction made in wine and drank, strengthens the back, and easeth the pains thereof. It helps bruises and falls, and is as gallant a remedy to drive out the smallpox and measles as any is; an ointment made of it is excellent for green wounds, pricks or thrusts."

ALLSPICE

Botanical: Pimento officinalis (LINDL.)
Family: N.O. Myrtaceae
Synonyms: Pimento. Jamaica Pepper.
Part Used: Fruit, particularly the shell.

Habitat

Pimento, or Jamaica Pepper, familiarly called Allspice, because it tastes like a combination of cloves, juniper berries, cinnamon and pepper, is the dried full-grown, but immature fruit of Pimento officinalis (Lindl.), or Eugenia Pimenta, an evergreen tree about 30 feet high, a member of the natural order Myrtaceae, indigenous to the West Indian Islands and South America, and extensively grown in Jamaica, where it flourishes best on limestone hills near the sea. In this country, it only grows as a stove plant.

It is also cultivated in Central America and surrounding states, but more than half the supply of the spice found in commerce comes from Jamaica, where the tree is so abundant as to form in the mountainous districts whole forests, which require little attention beyond clearing out undergrowth.

Description

The tree begins to fruit when three years old and is in full bearing after four years. The flowers appear in June, July and August and are quickly succeeded by the berries.

The special qualities of the fruit reside in the rind of the berries. It loses its aroma on ripening, owing to loss of volatile oil, and the berries are therefore collected as soon as they have attained their full size, in July and August, but while unripe and green.

Gathering is performed by breaking off the small twigs bearing the bunches; these are then spread out and exposed to the sun and air for some days, after which the stalks are removed and the berries are ready for packing into bags and casks for exportation.

The spice is sometimes dried in ovens (Kiln-dried Allspice), but the method by evaporation from sunheat produces the best article, though it is tedious and somewhat hazardous, requiring about twelve days, during which the fruit must be carefully guarded against moisture, being housed at night and during rainy and damp weather.

The green color of the fresh fruit changes on drying to reddish brown. If the fruit is allowed to ripen, it loses almost the whole of its aromatic properties, becoming fleshy sweet and of a purple-black color. Such pimento, to render it more attractive, is then often artificially coloured with bole or brown ochre, a sophistication which may be detected by boiling for a few seconds with diluted hydrochloric acid, filtering and testing with potassium ferrocyanide; the liquid should assume at most a bluish-green color.

The fruits as found in commerce are small nearly globular berries, about 3/10 inch in diameter, somewhat like black pepper in appearance, with a rough and brittle surface and crowned by the remains of the calyx teeth, surrounding the short style. The fruit is two-celled, each cell containing a single, kidney-shaped seed. The remains of the calyx crowning the fruit and the presence of two single-seeded cells are features that distinguish Pimento from Cubebs, the fruit of which is one-celled, one-seeded and grey and from Black Peppercorns, which are also one-celled and one-seeded.

The spice derives its name from the Portuguese pimenta, Spanish pimienta==pepper, which was given it from its resemblance to peppercorns.

Constituents

The chief constituent of Pimento is from 3 to 4.5 per cent of a volatile oil, contained in glands in the pericarp of the seeds and obtained by distillation from the fruit.

It occurs as a yellow or yellowish-red liquid, becoming gradually darker on keeping and having a pleasant aromatic odor, somewhat similar to that of oil of cloves, and a pungent, spicy taste. It has a slightly acid reaction. It is soluble in all proportions of alcohol. The specific gravity is 1.030 to 1.050. Its chief constituent is the phenol Eugenol, which is present to the extent of 60 to 75 per cent, and a sesquiterpene, the exact nature of which has not yet been ascertained. The specific gravity to some extent indicates the amount present; if lower than 1.030, it may be assumed that some eugenol has been removed, or that the oil has been adulterated with substitutes having a lower specific gravity than that of eugenol. The eugenol can be determined by shaking the oil with a solution of potassium hydroxide and measuring the residual oily layer. The United States Pharmacopoeia specifies that at least 65 per cent by volume of eugenol should be present. On shaking the oil with an equal volume of strong solution of ammonia, it should be converted into a semisolid mass of eugenol-ammonium.

The clove-like odor of the oil is doubtless due to the eugenol, but the characteristic odor is due to some other substance or substances as yet unknown. A certain amount of resin is also present, but the oil has not yet been fully investigated.

Bonastre obtained from the fruit, a volatile oil, a

green fixed oil, a fatty substance in yellowish flakes, tannin, gum, resin, uncrystallizable sugar, coloring matter, malic and gallic acids, saline matter and lignin. The green fixed oil has a burning, aromatic taste of Pimento and is supposed to be the acrid principle. Upon this, together with the volatile oil, the medicinal properties of the berries depend, and as these two principles exist most in the shell, this part is the most efficient. According to Bonastre, the shell contains 10 per cent of the volatile and 8 per cent of the fixed oil; the seeds only 5 per cent of the former and 2.5 of the latter. Berzelius considered the green fixed oil of Bonastre to be a mixture of the volatile oil, resin, fixed oil and perhaps a little chlorophyll.

On incineration, the fruits yield from 2.5 to 5 per cent of ash.

They impart their flavor to water and all their virtues to alcohol. The infusion is of a brown color and reddens litmus paper.

The leaves and bark abound in inflammable particles.

Medicinal Action and Uses

The chief use of Pimento is as a spice and condiment: the berries are added to curry powder and also to mulled wine. It is popular as a warming cordial, of a sweet odor and grateful aromatic taste.

The oil inaction resembles that of cloves, and is occasionally used in medicine and is also employed in perfuming soaps.

It was formerly official in both the British and United States Pharmacopoeias. Both Pimento Oil and Pimento Water were official in the British Pharmacopoeia of 1898, but Oil of Pimento was deleted from the British Pharmacopeia of 1914, though the Water still has a place in the British Pharmacopeia Codex.

Pimento has also been dropped from the United States Pharmacopoeia, but admitted to the National Formulary IV. Pimento is one of the ingredients in the Compound Tincture of Guaic of the National Formulary IV.

Pimento is an aromatic stimulant and carminative to the gastro-intestinal tract, resembling cloves in its action. It is employed chiefly as an addition to tonics and purgatives and as a flavoring agent.

The Essential Oil, as well as the Spirit and the distilled Water of Pimento are useful for flatulent indigestion and for hysterical paroxysms. Two or three drops of the oil on sugar are given to correct flatulence. The oil is also given on sugar and in pills to correct the griping tendencies of purgatives: it was formerly added to Syrup of Buckthorn to prevent griping.

Pimento Water (Aqua Pimentae) is used as a vehicle for stomachic and purgative medicines. It is made by taking 5 parts of bruised Pimento to 200 parts of water and distilling down to 100, the dose being 1 to 2 fluid ounces.

Concentrated Pimento Water of the British Pharmacopoeia Codex

Oil of Pimento 1 fl. oz.

Alcohol 12 fl. oz.

Purified Talc 1 oz.

Distilled Water up to 20 fl. oz.

Dissolve the oil in the alcohol, contained in a suitable bottle, add the water gradually shaking after each addition; add the talc shake, allow to stand for a few hours, occasionally shaking, and filter.

One part of this solution corresponds to about 40 parts of Pimento Water.

Other Preparations

The powdered fruit: dose, 10 to 30 grains. Fluid extract: dose, 1/2 to 1 drachm. Oil: dose, 2 to 5 drops.

Pimento is one of the ingredients of Spice Plaster. An extract made from the crushed berries by boiling them down to a thick liquor is, when spread on linen, a capital stimulating plaster for neuralgic or rheumatic pains.

The fruits of four other species of the genus Pimento, found in Venezuela, Guiana and the West Indies, are employed in their native countries as spices.

The 'Bay Rum," used as a toilet article, is a tincture scented with the oil of the leaves of an allied species, P. acris, commonly known as the Bayberry tree.

Adulterations

Although ground Pimento is sometimes used to adulterate powdered cloves, it is itself little subject to adulteration in the entire condition, though the ground article for household consumption as a spice is subject to the same adulteration as other similar substances, it is sometimes adulterated with the larger and less aromatic berries of the Mexican Myrtus Tobasco, Mocino called Pimienta de Tabasco.

At one time the fruit of the common American Spice Bush, 'Benzoin " was used for this purpose. The powdered berries of this American plant, a member of the natural order Lauracece, Lindera Benzoin, occurring in damp woods throughout the Eastern and Central States, were used during the War of Independence by the Americans as a substitute for Allspice and its leaves as a substitute for tea, hence the plant was often called 'Wild Allspice." All parts of the shrub have a spicy, agreeable flavor, which is strongest in the bark and berries. The leaves and berries are also used in decoction in domestic practice as a febrifuge and are considered to have tonic and also anthelmintic properties. A tincture prepared from the fresh young twigs before the buds have burst in the spring, is still used in homeopathy, but no preparation is employed officially.

The 'Carolina Allspice," or Sweet Bush (Calycanthis foridus, Lindl), is a shrub 6 to 8 feet high, which inhabits the low, shady woods along the mountains of Georgia and North Carolina and in Tennessee. The whole plant is aromatic, having the odor of strawberries when crushed.

It is asserted that the shrub is important as a source of poisoning to cattle and sheep. The alkaloid it contains exercises a powerfully depressant action upon the heart.

It has been used as an antiperiodic, in fluid extract.

ALMONDS

Family: N.O. Rosaceae

Habitat

The Almond tree is a native of the warmer parts of western Asia and of North Africa, but it has been extensively distributed over the warm temperate region of the Old World, and is cultivated in all the countries bordering on the Mediterranean. It was very early introduced into England, probably by the Romans, and occurs in the Anglo-Saxon lists of plants, but was not cultivated in England before 1562, and then chiefly for its blossom.

History

The tree has always been a favorite, and in Shakespeare's time, as Gerard tells us, Almond trees were 'in our London gardens and orchards in great plenty." There are many references to it in our early poetry. Spenser alludes to it in the Fairy Queen:

'Like to an Almond tree ymounted hye,
On top of greene Selinis all alone,
With blossoms brave bedecked daintly;
Whose tender locks do tremble every one
At everie little breath that under Heaven is blowne."

Shakespeare mentions it only once, very casually, in Troilus and Cressida: - 'The parrot will not do more for an Almond' - 'An Almond for a parrot' being an old simile in his days for the height of temptation.

The early English name seems to have been Almande: it thus appears in the Romaunt of the Rose. Both this old name and its more modern form came through the French amande, derived from the late Latin amandela, in turn a form of the Greek amygdalus, the meaning of which is obscure.

The tree grows freely in Syria and Palestine: it is

mentioned in Scripture as one of the best fruit trees of the land of Canaan, and there are many other biblical references to it. The Hebrew name, shakad, is very expressive: it signifies 'hasty awakening," or 'to watch for," hence 'to make haste," a fitting name for a tree, whose beautiful flowers appearing in Palestine in January, herald the wakening up of Creation. The rod of Aaron was an Almond twig, and the fruit of the Almond was one of the subjects selected for the decoration of the golden candlestick employed in the tabernacle. The Jews still carry rods of Almond blossom to the synagogues on great festivals.

As Almonds were reckoned among 'the best fruits of the land' in the time of Jacob we may infer they were not then cultivated in Egypt. Pliny, however, mentions the Almond among Egyptian fruit-trees; and it is not improbable that it was introduced between the days of Jacob and the period of the Exodus.

Almonds, as well as the oil pressed from them, were well known in Greece and Italy long before the Christian era. A beautiful fable in Greek mythology is associated with the tree. Servius relates that Phyllis was changed by the gods into an Almond tree as an eternal compensation for her desertion by her lover Demophoon, which caused her death by grief. When too late, Demophoon returned, and when the leafless, flowerless and forlorn tree was shown him, as the memorial of Phyllis, he clasped it in his arms, whereupon it burst forth into bloom - an emblem of true love inextinguishable by death.

During the Middle Ages, Almonds became an important article of commerce in Central Europe. Their consumption in medieval cookery was enormous. An inventory, made in 1372, of the effects of Jeanne d'Evreux, Queen of France, enumerates only 20 lb. of sugar, but 500 lb. of Almonds.

The ancients attributed many wonderful virtues to the Almond, but it was chiefly valued for its supposed virtue in preventing intoxication. Plutarch mentions a great drinker of wine, who by the use of Bitter Almonds escaped being intoxicated, and Gerard says: 'Five or six, being taken fasting, do keepe a man from being drunke." This theory was probably the origin of the custom of eating salted Almonds through a dinner.

Description

The Almond belongs to the same group of plants as the rose, plum, cherry and peach, being a member of the tribe Prunae of the natural order Rosaceae. The genus Amygdalus to which it is assigned is very closely allied to Prunus (Plum) in which it has sometimes been merged; the distinction lies in the fruit, the succulent pulp attached to the stone in the plum (known botanically as the mesocarp) being replaced by a leathery separable coat in the almond which is hard and juiceless, of a dingy green tinged with dull red, so that when growing it looks not unlike an unripe apricot. When fully ripe, this green covering dries and splits, and the Almond, enclosed in its rough shell (termed the endocarp) drops out. The shell of the Almond is a yellowish buff color and flattened-ovoid in shape, the outer surface being usually pitted with small holes; frequently it has a more or less fibrous nature. Sometimes it is thin and friable (soft-shelled Almond), sometimes extremely hard and woody (hard-shelled Almond). The seed itself is rounded at one end and pointed at the other, and covered with a thin brown, scurfy coat. The different sorts of Almonds vary in form and size, as well as in the firmness of the shell. The fruit is produced chiefly on the young wood of the previous year, and in part on small spurs of two and three years growth.

The tree is of moderate size, usually from 20 to 30 feet high, with spreading branches the leaves lance-shaped, finely toothed (or serrated) at the edges. The flowers are produced before the leaves - in this country early in March; and in great profusion. There are two principal forms of the Almond the one with entirely pink flowers, Amygdalus communis, var. dulcis, producing Sweet Almonds; the other, A. communis, var. amara, with flowers slightly larger, and the petals almost white towards the tips, deepening into rose at the base, producing Bitter Almonds. Botanically, they are considered merely variations of the one type, and the difference in variety has been supposed originally to be mainly owing to climate, the Bitter Almond being a native of Barbary. The Sweet Almond is the earliest to flower, and is cultivated more largely than the Bitter Almond. It is valuable as a food and for confectionery purposes, as well as in medicine, being rich in a bland oil, and sustaining as a nutriment: the staying power conferred by a meal of Almonds and raisins is well known. It is only the Bitter Almond in the use of which caution is necessary, especially with regard to children, as it possesses dangerous poisonous properties.

Cultivation

The early, delicate flowers of the Almond give it a unique position among ornamental trees, and it should have a place in every shrubbery, for it will flourish in any ordinary, well-drained soil, both in open and somewhat sheltered situations, and does well in town gardens.

There are several varieties, differing in color and size of the flowers: one dwarf variety, A. nana, a native of the Lower Danube, is especially decorative, and is often planted in the forefront of shrubberies. All the species are deciduous.

Sicily and Southern Italy are the chief Almond-producing countries; Spain, Portugal, the South of France, the Balearic Islands and Morocco also export considerable quantities.

In the southern counties of England it is not uncommon for the tree to produce a fair crop of fruit, though it is mostly very inferior to that which is imported, but in less favoured districts in this country the production of fruit is rare.

The tree is liable to destruction by frosts in many parts of Central Europe. In France and Belgium, when grown in gardens for its fruit, the tender-shelled varieties are preferred, and the cultivation is the same as for the peach.

SWEET ALMOND

Family: N.O. Rosaceae
Botanical: Amygdalus communis (LINN.) var. dulcis

There are numerous varieties of the Sweet Almond in commerce, the chief being: (1) the Jordan Almonds, the finest and best of the Sweet variety. These, notwithstanding their Oriental name (derived really from the French jardin), we receive from Malaga, imported without their shells. They are distinguished from all other Almonds by their large size, narrow, elongated shape and thin skin; (2) Valentia Almonds, which are broader and shorter than the Jordan variety, with a thicker dusty brown, scurfy skin, usually imported in their shell, and sometimes called in consequence, 'Shell Almonds'; (3) and (4) Sicilian and Barbary Almonds, which closely resemble the Valentia Almonds but are rather smaller and of an inferior quality. They occasionally contain an admixture of Bitter Almonds.

The annual import of Sweet Almonds into this country is normally over 500 tons.

Sweet Almonds have a bland taste, and the white emulsion formed when they are bruised with water is characterized by no marked odor, the seeds being thus distinguished from Bitter Almonds.

Medicinal Action and Uses

Fresh Sweet Almonds possess demulcent and nutrient properties, but as the outer brown skin sometimes causes irritation of the alimentary canal, they are blanched by removal of this skin when used for food. Though pleasant to the taste, their nutritive value is diminished unless well masticated, as they are difficult of digestion, and may in some cases induce nettlerash and feverishness. They have a special dietetic value, for besides containing about 20 per cent of proteids, they contain practically no starch, and are therefore often made into flour for cakes and biscuits for patients suffering from diabetes.

Sweet Almonds are used medicinally, the official preparations of the British Pharmacopoeia being Mistura Amygdalae, Pulvis Amygdalae Compositus and Almond Oil.

On expression they yield nearly half their weight in a bland fixed oil, which is employed medicinally for allaying acrid juices, softening and relaxing solids, and in bronchial diseases, in tickling coughs, hoarseness, costiveness, nephritic pains, etc.

When Almonds are pounded in water, the oil unites with the fluid, forming a milky juice - Almond Milk - a cooling, pleasant drink, which is prescribed as a diluent in acute diseases, and as a substitute for animal milk: an ounce of Almonds is sufficient for a quart of water, to which gum arabic is in most cases a useful addition. The pure oil mixed with a thick mucilage of gum arabic, forms a more permanent emulsion; one part of gum with an equal quantity of water being enough for four parts of oil. Almond emulsions possess in a certain degree the emollient qualities of the oil, and have this advantage over the pure oil, that they may be given in acute or inflammatory disorders without danger of the ill effects which the oil might sometimes produce by turning rancid. Sweet Almonds alone are employed in making emulsions, as the Bitter Almond imparts its peculiar taste when treated in this way.

Blanched and beaten into an emulsion with barley-water, Sweet Almonds are of great use in the stone, gravel, strangury and other disorders of the kidneys, bladder and biliary ducts.

By their oily character, Sweet Almonds sometimes give immediate relief in heartburn. For this, it is recommended to peel and eat six or eight Almonds.

Almonds are also useful in medicine for uniting substances with water. Castor oil is rendered palatable when rubbed up with pounded Almonds and some aromatic distilled water.

The fixed Oil of Almonds is extracted from both Bitter and Sweet Almonds. If intended for external use, it must, however, be prepared only from Sweet Almonds.

The seeds are ground in a mill after removing the reddish-brown powder adhering to them and then subjected to hydraulic pressure, the expressed oil being afterwards filtered and bleached, preferably by exposure to light.

Constituents

Almond oil is a clear, pale yellow, odourless liquid, with a bland, nutty taste. It consists chiefly of Olein, with a small proportion of the Glyceride of Linolic Acid and other Glycerides, but contains no Stearin. It is thus very similar in composition to Olive Oil (for which it may be used as a pleasant substitute), but it is devoid of Chlorophyll, and usually contains a somewhat larger proportion of Olein than Olive Oil.

It is used in trade, as well as medicinally, being most valuable as a lubricant for the delicate works of watches, and is much employed as an ingredient in toilet soap, for its softening action on the skin. It forms a good remedy for chapped hands.

Gerard says:

'The oil newly pressed out of Sweet Almonds is a mitigator of pain and all manner of aches, therefore it is good in pleurisy and colic. The oil of Almonds makes smooth the hands and face of delicate persons, and cleanseth the skin from all spots and pimples."

And Culpepper writes:

'The oil of both (Bitter and Sweet) cleanses the skin, it easeth pains of the chest, the temples being annointed therewith, and the oil with honey, powder of liquorice, oil of roses and white wax, makes a good ointment for dimness of sight."

Culpepper also tells us of Almond butter, saying:

'This kind of butter is made of Almonds with sugar and rose-water, which being eaten with violets is very wholesome and commodious for students, for it rejoiceth the heart and comforteth the brain, and qualifieth the heat of the liver."

BITTER ALMOND

Family: N.O. Rosaceae
Botanical: Amygdalus communis (LINN.) var. amara

There are several varieties of the Bitter Almond, the best being imported from the south of France, and others from Sicily and Northern Africa (Barbary), where it forms a staple article of trade. The annual imports of Bitter Almonds to this country amount normally to about 300 tons.

The seeds are used chiefly as a source of Almond Oil, but also yield a volatile oil, which is largely employed as a flavoring agent.

Bitter Almonds are usually shorter, proportionately broader and smaller, and less regular than the Sweet Almonds. They contain about 50 per cent of the same fixed oil which occurs in the Sweet Almond, and are also free from starch. The bitter taste is characteristic.

Constituents

The Bitter Almond differs from the Sweet Almond in containing a colorless, crystalline glucoside, Amygdalin, of which the Sweet are entirely destitute. This substance is left in the cake obtained after the oil has been expressed, and can be extracted from it by digestion with alcohol. Many other Rosaceous plants contain Amygdalin, such as the peach, apricot, plum, etc., not only in the seed, but also in the young shoots and flower-buds.

The Bitter Almond seed also contains a ferment Emulsin, which in presence of water acts on the soluble glucoside Amygdalin yielding glucose, prussic acid and the essential oil of Bitter Almonds, or Benzaldehyde, which is not used in medicine. Bitter Almonds yield from 6 to 8 per cent of Prussic Acid. About 5 lb. of the seeds yield on the average half an ounce of the essential oil.

The term 'prussic acid' owes its origin to the fact of its having been first obtained from Prussian blue. This acid is contained in small quantities in the leaves and seeds of some of our commonest fruits, especially in applepips. While it is a valuable remedy for some diseases, it is also a deadly poison and its action is extremely rapid.

The leaves of the Cherry-laurel (Prunus laurocerasus) owe their activity to the prussic acid they contain. The laurel water made by distillation is a dangerous poison, and is so variable in strength, that it is unsuited for administration as a medicinal agent. Several fatal cases have occurred from its injudicious use.

The once famous 'Macassor Oil' consisted chiefly of Oil of Almonds, coloured red with Alkanet root, and scented with Oil of Cassia.

This essential volatile oil of Bitter Almonds, under the name of 'Almond flavoring' and 'Spirit of Almonds," is used in confectionery and as a culinary flavoring, but on account of its poisonous nature, great care ought to be exercised in its use, and for the same reason, Bitter Almonds and ratifia biscuits and Marchpane (made largely of Bitter Almonds) should be eaten sparingly.

Bitter Almonds and their poisonous properties were well known to the ancients, who used them in intermittent fevers and as a vermifuge, and they were also employed by them, and in the Middle Ages as an aperient and diuretic, and as a cure for hydrophobia, but from the uncertainty of their operation and the risk attending it, we seldom see them administered now. Taken freely in substance they occasion sickness and vomiting, and to dogs, birds and some other animals, they are poisonous. A simple water, strongly impregnated by distillation with the volatile oil, will cause giddiness, headache and dimness of sight, and has been found also poisonous to animals, and there are instances of cordial spirits flavoured by them being poisonous to man.

Of the several varieties under which they exist, none in size and form resembles the long, sweet Jordan Almond, and it is to avoid Bitter Almonds being used instead of Sweet that the British Pharmacopoeia directs that Jordan Almonds alone shall be employed when Sweet Almonds are used medicinally.

Culpepper says that Bitter Almonds

'do make thin and open, they remove stoppings out of the liver and spleen, therefore they be good against pain in the sides.... The same doth likewise kill tetters in the outward parts of the body (as Dioscorides addeth) if it be dissolved in vinegar."

He also tells us that mixed with honey, these Almonds 'are good for bitings of a mad dog."

Adulterations and Substitutes

The adulteration of Bitter Almonds with Sweet Almonds is a frequent source of loss and annoyance to the pressers of Almond Oil, whose profit largely depends on the amount of volatile oil they are able to extract from the residual cake.

Apricot and peach kernels contain constituents similar to those of the Bitter Almonds. They are imported in large quantities from Syria and California, and are often used by confectioners in the place of Bitter Almonds.

The fixed oil expressed from them is known as Peach Kernel Oil (01. Amygdae Pers.). From the cake, an essential oil is distilled (01. Amygdae Essent. Pers.), as from Bitter Almond cake.

True Oil of Almonds is frequently distinguished from these by being described as 'English," since the bulk of it has hitherto been pressed in this country. The kernels of the peach and apricot are with difficulty distinguished from those of the Almond, and the oils obtained from them closely resemble the so-called English, and much more expensive oil.

Recipes

To make Almond Cake (Seventeenth Century)

'Take one pound of Jordan almonds, Blanch ym into cold water, and dry ym in a clean cloth: pick out these that are nought and rotten: then beat ym very fine in a stone mortar, puting in now and then a little rose water to keep ym from oyling: then put it out into a platter, and half a pound of loaf sugar beaten fine and mixt with ye almonds, ye back of a spoon, and set it on a chafing dish of coals, and let it stand till it be hott: and when it is cold then have ready six whites of eggs beaten with too spoonfuls of flower to a froth, and mix it well with ye almonds: bake ym on catt paper first done over with a feather dipt in sallet oyle."

Almond Butter (Seventeenth Century)

'Seeth a little French Barly with a whole mace and some anniseeds to sweeten but not to give any sensible tast: then blanch and beat the almonds with some of the clearest of the liquor to make the milke the thicker, and strain them, getting forth by often beating what milk you can: seeth the milke till it thicken and bee ready to rise, and turne it with the juice of a lemon or salt dissolved in rose water: spread the curd on a linnen cloath that the whey may run out, and let it hang till it leave dropping: then season the butter that is left with rose water, and sugar to your liking."

To make Almond Milk (Seventeenth Century)

'Take 3 pints of running water, a handfull of Raisins of the Sun stoned, halfe a handfull of Sorrell as much violet and strawberry leaves, halfe a handfull of the topps and flowers of burrage (borage), as much of Buglass, halfe a handfull of Endive, as much Succory, some Pauncys (Pansies), a little broad time and Orgamen (Marjoram), and a branch or two of Rosemary, lett all these boyle well together; then take a good handfull of French Barley, boyling it in three waters, put it to the rest, and lett them boyle till you think they are enough, then pour the liquor into a basin, and stampe the barley and reasons, straining them thereto; then take a quarter of a pound of Sweet Almonds, blanch them and pound them thrice, straining them to the other liquor; then season it with damask rosewater to your liking."

A Paste for ye Hands (Seventeenth Century)

'Take a pound of sun raysens, stone and take a pound of bitter Almonds, blanch ym and beat ym in stone morter, with a glass of sack take ye peel of one Lemond, boyle it tender; take a quart of milk, and a pint of Ale, and make therewith a Possett; take all ye Curd and putt it to ye Almonds: yn putt in ye Rayson: Beat all these till they come to a fine Past, and putt in a pott, and keep it for ye use."

ALOES

Botanical: Aloe Perryi (J. G. BAKER), Aloe vera (LINN)

Family: N.O. Liliaceae
Part Used: Leaves.

Habitat

Aloes are indigenous to East and South Africa, but have been introduced into the West Indies (where they are extensively cultivated) and into tropical countries, and will even flourish in the countries bordering on the Mediterranean.

The drug Aloes consists of the liquid exuded from the transversely-cut bases of the leaves of various species of Aloes, evaporated to dryness.

Description

They are succulent plants belonging to the Lily family, with perennial, strong and fibrous roots and numerous, persistent, fleshy leaves, proceeding from the upper part of the root, narrow, tapering, thick and fleshy, usually beset at the edges with spiney teeth. Many of the species are woody and branching. In the remote districts of S.W. Africa and in Natal, Aloes have been discovered 30 to 60 feet in height, with stems as much as 10 feet in circumference.

The flowers are produced in erect, terminal spikes. There is no calyx, the corolla is tubular, divided into six narrow segments at the mouth and of a red, yellow or purplish color. The capsules contain numerous angular seeds.

The true Aloe is in flower during the greater part of the year and is not to be confounded with another plant, the Agave or American Aloe (Agave Americana), which is remarkable for the long interval between its periods of flowering. This is a succulent plant, without stem, the leaves being radical, spiney, and toothed. There is a variety with variegated foliage. The flower-stalk rises to many feet in height, bearing a number of large and handsome flowers. In cold climates there is usually a very long interval between the times of its flowering, though it is a popular error to suppose that it happens only once in a hundred years for when it obtains sufficient heat and receives a culture similar to that of the pineapple, it is found to flower much more frequently. Various species of Agave, all of which closely resemble each other, have been largely grown as ornamental plants since the first half of the sixteenth century in the south of Europe, and are completely acclimatized in Spain, Portugal and Southern Italy, but though often popularly called Aloes all of them are plants of the New World whereas the true Aloes are natives of the Old World. From a chemical point of view there is also no analogy at all between Aloes and Agaves.

Although the Agave is not employed medicinally, the leaves have been used in Jamaica as a substitute for soap, the expressed juice (a gallon of the juice yields about 1 lb. of the soft extract), dried in the sun, being made into balls with wood ash. This soap lathers with salt water as well as fresh. The leaves have also been used for scouring pewter and kitchen utensils. The inner spongy substance of the leaves in a decayed state has been employed as tinder and the fibres may be spun into a strong, useful thread.

The fleshy leaves of the true Aloe contain near the epidermis or outer skin, a row of fibrovascular bundles, the cells of which are much enlarged and filled with a yellow juice which exudes when the leaf is cut. When it is desired to collect the juice, the leaves are cut off close to the stem and so placed that the juice is drained off into tubs. This juice thus collected is concentrated either by spontaneous evaporation, or more generally by boiling until it becomes of the consistency of thick honey. On cooling, it is then poured into gourds, boxes, or other convenient receptacles, and solidifies.

Aloes require two or three years' standing before they yield their juice. In the West Indian Aloe plantations they are set out in rows like cabbages and cutting takes place in March or April, but in Africa the drug is collected from the wild plants.

Constituents

The most important constituents of Aloes are the two Aloins, Barbaloin and Isobarbaloin, which constitute the so-called 'crystalline' Aloin, present in the drug at from 10 to 30 per cent. Other constituents are amorphous Aloin, resin and Aloe-emodin. The proportion in which the Aloins are present in the respective Aloes is not accurately known.

The manner in which the evaporation is conducted has a marked effect on the appearance of the Aloes, slow and moderate concentration tending to induce crystallization of the Aloin, thus causing the drug to appear opaque. Such Aloes is termed 'livery' or hepatic, and splinters of it exhibit minute crystals of Aloin when examined under the microscope. If, on the other hand, the evaporation is carried as far as possible, the Aloin does not crystallize and small fragments of the drug appear transparent; it is then termed 'glassy,'' 'vitreous,'' or 'lucid' Aloes and exhibits no crystals of Aloin under the microscope.

Varieties

The chief varieties of Aloes are Curacao or Barbados, Socotrine (including Zanzibar) and Cape. Other varieties of Aloes, such as black 'Mocha' Aloes, occasionally find their way to the London market. Jafferabad Aloes, supposed to be the same as 'Mocha' Aloes, is of a black, pitch-like color and a glassy, somewhat porous fracture; it is the product of Aloe Abyssinica and is imported to Bombay from Arabia. It does not enter into English commerce. Musambra Aloes is made in India from A. vulgaris. Uganda Aloes, imported from Mossel Bay, not from Uganda, is a variety of Cape Aloes produced by careful evaporation. Natal Aloes, another South African variety, is no longer a commercial article in this country. The A. Purificata of the United States Pharmacopoeia is prepared by adding Alcohol to melted Aloes, stirring thoroughly, straining and evaporating the strained liquid. The product occurs in irregular, brittle, dull-brown or reddish pieces and is almost entirely soluble in Alcohol.

Curacoa Aloes is obtained from A. chinensis (Staud.) A. vera (Linn.) and probably other species. It was formerly produced on the island of Barbados, where it was largely cultivated, having been introduced at the beginning of the sixteenth century, and is still frequently, but improperly called Barbados Aloes. It is now almost entirely made on the Dutch islands of Curacoa, Aruba and Bonaire by boiling the Aloe juice down and pouring the viscid residue into empty spirit cases, in which it is allowed to solidify. Formerly gourds of various sizes were used (usually containing from 60 to 70 lb.) but Aloes in gourds is now seldom seen. It is usually opaque and varies in color from bright yellowish or rich reddish brown to black. Sometimes it is vitreous and small fragments are then of a deep garnet-red color and transparent. It is then known as 'Capey Barbados' and is less valuable, but may become opaque and more valuable by keeping. Curacoa Aloes possesses the nauseous and bitter taste that is characteristic of all Aloes and a disagreeable, penetrating odor. It is almost entirely soluble in 60 per cent alcohol and contains not more than 30 per cent of substances insoluble in water and 12 per cent of moisture. It should not yield more than 3 per cent of ash.

Commercial Aloin is obtained usually from Curacoa Aloes.

Solutions of Curacoa and other Aloes gradually undergo change, and may after a month no longer react normally, and may also lose the bitterness natural to Aloes.

Socotrine Aloes is prepared to a certain extent on the island of Socotra, but probably more largely on the African and possibly also on the Arabian mainland, from the leaves of A. Perryi (Baker). It is usually imported in kegs in a pasty condition and subsequent drying is necessary. It may be distinguished principally from Curacoa Aloes by its different odor. Much of the dry drug is characterized by the presence of small cavities in the fractured surface, but the variety of Socotrine Aloes distinguished as Zanzibar Aloes often very closely resembles Curacoa in appearance and is usually imported in liver-brown masses which break with a dull, waxy fracture, differing from that of Socotrine Aloes in being nearly smooth and even. When it is prepared, it is commonly poured into goat skins, which are then packed into cases.

Constituents

The name 'Socotrine' Aloes is officially applied to both Socotrine and Zanzibar Aloes. Its chief constituents are Barbaloin (formerly called Socaloin and Zanaloin) and B. Barbaloin, no Isobarbaloin being present in this variety of Aloes. Resin water-soluble substances other than Aloin and Aloe-emodin are also present.

Socotrine Aloes should be of a dark, reddish-brown color, and almost entirely soluble in alcohol. Not more than 50 per cent should be insoluble in water and it should yield not more than 3 per cent of ash. Garnet-coloured, translucent Socotrine Aloes is not now found in commerce, though fine qualities of Zanzibar Aloes are sometimes slightly translucent. Samples of the drug which are nearly black are unfit for pharmaceutical purposes. The odor of Zanzibar Aloes is strong and characteristic, and its taste nauseous and bitter.

Cape Aloes is prepared in Cape Colony from A. ferou (Linn.), A. spicata (Thumb.) A. Africana, A. platylepia and other species of Aloe. It possesses more powerfully purgative properties than any other variety of the drug and is preferred to other varieties on the Continent, but is chiefly employed in this country for veterinary purposes only though for this purpose the Curacoa Aloes is as a rule preferred. Another form of the drug used for veterinary purposes, called Caballine or Horse Aloes, usually consists of the residue from the purification of the more valuable sorts.

Cape Aloes almost invariably occurs in the vitreous modification; it forms dark coloured masses which break with a clean glassy fracture and exhibit in their splinters a yellowish, reddish-brown or greenish tinge. Its translucent, glossy appearance and very characteristic, red-currant like odor sufficiently distinguish it from all other varieties of Aloes.

Uganda Aloes is also obtained from A. ferox. It occurs in bricks or fragments of hepatic, yellowish-brown color, with a bronze gold fracture and its odor resembles that of Cape Aloes.

Cape Aloes contains 9 per cent or more of Barbaloin (formerly known as Capaloin) and B. Barbaloin. Only traces of Capalores not annol combined with paracumaric acid. Cape Aloes should not contain more than 12 per cent of water; it should yield at least 45 per cent of aquoeus extract but not more than 2 per cent of ash Uganda Aloes yields about 6 per cent of Aloin, part of which is B. Barbaloin. The leaves of the plants from which Cape Aloes is obtained are cut off near the stem and arranged around a hole in the ground, in which a sheepskin is spread, with smooth side upwards. When a sufficient quantity of juice has drained from the leaves it is concentrated by heat in iron cauldrons and subsequently poured into boxes or skins in which it solidifies on cooling. Large quantities of the drug are exported from Cape Town and Mossel Bay.

Natal Aloes. The source of this variety which is seldom imported, is not yet definitely ascertained, but it is probably prepared from one or more species of Aloe, probably including A. ferox. Natal Aloes is prepared with greater care than Cape Aloes the leaves being cut obliquely into slices and the juice allowed to exude in the hot sunshine, after which it is boiled down in iron pots the liquid being stirred until it becomes thick and then poured into wooden cases to solidify. Natal Aloes is much weaker than any other variety, having little purgative action on human beings, apparently because it contains no Emodin. It is no longer of commercial importance. It resembles Cape Aloes in odor and occurs in irregular pieces which are almost always opaque and have a characteristic, dull greenish-black or brown color. It is much less soluble than Cape Aloes. It has not a glassy fracture like that of Cape Aloes and when powdered is of a greenish color.

Good Aloes should yield 40 per cent of soluble matter to cold water.

Both Curacoa and Cape Aloes in powder give a crimson color with nitric acid, Socratine Aloes powder touched with nitric acid does not give a crimson color.

History

The Mahometans, especially those in Egypt, regard the Aloe as a religious symbol, and the Mussulman who has made a pilgrimage to the shrine of the Prophet is entitled to hang the Aloe over his doorway. The Mahometans also believe that this holy symbol protects a householder from any malign influence.

In Cairo, the Jews also adopt the practice of hanging up the Aloe.

In the neighborhood of Mecca, at the extremity of every grave, on a spot facing the epitaph, Burckhardt found planted a low shrubby species of Aloe whose Arabic name, saber, signifies patience. This plant is evergreen and requires very little water. Its name refers to the waiting-time between the burial and the resurrection morning.

All kinds of Aloes are admirably provided by their succulent leaves and stems against the drought of the countries where they flourish. The cuticle which covers every part of the plant is, in those which contain a great quantity of pulpy material, formed so as to imbibe moisture very easily and to evaporate it very slowly. If the leaf of an Aloe be separated from the parent plant, it may be laid in the sun for several weeks without becoming entirely shrivelled; and even when considerably dried by long exposure to heat, it will, if plunged into water, become in a few hours plump and fresh.

Medicinal Action and Uses

The drug Aloes is one of the safest and best warm and stimulating purgatives to persons of sedentary habits and phlegmatic constitutions. An ordinary small dose takes from 15 to 18 hours to produce an effect. Its action is exerted mainly on the large intestine, for which reason, also it is useful as a vermifuge. Its use, however, is said to induce Piles.

From the Chemist and Druggist (July 22, 1922):

'Aloes, strychnine and belladonna in pill form was criticized by Dr. Bernard Fautus in a paper read before the Chicago branch of the American Pharmaceutical Society. He pointed out that when given at the same time they cannot possibly act together because of the different speed and duration of the three agents. Aloin is slow in action, requiring from 10 to 12 hours. Strychnine and Atropine, on the other hand, are rapidly absorbed, and have but a brief duration of action."

Preparations of Aloes are rarely prescribed alone, they require the addition of carminatives to moderate the tendency to griping. The compound preparations of Aloes in use generally contain such correctives, but powdered Aloes and the extracts of Aloes represent the crude drug.

Aloes in one form or another is the commonest domestic medicine and is the basis of most proprietary or so-called 'patent' pills.

There is little to choose medicinally between the Curacoa and Socotrine varieties, but the former is somewhat more powerful, 2 grains of Curacoa Aloes being equal to 3 grains of Socotrine Aloes in purgative action. The latter is more expensive, but varies much in quality.

Aloes is the purgative in general uses for horses, it is also used in veterinary practice as a bitter tonic in small doses, and externally as a stimulant and desiccant.

Aloes was employed by the ancients and was known to the Greeks as a production of the island of Socotra as early as the fourth century B.C. The drug was used by Dioscorides, Celsus and Pliny, as well as by the later Greek and Arabian physicians, though it is not mentioned either by Hippocrates or Theophrastus.

From notices of it in the Anglo-Saxon leech-books and a reference to it as one of the drugs recommended to Alfred the Great by the Patriarch of Jerusalem, we may infer that its use was not unknown in Britain as early as the tenth century. At this period the drug was imported into Europe by way of the Red Sea and Alexandria. In the early part of the seventeenth century, there was a direct trade in Aloes between England and Socotra, and in the records of the East Indian Company there are notices of the drug being bought of the King of Socotra, the produce being a monopoly of the Sultan of the island.

The word Aloes, in Latin Lignum Aloes, is used in the Bible and in many ancient writings to designate a substance totally distinct from the modern Aloes, namely the resinous wood of Aquilaria agallocha, a large tree growing in the Malayan Peninsula. Its wood constituted a drug which was, down to the beginning of the present century, generally valued for use as incense, but now is esteemed only in the East.

A beautiful violet color is afforded by the leaves of the Socotrine Aloe, and it does not require a mordant to fix it.

Preparations

Fluid extract: dose, 5 to 30 drops. Powdered extract: dose, 1 to 5 grains. Comp decoc., B.P.: dose, 1/2 to 2 OZ. Tincture B.P.: dose, 1/4 to 2 drachms. Tincture aloes myrrh, U.S.P.: dose, 30 drops.

ALSTONIA

Botanical: Alstonia scholaris (R. BR.)
Family: N.O. Apocynaceae
Synonyms: Echites scholaris (Linn.). Dita Bark. Bitter Bark. Devil Tree. Pale Mara.
Part Used: The bark.
Habitat: India and the Philippines.

Description

The tree grows from 50 to 80 feet high, has a furrowed trunk, oblong stalked leaves up to 6 inches long and 4 inches wide, dispersed in four to six whorls round the stem, their upper side glossy, under side white, nerves running at right angles to the mid-rib. The bark is almost odourless and very bitter, in commerce it is found in irregular fragments 1/8 to 1/2 inch thick, texture spongy, fracture coarse and short, outside layer rough uneven fissured brownish grey and sometimes blackish spots; inside layer bright buff, transverse section shows a number of small medullary rays in inner layer.

Constituents

It contains three alkaloids, Ditamine, Echitamine or Ditaine, and Echitenines, and several fatty and resinous substances- the second is the strongest base and resembles ammonia in chemical characters.

Medicinal Action and Uses

The bark is used in homeopathy for its tonic bitter and astringent properties; it is particularly useful for chronic diarrhea and dysentry.

Preparations and Dosages

Infusion of Alstonia, 5 parts to 100 parts water. Dose, 1 fluid ounce. Powdered bark, 2 to 4 grains.

In India the natives use the bark for bowel complaints. In Ceylon its light wood is used for coffins. In Borneo the wood close to the root of the same species is very light and of white color and is used for net floats, household utensils, trenchers, corks, etc.

Other Species

A bark called Poele is obtained from Alstonia spectabilis, habitat Java; it contains the same alkaloids as dita and an additional crystalline, Alstonamine.

ALSTONIA BARK

Botanical: Alstonia constricta (F. MUELL.)
Family: N.O. Apocynaceae
Synonyms: Fever Bark. Australian Quinine.
Part Used: The dried bark.
Habitat: New South Wales and Australia.

Description

The name is derived from Alston, a professor of botany in Edinburgh. In commerce the bark is usually in curved pieces or quills 2 1/2 inches wide and 1/2, inch thick. Periderm 1/10 to 1/4 of an inch; rusty brown, rugose, deeply fissured recticulations; internally the bark is cinnamon brown with strong coarse longitudinal stripes. Transverse section shows dark brown periderm covering the inner orange-brown tissues. Fracture short granular in outer layers and fibrous inner ones, slight aromatic odor, very bitter taste.

Constituents

Contains three alkaloids Alstonine, Porphrine and Astonidine, and traces of others.

Medicinal Action and Uses

Used for chronic diarrhea, dysentery and in intermittent fever; also as an anthelmintic. Scientific investigation has failed to show why it is of such service in malaria, but herbalists consider it superior to quinine and of great use in convalescence, also much used by homeopaths.

Preparations and Dosages

Powdered bark 2 to 8 grains. Fluid extract, 4 to 40 minims.

AMARANTHS

Botanical: Amaranthus hypochondriacus (LINN.)
Family: N.O. Amaranthaceae
Synonyms: Love-Lies-Bleeding. Red Cockscomb. Velvet Flower.

Habitat

The Amaranths are met with most abundantly in the tropics, especially in tropical America, but are not plentiful in cold countries.

Many species are widely distributed as pernicious weeds. Their economic importance is slight, their properties chiefly proteid nutrient. Many abound in mucilage and sugar and many species are used as pot-herbs, resembling those of Chenopodiaceae. Many, also, are excellent fodder-plants, though not cultivated.

Constituents

Their constituents are indefinite; none are poisonous, none possess very distinct medicinal properties, though many have use in native practice as alteratives, and as antidotes to snake-bite, etc.

Medical Action and Uses

Some species have slightly astringent properties, others are diaphoretics and diuretics, and a few are tonics and stimulants.

In ancient Greece, the Amaranth was sacred to Ephesian Artemis: it was supposed to have special healing properties and as a symbol of immortality was used to decorate images of the gods and tombs. The name, from the Greek signifying unwithering, was applied to certain plants which from their lasting for ever, typified immortality.

Some of the species are old favorites as garden flowers, viz., Amaranthus hypochondriacus, known as Prince's Feather, an Indian annual - with deeply-veined, lance-shaped leaves, purple on the under side with deep crimson flowers, densely packed on erect spikes, and A. caudatus (Jacq.) (Love-lies-bleeding), a native of Africa and Java, a vigorous hardy annual with dark purplish flowers crowded in handsome drooping spikes. It is considered astringent and a decoction of the flowers has been administered in spitting of blood and various hemorrhages and has been said to be so energetic that it may be used in cases of menorrhagia. With several other species belonging to the closely allied genus Aeva, natives of India, it has also been used as an anthelmintic.

A. spinosa (Linn.), A. campestris (Willd.) and many others are used in India as diuretics. A. oleraceus (Linn.) is used in India in diarrhea and menstrual disorders and the young leaves and shoots are also eaten as a vegetable, similarly to spinach. A. polygonoides, a common garden weed in India, is also used as a pot-herb and considered so wholesome that convalescents are ordered it in preference to all other kinds.

AMARANTH, WILD

Botanical: Amaranthum blitum (LINN.)
Family: N.O. Amaranthaceae
Synonym: Strawberry Blite.

Amaranthum blitum (Linn.), the wild Amaranth admitted to the list of British plants, is an inconspicuous weed, often mistaken for an Orache or Goosefoot, sometimes found on rubbish-heaps near towns and probably a remnant of ancient cultivation as a pot-herb.

It is an annual, with trailing stems a foot or two in length and more or less oval leaves with long stalks. The numerous green flowers are clustered in the angles between leaf and stem and are unisexual, without petals, both male and female flowers occurring on the same plant.

The female flower develops into a juicy, crimson capsule containing a single seed. The clusters of these fruits have in some localities suggested the name of Strawberry Blite for the plant.

It flowers in August.

In France, its leaves are still eaten in the same way as spinach.

Culpepper, speaking of the garden Amaranths and especially of the Love-lies-bleeding, which he calls Flower Gentle, Flower Velure, Floramor and Velvet flower, says:

'The flowers dried and beaten into powder stops the terms in women, and so do almost all other red things. And by the icon or image of every herb, the ancients at first found out their virtues. Modern writers laugh at them for it- but I wonder how the virtues of herbs came at first to be known, if not by their signatures, the moderns have them from the writings of the ancients; the ancients had no writings to have them from. -The flowers stop all fluxes of blood, whether in man or woman, bleeding either at the nose or wound."

Medicinal Uses

In modern herbal medicine, a fluid extract is employed, the dose being 1/2 to 1 drachm and also a decoction taken in wine glassful doses, which is used externally as an application in ulcerated conditions of the throat and mouth and as an injection in leucorrhoea, and as a wash for ulcers, sores, etc. For its astringency it is much recommended in diarrhea, dysentery and hemorrhages from the bowels.

AMMONIACUM

Botanical: Dorema ammoniacum (D. DON.)
Family: N.O. Umbelliferae
Synonyms: Gum Ammoniac.
Part Used: The gum resin exuding from the flowering and fruiting stem of Dorema ammoniacum and probably other species.
Habitat: Persia, extending into Southern Siberia.

Description

The plant grows to height of about 7 feet and in spring and early summer contains a milky juice. It is visited by numbers of beetles which puncture the stem and thus cause an exudation, part of which dries on the stem, the rest falling to the ground where it becomes mixed with stones and other impurities found in the gum collected by the natives. The gum resin is found in special cavities in the tissues of the stem, root and petioles of the leaves. The name of the drug is said to be derived from the Temple of Jupiter Ammon in the Libyan Desert where it was collected by the ancients. The gum resin occurs in commerce in two forms, tear ammoniacum and lump or block ammoniacum. The former alone is official in England and consists of pale yellow nodular masses varying in size from a pea to a walnut, brittle when cold but softens on warming, fractured surface, milky white or pale brown in color. The lump ammoniacum, which is that collected from the ground, is used sometimes but is not official in medicine. The odor of the drug is slight, taste acrid and persistent.

Constituents

The drug contains volatile oil resin and gum. The resin consists of an indifferent resene associated with ammoresinotannol combined with salicylic acid.

Medicinal Action and Uses

Taken internally, it acts by facilitating expectoration and is of value in chronic bronchitis, especially in the aged when the secretion is tough and viscid. The resin has a mild diuretic action. It is antispasmodic and stimulant and is given sometimes as a diaphoretic and emmenagogue, used as a plaster for white swellings of the joints and for indolent tumors. Its use is of great antiquity and is mentioned by Hippocrates.

Preparations and Dosages

Ammoniacum mixture, B.P. 4 to 8 drachms. Ammoniacum in powder, 1 part; syrup of balsam of tolu, 2 parts; distilled water, 30 parts. Dose, 1/2 to 1 fluid ounce. Dose of the powdered gum, 5 to 15 grains, B.P.C. Dose of the powdered gum, 10 to 30 grains, U.S.P.

Other Species

African Ammoniacum or 'feshook," from Ferula Communis is not a commercial article. The Mahommedans use if for incense; this variety grows well in the author's garden at Chalfont St. Peter.

ANEMONES

Family: N.O. Ranunculaceae

The Anemones are represented in our native British flora by only two species, the dainty little Wood Anemone (Anemone nemorosa) and the Pasque Flower (A. pulsatilla), both possessing medicinal properties, though the former is little used now.

There are, however, about seventy species in the genus Anemone, including the subgenus Hepatica, now also reckoned as Anemones, though formerly ranking as a separate genus, the chief representative of which, A. hepatica, is of some considerable medicinal value. A. pratensis, a continental species, is employed medicinally for the same purposes as A. pulsatilla, and the number of species familiar to us as garden flowers is very great, the most popular among these being, perhaps, the Poppy or Garden Anemone, A. coronavria a native of the Levant and Southern Europe, introduced here in 1596, and the Star Anemone, A. hortensis, a native of Italy, brought to England from Holland about the same time. A. apennina and A. blanda are also particularly charming the latter with large flowers of various shades of blue being the earliest to open.

Description

The distinguishing characteristics of the genus Anemone are the presence of three entire leaflets arranged in a whorl just under the flowers, forming an involucre, and the fact that the flowers themselves have no real petals, but a calyx of six to eight petal-like sepals. All species share the acrid and bitter nature of almost all plants of the Ranunculus order to which they belong, and the leaves and flowers should not be eaten. The toxic principle has been extracted from three species: the two British species and one foreign one, though no actually fatal results have been recorded. A yellow-flowered foreign species, A. ranunculoides, found in almost all parts of the Continent, has been used for poisoning arrows, and in France, swelling and blistering of the hands has resulted from using the juice as a stimulant to ulceration.

Cultivation

Anemones flourish best in a rich, sandy loam, but will thrive in any garden soil which is well-drained and tolerably light, it should also be enriched with decayed manure. Sea sand, or a little salt mixed with the soil is a good preventive of mildew.

Propagation is by division of the rootstocks and cuttings of the root in autumn and early spring - from October to the end of March - and also from seed, which should be sown within a month of ripening, as it deteriorates with keeping. Sow thinly in lines on the surface and merely rake the seeds in with a very light hand. Germination is slow. Thin the plants to 6 inches apart. Thinnings will bear transplanting if carefully handled and helped with water afterwards. The first flowers are generally produced the first spring after sowing, but soil and situation have always a great effect on them.

Some persons take up Anemone tubers as soon as the leaf has died down, and replant in the early part of the year, but this is not necessary: those that have been two or three years in the ground attain a large size - they are solid, flattened masses, not unlike ginger. When planting, cover with soil to the depth of 3 inches.

Most garden Anemones can be treated in this way. The best time for transplanting A. pulsatilla is considered to be directly after it has flowered, or at any rate during the summer, while it is in growth; autumn is a bad time and early spring not much better.

ANEMONE PULSATILLA

Botanical: Anemone pulsatilla (LINN.)
Family: N.O. Ranunculaceae
Synonyms: Pasque Flower. Wind Flower. Meadow

Anemone. Passe Flower. Easter Flower.
Part Used: Whole herb.

Habitat

Anemone pulsatilla is found not in woods, but in open situations. It grows wild in the dry soils of almost every Central and Northern country of Europe, but in England is rather a local plant, abounding on high chalk downs and limestone pastures, mostly in Yorkshire, Berkshire, Oxford and Suffolk, but seldom found in other situations and other districts in this country.

Description

It has a thick and somewhat woody root-stock, from which arises a rosette of finely-divided, stalked leaves, covered with silky hairs, especially when young, the foot-stalk often being purplish. The flowers, which are about 1 1/2 inches across, are borne singly on stalks 5 to 8 inches in height, with an involucre of three sessile (i.e stalkless) deeply-cut leaflets or bracts. The sepals are of a dull violet-purple color, very silky on the under surfaces. The seed- vessels are small, brown hairy achenes, with long, feathery tails, like those of the Traveller's Joy or Wild Clematis.

The whole plant, especially the bases of the foot-stalks, is covered with silky hairs. It is odourless, but possesses at first a very acrid taste, which is less conspicuous in the dried herb and gradually diminishes on keeping. The majority of the leaves develop after the flowers; they are two to three times deeply three-parted or pinnately cleft to the base, in long, linear, acute segments.

The juice of the purple sepals gives a green stain to paper and linen, but it is not permanent. It has been used to color the Paschal eggs in some countries, whence it has been supposed the English name of the plant is derived. Gerard, however, expressly informs us that he himself was 'moved to name' this the Pasque Flower, or Easter Flower, because of the time of its appearance, it being in bloom from April to June. The specific name, pulsatilla, from pulsc, I beat, is given in allusion to its downy seeds being beaten about by the wind.

Varieties of pulsatilla when cultivated in this country like a well-drained, light, but deep soil, and will flourish in a peat or leaf soil, with the addition of lime rubble.

Part used Medicinally

The drug Pulsatilla, which is of highly valuable modern curative use as a herbal simple, is obtained not only from the whole herb of A. pulsatilla, but also from A. pratensis, the Meadow Anemone, which is closely allied to the Pasque Flower, differing chiefly in having smaller flowers with deeper purple sepals, inflexed at the top. It grows in Denmark, Germany and Italy, but not in England. It is recommended for certain diseases of the eye, like Pulsatilla, and is used in homeopathy, but has been considered somewhat dangerous. The whole plant has a strong acrid taste, but is eaten by both sheep and goats, though cows and horses will not touch it. The leaves when bruised and applied to the skin raise blisters. A. patens, var. Nutalliana is also used for the same purpose as A. pulsatilla.

In each case, the whole herb is collected, soon after flowering, and should be carefully preserved when dried; it deteriorates if kept longer than one year.

Constituents

The fresh plant yields by distillation with water an acrid, oily principle, with a burning, peppery taste, Oil of Anemone. A similar oil is obtained from Ranunculus bulbosus, R. flammula and R. sceleratus, which belong to the same order of plants. Its therapeutic value is not considered great. When kept for some time,this oily substance becomes decomposed into Anemonic acid and Anemonin. Anemonin is crystalline, tasteless and odourless when pure and melts at 152ø. The action of Pulsatilla is virtually that of this crystalline substance Anemonin, which is a powerful irritant, like cantharides, in overdoses causing violent gastro-enteritis. It is volatile in water vapor and is then irritative to the eyes and mouth. The Oil acts as a vescicant when applied to the skin. Anemonicacid appears to be inert. Anemonin sometimes causes local inflammation and gangrene when subcutaneously injected, vomiting and purging when given internally.

It is, however, uncertain whether these symptoms are due to Anemonin itself or to some impurity in it. The chief action of pure Anemonin is a depressant one on the circulation, respiration and spinal cord, to a certain extent resembling that of Aconite. The symptoms are slow and feeble pulse, slow respiration, coldness, paralysis and death without convulsions. In poisoning by extract of Pulsatilla, convulsions are always present. Their absence in poisoning by pure Anemonin appears to be due to its paralysing action on motor centres in the brain.

Medicinal Action and Uses

Nervine, antispasmodic, alterative and diaphoretic. The tincture of Pulsatilla is beneficial in disorders of the mucous membrane, of the respiratory and of the digestive passages. Doses of 2 to 3 drops in a spoonful of water will allay the spasmodic cough of asthma, whooping-cough and bronchitis.

For catarrhal affection of the eyes, as well as for catarrhal diarrhea, the tincture is serviceable. It is also valuable as an emmenagogue, in the relief of headaches and neuralgia, and as a remedy for nerve exhaustion in women.

It is specially recommended for fair, blue-eyed women.

It has been employed in the form of extract in some cutaneous diseases with much success; it is included in the British Pharmacopoeia and was formerly included in the United States Pharmacopoeia.

In homeopathy it is considered very efficacious and even a specific in measles. It is prescribed as a good remedy for nettlerash and also for neuralgic toothache and earache, and is administered in indigestion and bilious attacks.

Preparation

Fluid extract, 5 to 10 drops. Parkinson says of this species: 'There are five different kinds of Pulsatilla, which flower in April: they are sometimes used for tertian ague and to help obstructions."

ANEMONE (WOOD)

Botanical: Anemone nemorosa (LINN.)
Family: N.O. Ranunculaceae
Synonyms: Crowfoot. Windflower. Smell Fox.
Parts Used: Root, leaves, juice.

The Wood Anemone is one of the earliest spring flowers.

Description

It has a long, tough, creeping root-stock, running just below the surface; it is the quick growth of this root-stock that causes the plant to spread so rapidly, forming large colonies in the moist soil of wood and thicket. The deeply-cut leaves and star-like flowers rise directly from it on separate unbranched stems. Some distance below the flower are the three leaflets, often so deeply divided as to appear more than three in number and very similar to the true leaves. They wrap round and protect the flower-bud before it unfolds, but as it opens, its stalk lengthens and it is carried far above them.

The flower has no honey and little scent, and apparently relies little on the visits of insects for the fertilization of its one-celled seed-vessels, which are in form like those of the butter-cup, arranged in a mass in the centre of the many stamens, and are termed achenes. As in all the Anemones, there are no true petals, what seem so are really the sepals, which have assumed the coloring and characteristics of petals. They are six in number, pure white on the upper surfaces and pale rose-colored beneath.

In sunshine, the flower is expanded wide, but at the approach of night, it closes and droops its graceful head so that the dew may not settle on it and injure it. If rain threatens in the daytime, it does the same, receiving the drops upon its back, whence they trickle of harmlessly from the sepal tips. The way the sepals then fold over the mass of stamens and undeveloped seed-vessels in their centre has been likened to a tent, in which, as used fancifully to be said by country-folk, the fairies nestled for protection, having first pulled the curtains round them.

The plant is very liable to attack from certain fungi:

at times, a species of Puccinia settles on it, the result being that the stalks of infected leaves grow rapidly, high above the others, though the leaves themselves dwindle and lose their divisions. A species of Sclerotinia attacks the swollen tubers of the root, doing still more harm, for in the spring there arise not the delicate white flowers, but the ugly fructifications of the fungus.

Though so innocent in appearance, the Wood Anemone possesses all the acrid nature of its tribe and is bitter to the tongue and poisonous. Cattle have been poisoned, Linnaeus tells us, by eating it in the fresh state after having been underfed and kept on dry food during the winter, so that they were ready to browse on the first leaves they saw. A vinegar made from the leaves retains all the more acrid properties of the plant, and is put in France to many domestic purposes: its rubifacient effects have caused it to be used externally in the same way as mustard.

The Egyptians held the Anemone as the emblem of sickness, perhaps from the flush of color upon the backs of the white sepals. The Chinese call it the 'Flower of Death." In some European countries it is looked on by the peasants as a flower of ill-omen, though the reason of the superstition is obscure. The Romans plucked the first Anemones as a charm against fever, and in some remote districts this practice long survived, it being considered a certain cure to gather an Anemone saying, 'I gather this against all diseases," and to tie it round the invalid's neck.

Greek legends say that Anemos, the Wind, sends his namesakes the Anemones, in the earliest spring days as the heralds of his coming. Pliny affirmed that they only open when the wind blows, hence their name of Windflower, and the unfolding of the blossoms in the rough, windy days of March has been the theme of many poets:

'Coy anemone that ne'er uncloses
Her lips until they're blown on by the wind."

Culpepper also uses the word 'windflower." In Greek mythology it sprang from the tears of Venus, as she wandered through the woodlands weeping for the death of Adonis -

'Where streams his blood there blushing springs a rose
And where a tear has dropped, a wind-flower blows."

The old herbalists called the Wood Anemone the Wood Crowfoot, because its leaves resemble in shape those of some species of Crowfoot. We also find it called Smell Fox. The specific name of nemorosa refers to its woodland habits.

['Anemone nemorosa, Varieties in," by E. J. Salisbury (Ann. Bot., October 1916, Vol. XXXX, No. CXX: figs.) - Two varieties distinct from the common form are mentioned as being fairly numerous in some of the Hertfordshire woodlands, and for which the author has proposed the names A. nemorosa, var. robusta and A. nemorosa, var. apetala. The former differs from the normal type in the lighter green color and larger size of the vegetative organs and in the perianth segments, which are broadest above the middle and rounded towards the apex. The latter bears inconspicuous flowers, which are small purplish-green structures, and it is noted that these plants are usually associated with the more deeply shaded situations, but as this character is maintained when the coppice in which the variety grows is felled, it is not considered a mere effect of inadequate illumination. - G.D.L.]

Medicinal Action and Uses

Though this species of Anemone has practically fallen out of use, the older herbalists recommended application of various parts of the plant for headaches, tertian agues and rheumatic gout. Culpepper practically copies verbatim the some half-dozen uses of the Anemone that Gerard gives, saying:

'The body being bathed with the decoction of the leaves cures the leprosy: the leaves being stamped and the juice snuffed up the nose purgeth the head mightily; so doth the root, being chewed in the mouth, for it procureth much spitting and bringeth away many watery and phlegmatic humours, and is therefore excellent for the lethargy.... Being made into an ointment and the eyelids annointed with it, it helps inflammation of the eyes. The same ointment is excellent good to cleanse malignant and corroding ulcers."

Culpepper also advises the roots to be chewed because it 'purgeth the head mightily'; he adds, 'And when all is done let physicians prate what they please, all the pills in the dispensary purge not the head like to hot things held in the mouth."

Parkinson writes:

'there is little use of these (the Anemones) in physic in our days, either for inward or outward diseases; only the leaves are used in the ointment called Marciatum, which is composed of many other hot herbs.... The root by reason of the sharpness is apt to draw down rheum if it be tasted or chewed in the mouth."

Modern authorities would, however, hesitate to recommend the chewing of the root on account of the acrid, irritant poison known to be present in it.

Linnaeus noticed that in Sweden the Wood Anemone flowered at the same time as the return of the swallow, and that the Marsh Marigold was contemporaneous with the cuckoo. A British naturalist in this country has also remarked this. Another naturalist who took an annual account of the days on which various flowers came into bloom in spring, found that the Wood Anemone never blossomed earlier than March 16, and never later than April 22. His observations were made each spring during thirty years.

The English name is derived from its Greek signification (wind) and is due to the fact that so many of its species grow on elevated places exposed to high winds; other writers attribute the name to the trembling of the flower before the blasts of spring.

ANGELICA

Botanical: Angelica Archangelica (LINN.)
Family: N.O. Umbelliferae
Synonyms: Garden Angelica. Archangelica officinalis.
Parts Used: root, leaves, seeds.

Habitat

By some botanists, this species of Angelica is believed to be a native of Syria from whence it has spread to many cool European climates, where it has become naturalized. It is occasionally found native in cold and moist places in Scotland, but is more abundant in countries further north, as in Lapland and Iceland. It is supposed to have come to this country from northern latitudes about 1568, There are about thirty varieties of Angelica, but this one is the only one officially employed in medicine.

Parkinson, in his Paradise in Sole, 1629, puts Angelica in the forefront of all medicinal plants, and it holds almost as high a place among village herbalists to-day, though it is not the native species of Angelica that is of such value medicinally and commercially. but an allied form, found wild in most places in the northern parts of Europe. This large variety, Angelica Archangelica (Linn.), also known as Archangelica officinalis, is grown abundantly near London in moist fields, for the use of its candied stems. It is largely cultivated for medicinal purposes in Thuringia, and the roots are also imported from Spain.

History

Its virtues are praised by old writers, and the name itself, as well as the folk-lore of all North European countries and nations, testify to the great antiquity of a belief in its merits as a protection against contagion, for purifying the blood, and for curing every conceivable malady: it was held a sovereign remedy for poisons agues and all infectious maladies. In Couriand, Livonia and the low lakelands of Pomerania and East Prussia, wild-growing Angelica abounds; there, in early summer-time, it has been the custom among the peasants to march into the towns carrying the Angelica flower-stems and to offer them for sale, chanting some ancient ditty in Lettish words, so antiquated as to be unintelligible even to the singers themselves. The chanted words and the tune are learnt in childhood, and may be attributed to a survival of some Pagan festival with which the plant was originally associated. After the introduction of Christianity, the plant became linked in the popular mind with some archangelic patronage, and associated with the spring-time festival of the Annunciation. According to one legend, Angelica was revealed in a dream by an angel to cure the plague. Another explanation of the name of this plant is that it blooms on the day of Michael the Archangel (May 8, old style), and is on that account a preservative against evil spirits and witchcraft: all parts of the plant were believed efficacious against spells and enchantment. It was held in such esteem that it was called 'The Root of the Holy Ghost."

Angelica may be termed a perennial herbaceous plant. It is biennial only in the botanical sense of that term, that is to say, it is neither annual, nor naturally perennial: the seedlings make but little advance towards maturity within twelve months, whilst old plants die off after seeding once, which event may be at a much more remote period than in the second year of growth. Only very advanced seedlings flower in their second year, and the third year of growth commonly completes the full period of life. There is another species, Angelica heterocarpa, a native of Spain, which is credited as truly perennial; it flowers a few weeks later than the biennial species, and is not so ornamental in its foliage.

Description

The roots of the Common Angelica are long and spindle-shaped, thick and fleshy - large specimens weighing sometimes as much as three pounds - and are beset with many long, descending rootlets. The stems are stout fluted, 4 to 6 feet high and hollow. The foliage is bold and pleasing, the leaves are on long stout, hollow footstalks, often 3 feet in length, reddish purple at the much dilated, clasping bases; the blades, of a bright green color, are much cut into, being composed of numerous small leaflets, divided into three principal groups, each of which is again subdivided into three lesser groups. The edges of the leaflets are finely toothed or serrated. The flowers, small and numerous, yellowish or greenish in color, are grouped into large, globular umbels. They blossom in July and are succeeded by pale yellow, oblong fruits, 1/6 to a 1/4 inch in length when ripe, with membraneous edges, flattened on one side and convex on the other, which bears three prominent ribs. Both the odor and taste of the fruits are pleasantly aromatic.

Our native form, A. sylvestris (Linn.), is hairy in stalk and stem to a degree which makes a well-marked difference. Its flowers differ, also, in being white, tinged with purple. The stem is purple and furrowed. This species is said to yield a good, yellow dye.

Angelica is unique amongst the Umbelliferae for its pervading aromatic odor, a pleasant perfume, entirely differing from Fennel, Parsley, Anise, Caraway or Chervil. One old writer compares it to Musk, others liken it to Juniper. Even the roots are fragrant, and form one of the principal aromatics of European growth- the other parts of the plant have the same flavor, but their active principles are considered more perishable.

In several London squares and parks, Angelica has continued to grow, self-sown, for several generations as a garden escape; in some cases it is appreciated as a useful foliage plant, in others, it is treated rather as an intruding weed. Before the building of the London Law Courts and the clearing of much slum property between Holywell Street and Seven Dials, the foreign population of that district fully appreciated its value, and were always anxious to get it from Lincoln's Inn Fields, where it abounded and where it still grows. Until very recent years, it was exceedingly common on the slopes bordering the Tower of London on the north and west sides; there, also, the inhabitants held the plant in high repute, both for its culinary and medicinal use.

Cultivation

Cultivate in ordinary deep, moist loam, in a shady position, as the plant thrives best in a damp soil and loves to grow near running water. Although the natural habitat is in damp soil and in open quarters, yet it can withstand adverse environment wonderfully well, and even endure severe winter frost without harm. Seedlings will even successfully develop and flower under trees, whose shelter creates an area of summer dryness in the surface soil, but, of course, though such conditions may be allowable when Angelica is grown merely as an ornamental plant, it must be given the best treatment as regards suitable soil and situation when grown for its use commercially. Insects and garden pests do not attack the plant with much avidity: its worst enemy is a small twowinged fly, of which the maggots are leafminers, resembling those of the celery plant and of the spinach leaf.

Propagation

should not be attempted otherwise than by the sowing of ripe, fresh seed, though division of old roots is sometimes recommended, and also propagation by offshoots, which are thrown out by a twoyearold plant when cut down in June for the sake of the stems, and which transplanted to 2 feet or more apart, will provide a quick method of propagation, considered inferior, however, to that of raising by seed. Since the germinating capacity of the seeds rapidly deteriorates, they should be sown as soon as ripe in August or early September. If kept till March, especially if stored in paper packets, their vitality is likely to be seriously impaired. In the autumn, the seeds may be sown where the plants are to remain, or preferably in a nursery bed, which as a rule will not need protection during the winter. A very slight covering of earth is best. Young seedlings, but not the old plants, are amenable to transplantation. The seedlings should be transplanted when still small, for their first summer's growth, to a distance of about 18 inches apart. In the autumn they can be removed to permanent quarters, the plants being then set 3 feet apart.

Parts Used

The roots and leaves for medicinal purposes, also the seeds.

The stems and seeds for use in confectionery and flavoring and the preparation of liqueurs.

The dried leaves, on account of their aromatic qualities, are used in the preparation of hop bitters.

The whole plant is aromatic, but the root only is official in the Swiss, Austrian and German Pharmacopoeias.

Angelica roots should be dried rapidly and placed in air-tight receptacles. They will then retain their medicinal virtues for many years.

The root should be dug up in the autumn of the first year, as it is then least liable to become mouldy and worm-eaten: it is very apt to be attacked by insects. Where very thick, the roots should be sliced longitudinally to quicken the drying process.

The fresh root has a yellowish-grey epidermis, and yields when bruised a honeycoloured juice, having all the aromatic properties of the plant. If an incision is made in the bark of the stems and the crown of the root at the commencement of spring, this resinous gum will exude. It has a special aromatic flavor of musk benzoin, for either of which it can be substituted.

The dried root, as it appears in commerce, is greyish brown and much wrinkled externally, whitish and spongy within and breaks with a starchy fracture, exhibiting shining, resinous spots. The odor is strong and fragrant, and the taste at first sweetish, afterwards warm, aromatic, bitterish and somewhat musky. These properties are extracted by alcohol and less perfectly by water.

If the plants are well grown, the leaves may be cut for use the summer after transplanting. Ordinarily, it is the third or fourth year that the plant develops its tall flowering stem, of which the gathering for culinary or confectionery use prolongs the lifetime of the plant for many seasons. Unless it is desired to collect seed, the tops should be cut at or before flowering time. After producing seed, the plants generally die, but by cutting down the tops when the flower-heads first appear and thus preventing the formation of seed, the plants may continue for several years longer, by cutting down the stems right at their base, the plants practically become perennial, by the development of side shoots around the stool head.

The whole herb, if for medicinal use, should be collected in June and cut shortly above the root.

If the stems are already too thick, the leaves may be stripped off separately and dried on wire or netting trays.

The stem, which is in great demand when trimmed

and candied, should be cut about June or early July.

If the seeds are required, they should be gathered when ripe and dried. The seedheads should be harvested on a fine day, after the sun has dried off the dew, and spread thinly on sailcloth in a warm spot or open shed, where the air circulates freely. In a few days the tops will have become dry enough to be beaten out with a light flail or rod, care being taken not to injure the seed. After threshing, the seeds (or fruits) should be sieved to remove portions of the stalks and allowed to remain for several days longer spread out in a very thin layer in the sun, or in a warm and sunny room, being turned every day to remove the last vestige of moisture. In a week to ten days they will be dry. Small quantities of the fruits can be shaken out of the heads when they have been cut a few days and finished ripening, so that the fruits divide naturally into the half-fruits or mericarps which shake off readily when quite ripe, especially if rubbed out of the heads between the palms of the hands. It is imperative that the seeds be dry before being put into storage packages or tins.

Constituents

The chief constituents of Angelica are about 1 per cent. of volatile oil, valeric acid, angelic acid, sugar, a bitter principle, and a peculiar resin called Angelicin, which is stimulating to the lungs and to the skin. The essential oil of the roots contains terebangelene and other terpenes; the oil of the 'seeds' contains in addition methyl-ethylacetic acid and hydroxymyristic acid.

Angelica balsam is obtained by extracting the roots with alcohol, evaporating and extracting the residue with ether. It is of a dark brown color and contains Angelica oil Angelica wax and Angelicin.

Uses

Angelica is largely used in the grocery trade, as well as for medicine, and is a popular flavoring for confectionery and liqueurs. The appreciation of its unique flavor was established in ancient times when saccharin matter was extremely rare. The use of the sweetmeat may probably have originated from the belief that the plant possessed the power of averting or expelling pestilence.

The preparation of Angelica is a small but important industry in the south of France, its cultivation being centralized in ClermontFerrand. Fairly large quantities are purchased by confectioners and high prices are easily obtainable. The flavor of Angelica suggests that of Juniper berries, and it is largely used in combination with Juniper berries, or in partial substitution for them by gin distillers. The stem is largely used in the preparation of preserved fruits and 'confitures' generally, and is also used as an aromatic garnish by confectioners. The seeds especially, which are aromatic and bitterish in taste, are employed also in alcoholic distillates, especially in the preparation of Vermouth and similar preparations, as well as in other liqueurs, notably Chartreuse. From ancient times, Angelica has been one of the chief flavoring ingredients of beverages and liqueurs, but it is not a matter of general knowledge that the Muscatel grape-like flavor of some wines, made on both sides of theRhine, is (or is suspected to be) due to the secret use of Angelica. An Oil of Angelica, which is very expensive, was prepared in Germany some years ago: it is obtained from the seeds by distillation with steam, the vapor being condensed and the oil separated by gravity. One hundred kilograms of Angelica seeds yield one kilolitre of oil, and the fresh leaves a little less, the roots yielding only 0.15 to 0.3 kilograms. Like the seeds themselves, the oil is used for flavoring. Besides being employed as a flavoring for beverages and medicinally, Angelica seeds are also used to a limited extent in perfumery.

Medicinal Action and Uses

The root stalks, leaves and fruit possess carminative, stimulant, diaphoretic, stomachic, tonic and expectorant properties, which are strongest in the fruit, though the whole plant has the same virtues.

Angelica is a good remedy for colds, coughs, pleurisy, wind, colic, rheumatism and diseases of the urinary organs, though it should not be given to patients who have a tendency towards diabetes, as it causes an increase of sugar in the urine.

It is generally used as a stimulating expectorant, combined with other expectorants the action of which is facilitated, and to a large extent diffused, through the whole of the pulmonary region.

It is a useful agent for feverish conditions, acting as a diaphoretic.

An infusion may be made by pouring a pint of boiling water on an ounce of the bruised root, and two tablespoonsful of this should be given three or four times a day, or the powdered root administered in doses of 10 to 30 grains. The infusion will relieve flatulence, and is also of use as a stimulating bronchial tonic, and as an emmenagogue. It is used much on the Continent for indigestion, general debility and chronic bronchitis. For external use, the fresh leaves of the plant are crushed and applied as poultices in lung and chest diseases.

The following is extracted from an old family book of herbal remedies:

'Boil down gently for three hours a handful of Angelica root in a quart of water; then strain it off and add liquid Narbonne honey or best virgin honey sufficient to make it into a balsam or syrup and take two tablespoonsful every night and morning, as well as several times in the day. If there be hoarseness or sore throat, add a few nitre drops."

A somewhat similar drink, much in use on the Continent in the treatment of typhus fever, is thus prepared:

'Pour a quart of boiling water upon 6 oz. of Angelica root cut up in thin slices, 4 oz. of honey, the juice of 2 lemons and 1/2 gill of brandy. Infuse for half an hour."

Formerly a preparation of the roots was much used as a specific for typhoid.

Angelica stems are also grateful to a feeble stomach, and will relieve flatulence promptly when chewed. An infusion of Angelica leaves is a very healthful, strengthening tonic and aromatic stimulant, the beneficial effect of which is felt after a few days' use.

The yellow juice yielded by the stem and root becomes, when dry, a valuable medicine in chronic rheumatism and gout.

Taken in medicinal form, Angelica is said to cause a disgust for spirituous liquors.

It is a good vehicle for nauseous medicines and forms one of the ingredients in compound spirit of Aniseed.

Gerard, among its many virtues that he extols, says 'it cureth the bitings of mad dogs and all other venomous beasts."

Preparations

Fluid extract, herb: dose, 1 drachm. Fluid extract, root: dose, 1/4 to 1 drachm.

Recipes

To Preserve Angelica.

Cut in pieces 4 inches long. Steep for 12 hours in salt and water. Put a layer of cabbage or cauliflower leaves in a clean brass pan, then a layer of Angelica, then another layer of leaves and so on, finishing with a layer of leaves on the top. Cover with water and vinegar. Boil slowly till the Angelica becomes quite green, then strain and weigh the stems. Allow 1 lb. loaf sugar to each pound of stems. Put the sugar in a clean pan with water to cover; boil 10 minutes and pour this syrup over the Angelica. Stand for 12 hours. Pour off the syrup, boil it up for 5 minutes and pour it again over the Angelica. Repeat the process, and after the Angelica has stood in the syrup 12 hours, put all on the fire in the brass pan and boil till tender. Then take out the pieces of Angelica, put them in a jar and pour the syrup over them, or dry them on a sieve and sprinkle them with sugar: they then form candy.

Another recipe (from Francatelli's Cook's Guide)

'Cut the tubes or stalks of Angelica into sixinch lengths; wash them, then put them into a copper preserving-pan with hot syrup; cover the surface with vine-leaves, and set the whole to stand in the larder till next day. The Angelica must then be drained on a sieve, the vine-leaves thrown away, half a pint of water added to the syrup, in which, after it has been boiled, skimmed, and strained into another pan, and the copper-pan has been scoured clean, both the Angelica and the boiling syrup are to be replaced and the surface covered with fresh vine-leaves, and again left to stand in this state till the next day- this process must be repeated 3 or 4 days running: at the end of which time the Angelica will be sufficiently green and done through, and should be put in jars without breaking the tubes. After the syrup has been boiled and skimmed, fill up the jars, and when they are become cold, cover them over with bladder and paper, and let them be kept in a very cool temperature."

Another way of preserving Angelica:

Choose young stems, cut them into suitable lengths, then boil until tender. When this stage is reached, remove from the water, and strip off the outer skin, then return to the water and simmer slowly until the whole has become very green. Dry the stems and weigh them, allowing one pound of white sugar to every pound of Angelica. The boiled stalks should be laid in an earthenware pan and the sugar sprinkled over them, allowing the whole to stand for a couple of days- then boil all together. When well boiling, remove from the fire and turn into a colander to drain off the superfluous syrup. Take a little more sugar and boil to a syrup again, then throw in the Angelica, and allow it to remain for a few minutes, and finally spread on plates in a cool oven to dry.

If a small quantity of the leaf-stalks of Angelica be cooked with 'sticks' of rhubarb, the flavor of the compound will be acceptable to many who do not relish plain rhubarb. The quantity of Angelica used may be according to circumstances, conditions and individual taste. If the stems are young and juicy, they may be treated like rhubarb and cut up small, the quantity used being in any proportion between 5 and 25 per cent. If the stalks are more or less fully developed, or even rather old and tough, they can be excellently used in economically small quantities for flavoring large quantities of stewed rhubarb, or of rhubarb jam, being added in long lengths before cooking and removed before sending to table. The confectioner's candied Angelica may be similarly utilized, but is expensive and not so good, whilst the home-garden growth in spring-time of fresh Angelica, with thick, stout leaf-stalks, and of still stouter flowering stems, is very easy to use and cheap. If this flowering stem be cut whilst very tender, early in May, later leafstalks will be plentifully available for use with the latter part of the rhubarb crop.

A well-known jam maker and confectioner, the late Mr. Robertson, of Chelsea, won considerable reputation by reason of his judicious blending of Angelica in jam-making and its combination in other confections, including temperance beverages. A pleasant form of Hop Bitters is made by taking 1 OZ. of dried Angelica herb, combined with 1 OZ. of Holy Thistle, and 1/2 oz. of hops, infused with 3 pints of boiling water and strained off when cold, a wine glassful being taken several times a day before meals, forming a good appetiser.

A delicious liqueur which is also a digestive, preserving all the virtues of the plant, is made in this way: 1 OZ. of the freshly gathered stem of Angelica is chopped up and steeped in 2 pints of good brandy during five days 1 OZ. of skinned bitter almonds reduced to a pulp being added. The liquid is then strained through fine muslin and a pint of liquid sugar added to it.

Angelica is used in the preparation of Vermouth and Chartreuse

Though the tender leaflets of the blades of the leaves have sometimes been recommended as a substitute for spinach, they are too bitter for the general taste, but the blanched mid-ribs of the leaf, boiled and used as celery, are delicious, and Icelanders eat both the stem and the roots raw, with butter. The taste of the juicy raw stems is at first sweetish and slightly bitter in the mouth and then gives a feeling of glowing warmth. In Lapland, the inhabitants regard the stalks of Angelica as a great delicacy. These are gathered before flowering, the leaves being stripped off and the peel removed, the remainder is eaten with much relish. The Finns eat the young stems baked in hot ashes, and an infusion of the dried herb is drunk either hot or cold: the flavor of the decoction is rather bitter, the color is a pale greenish grey and the odor greatly resembles China Tea. It was formerly a practice in this country to put a portion of the fresh herb into the pot in which fish is boiled.

The Norwegians make bread of the roots.

Angelica may be made much use of in the garden by cutting the hollow stalks into convenient lengths and placing them amongst shrubs as traps for earwigs.

A drink much in use on the Continent for typhus fever: Pour a quart of boiling water on 6 oz. of Angelica root sliced thin, infuse for half an hour, strain and add juice of 2 lemons, 4 oz. of honey and 1/2 gill of brandy.

Other Angelicas

AMERICAN ANGELICA or Masterwort (A. atropurpurea, Linn.), also used in herbal medicine in North America, grows throughout the eastern United States. The root has a strong odor and a warm aromatic taste. The juice of the fresh root is acrid and said to be poisonous, but the acridity is dissipated by drying.

The root, though lighter and less branched, is similar in appearance to that of A. Archangelica, with nearly allied constituents and properties, and the medicinal virtues of the whole plant are similar, so that it has been employed as a substitute, but it is inferior to the European Angelica, being less aromatic.

WILD ANGELICA (A. sylvestris, Linn.), yields a yellow dye.

The Angelica Tree of America (Xanthoxylum Americanum, Mill), the Prickly Ash, as it is more generally named, is not allied to the umbelliferous Angelicas. Its berries and bark are employed to prepare a tonic, and it is used in the treatment of rheumatism and skin diseases.

ANGELICA TREE

Botanical: Aralia spinosa
Family: N.O. Araliaceae
Synonyms: Hercules Club. Toothache Tree. Prickly Elder. Prickly Ash, though not to be confused with the better-known Prickly Ash.
Parts Used: Bark, root and berries.
Habitat: Virginia and Japan.

Description

Grows from 8 to 12 feet high stem and leaves prickly, leaves doubly and triply pinnate, ovate, serrated leaflets, panicles much branched, downy, numerous umbels of white flowers, blooming in August and September, berries juicy and blackish.

The bark is used officially (is thin and ashcoloured), but other parts of the plant possess medical properties- odor fragrant and peculiar, slightly bitter taste.

Constituents

Aralia spinosa contains a glucoside Araliin.

Medicinal Action and Uses

Fresh bark causes/vomiting and purging, but dried is a stimulating alterative. A tincture made from the bark is used for rheumatism, skin diseases and syphilis. The berries in tincture form, lull pain in decayed teeth and in other parts of the body, violent colic and rheumatism, useful in cholera when a cathartic is required in the following compound: 1 drachm compound powdered Jalap, 1 drachm Aralia spinosa, 2 drachms compound rhubarb powder or infused in 1/2, pint boiling water and when cold taken in tablespoonful doses every half-hour. This does not produce choleric discharges. Also a powerful sialogogue and valuable in diseases where mouth and throat get dry, and for sore throat; will relieve difficult breathing and produce moisture if given in very small doses of the powder. The bark, root, and berries can all be utilized.

ANGOSTURA (TRUE)

Botanical: Cusparia febrifuga (D. C.)
Family: N.O. Rutaceae

Synonyms: Cusparia Bark. Galipea officinalis.
Part Used: The dried bark.
Habitat: Tropical South America.

Description

A small tree with straight stem irregularly branched, covered with a smooth grey bark, leaves alternate, petiolate and composed of three leaflets oblong and pointed, smooth, glossy and vivid green, sometimes with small white spots on them and in their first state having a tobacco-like aroma, this odor is one of the characteristics distinguishing the true Angostura from the false which is odourless. The flowers also have a peculiar nauseous smell; salver-shaped corollas and arranged in axillary, terminal, peduncled racemes. Fruit has five two-valved capsules, two or three of which are often abortive; two seeds in each capsule, round and black, one only is generally fertile. The tree was given the name of Galipea officinalis to denote the true variety of Angostura and thus distinguish it from the very dangerous substitute and adulterant. The characteristics of the true commercial bark are flattened curved pieces or quills 4 to 5 inches long, 1 inch wide and 1/12 of an inch thick. The outer layer of bark is a yellowishgrey cork which is easily removed, often being soft, the inner surface is lighter brown and sometimes laminated, fracture short and resinous white, points being visible on broken surface; the transverse section shows numerous cells filled with circular crystals of Calcium Oxalate, small oil glands, small groups of bast fibres with a musty smell and bitte taste.

Constituents

The chief bitter principle of Angostura bark is Angosturin, a colorless crystalline substance readily soluble in water alcohol or ether. The bark also contains about 2.4 per cent of the bitter crystalline alkaloids Galipine, Cusparine, Galipidine Cusparidine and Cuspareine, about 1.5 per cent. of volatile oil and a glucoside which yields a fluorescent substance when hydrolysed by heating with dilute sulphuric acid.

Medicinal Action and Uses

The bark has long been known and used by the natives of South America and West Indies as a stimulant tonic. In large doses it causes diarrhea and is often used as a purgative. Most useful in bilious diarrhea, dysentery, and diseases which require a tonic. Commercially it is an ingredient of bitter liqueurs. The natives also employ it to stupefy fish in the same manner as Cinchona is used by the Peruvians. Some doctors prefer Angostura Bark to Cinchona for use in fever cases; it is also used in dropsy.

Dosages and Preparations

Infusion Cuspariae, B.P.: Angostura Bark in powder,5 parts; distilled water, boiling, 100 parts; infuse for 15 minutes in a covered vessel and strain. Dose, 1 to 2 fluid ounces. This infusion is the most satisfactory way of taking the bark, but to obviate nausea it should be combined with aromatics. It may be given in powder, tincture or fluid extract. Dose of the powder, 5 to 15 grains. Fluid extract, 5 to 30 minims.

Other Species

Dangerous substitutions are: The bark of the Nux Vomica Tree; this is known as False Angostura Bark; it is much more twisted and bent than the true, has no unpleasant smell, is not so heavy, and is more easily broken.

Copalchi Bark from Mexico, composition similar to Cascarilla Esenbeckia febrifuga (N.O. Rutaceae), contains Ovodine.

ANISE

Botanical: Pimpinella anisum (LINN.)
Family: N.O. Umbelliferae
Part Used: Seeds.

Habitat

It is a native of Egypt, Greece, Crete and Asia Minor and was cultivated by the ancient Egyptians. It was well known to the Greeks, being mentioned by Dioscorides and Pliny and was cultivated in Tuscany in Roman times. In the Middle Ages its cultivation spread to Central Europe.

Description

Anise is a dainty, white-flowered urnbelliferous annual, about 18 inches high, with secondary feather-like leaflets of bright green, hence its name (of mediaeval origin), Pimpinella, from dipinella, or twicepinnate, in allusion to the form of the leaves.

History

In this country Anise has been in use since the fourteenth century, and has been cultivated in English gardens from the middle of the sixteenth century, but it ripens its seeds here only in very warm summers, and it is chiefly in warmer districts that it is grown on a commercial scale, Southern Russia, Bulgaria, Germany, Malta, Spain, Italy, North Africa and Greece producing large quantities. It has also been introduced into India and South America. The cultivated plant attains a considerably larger size than the wild one.

In the East Anise was formerly used with other spices in part payment of taxes. 'Ye pay tithe of Mint, Anise and Cummin," we read in the 23rd chapter of St. Matthew, but some authorities state that Anise is an incorrect rendering and should have been translated 'Dill."

In Virgil's time, Anise was used as a spice. Mustacae, a spiced cake of the Romans introduced at the end of a rich meal, to prevent indigestion, consisted of meal, with Anise, Cummin and other aromatics. Such a cake was sometimes brought in at the end of a marriage feast, and is, perhaps, the origin of our spiced wedding cake.

On the Continent, especially in Germany, many cakes have an aniseed flavoring, and Anise is also used as a flavoring for soups.

It is largely employed in France, Spain Italy and South America in the preparation of cordial liqueurs. The liqueur Anisette added to cold water on a hot summer's day, makes a most refreshing drink.

Anise is one of the herbs that was supposed to avert the Evil Eye.

The oil extracted from the seed is said to prove a capital bait for mice, if smeared on traps. It is poisonous to pigeons.

Turner's Herbal, 1551, says that 'Anyse maketh the breth sweter and swageth payne." 'The seeds," says Delamer, Kitchen Garden, 1861, 'are much used by distillers to give flavor to cordial liqueurs." Anisette is a liqueur flavoured with aniseed. Langham, Garden Health, 1683, says: 'For the dropsie, fill an old cock with Polipody and Aniseeds and seethe him well, and drink the broth." The leaves are useful for seasoning some dishes. The essential oil of Anise is a good preventive of mould in paste. The ground seeds form an ingredient of sachet powders.

Cultivation

Sow the seed in dry, light soil, on a warm, sunny border, early in April, where the plants are to remain. When they come up, thin them and keep them clean from weeds. Allow about a foot each way. The seeds may also be sown in pots in heat and removed to a warm site in May.

The seeds will ripen in England in good seasons if planted in a warm and favourable situation, though they are not successful everywhere, and can hardly be looked upon as a remunerative crop. The plant flowers in July, and if the season prove warm, will ripen in autumn, when the plants are cut down and the seeds threshed out.

Part Used

The fruit, or so-called seeds. When threshed out, the seeds may be easily dried in trays, in a current of air in half-shade, out-of-doors, or by moderate heat. When dry, they are greyish brown, ovate, hairy, about one-fifth of an inch long, with ten crenate ribs and often have the stalk attached. They should be free from earthy matter. The taste is sweet and spicy, and the odor aromatic and agreeable.

The commercial varieties differ considerably in size, but the larger varieties alone are official. The Spanish Anise, sold as Alicante Anise, are the largest and the best adapted for pharmaceutical use, yielding about 3 per cent. of oil. Russian and German fruits are smaller and darker and are the variety generally used for distillation of the volatile oil. Italian Anise is frequently adulterated with Hemlock fruit.

Constituents

Anise fruit yields on distillation from 2.5 to 3.5 per cent. of a fragrant, syrupy, volatile oil, of which anethol, present to about 90 per cent., is the principal aromatic constituent. It has a strong Anise odor and separates in the form of shining white crystalline scales on cooling the oil. Other constituents of the fruit are a fixed oil, choline, sugar and mucilage.

Oil of Anise, distilled in Europe from the fruits of Pimpinella anisum, Anise, and in China from the fruits of Illicium anisatum, Star Anise, a small tree indigenous to China, is colorless, or very pale yellow, with taste and odor like the fruit. The oils obtainable from these two fruits are identical in composition, and nearly the same in most of their characters, but that from Star Anise fruit congeals at a lower temperature. The powdered drug from Star Anise is administered in India as a substitute for the official fruit, and the oil is employed for its aromatic, carminative and stimulant properties. The bulk of the oil in commerce is obtained from the Star Anise fruit in China. The fruits are also often imported into France and the oil extracted there. Chinese Anise oil is harsh in taste.

Medicinal Action and Uses

Carminative and pectoral. Anise enjoys considerable reputation as a medicine in coughs and pectoral affections. In hard, dry coughs where expectoration is difficult, it is of much value. It is greatly used in the form of lozenges and the seeds have also been used for smoking, to promote expectoration.

The volatile oil, mixed with spirits of wine forms the liqueur Anisette, which has a beneficial action on the bronchial tubes, and for bronchitis and spasmodic asthma, Anisette, if administered in hot water, is an immediate palliative.

For infantile catarrh, Aniseed tea is very helpful. It is made by pouring half a pint of boiling water on 2 teaspoonsful of bruised seed. This, sweetened, is given cold in doses of 1 to 3 teaspoonsful frequently.

Gerard said:

'Aniseed helpeth the yeoxing or hicket (hiccough) and should be given to young children to eat, which are like to have the falling sickness (epilepsy), or to/ such as have it by patrimony or succession."

The stimulant and carminative properties of Anise make it useful in flatulency and colic. It is used as an ingredient of cathartic and aperient pills, to relieve flatulence and diminish the griping of purgative medicines, and may be given with perfect safety in convulsions. For colic, the dose is 10 to 30 grains of bruised or powdered seeds infused in distilled water, taken in wine glassful doses, or 4 to 20 drops of the essential oil on sugar. For the restlessness of languid digestion, a dose of essence of aniseed in hot water at bedtime is much commended.

In the Paregoric Elixir (Compound Tincture of Camphor), prescribed as a sedative cordial by doctors, oil of Anise is also included - 30 drops in a pint of the tincture.

Anise oil is a good antiseptic and is used, mixed with oil of Peppermint or Gaultheria (Wintergreen) to flavor aromatic liquid dentrifrices.

Oil of Anise is used also against insects especially when mixed with oil of Sassafras and Carbolic oil.

ANISE (STAR)

Botanical: Illicuim verum (HOOK, F.)
Family: N.O. Magnoliaceae
Synonyms: Chinese Anise. Aniseed Stars. Badiana.
Parts Used: Seeds, oil.

Star Anise is so named from the stellate form of its fruit. It is often chewed in small quantities after each meal to promote digestion and sweeten the breath.

Medicinal Action and Uses

Carminative, stimulant, diuretic.

The fruit is used in the East as a remedy for colic and rheumatism, and in China for seasoning dishes, especially sweets.

The Japanese plant the tree in their temples and on

tombs; and use the pounded bark as incense.

The homeopaths prepare a tincture from the seeds.

APPLE

Botanical: Pyrus malus
Family: N.O. Pomaceae
Synonyms: Wild Apple. Malus communis.
Parts Used: The fruit and the bark.
Habitat: Temperate regions of the Northern Hemisphere.

History

The Apple is a fruit of the temperate zones and only reaches perfection in their cooler regions. It is a fruit of long descent and in the Swiss lake-dwellings small apples have been found, completely charred but still showing the seed-valves and the grain of the flesh. It exists in its wild state in most countries of Europe and also in the region of the Caucasus: in Norway, it is found in the lowlands as far north as Drontheim.

The Crab-tree or Wild Apple (Pyrus malus), is native to Britain and is the wild ancestor of all the cultivated varieties of apple trees. It was the stock on which were grafted choice varieties when brought from Europe, mostly from France. Apples of some sort were abundant before the Norman Conquest and were probably introduced into Britain by the Romans. Twenty-two varieties were mentioned by Pliny: there are now about 2,000 kinds cultivated. In the Old Saxon manuscripts there are numerous mentions of apples and cider. Bartholomeus Anglicus, whose Encyclopedia was one of the earliest printed books containing botanical information (being printed at Cologne about 1470), gives a chapter on the Apple. He says:

'Malus the Appyll tree is a tree yt bereth apples and is a grete tree in itself. . . it is more short than other trees of the wood wyth knottes and rinelyd Rynde. And makyth shadowe wythe thicke bowes and branches: and fayr with dyurs blossomes, and floures of swetnesse and Iykynge: with goode fruyte and noble. And is gracious in syght and in taste and vertuous in medecyne . . . some beryth sourysh fruyte and harde, and some ryght soure and some ryght swete, with a good savoure and mery."

Description

The Crab-tree is a small tree of general distribution in Britain south of Perthshire. In most respects it closely resembles the cultivated Apple of the orchard differing chiefly only in the size and flavor of the fruit. Well-grown specimens are not often met with, as in woods and copses it is cramped by other trees and seldom attains any considerable height, 30-foot specimens being rare and many being mere bushes. Those found in hedgerows have often sprung from the seeds of orchard apples that have reverted to ancestral type. The branches of the Crab-tree become pendant, with long shoots which bear the leaves and flowers. The leaves are dark green and glossy and the flowers, in small clusters on dwarf shoots are produced in April and May. The buds are deeply tinged with pink on the outside the expanded flowers an inch and a half across, and when the trees are in full bloom, they are a beautiful sight.

The blossoms, by their delightful fragrance and store of nectar, attract myriads of bees, and as a result of the fertilization effected by these visitors in their search for the buried nectar, the fruit develops and becomes in autumn the beautiful little Crab Apple, which when ripe is yellow or red in color and measures about an inch across. It has a very austere and acid juice, in consequence of which it cannot be eaten in the raw condition, but a delicious jelly is made from it, which is always welcome on the table, and the fruit can also be used for jammaking, with blackberries, pears or quinces. In Ireland, it is sometimes added to cider, to impart a roughness. The fruit in some varieties is less acid than in others: in the variety in which the fruit hangs down from the shoots, the little apples are exceedingly acid, but in another kind, they stand more or less erect on their stalks and these are so much less acid as to give almost a suggestion of sweetness. The fruit of the Siberian Crab, or Cherry-apple, grown as an ornamental tree, makes also a fine preserve.

Cider Apples may be considered as a step in development from the Wild Apple to the Dessert Apple. Formerly every farmhouse made its cider. The apples every autumn were tipped in heaps on the straw-strewn floor of the pound house, a building of cob, covered with thatch, in which stood the pounder and the press and vats and all hands were busy for days preparing the golden beverage. This was the yearly process - still carried out on many farms of the west of England, though cider-making is becoming more and more a product of the factories. One of the men turned the handle of the pounder, while a boy tipped in the apples at the top. A pounder is a machine which crushes the apples between two rollers with teeth in them. The pulp and juice are then taken to the press in large shovels which have high sides and are scored bright by the acid. The press is a huge square tray with a lip in the centre of the front side and its floor slopes towards this opening. On either side are huge oaken supports on which rests a square baulk of the same wood. Through this works a large screw. Under the timber is the presser Directly the pulp is ready, the farmer starts to prepare the 'cheese." First of all goes a layer of straw, then a layer of apples, and so on until the 'cheese' is a yard high, and sometimes more. Then the ends of straw which project are turned up to the top of the heap. Now the presser is wound down and compresses the mound until the clear juice runs freely. Under the lip in the front of the cider press is put a vat. The juice is dipped from this into casks. In four months' time the cider will be ready to drink.

The demand for cider has increased rapidly of late years, chiefly on account of the dry varieties being so popular with sufferers from rheumatism and gout. As very good prices have been paid in recent seasons for the best cider apples, and as eight tons per acre is quite an average crop from a properly-managed orchard in full bearing, it is obvious to all progressive and up-to-date farmers and apple-growers that this branch of agriculture is well worthy of attention. In the last few years, with the object of encouraging this special Applegrowing industry, silver cups have been awarded to the owners of cider-apple orchards in Devon who make the greatest improvement in the cultivation of their orchards during the year, and it is hoped this will still further stimulate the planting of new orchards and the renovation of the old ones.

The peculiar winy odor is stimulating to many. Pliny, and later, Sir John Mandeville, tell of a race of little men in 'Farther India' who 'eat naught and live by the smell of apples." Burton wrote that apples are good against melancholy and Dr. John Caius, physician to Queen Elizabeth, in his Boke of Counseille against the Sweatynge Sicknesse advises the patient to 'smele to an old swete apple to recover his strengthe." An apple stuck full of cloves was the prototype of the pomander, and pomatum (now used only in a general sense) took its name from being first made of the pulp of apples, lard and rosewater.

In Shakespeare's time, apples when served at dessert were usually accompanied by caraway, as we may read in Henry IV, where Shallow invites Falstaff to 'a pippin and a dish of caraway," In a still earlier Booke of Nurture, it is directed 'After mete pepyns, caraway in comfyts." The custom of serving roast apples with a little saucerful of Carraways is still kept up at Trinity College, Cambridge, and at some of the old-fashioned London Livery dinners, just as in Shakespeare's days.

The taste for apples is one of the earliest and most natural of inclinations; all children love apples, cooked or uncooked. Apple pies, apple puddings, apple dumplings are fare acceptable in all ages and all conditions.

Apple cookery is very early English: Piers Ploughman mentions 'all the povere peple' who 'baken apples broghte in his lappes' and the ever popular apple pie was no less esteemed in Tudor times than it is to-day, only our ancestors had some predilections in the matter of seasonings that might not now appeal to all of us, for they put cinnamon and ginger in their pies and gave them a lavish coloring of saffron.

Apple Moyse is an old English confection, no two recipes for which seem to agree. One Black Letter volume tells us to take a dozen apples, roast or boil them, pass them through a sieve with the yolks of three or four eggs, and as they are strained temper them with three or four spoonfuls of damask (rose) water; season them with sugar and half a dish of sweet butter, and boil them in a chafing dish and cast biscuits or cinnamon and ginger upon them.

Halliwell says, upon one authority, that apple moyse was made from apples after they had been pressed for cider, and seasoned with spices.

Probably the American confection, Apple Butter, is an evolution of the old English dish? Apple butter is a kind of jam made of tart apples, boiled in cider until reduced to a very thick smooth paste, to which is added a flavoring of allspice, while cooking. It is then placed in jars and covered tightly.

The once-popular custom of wassailing the orchard-trees' on Christmas Eve, or the Eve of the Epiphany, is not quite extinct even yet in a few remote places in Devonshire. More than three centuries ago Herrick mentioned it among his 'Ceremonies of Christmas Eve':

'Wassaile the trees, that they may beare
You many a Plum and many a Peare:
For more or lesse fruits they will bring,
As you do give them Wassailing."

The ceremony consisted in the farmer, with his family and labourers, going out into the orchard after supper, bearing with them a jug of cider and hot cakes. The latter were placed in the boughs of the oldest or best bearing trees in the orchard, while the cider was flung over the trees after the farmer had drunk their health in some such fashion as the following:

'Here's to thee, old apple-tree!
Whence thou may'st bud, and whence thou may'st blow,
Hats full! Caps full!
Bushel - bushel-bags full!
And my pockets full too! Huzza!"

The toast was repeated thrice, the men and boys often firing off guns and pistols, and the women and children shouting loudly.

Roasted apples were usually placed in the pitcher of cider, and were thrown at the trees with the liquid. Trees that were bad bearers were not honoured with wassailing but it was thought that the more productive ones would cease to bear if the rite were omitted. It is said to have been a relic of the heathen sacrifices to Pomona. The custom also prevailed in Somersetshire and Dorsetshire.

Roast apples, or crabs, formed an indispensable part of the old-fashioned 'wassailbowl," or 'good brown bowl," of our ancestors.

'And sometime lurk I in a gossip's bowl
In very likeness of a roasted Crab'

Puck relates in Midsummer's Night's Dream.

The mixture of hot spiced ale, wine or cider, with apples and bits of toast floating in it was often called 'Lamb's wool," some say from its softness, but the word is really derived from the Irish 'la mas nbhal," 'the feast of the apple-gathering' (All Hallow Eve), which being pronounced somewhat like 'Lammas-ool," was corrupted into 'lamb's wool." It was usual for each person who partook of the spicy beverage to take out an apple and eat it, wishing good luck to the company.

Constituents

Various analyses show that the Apple contains from 80 to 85 per cent. of water, about 5 per cent. of proteid or nitrogenous material, from 10 to 15 per cent. of carbonaceous matter, including starch and sugar, from 1 to 1.5 per cent. of acids and salts. The sugar content of a fresh apple varies from 6 to 10 per cent., according to the variety. In spite of the large proportion of water, the fresh Apple is rich in vitamins, and is classed among the most valuable of the anti-scorbutic fruits for relieving scurvy. All apples contain a varying amount of the organic acids, malic acid and gallic acid, and an abundance of salts of both potash and soda, as well as salts of lime, magnesium, and iron.

It has been calculated that in 100 grams of dried apples, there are contained 1.7 milligrams of iron in sweet varieties and 2.1 milligrams in sour varieties. It has also been proved by analysis that the Apple contains a larger quantity of phosphates than any other vegetable or fruit.

The valuable acids and salt of the Apple exist to a special degree in and just below the skin, so that, to get the full value of an apple, it should be eaten unpeeled.

The bark of the Apple-tree which is bitter, especially the root-bark, contains a principle called Phloridzin, and a yellow coloring matter, Quercetin, both extracted by boiling water. The seeds give Amygdaline and an edible oil.

Apple oil is Amyl Valerate or Amylvaleric Ester. An alcoholic solution has been used as a flavoring liquid, called Apple Essence.

Fresh apple-juice is employed for the N.F. Ferrated Extract of Apples.

Medicinal Uses

The chief dietetic value of apples lies in the malic and tartaric acids. These acids are of signal benefit to persons of sedentary habits, who are liable to liver derangements, and they neutralize the acid products of gout and indigestion. 'An apple a day keeps the doctor away' is a respectable old rhyme that has some reason in it.

The acids of the Apple not only make the fruit itself digestible, but even make it helpful in digesting other foods. Popular instinct long ago led to the association of apple sauce with such rich foods as pork and goose, and the old English fancy for eating apple pie with cheese, an obsolete taste, nowadays, is another example of instinctive inclination, which science has approved.

The sugar of a sweet apple, like most fruit sugars, is practically a predigested food, and is soon ready to pass into the blood to provide energy and warmth for the body.

A ripe raw apple is one of the easiest vegetable substances for the stomach to deal with, the whole process of its digestion being completed in eighty-five minutes.

The juice of apples, without sugar, will often reduce acidity of the stomach; it becomes changed into alkaline carbonates, and thus corrects sour fermentation.

It is stated on medical authority that in countries where unsweetened cider is used as a common beverage, stone or calculus is unknown, and a series of inquiries made of doctors in Normandy, where cider is the principal drink, brought to light the fact that not a single case of stone had been met with during forty years.

Ripe, juicy apples eaten at bedtime every night will cure some of the worst forms of constipation. Sour apples are the best for this purpose. Some cases of sleeplessness have been cured in this manner. People much inclined to biliousness will find this practice very valuable. In some cases stewed apples will agree perfectly well, while raw ones prove disagreeable. There is a very old saying:

'To eat an apple going to bed
Will make the doctor beg his bread."

The Apple will also act as an excellent dentifrice, being a food that is not only cleansing to the teeth on account of its juices, but just hard enough to mechanically push back the gums so that the borders are cleared of deposits.

Rotten apples used as a poultice is an old Lincolnshire remedy for sore eyes, that is still in use in some villages.

It is no exaggeration to say that the habitual use of apples will do much to prolong life and to ameliorate its conditions. In the Edda, the old Scandinavian saga, Iduna kept in a box, apples that she gave to the gods to eat, thereby to renew their youth.

A French physician has found that the bacillus of typhoid fever cannot live long in apple juice, and therefore recommends doubtful drinking water to be mixed with cider.

A glucoside in small crystals is obtainable from the bark and root of the apple, peach and plum, which is said to induce artificial diabetes in animals, and thus can be used in curing it in human beings.

The original pomatum seems to date from Gerard's days, when an ointment for roughness of the skin was made from apple pulp, swine's grease, and rosewater.

The astringent verjuice, rich in tannin, of the Crab, is helpful in chronic diarrhea.

The bark may be used in decoction for intermittent and bilious fevers.

Cider in which horse-radish has been steeped has been found helpful in dropsy.

Cooked apples make a good local application for sore throat in fevers, inflammation of the eyes, erysipelas, etc.

Stewed apples are laxative; raw ones not invariably so.

Dosages

Of infusion of the bark, 1 to 4 fluid ounces. Of phloridzin, 5 to 20 grains.

Other Species

APPLE OF SODOM (Solanum sosomeum). This is a prickly species found near the Dead Sea, full of dust when ripe, the result of insects' eggs deposited in the young fruit. Some regard the name as referring to Colocynth, and others again to Calatropis procera.

ADAM'S APPLE is a variety of the Lime (Citrus limetta). Superstition relates that a piece of the forbidden apple stuck in Adam's throat, and his descendants ever after had the lump in the front of the neck which is so named.

MAY APPLE. American Mandrake, Racoonberry, Hog-apple, Devil's Apple, Indian Apple, or Wild Lemon, a purgative used in liver complaints.

THORN-APPLE. Datura stramonium, Jamestown Weed, Stinkweed, or Apple of Peru has narcotic, anodyne leaves and seeds.

CUSTARD APPLES, or Annonas, grow in hotter countries than common apples. Several species are edible, especially Annona tripetela, A. squamosa and A. glabra. A. palustris of Jamaica, also called Shiningleaved Custard Apple or Alligator Apple, is said to be a strong narcotic. The wood is so soft that it is used for corks.

PINE APPLE is the fruit of Bromelia ananas, deriving its name from its pine-cone shape.

LOVE APPLE, or Tomato Plant, is the fruit of Solanum lycopersicum or Lycopersicum esculentum.

MAD, or JEW'S APPLE is the fruit of S. esculentum.

RED ASTRACEIAN APPLE is var. Astracanica of P. malus. Var. Paradisiaca and var. Pendula are also well-known.

Varieties of Crabs are Dartmouth or Hyslop, Fairy, John Downie, Orange, Transcendent and Transparent.

MALAY APPLE is the fruit of Eugenia malaccensis.

ROSE APPLE, or Jamrosade, is the fruit of E. jambos. The bark and seeds arc employed in diarrhea and diabetes. Dose, of fluid extract, 10 minims or more, in hot water.

THE STAR APPLE (Chrysophyllum cainito) of the West Indies has an astringent, milky juice.

APPLE OF ACAJOU is a name of Anacardium occidentale, which yields a caustic oil used like croton oil. It is used in marking-ink. It also supplies a gum like gum-arabic.

CEDAR APPLES are excrescences on the trunk of Juniperus virginiana, used as an anthelmintic in the dose of from 10 to 20 grains three times a day.

ELEPHANT APPLE is the fruit of Feronia elephantum.

KANGAROO APPLE is the fruit of S. laciniatum.

KAU, or KEL APPLE is the South African name for the fruit of Abaria Kaffra.

MAMMEE APPLE is the fruit of Mammea americana.

MANDRAKE APPLE is the fruit of Mandragora officinalis.

MONKEY APPLE is the West Indian name for Clusia flava.

OAK-APPLES are spongy excrescences on the branches of oak-trees.

OATAHETTE APPLE is the fruit of Spondias dulcis.

PERSIAN APPLE is the name by which the peach was first known in Europe.

PRAIRIE APPLE is Psoralea esculenta.

WILD BALSAM APPLE is Ehinocystis lobata.

Recipes

Plain Apple Marmalade, unspiced, is made by peeling, and coring and cutting up 12 lb. of apples and cooking very gently with 6 lb. of sugar and 1 quart of cider till the fruit is very soft. Then pour through a sieve and place in glass jars. This is delicious with cream as a sweet.

It is also possible to make a very delicious preserve called Apple Honey, by boiling apples slowly for a very long time without any addition of sugar. The people of Denmark make this in hayboxes, thus saving fuel. When cooked long enough it is thick and brown, and very sweet, and will keep any length of time.

Spiced Apples

Peel some nice-shaped firm apples, and for every 3 lb. allow 1 quart of vinegar, 4 lb. of sugar, 1 OZ. of stick cinnamon, and 1/2 oz. of cloves. Boil sugar, vinegar, and spices together, then put in the apples, and let them cook until tender. Put them into a jar; boil down the syrup quite thick, and pour it over. Cover and keep for a few months in a cool place.

Apple Ginger

4 lb. apples. 3 pt. water.

4 lb. sugar. 2 OZ. essence of ginger.

Boil sugar and water until they form a syrup. Add ginger. Pare, core and quarter apples, boil them in the syrup until transparent. Place in warm, clean, dry jars. Tie down at once.

Another recipe. 3 lb. of apples, 1/4 lb. of preserved ginger. Pare apples and cut up in small pieces. Put in a basin of water till required; then put skins and cores into preserving pan, cover with water and boil till tender; strain and measure juice. To 3 pints of juice allow 2 lb. of sugar. Take next the cut apples and weigh them. To every 3 lb. allow 2 lb. of sugar. Put apples, juice, sugar and ginger all together into pan, and boil till ready.

Apple Jelly

6 lb. apples (any kind).

1 lemon.

Wipe and cut apples in four, remove bad parts. Place in preserving pan with lemon, well cover with water. Boil to a pulp. Place in a bag, allow to drip into a clean basin all night. Return to pan, adding 1 lb. sugar to each pint of juice. Boil for 3/4 hour or until jelly will set. Pour into clean, dry, warm jar. Tie down at once.

Crab-apple Jelly

Cook the Crab-apples with 6 cloves and an inch of ginger until the fruit is soft. Strain, boil again and add 3/4 lb. of sugar to a pint of liquid. Let boil until it jells. To make a successful jelly, the fruit should not be cooked too long, and the sugar should be added just before the strained liquid boils.

Apples Stewed Whole

Take 6 large Red apples, wash carefully and put in a fruit kettle, with just enough boiling water to cover. Cover the kettle, and cook slowly until the apples are soft, with the skins broken and the juice a rich red color. After removing the apples, boil the juice to a syrup, sweeten, and pour over the apples. A better plan is to make a syrup with sugar and water in which apples are stewed whole or sliced. Some add a clove, others the rind of lemon to improve the flavor.

Apples with Raisins

Pare, core, and quarter a dozen or more medium-sized apples. Clean thoroughly one fourth the weight of apples in raisins, and pour over them a quart of boiling water. Let them steep until well swollen, then add the apples, and cook until tender. Sugar to sweeten may be added if desired, although little will be needed unless the apples are very tart. Dried apples soaked overnight may be made much more palatable by stewing with raisins or English currants in the same way for about 40 minutes.

Apple Sandwiches

Cut apples into very thin slices, and lay between slices of bread and butter.

Apple and Egg Cream

Stew and strain 1 large tart apple, when cold add the well-beaten white of an egg. Serve with cream.

Apple Water

The following is an excellent recipe for a suitable drink for all fevers and feverish conditions:

Slice thinly 3 or 4 apples without peeling. Boil in a saucepan with a quart of water and a little sugar until the slices become soft. The apple water must then be strained and taken cold.

Mutton Baked with Apples and Onions

2 lb. of mutton cutlets from neck, salt,1 onion, 4 medium-sized apples. Prepare the meat by removing the bone and superfluous fat. Season with salt and lay in a baking dish. Cover the meat with finely-sliced sour apples and finely-chopped onions. Bake in a moderate oven until the meat is tender, which will be about 1 hour.

There is an old recipe for Apple Bread, wherein to the sponge was added one-third as much grated apple, which is perhaps worth reviving.

In some years, especially in a drought, the number of windfalls in the orchard is unusually large. They should never be allowed to lie on the ground, as most of them contain grubs which will hatch out into insect pests that ruin the fruit trees. But not a single windfall need be wasted. Those which are big enough to peel can be used for puddings or tarts. The small fruit can be used for making jelly, by cutting each in half so as to remove any grub that may be present, and then proceeding in the usual manner, as given above. The jelly will be a brilliant red color, equal to Crab-apple Jelly in taste and appearance.

Excellent chutneys, syrups, and jams can also be made from windfalls, which curiously enough so many housewives use only for stewing and baking, neglecting less humdrum methods, of which there are quite a number, of using the fruit. We give a few recipes:

Apple Fool

2 lb. of windfall apples, 4 oz. of brown sugar, 1 gill of water, a strip of lemon peel or z or 3 cloves or an inch of stick cinnamon, 1/2 pint of custard or cream.

Wash and wipe the fruit, remove any damaged portions, and cut into quarters without peeling or coring. Put it into a pan with the sugar, water, and flavoring, bring to the boil, and simmer until the fruit is soft. If too dry add a little more water. Rub through a sieve, and mix the puree with custard or cream.

Pears (windfall) or plums of any kind may be used in the same way, or apples and pears mixed.

Apple, Pear and Plum Jam

8 lb. of each fruit, 1/2, pint of cider, 1/4 oz. of powdered cloves (no sugar is required).

Cut the windfall apples and pears in quarters (do

not peel or core), put into a preserving pan with the plums, and add enough water to cover the bottom of the pan. Bring to the boil, then simmer until soft. Press out all the juice by pouring the fruit on to a fine hair sieve. Strain the juice through muslin, and boil it quickly in an uncovered pan until thick like a syrup. Put the syrup into bottles and cork well. Tie bladder or run sealing wax over the corks, and store in a dry, cool place.

Apple Chutney

About 30 windfall apples, 2 OZ. of salt, 3/4 Ib. of brown sugar, 4 oz. of onions, 1 clove of garlic, 3 oz. of powdered ginger, 1/2 oz. of dried chillies, 1 OZ. of mustard seeds, 4 oz. of raisins, 1 quart of vinegar.

Peel, core and slice the apples, put them into a pan with the sugar and vinegar and simmer until the apples are soft. Wash the mustard seed with vinegar and dry in a cool oven. Stone and chop the raisins. Peel and slice the garlic and onions, slice the chillies and pound them all in a mortar with the ginger and mustard seeds. When the apples are soft add the rest of the ingredients and let the mixture become cold. Mix well and put into bottles. Cork and cover like jam.

Note - Some prefer not to pound the chillies, but to add them just before putting the chutney into the bottles.

APPLE (BALSAM)

POISON
Botanical: Momordica balsamina
Family: N.O. Cucurbitaceze
Synonyms: Balsamina.
Part Used: The fruit deprived of the seeds.
Habitat: East India.

Description

A climbing annual plant cultivated in gardens for the sake of its ornamental fruit, which is of a rich orange red color, ovate attenuated towards each extremity, angular, warty, not unlike a cucumber. The name is derived from Mordio, to bite, so called from the bitten appearance.

Constituents

Has not been examined qualitatively.

Medicinal Action and Uses

A liniment is made by adding the pulped fruit (without the seeds) to almond oil. This is useful for piles, burns, chapped hands, etc. The pulp is also used as a poultice. The fluid extract is used for dropsy.

Caution is required in administering - large doses resulting in death.

Dosage and Preparation

Dose, 6 to 15 grains.

Poisons and Antidotes

As for Bitter Apple.

Other Species

Momordica charantia and East Indian species with bright orange yellow oblong fruits. Momordica mixta has fruit shaped like a bullock's heart, bright red in color.

APPLE (BITTER)

POISON
Botanical: Citrullus colocynthis (SCHRAD.)
Family: N.O. Cucurbilaceae
Synonyms: Colocynth Pulp. Bitter Cucumber.
Part Used: The dried pulp.

Habitat

Native of Turkey abounding in the Archipelago; also found in Africa (Nubia especially), Asia, Smyrna and Trieste.

Description

The Colocynth collected from the Maritime Plain between the mountains of Palestine and the Mediterranean, is mainly shipped from Jaffa and known as Turkish Colocynth. This is the best variety. It is an annual plant resembling the common watermelon. The stems are herbaceous and beset with rough hairs; the leaves stand alternately on long petioles. They are triangular, manycleft, variously sinuated, obtuse, hairy, a fine green on upper surface, rough and pale under. Flowers yellow, appearing singly at axils of leaves; fruit globular, size of an orange, yellow and smooth, when ripe contains within a hard coriaceous rind, a white spongy pulp enclosing numerous ovate compressed white or brownish seeds.

Constituents

The pulp contains Colocynthin, extractive, a fixed oil, a resinous substance insoluble in ether, gum, pectic acid or pectin, calcium and magnesium phosphates, lignin and water.

Medicinal Action and Uses

It is a powerful drastic hydragogue cathartic producing, when given in large doses, violent griping with, sometimes, bloody discharges and dangerous inflammation of the bowels. Death has resulted from a dose of 1 1/2 teaspoonsful of the powder. It is seldom prescribed alone. It is of such irritant nature that severe pain is caused if the powdered drug be applied to the nostrils; it has a nauseous, bitter taste and is usually given in mixture form with the tinctures of podophylum and belladonna. Colocynth fruits broken small are useful for keeping moth away from furs, woollens, etc.

Dosage and Preparation

Dose of the powder, 2 to 5 grains.

It is an important ingredient in Extractum Colocynthidis Compositum, Pilula Colocynthidis Composita, and Pilula Colocynthidis et Hyosiyami.

Poison and Antidotes

In case of poisoning by Colocynth the stomach should be emptied, opium given by mouth or rectum followed by stimulants and demulcent drinks.

APLOPPAS

Botanical: Bixa orillana

Description

Bixa orillana is a small tree 20 to 30 feet high, leaves broad, heartshape, pointed, flowers in bunches, rosecoloured fruit, heart-shaped, 1 1/4 inches long, reddish brown, covered with stiff prickles. Annatto is obtained by pulping the seeds, allowing the pulp to dry spontaneously and pressing it into cakes, or the seeds are soaked in water, allowed to ferment, and when the coloring matter subsides are collected and formed into cakes. There are two forms of Annatto used in commerce, the Spanish made in Brazil, which is hard, brittle, odourless, and is usually sent over in rolls; and the French, or flag, Annatto which comes from Cayenne, and is bright yellow in color, firm, sort, and evil-smelling, owing to the fermentive process used in which urine is utilized. The French is superior as a dye. Annatto has a dull fracture, a sweetish odor and a very disagreeable saline bitterish taste. It is inflammable, but does not melt with heat; insoluble in water, though it colors it yellow.

Constituents

The chief constituent is a red resinous substance named Bixin.

Medicinal Action and Uses

In the past it was used internally as medicine, but is now only employed as a coloring agent for ointments and plasters, and sometimes as a substitute for saffron. In South America it is largely used by the Caribs and other Indian tribes to paint their bodies. South American Indians are said to produce directly from the seeds, without fermentation, a brilliant carmine-like color.

In this country it is used for coloring cheese, inferior chocolate, etc., and by the Dutch as a butter coloring. It is also used as a dye for fabrics and in the manufacture of varnishes and lacquers.

Adulterants

Annatto is adulterated with ochre, sand gypsum, and a farinaceous matter.

APRICOT

Botanical: Prunus Armeniaca (LINN.)
Family: N.O. Rosaceae

Synonyms: Apricock. Armeniaca vulgaris.
Parts Used: Kernels, oil.

Habitat

Although formerly supposed to come from Armenia, where it was long cultivated, hence the name Armeniaca, there is now little doubt that its original habitat is northern China, the Himalaya region and other parts of temperate Asia. It is cultivated generally throughout temperate regions. Introduced into England, from Italy, in Henry VIII's reign.

Description

A hardy tree, bearing stone fruit, closely related to the peach. The leaves are broad and roundish, with pointed apex; smooth; margin, finely serrated; petiole 1/2 inch to an inch long, generally tinged with red. The flowers are sessile, white, tinged with the same dusky red that appears on the petiole, with five regular sepals and petals and many stamens, and open very early in the spring. The fruit, which ripens end of July to mid-August, according to variety, is a drupe, like the plum, with a thin outer, downy skin enclosing the yellow flesh (mesocarp), the inner layers becoming woody and forming the large, smooth, compressed stone, the ovule ripening into the kernel, or seed. As a rule in Britain, the fruit rarely ripens unless the tree is trained against a wall; when growing naturally, it is a medium-sized tree. It is propagated by budding on the musselplum stock. A great number of varieties are distinguished by cultivators. Large quantities of the fruit are imported from France. The kernels of several varieties are edible and in Egypt, those of the Musch-musch variety form a considerable article of commerce. Like those of the peach, apricot kernels contain constituents similar to those of the bitter almond: they are imported in large quantities from Syria and California and are oftenused by confectioners in the place of bitter almonds, which they so closely resemble as to be with difficulty distinguished.

The French liqueur Eau de Noyaux is prepared from bitter apricot kernels.

Constituents

Apricot kernels yield by expression 40 to 50 per cent. of a fixed oil, similar to that which occurs in the sweet almond and in the peach kernel, consisting chiefly of Olein, with a small proportion of the Glyceride of Linolic acid, and commonly sold as Peach Kernel oil (O1. Amygdae Pers.). From the cake is distilled, by digestion with alcohol, an essential oil (01. Amygdae Essent. Pers.) which contains a colorless, crystalline glucoside, Amygdalin, and is chemically identical with that of the bitter almond. The essential oil is used in confectionery and as a culinary flavoring.

Medicinal Action and Uses

Apricot oil is used as a substitute for Oil of Almonds, which it very closely resembles. It is far less expensive and finds considerable employment in cosmetics, for its softening action on the skin. It is often fraudulently added to genuine Almond oil and used in the manufacture of soaps, cold creams and other preparations of the perfumery trade.

ARAROBA

Botanical: Andira araroba (AGUIAR.)
Family: N.O. Leguminosae
Synonyms: Goa Powder. Crude Chrysarobin. Bahia Powder. Brazil Powder. Ringworm Powder. Chrysatobine. Goa. Araroba Powder. Voucapoua Araroba.
Parts Used: The medullary matter of the stem and branches, dried and powdered.
Habitat: Brazil.

Description

The powder is named Goa, after the Malabar port, and it was not realized until 1875 that the drug was Brazilian Araroba, and reached the East Indies through Portugal and her colonies. The tree from which it is obtained, Andira Araroba, is large, smooth, and quite commonly found in Bahia, Brazil. The yellowish wood has longitudinal canals and interspaces in which the powder is deposited in increasing quantity as the tree ages. It is probably due to a pathological condition. It is scraped out with an axe, after felling, sawing, and splitting the trunk, and is thus inevitably mixed with splinters and debris, so that it needs sifting, and is sometimes ground, dried, boiled, and filtered.

It irritates the eyes and face of the woodmen.

As it darkens quickly, the crude chrysarobin is changed from primrose yellow to shades of dark brown before it is met with in commerce, when it often contains a large percentage of water, added to prevent the dust from rising.

An amber skin-varnish is made with 20 parts of amber to 1 of chrysarobin in turpentine.

Constituents

The powder is insoluble in water, but yields up to 80 per cent. of its weight to solutions of caustic alkalies and to benzene. It contains 80 to 84 per cent. of chrysarobin (easily convertible into chrysophanic acid), resin, woody fibre, and bitter extractive. Goa Powder is usually regarded as crude chrysarobin, while the purified chrysarobin, or Araroba, is a mixture extracted by hot benzene, which melts when heated, and leaves not more than 1 per cent. of ash when it finally burns.

Chrysarobin is a reduced quinone, and chrysophanic acid (also found in rhubarb yellow lichen, Buckthorn Berries, Rumox Eckolianus, a South African dock, etc., etc.), is a dioxymethylanthraquinone.

Chrysarobin contains at least five substances, and owes its power to one of these, chrysophanol-anthranol.

Lenirobin, a tetracetate,, and eurobin, a triacetate, are recommended as substitutes for chrysarobin, as they do not stain linen indelibly. (Benzin helps to remove the stains of chrysarobin.)

The action of chrysarobin on the skin is not due to germicidal properties, but to its chemical affinity for the keratin elements of the skin. The oxygen for its oxidation is abstracted from the epithelium by the drug.

Oxidized chrysarobin, obtained by boiling chrysarobin in water with sodium peroxide, can be used as an ointment for forms of eczema which chrysarobin would irritate too much.

Medicinal Action and Uses

The internal dose in pill or powder is a gastrointestinal irritant, producing large, watery stools and vomiting. It is used in eczema, psoriasis, acne, and other skin diseases.

In India and South Ameriea it has been esteemed for many years for ringworm, psoriasis, dhobi's itch, etc., as ointment, or simply moistened with vinegar or saliva. The application causes the eruption to become whitish, while the skin around it is stained dark.

In the crude form it should never be applied to the head, as it may cause erythema and oedema of the face. The 2 per cent. ointment is good in ecezema (after exudation has ceased), fissured nipples, and tylosis of the palms and soles after the skin has been removed by salicylic acid plaster, etc.

A drachm of chrysarobin may be dissolved in a fluid ounce of official flexible collodion, painted over the parts with a camel's-hair brush, and the part coated with plain collodion to avoid staining the clothing; or chrysarobin may be dissolved in chloroform and the solution painted on the skin. For hemorrhoids, an ointment mixed with iodoform, belladonna, and petrolatum is recommended.

It is said to have been used as a taenifuge.

Dosage

One-half grain.

Other Species

A. Inermis, or Cabbage Tree of South America and Senegambia, has a narcotic, anthelmintic bark, known as Bastard Cabbage Bark or Worm Bark. The powder, in doses of 3 to 4 grains, purges like jalap. The decoction is usually preferred.

The symptoms of an overdose are feverish delirium and vomiting, which should be counteracted with lime-juice or castor oil.

It is no longer officially used in England.

ARBUTUS (STRAWBERRY TREE)

Botanical: Arbutus unede
Family: N.O. Ericaceae

Habitat

In the woods at Killarney and Bantry is found growing wild the beautiful evergreen shrub, known as the Arbutus, or Strawberry Tree (Arbutus unede), which for its attractiveness should gain a place in every well-planted garden. It would, indeed, be hard to find any other ornamental shrub or tree that has such a cheerful appearance throughout the autumn and early winter, when its dense mass of greenery is mingled with a profusion of flower clusters and ruddy, round fruit resembling small strawberries. The creamy-white, bell-shaped flowers, often tinged with pink, are intermixed with the orange-scarlet rough fruit, which owing to the length of time it takes to ripen, remains on the tree for twelve months, not maturing until the autumn succeeding that in which the flower is produced.

Although a native of South Europe, and only growing wild here in the South of Ireland on the rocks at Killarney, the Arbutus will thrive almost anywhere in this country, especially in warm and coast regions, where it will grow 20 feet high, making huge, globular masses of green, though ordinarily its height is only from 8 to 10 feet. In inland districts it is liable to be cut down during exceptionally severe winters, but this rarely happens, and if large bushes are apparently killed by cold, they almost invariably send up strong shoots again. When young, it requires in order to get it established, a slight protection during winter. It grows quickly in sheltered places but dislikes shade, and seems to be most at home in a deep, light soil, flourishing best in a sandy loam.

When eaten in quantities this fruit is said to be narcotic, and the wine made from it in Spain has the same property.

The tree is common in the Mediterranean region, and the fruit was known to the ancients, but according to Pliny (who gave the tree the name of Arbutus) was not held in much esteem, as the name implies (un ede=one 1 eat), the fruits being considered so unpalatable, that no one tasting them for the first time would be tempted to repeat the experiment. Nevertheless, there is some evidence that at one time the fruit was an article of diet with the ancients. Horace praises the tree for its shade and Ovid for its loads of 'blushing fruit." Virgil recommends the young shoots as winter food for goats and for basket-work.

Gerard speaks of it in his time as growing in 'some few gardens," and says, 'the fruit being ripe is of a gallant red color, in taste somewhat harsh, and in a manner without any relish, of which thrushes and blackbirds do feed in winter ."

In Spain, a sugar and spirit have been extracted from the fruit and a wine made from it in Corsica.

In the neighborhood of Algiers it forms hedges, and in Greece and Spain the bark has been used for tanning. The wood of the tree makes good charcoal.

ARBUTUS, TRAILING

Botanical: Epigaea repens (LINN.)
Family: N.O. Ericaceae
Synonyms: Mountain Pink. May Flower. Gravel Plant. Ground Laurel. Winter Pink.
Part Used: The leaves, used dried to make an infusion, and fresh to make a tincture.

Habitat

The Trailing Arbutus (Epigaea repens, Linn.) is a small evergreen creeping shrub, found in sandy soil in many parts of North America, in the shade of pines. Its natural home is under trees, and it will thrive in this country only in moist, sandy peat in shady places. It has long been known in cultivation here as an ornamental plant, having been introduced into Great Britain in 1736. Like the common Arbutus, or the Strawberry Tree and the Bearberry, it belongs to the order Ericacece, the family of the heaths.

Description

It grows but a few inches high, with a trailing, shrubby stalk, which puts out roots at the joints, and when in a proper soil and situation multiplies very fast. The evergreen leaves are stalked, broadly ovate, 1 to 1 1/2 inches long, rough and leathery, with entire, wavy margins and a short point at the apex. Branches, leaf-stalks and nerves of the leaves are very hairy. The flowers are produced at the end of the branches in dense clusters. They are white, with a reddish tinge and very fragrant, divided at the top into five acute segments, which spread open in the form of a star. The plant flowers in April and May, but rarely produces fruit in England. It is stated to be injurious to cattle when eaten by them.

The name of the genus, Epigaea, derived from Greek words signifying 'upon the ground," expresses the mode of growth and trailing habit of the species.

Cultivation

The Trailing Arbutus generally does not do well when attempts are made to take it from its natural surroundings and place it under garden conditions. It needs partial shade and very free soil, composed mainly of decayed leaves, and perfect shelter from cold winds. In short grass, just within the shelter of oak trees, the overhanging boughs of which give a certain amount of shade, it will do well and is usually found at its best in sandy loam, on a gravelly, well-drained subsoil.

In removing it from its native haunts, dense tufts of low-growing and apparently young plants should be selected. These should be lifted intact, and to such a depth, that the roots are not disturbed, and placed in conditions in the home garden exactly similar to those from which they are taken. To plant in an ordinary herbaceous border means failure. They must not be choked out with long grass or coarse weeds. In dry weather water the plants occasionally, and in winter give a little mulching of leaves .

It may be increased by seeds, but they are slow in sprouting. By carefully dividing the well-established tufts in autumn, or by layering the branches, good plants are sometimes obtained. The trailing stalks, which put out roots at the joints, may be cut off from the old plant and placed in a shady situation and a moist soil. If done in autumn, the plants may be well rooted before the spring. Cuttings of previous year's wood are more successful inserted in sandy soil, under a glass in gentle heat in spring. As soon as rooted, plants should be grown on in pots until well established, and then transferred in early autumn, or spring, to their permanent positions outside, but they will never grow so well in the open (where they will always be more or less stunted specimens), as they will under conditions which closely imitate those which the plant enjoys in the woods of New England.

Medicinal Action and Uses

Astringent and diuretic. Used in the same way as Buchu and Uva ursi for bladder and urinary troubles: of special value when the urine contains blood or pus, and when there is irritation.

The infusion of 1 OZ. of the leaves to a pint of boiling water may be taken freely.

ARECA NUT

Botanical: Areca catechu (LINN.)
Family: N.O. Palmacea
Synonyms: Betel Nut. Pinang.
Part Used: The seed.
Habitat: East Indies, cultivated in India and Ceylon.

Description

A handsome tree cultivated in all the warmer parts of Asia for its yellowish-red fruits the size of a hen's egg, containing the seed about the size of an acorn, conical shape with flattened base and brownish in color externally; internally mottled like a nutmeg. The seeds are cut into narrow pieces and rolled inside Betel Pepper leaf, rubbed over with lime and chewed by the natives. They stain the lips and teeth red and also the excrement, they are hot and acrid when chewed.

Constituents

Areca Nut contains a large quantity of tannin, also gallic acid, a fixed oil gum, a little volatile oil, lignin, and various saline substances. Four alkaloids have been found in Areca Nut - Arecoline, Arecain, Guracine, and a fourth existing in very small quantity. Arecoline resembles Pilocarpine in its effects on the system. Arecaine is the active principle of the Areca

Nut.

Medicinal Actions and Uses

Areca Nut is aromatic and astringent and is said to intoxicate when first taken. The natives chew these nuts all day. Whole shiploads are exported annually from Sumatra, Malacca, Siam and Cochin China. In this country Areca Nut is made into a dentrifrice on account of its astringent properties. Catechu is often made by boiling down the seeds of the plant to the consistency of an extract, but the proper Catechu used in Britain is produced from the Acacia catechu. The flowers are very sweet-scented and in Borneo are used in medicines as charms for the healing of the sick. In India the nut has long been used as a taenifuge for tapeworm. The action of Arecain resembles that of Muscarine and Pilocarpine externally, internally used it contracts the pupils.

Arecoline Hydrobromide, a commercial salt, is a stronger stimulant to the salivary glands than Pilocarpine and a more energetic laxative than Eserine. It is used for colic in horses.

Dosages and Preparations

Of the powdered nut for tapeworm 1 to 2 teaspoonsful. Of the Fluid Extract of Areca Nut, 1 drachm. Of the Arecoline Hydrobromide, for colic in horses, 1 to 1 1/2 grains. Of the Arecoline Hydrobromide, for human use, 1/15 to 1/10 grains .

Other Species

In Malabar Areca Dicksoni is found growing wild and is used by the poor as a substitute for the true Betel Nut (A. aleraceae). The Cabbage Palm, which grows profusely in the West Indies, derives its name from the bud topping the tall stem; this consists of leaves wrapped round each other as in the cabbage, the heart of which is white inside. It has a delicate taste and is cut and cooked as a vegetable, many of these beautiful palms being destroyed in this way. It is said that in the empty cavity a beetle lays its eggs. These turn into maggots which are eaten with great relish by the negroes of Guiana.

ARNICA

Botanical: Arnica montana (LINN.)
Family: N.O. Compositae
Synonyms: Mountain Tobacco. Leopard's Bane.
Parts Used: Root, flowers.

Habitat

Arnica montana or Leopard's Bane is a perennial herb, indigenous to Central Europe, in woods and mountain pastures. It has been found in England and Southern Scotland. but is probably an escape.

Description

The leaves form a flat rosette, from the centre of which rises a flower stalk, 1 to 2 feet high, bearing orange-yellow flowers. The rhizome is dark brown, cylindrical, usually curved, and bears brittle wiry rootlets on the under surface.

Cultivation

Arnica thrives in a mixture of loam, peat, and sand. It may be propagated by root division or from seed. Divide in spring. Sow in early spring in a cold frame, and plant out in May.

The flowers are collected entire and dried, but the receptacles are sometimes removed as they are liable to be attacked by insects.

The root is collected in autumn after the leaves have died down.

Constituents

A bitter yellow crystalline principle, Arnicin, and a volatile oil. Tannin and phulin are also present. The flowers are said to contain more Arnicin than the rhizome, but no tannin.

Medicinal Action and Uses

In countries where Arnica is indigenous, it has long been a popular remedy. In the North American colonies the flowers are used in preference to the rhizome. They have a discutient property. The tincture is used for external application to sprains, bruises, and wounds, and as a paint for chilblains when the skin is unbroken. Repeated applications may produce severe inflammation. It is seldom used internally, because of its irritant effect on the stomach. Its action is stimulant and diuretic, and it is chiefly used in low fevers and paralytie affections.

Arnica flowers are sometimes adulterated with other composite flowers, especially Calendula officinalis, Inula brittanica, Kragapogon pratensis, and Scorzonera humilis.

A homeopathic tincture, X6, has been used successfully in the treatment of epilepsy; also for seasickness, 3 X before sailing, and every hour on board till comfortable.

For tender feet a foot-bath of hot water containing 1/2 oz. of the tineture has brought great relief. Applied to the scalp it will make the hair grow.

Great care must be exercised though, as some people are particularly sensitive to the plant and many severe cases of poisoning have resulted from its use, especially if taken internally.

British Pharmacopoeia Tincture, root, 10 to 30 drops. United States Pharmacopoeia Tincture, flowers, 10 to 30 drops.

ARRACHS OR ORACHES

Botanical: Chenopodium olidum (LINN.)
Chenopodium vulvaria (S. WATS.)
Family: N.O. Chenopodiaceae
Synonyms: Stinking Motherwort. Wild Arrach. Stinking Arrach. Stinking Goosefoot. Netchweed. Goat's Arrach.
Part Used: Herb.

Habitat

The Wild Arrach, or Netchweed (Chenopodium olidum, Linn.), (syn. C. vulvaria S. Wats.), one of the common Goosefoots, is an annual herb, found on roadsides and dry waste ground near houses, from Edinburgh southward.

Description

Its stem is not erect, but partly Iying, branched from the base, the opposite branches spreading widely, a foot or more in length.

The stalked leaves are oval, wedge-shaped at the base, about 1/2 inch long, the margins entire.

The small, insignificant green flowers are borne in spikes from the axils of the leaves and consist of five sepals, five stamens and a pistil with two styles. There are no petals and the flowers are wind-fertilized. They are in bloom from August to October.

The whole plant is covered with a white, greasy mealiness, giving it a grey-green appearance which when touched, gives out a very objectionable and enduring odor, like that of stale salt fish, and accounts for its common popular name: Stinking Goosefoot.

Medicinal Action and Uses

The name of 'Stinking Motherwort' refers to the use of its leaves in hysteria and nervous troubles connected with women's ailments: it has emmenagogue and anti-spasmodic properties. In former days, it was supposed even to cure barrenness and in certain cases, the mere smelling of its foetid odor was held to afford relief.

An infusion of 1 OZ. of the dried herb in a pint of boiling water is taken three or four times daily in wine glassful doses as a remedy for menstrual obstructions. It is also sometimes used as a fomentation and injection, but is falling out of use, no doubt on account of its unpleasant odor and taste.

The infusion has been employed in nervous debility and also for colic.

A fluid extract is prepared, the dose being 1/2, to 1 drachm.

The leaves have also been made into a conserve with sugar. Dr. Fuller's famous Electuarium hystericum was compounded by adding 48 drops of oil of Amber (Oleum Succini) to 4 oz. of the conserve of this Chenopodium. A piece of the size of a chestnut was prescribed to be taken when needed and repeated as often as required.

Constituents

Chemical analysis has proved Trimethylamine to be a constituent, together with Osmazome and Nitrate of Potash.The plant gives off free Ammonia.

Culpepper speaks of two kinds of 'Arrach." One he calls Garden Arrach, 'called also Orach; and Arage," giving its Latin name as Atriplex hortensis. The other kind he calls 'Wild and Stinking Arrach' (A. olida), 'called also Vulvaria, Dog's Arrach, Goat's Arrach and Stinking Motherwort." He is emphatic in his commendation of this 'Stinking Arrach' for every kind of women's diseases and troubles, though he describes its odor in his usual unvarnished language, saying: 'It smells like rotten fish, or something worse."

The names 'Dog's Arrach," 'Goat's Arrach' and 'Dog's Orache' point to a contemptuous scorn of its unfitness as a pot-herb compared with the true Orache (Atriplex), closely allied to it.

ARRACH (GARDEN)

Botanical: Atriplex hortensis
Synonyms: Mountain Spinach. Garden Orache.

The Garden Orache, or Mountain Spinach (Atriplex hortensis), is a tall, erect-growing hardy annual, a native of Tartary, introduced into this country in 1548. It is not much cultivated here now, but is grown a good deal in France, under the name of Arroche, for its large and succulent leaves, as a substitute for Spinach and to correct the acidity of Sorrel.

The quality of the spinach yielded by Orache is, however, far inferior to that of Common Spinach, or even of the New Zealand Spinach.

There are several varieties of Orache of various colourings. The White and the Green are the most desirable kinds.

The plants should be grown quickly, in rich soil. They may be sown in rows, 2 feet apart, and thinned out to the same distance apart in the rows, sowings being in May, and for succession, again in June. If dry, water must be freely given so as to maintain a rapid growth.

'Orache is cooling," says Evelyn, 'and allays the pituit humours." Being set over the fire, neither this nor the lettuce needs any other water than their own moisture to boil them in.

The name Orache, given to this Goosefoot and others of the same tribe, is a corruption of aurum, gold, because their seeds, mixed with wine, were supposed to cure the ailment known popularly as the 'yellow jaundice." They excite vomiting.

Uses

Heated with vinegar, honey and salt and applied, the Orache was considered efficacious to cure an attack of gout.

ARRACH (HALBERD-LEAVED)

Botanical: Atriplex hastata

The Halberd-leaved Wild Orache (Atriplex hastata) closely resembles the Spreading Orache and is often regarded merely as a sub-species, but is, however, of a more erect character and the lower leaves are broadly triangular, the lobes widely spread.

It is a troublesome weed in gardens and cultivated ground.

The leaves have been frequently eaten instead of spinach, but Culpepper says its chief virtues lie in the seed, employed in the same manner as that of the Garden Orache.

ARRACH (WILD)

Botanical: Atriplex patula
Synonym: Spreading Orache.

The Wild Orache (Atriplex patula) is a common native weed on clays and heavy ground. It has spreading stems, 2 to 3 feet long, sometimes prostrate, only occasionally erect (hence often called the Spreading Orache).

The leaves are triangular in outline, rather narrow, the lower ones in opposite pairs. The very small, green flowers are in dense clusters.

The whole plant is more or less covered with a powdery meal, often tinged red. It is distinguished from the Goosefoot genus Chenopodium, by the solitary seeds being enclosed between two triangular leaf-like valves.

'These are to be gathered when just ripe for if suffered to stand longer, they lose part of their virtue. A pound of these bruised, and put into three quarts of spirit, of moderate strength, after standing six weeks, afford a light and not unpleasant tincture; a tablespoonful of which, taken in a cup of water-gruel, has the same effect as a dose of ipecacuanha, only that its operation is milder and does not bind the bowels afterwards.... It cures headaches, wandering pains, and the first attacks of rheumatism."

ARROWHEAD

Botanical: Sagittaria sagittifolia (LINN.)
Family: N.O. Alismaceae
Medicinal Action and Uses
Synonyms: Wapatoo. Is'-ze-kn.

The Alismaceae group of plants in general contain acrid juices, on account of which, a number of species, besides the Water Plantain, have been used as diuretics and antiscorbutic.

Several species of Sagittaria, natives of Brazil, are astringent and their expressed juice has been used in making ink.

The rhizome of Sagittaria sagittifolia (Linn.), the Arrowhead, Wapatoo, and S. Chinensis (Is'-ze-kn) are used respectively by the North American Indians and the Chinese as starchy foods, as are some other species.

The Arrowhead is a water plant widely distributed in Europe and Northern Asia, as well as North America, and abundant in many parts of England, though only naturalized in Scotland.

The stem is swollen at the base and throws out creeping stolons or runners, which produce globose winter tubers, 1/2 inch in diameter, composed almost entirely of starch.

The leaves are borne on triangular stalks that vary in length with the depth of the water in which the plant is growing. They do not lie on the water, like those of the Water Lily, but stand boldly above it. They are large and arrow-shaped and very glossy. The early, submerged leaves are ribbonlike.

The flower-stem rises directly from the root and bears several rings of buds and blossoms, three in each ring or whorl, and each flower composed of three outer sepals and three large, pure white petals, with a purple blotch at their base. The upper flowers are stamen-bearing, the lower ones generally contain the seed vessels only.

The root tubers are about the size of a small walnut. They grow just below the surface of the mud. The Chinese and Japanese cultivate the plant for the sake of these tubercles, which are eaten as an article of wholesome food. Bryant, in Flora Dietetica, writes of them:

'I cured some of the bulbs of this plant in the same manner that saloop is cured, when they acquired a sort of pellucidness, and on boiling afterwards, they broke into a gelatinous meal and tasted like old peas boiled."

The tubers, it has been stated, may also be eaten in the raw state.

Medicinal Action and Uses

Diuretic and antiscorbutic.

ARROWROOT

Botanical: Maranta arundinaceae (LINN.)
Family: N.O. Marantaceae
Synonyms: Indian Arrowroot. Maranta Indica. Maranta ramosissima. Maranta Starch or Arrowroot. East or West Indian Arrowroot. Araruta. Bermuda Arrowroot.
Part Used: The fecula or starch of the rhizome.

Habitat

Indigenous in the West Indian Islands and possibly Central America. Grows in Bengal, Tava. Philippines, Mauritius. Natal. West Africa.

Description

The name of the genus was bestowed by Plumier in memory of Bartommeo Maranto (d. 1559, Naples), a physician of Venosa in Basilicata. The popular name is a corruption of the Aru-root of the Aruac Indians of South America, or is derived from the fact that the plant is said to be an antidote to arrow-poison.

The product is usually distinguished by the name of the place from which it is imported. Bermuda Arrowroot was formerly the finest, but it is now rarely produced, and the name is applied to others of high standard.

It was introduced into England about 1732 though it will only grow as a stove plant, with tanners' bark. The plant is an herbaceous perennial, with a creeping rhizome with upward-curving, fleshy, cylindrical tubers covered with large, thin scales that leave rings of scars. The flowering stem reaches a height of 6 feet, and bears creamy flowers at the ends of the slender branches that terminate the long peduncles. They grow in pairs. The numerous, ovate, glabrous leaves are from 2 to 10 inches in length, with long sheaths often enveloping the stem.

The starch is extracted from rhizomes not more than a year old. They are washed, pulped in wooded mortars, stirred in clean water, the fibres wrung out by hand, and the milky liquor sieved, allowed to settle, and then drained. Clean water is again added, mixed, and drained, after which the starch is dried on sheets in the sun, dust and insects being carefully excluded. The starch yield is about one-fifth of the original weight of the rhizomes. It should be odourless and free from unpleasant taste, and when it becomes mouldy, should be rejected. It keeps well if quite dry. The powder creaks slightly when rubbed, and feels firm. Microscopical examination of the starch granules is necessary for certainty of purity. Potato starch, which corresponds in chemical and nutritive qualities, is sometimes substituted, but it has a somewhat unpleasant taste, and a test with hydrochloric acid brings out an odor like French beans. Sago, rice and tapioca starches are also found occasionally as substitutes.

The jelly is more tenacious than that of any other starch excepting Tous-les-mois.

Arrowroot is often used simply in the form of pudding or blanc-mange. The roots could be candied like Eryngo.

Constituents

An 1887 analysis of the root of the St. Vincent Arrowroot gave starch 27.17 per cent, fibre, fat, albumen, sugar, gum, ash, and 62.96 per cent water.

Of the starch was given: starch 83'70 per cent., fibre, fat, sugar, gum, ash and sand, and water 15.87 per cent.

The official granules, according to Pereira, are 'rarely oblong, somewhat ovate-oblong, or irregularly convex, from 10 to 70 microns in diameter, with very fine lamellae, a circular hilium which is fissured in a linear or stellate manner."

Medicinal Auction and Uses

Arrowroot is chiefly valuable as an easily digested, nourishing diet for convalescents, especially in bowel complaints, as it has demulcent properties. In the proportion of a tablespoonful to a pint of water or milk, it should be prepared by being first made into a smooth paste with a little cold milk or water, and then carefully stirred while the boiling milk is added. Lemon-juice, sugar, wine, or aromatics may be added. If thick, it will cool into a jelly that usually suits weaning infants better than other farinaceous foods.

It is said that the mashed rhizomes are used for application to wounds from poisoned arrows, scorpion and black spider bites, and to arrest gangrene.

The freshly-expressed juice, mixed with water, is said to be a good antidote, taken internally, for vegetable poisons, such as Savanna.

Other Species

Maranta ramosissima is the M. arundinaceae of the East Indies.

M. allouya and M. nobilis are also West Indian species. The term arrowroot is applied to other starches.

BRAZILIAN ARROWROOT, or Tapioca Meal, is obtained from Manihot utilissima (bitter) and M. palmata (sweet) . It is also called Bahia Rio, or Para-Arrowroot. See MANDIOCA.

TAHITI ARROWROOT is from Tacca oceanica (pinnatifida). It is a favorite article of diet in the tropics, being found in the Sandwich and South Sea Islands, and is said to be the best arrowroot for dysentery.

EAST INDIAN ARROWROOT is from Curcuma augustifolia, or longa.

TOUS-LES-MOIS is from Canna edulis and C. achiras, of the West Indies, called Indian Shot, from their hard, black seeds, used as beads, and Balisier, from the use of their leaves for packing, in Brazil.

OSWEGO ARROWROOT, used in America, is from Zea Mays, Indian Corn.

MEXICAN ARROWROOT is from the seeds of Dion edule.

CHINESE ARROWROOT is said to be from the tubers of Nelumbium speciosum.

PORTLAND ARROWROOT was formerly obtained from Arum maculatum, but it was acrid and not very satisfactory.

M. dichotoma has stems used, when split, for making shade mats in India.

M. Malaccensis has poisonous roots used as an ingredient in a Borneo arrow-poison.

ARTICHOKE, JERUSALEM

Botanical: Helianthus tuberosus

Family: N.O. Compositae

Synonym: Sunflower Artichoke.

Habitat

The Jerusalem Artichoke (Helianthus tuberosus, Linn.), now commonly cultivated in England for its edible tubers, another of the numerous Sunflowers, is a native of the North American plains, being indigenous in the lake regions of Canada, as far west as Saskatchewan, and from thence southward to Arkansas and the middle parts of Georgia.

Though it rarely blossoms in England, it flowers profusely in its native country (blooming also freely in South Africa), the flowers, however, being small and inconspicuous, produced just above the last leaves. Its name, Jerusalem Artichoke, does not, as it seems, imply that it grows in Palestine, but is a corruption of the Italian Girasola articiocco, the Sunflower Artichoke, Girasola meaning 'turning to the sun," an allusion to the habit it is supposed to have in common with many of the Sunflower tribe. The North Italian word articiocco - modern carciofo - comes through the Spanish, from the Arabic Al-Kharshuf. False etymology has corrupted the word in many languages: it has been derived (though wrongly) in English from 'choke' and 'heart," or the Latin hortus, a garden, and in French, the form artichaut has been connected with chaud, hot, and chou, a cabbage.

History

It appears to have been cultivated as an article of food by the Indians of North America before the settlement in that country of Europeans, and very soon attracted the attention of travellers. Sir J. D. Hooker, in the Botanical Magazine, July, 1897, gives the following account of its introduction:

'In the year 1617, Mr. John Goodyer, of Mapledurham, Hampshire, received two small roots of it from Mr. Franqueville of London, which, being planted, enablel him before 1621 "to store Hampshire." In October of the same year, Mr. Goodyer wrote an account of it for T. Johnson, who printed it in his edition of Gerard's "Herball," which appeared in 1636, where it is called Jerusalem Artichoke. Previous to which, in 1629, it had been figured and described under that name by Parkinson in his "Paradisus," and he also mentions it in his "Theatrum" in 1640. From the lastgiven date to the present time, the Jerusalem

Artichoke has been extensively cultivated in Europe, but rather as a garden vegetable than a field crop, and has extended into India, where it is making its way amongst the natives under Hindoo, Bengali, and other native names."

Parkinson speaks of it as 'a dainty for a queen." When first introduced, the mode of preparation of the tubers was to boil them till tender, and after peeling, they were eaten sliced and stewed with butter, wine and spices. They were also baked in pies, with marrow, dates, ginger, raisins, sack, etc. Parkinson called them 'Potatoes of Canada," because the French brought them first from Canada. Their flavor is somewhat sooty when cooked and not agreeable to everyone but they are very nutritious, and boiled in milk form an excellent accompaniment to roast beef.

The tuber, instead of containing starch like the potato, has the allied substance Inulin. The chief ingredients are water, 80 per cent. albuminoids, 2 per cent.; gum, known as Laevulin, 9.1 per cent.; sugar, 4.2 per cent.; inulin, 1.1 per cent.

Cultivation

In any odd bit of ground shaded or open, that is unsuitable for other vegetables, a crop of the tubers of Jerusalem Artichoke will always be obtained, though like other things, it pays for a good position and generous culture and the largest tubers will be produced in a light, rich soil.

The ground should be well dug over and if at all heavy, or poor, should be lightened by incorporating some sand with it enriched with well-rotted manure.

For planting, which may be done in February, but not later than March, small tubers should be chosen and indeed reserved for this purpose when the crop is taken up, but almost any part of a tuber will grow and form a plant. The sets should be planted in rows, 3 feet apart and at a distance of 18 inches from each other in the rows, they should be set at least 6 inches deep. As a rule, a great number of plants is produced from one tuber.

The ground should be kept clean by hoeing and as the plants grow in height, a little earth should be drawn up around the stem.

Cut the plants down when the leaves are decayed, but not before, otherwise the tubers will cease to grow. The tubers may be left in the ground till wanted for use. If taken up towards the end of November, they may be stored in sand or earth, but they must be covered, so that the light and air may be effectually excluded, otherwise they will be of a dark color when cooked.

The white-skinned variety, 'New White Mammoth," is to be recommended. The tubers have a clean, white skin, instead of the purplish-red tint of the old variety. They are also rounder in shape and not so irregular in form as the tubers of the red sort. This variety is equally hardy, being in no way liable to injury from frost.

Jerusalem Artichokes afford a useful screen for a wooden fence, when planted along the foot of it, but the more open the spot, the more likely they are to prosper. When once planted, the difficulty is to get the ground clear of them again, for the smallest tuber will grow. It is desirable to change the ground allotted to their culture about once in three years, for when they are permitted to remain too long on the same spot, the tubers deteriorate in size and quality.

ARTICHOKE, GLOBE

Botanical: Cynara Scolymus
Family: N.O. Compositae

Cultivation

The Globe Artichoke (Cynara Scolymus, Linn.) also has a tuberous root, but it is the large flower-buds that form the edible portion of the plant, and it is from a similarity in the flavor of the tuber of the Jerusalem Artichoke to that of the fleshy base of this flower that the Jerusalem Artichoke has obtained its name.

The expanded flower has much resemblance to a large thistle- the corollas are of a rich blue color.

It is one of the world's oldest cultivated vegetables,

grown by the Greeks and the Romans in the heyday of their power. It was introduced into this country in the early sixteenth century both as a vegetable and an ornamental plant in monastery gardens.

Gerard (1597) gives a good figure of the Artichoke. Parkinson (1640) alludes to a statement of Theophrastus (fourth century B.C.) that 'the head of Scolymus is most pleasant, being boyled or eaten raw, but chiefly when it is in flower, as also the inner substance of the heads is eaten." Though this 'inner substance' - botanically the 'receptacle' - has a delicate flavor, it contains little nutritive matter.

Tournefort (1730) says:

'The Artichoke is well known at the table. What we call the bottom is the thalamus on which the embryos of the seeds are placed. The leaves are the scales of the empalement. The Choak is the florets, with a chaffy substance intermixt (the pappus). The French and Germans boil the heads as we do, but the Italians generally eat them raw with salt, oil and pepper."

In Italy the receptacles, dried, are also largely used in soups.

The whole plant has a peculiar smell and a strong bitter taste. It was reputed to be aperient.

Cultivation

It is grown either from seed sown in March, in a deep, moist, rich soil which may be greatly aided by wood-ashes and seaweed (for it is partial to saline manures, its home being the sandy shores of Northern Africa); or by planting suckers in April; the latter is preferable for a permanent plantation. Strong plants may be ensured by inserting them 4 feet each way, but market growers usually put out suckers in rows 4 1/2, feet apart, and 2 feet distant in the rows. Suckers should be planted when about 9 inches high; put in rather deep in soil and planted firmly and covered with rough mulch. If the weather be dry, they will need watering, and during hot weather water and liquid manure should be given freely to ensure a good supply of large heads.

Seedlings that are started well in a suitable bed do better than plants from suckers, especially in a dry season.

Vigorous seedlings send down their roots to a great depth. To get large heads, all lateral heads should be removed when they are about the size of a large egg. After the heads are used, the plant should be cut down.

The Artichoke is hardy on dry soils in winters of only average severity. But on moist soils - so favourable to fine heads - a severe winter will kill the plantations unless they have some kind of protection. This is usually ensured by cutting down the stems and large leaves without touching the smaller central leaves, and when severe frost threatens, to partially earth up the rows with soil taken from between, also adding dry, light litter loosely thrown over; the latter is removed in the spring and the earth dug back, and a liberal supply of manure dug in. At the end of five years a plantation is worn out; the best method being to sow a bed annually and allow it to stand for two years.

The flower-stems grow erect and attain the height of 4 to 6 feet. They are each terminated by a large globular head of imbricated oval spiny scales of a purplish-green color. These envelop a mass of flowers in the centre. These flowerheads in an immature state contain the parts that are eatable, which comprise the fleshy receptacle usually called the 'bottom," freed from the bristles and seed-down, commonly called the 'choke," and the thick lower part of the imbricated scales or leaves of the involucre.

Although Artichokes are a common vegetable, they are not so much in request with us as on the Continent.

In France, the bottoms are often fried in paste, and enter largely into ragouts. They are occasionally used for pickling, but for this purpose the smaller heads which are formed on the lateral shoots that spring in succession from the main stem, are generally preferred when about the size of a large egg.

The chard of Artichokes, or the tender central leaf-stalks, blanched, is by some considered to be equal to the Cardoon.

The flowers are very handsome, and are said to possess the property of coagulating milk.

ARTICHOKE, CHINESE

Botanical: Stachvs Sieboldii

Cultivation

The Chinese Artichoke (Stachys Sieboldii), is a comparatively new variety of vegetable of which the edible portion is the tuber.

This plant has nothing to do with either of the well-known Artichokes both of which belong to the Compositae family, whereas this belongs to the Mint family, Labiatae, and to the same genus that is represented here by the Woundworts and Wood Betony. This species occurs wild in Northern China, where it is also cultivated, its native name being Tsanyungtzu, while in Japan it is called Chorogi. It was introduced as a culinary vegetable by the late Dr. M. T. Masters, F.R.S., in 1888. The tubers are eaten more in France than in this country.

The dietetic value resides especially in a carbonaceous substance, which reaches 16.6 per cent.; the nitrogenous ingredients amount to 3.2 per cent.; water forming 78.3 per cent. of the bulk.

Cultivation

It is perfectly hardy and may be left in the ground until required for use. Planting should take place in the spring and the tubers dug through the winter as required. The plants are perfectly easily grown and extraordinarily productive.

ARTICHOKE, CARDOON

Botanical: Carduncculus (LINN.)
Family: N.O. Compositae

The Cardoon (Scolymus Carduncculus, Linn.) is by some botanists regarded as merely a variety of this plant, but by others as a distinct species. The blanched inner leafstalks and the top of the stalk, the receptacle, are the only parts eaten, used in soups, stews and salads. It is more cultivated on the Continent than here. Dioscorides refers to its cultivation on a large scale near Great Carthage, and Pliny speaks of its medicinal virtues. Dodoens, in his History of Plants (1559), describes it as much more spinescent than the Articoca of Italy and less used as food.

Cultivation

It requires so much room that it is little grown in small gardens, and as a crop can hardly pay for the enormous extent of ground that it claims.

Its culture is very similar to that of celery, only on a rather larger scale, the trenches being made wider and slightly deeper than those for the latter, and the plants being placed about 18 inches to 2 feet apart in the rows and 6 feet between the rows. The trenches are prepared in just the same way as those for celery.

Sow three or four seeds in a 'large sixty' pot, in April, placing the pots in a gentle warmth, or in a cold frame, when the seed will soon germinate. Mice are very fond of the seed, consequently the frame must be kept close enough to prevent their entry, or the whole will be destroyed.

When the little plants appear, select the strongest plant in each pot and pull out all the others. In due course the plants are hardened off and planted out, usually in July, before they become potbound, in the previously prepared trenches, which have been well manured, about 18 inches or more apart, keeping them well supplied with water. Occasionally forking or hoeing between the plants to encourage growth and destroy weeds will be all that is required besides watering, until September or October, when they will be ready to earth up in order to blanch them.

Before doing this, it is usual to arrange the stalks upright and wind a hay-band round them closely, to within about a foot of the tops. This soil must then be earthed up nearly as high as the hay-bands. It is important that this operation should be performed on a dry day, when the hearts are free from water, or they will probably decay. No earth, also, must be allowed to fall between the leaves. When the plants have grown still further, the earthing up should be increased.

The plants will be fit for use in about a month after earthing up and may be taken up as required. Should Cardoons be in great demand, an earlier or later sowing may be made for successional crops; for spring crop, sow at midsummer. If the plants have to be kept for any length of time during winter, they must be protected from rain and frost by means of a covering of litter, or may be dug up and stored in a cool, dry place, the hay-bands being allowed to remain.

When taking up, remove the earth carefully and take up the plants by the roots, which must be cut off. The points of the leaves are also cut off to where they are solid and blanched. These latter are washed, the parts of the leaf-stalks remaining on the stem are tied to it, and they are ready for cooking.

The SPANISH CARDOON, with large solid ribs and spineless leaves, is the one most generally grown. It is not so liable to run to seed as the common variety.

In France, the TOURS CARDOON is much cultivated, but, on account of the long, sharp spines on the leaves, great care has to be exercised in working amongst them.

Uses

Cardoons are said to yield a good yellow dye, and in some parts of Spain they substitute the down of this plant for rennet in making cheese; a strong infusion is made overnight and the next morning, when the milk is warm from the cow, they put nearly half a pint of the infusion to about 14 gallons of milk.

Recipes

Artichoke Bottoms

If dried, they must be soaked, then stewed in weak gravy, and served with or without forcemeat in each. Or they may be boiled in milk, and served with cream sauce; or added to ragouts, French pies, etc.

To Dress Artichokes

Trim a few of the outside leaves off, and cut the stalk even. If young, half an hour will boil them. They are better for being gathered two or three days, first. Serve them with melted butter, in as many small cups as there are Artichokes, to help with each.

To keep Artichokes for the Winter

Artichoke bottoms, slowly dried, should be kept in paper bags.

Artichokes à la Barigoule

Trim some small Artichokes, and with the handle of an iron tablespoon scoop out all the fibrous part inside, Put about a pound of clean hog's-lard into a frying-pan on the fire, and when quite hot, fry the bottom of the Artichokes in it for about 3 minutes; then turn them upside down, and fry the tips of the leaves also, drain them upon a cloth to absorb all the grease, and fill them with a similar preparation to that directed for tomatoes a la Provencale; tie them up with a string, and place them in a large stewpan or fricaudeaupan; moisten with a little good stock; put the lid on; place them in the oven to simmer for about an hour; remove the strings, fill the centre of each Artichoke with some Italian sauce; dish them up with some of the sauce, and serve.

Artichokes à la Lyonnaise

Pull off the lower leaves without damaging the bottoms of the Artichokes, which must be turned smooth with a sharp knife; cut the Artichokes into quarters, remove the fibrous parts, trim them neatly, and parboil them in water with a little salt. Then put them in a saucepan on a slow fire to simmer very gently for about three-quarters of an hour, taking care that they do not burn; when done they should be of a deep yellow color and nicely glazed. Dish them up in the form of a dome, showing the bottom of the Artichokes only; remove any leaves that may have broken off in the sautapan; add a spoonful of brown gravy or sauce, 2 pats of butter and some lemon-juice, simmer this over the fire, stirring it meanwhile with a spoon; and when the butter has been mixed in with the sauce, pour it over the Artichokes, and serve.

ASAFETIDA

Botanical: Ferula foetida (REGEL.)
Family: N.O. Umbelliferae
Synonyms: Food of the Gods. Devil's Dung.
Part Used: An oleogum-resin obtained by incision of root.
Habitat: Afghanistan and Eastern Persia.

Description

A coarse umbelliferous plant growing up to 7 feet high, large fleshy root covered with bristly fibres, has been for some time successfully cultivated in Edinburgh Botanical Gardens; stem 6 to 10 feet, numerous stem leaves with wide sheathing petioles; flowers pale greeny yellow, fruit oval, flat thin, foliaceous, reddish brown with pronounced vittae, it has a milky juice and a strong foetid odor; was first found in the sandy desert of Aral in 1844, but has been known since the twelfth century. Several species of Ferula yield Asafetida. The bulk of the drug comes from the official plant, which is indigenous to Afghanistan and grows from two to four thousand feet above sealevel. These high plains are arid in winter but are thickly covered in summer with a luxuriant growth of these plants. The great cabbage-like folded heads are eaten raw by the natives. June is the month the juice is collected from plants about four years old. The roots of plants which have not flowered are exposed and slashed, then shaded from the sun for five or six weeks and left for the gummy oleoresin to leak out and harden. It is then scraped off in reddish lumps and put into leather bags and sent to Herat, where it is adulterated before being placed on the market. The fruit is sent to India for medicinal use. A very fine variety of Asafetida is obtained from the leaf bud in the centre of the root, but this does not come into European commerce, and is only used in India, where it is known in the Bazaars as Kandaharre Hing. It appears in reddish-yellow flakes and when squeezed gives out an oil.

Constituents

Its chief constituent is about 62 per cent of resin, 25 per cent. of gum and 7 per cent oil. The drug also contains free ferulic acid, water, and small quantities of various impurities.

Medicinal Action and Uses

The odor of Asafetida is stronger and more tenacious than that of the onion, the taste is bitter and acrid; the odor of the gum resin depends on the volatile oil. It is much used in India and Persia in spite of its offensive odor as a condiment and is thought to exercise a stimulant action on the brain. It is a local stimulant to the mucous membrane, especially to the alimentary tract, and therefore is a remedy of great value as a carminative in flatulent colic and a useful addition to laxative medicine. There is evidence that the volatile oil is eliminated through the lungs, therefore it is excellent for asthma bronchitis, whooping-cough, etc. Owing to its vile taste it is usually taken in pill form, but is often given to infants per rectum in the form of an emulsion. The powdered gum resin is not advocated as a medicine, the volatile oil being quickly dissipated.

Dosages and Preparations

Emulsion, Asafetida 4 parts, water 100 parts. Tincture, 1/2 to 1 fluid drachm. In pills, 3 grains of the oleogum-resin to a pill

Adulterants

Asafetida is admittedly the most adulterated drug on the market. Besides being largely admixed with inferior qualities of Asafetida, it has often red clay, sand, stones and gypsum added to it to increase the weight.

Other Species

The Thibetan Asafetida (Narthex Asafetida) is closely allied to the Ferulas. The umbels have no involucre, the limb of the calyx is suppressed, the stylopods depressed and cup-shaped, styles recurved, fruit compressed at back, dilated at margin. This variety produces some of the Asafetida used in commerce.

Scorodosma foetida, another gigantic umbelliferous plant found on the sandy steppes of the Caspian, also supplies the market. The Persian Sagapenum, or Serapinum, a species of Ferula which was formerly imported from Bombay, is in appearance very similar to Asafetida, but does not go pink when freshly fractured, and in smell is less disagreeable than Asafetida. This species is an ingredient of Confection Rutea, British Pharmacopeia Codex.

ASARABACCA

Botanical: Asarum europaeum (LINN.)
Family: N.O. Aristolochiaceae
Synonyms: Hazelwort. Wild Nard.
Parts Used: Root and Herb.

Asarabacca is the only British species of the Birthwort family (and perhaps not indigenous). It is a curious plant consisting of a very short fleshy stem, bearing two large, dark-green, kidney-shaped evergreen leaves, and a solitary purplish-green drooping flower.

Found in woods and very rare. Flowering in May - Perennial.

The herbs belonging to this order are chiefly plants or shrubs of a tropical habitat, very abundant in South America; but rare elsewhere.

Medicinal Action and Uses

Tonic and stimulant, sometimes acrid or aromatic. The dried and powdered leaves of Asarabacca (Asarum Europaeum) are used in the preparation of cephalic snuffs, exciting sneezing and giving relief to headache and weak eyes.

Mixed with Ribwort, this herb is used to remove mucous from the respiratory passages.

Virginian Snake-root (Aristolochia serpentaria) and other allied species are used as antidotes to the bite of venomous snakes.

The juice extracted from a South American species is said to have the power of stupefying serpents if placed in their mouths; and African species are used by Egyptian jugglers for this purpose.

The British variety is said to be found wild in Westmorland and other places in the north of England.

Culpepper says of the European species:

'This herb, being drunk, not only provoketh vomiting but purgeth downward . . . both choler and phlegm. If you add to it some spikenard, with the whey of goat's milk, or honeyed water, it is made more strong; but it purgeth phlegm more manifestly than choler, and therefore doth much help pains in the hips and other parts; being boiled in whey they wonderfully help the obstructions of the liver and spleen, and are therefore profitable for the dropsy and jaundice: being steeped in wine and drank it helps those continual agues that come by the plenty of stubborn tumors; an oil made thereof by setting in the sun, with some laudanum added to it, provoketh sweating (the ridge of the back anointed therewith) and thereby driveth away the shaking fits of the ague. It will not abide any long boiling, for it loseth its chief strength thereby; nor much beating, for the finer powder doth provoke vomit and urine, and the coarser purgeth downwards. The common use hereof is to take the juice of five or seven leaves in a little drink to cause vomiting; the roots have also the same virtue, though they do not operate forcibly, they are very effectual against the biting of serpents, and therefore are put in as an ingredient both into Mithridate and Venice treacle. The leaves and root being boiled in Iye, and the head often washed therewith while it is warm, comforteth the head and brain that is ill affected by taking cold, and helpeth the memory.

'I shall desire ignorant people to forbear the use of the leaves- the roots purge more gently, and may prove beneficial to such as have cancers, or old putrefied ulcers, or fistulas upon their bodies, to take a dram of them in powder in a quarter of a pint of white wine in the morning. The truth is, I fancy purging and vomiting medicines as little as any man breathing doth, for they weaken nature, nor shall ever advise them to be used unless upon urgent necessity. If a physician be nature's servant, it is his duty to strengthen his mistress as much as he can and weaken her as little as may be."

Constituents

The root and leaves are acrid and contain a volatile oil, a bitter matter, and a substance like camphor. Asarabacca was formerly used as a purgative and emetic also to promote sneezing - but it is now rarely used, having been supplanted by safer and more certain remedies.

ASCLEPIAS

Family: N.O. Asclepiadaceae

This genus consists of herbaceous plants with a milky juice, which are for the most part natives of America. Several species are cultivated for the sake of their showy flowers. All of them are more or less poisonous. Asclepias curassavica is employed in the West Indies as an emetic, and goes by the name of Ipecacuanha: the drug known in medicine by that name is derived from quite a different plant and must not be confused with it. A. tuberosa, the Butterfly-weed, has mild purgative properties, and promotes perspiration and expectoration. A. syriaca, a plant misnamed, as it is a native of America and Canada, is frequently to be met with in gardens; its dull red flowers are very fragrant, and the young shoots are eaten as asparagus in Canada, where a sort of sugar is also prepared from the flowers, while the silk-like down of the seeds is employed to stuff pillows. Some of the species furnish excellent fibre, which is woven into muslins, and in certain parts of India is made into paper.

In Hindu mythology, Soma - the Indian Bacchus- and one of the most important of the Vedic gods, is a personification of the Soma plant, A. acida, from which an intoxicating milky juice is squeezed. All the 114 hymns of the ninth book of the Rig Veda are in his praise. The preparation of the Soma juice was a very sacred ceremony and the worship of the god is very old. The true home of the plant was fabled to be in heaven, Soma being drunk by gods as well as men, and it is under its influence that Indra is related to have created the universe and fixed the earth and sky in their place. In postVedic literature, Soma is a regular name for the moon, which is regarded as being drunk by the gods and so waning, till it is filled up again by the Sun. In both the Rig Veda and Zend Avesta, Soma is the king of plants; in both, it is a medicine which gives health, long life and removes death.

The three species of Asclepias most used in medicine are the Calotropis procera, A. tuberosa (Pleurisy root) and A. Incarnata (Swamp Milkweed).

It is a very common roadside weed in the eastern and central states of North America, where it is called 'Silkweed," from the silky down which surmounts the seed, being an inch or two in length, and which has been used for making hats and for stuffing beds and pillows. Attempts have been made to use it as a cotton substitute. Both in France and Russia it has had textile use. The fibres of the stem, prepared in the same manner as those of hemp and flax, furnish a very long, fine thread, of a glossy whiteness.

Medicinal Action and Uses

The plant is used medicinally in the United States for the anodyne properties of its root and its rhizome and root have been employed successfully, like those of A. tuberosa, both in powder and infusion, in cases of asthma and typhus fever attended with catarrh, producing expectoration and relieving cough and pain. It has also been used in scrofula with great success.

Constituents

It has a very milky juice, which is used as a domestic application to warts. The juice has a faint smell and subacid taste and an acid reaction. It contains a crystalline substance of a resinous character, closely allied to lactucone and called Asclepione; also wax-like, fatty matter, caoutchouc, gum, sugar, salts of acetic acid and other salts.

Besides the above-named species, various other species of the genus have been used medicinally.

An indigenous North American species A. verticillata (Linn.), is used in the Southern States as a remedy in snake bites and the bites of venomous insects. Twelve fluid ounces of a saturated decoction are said to cause an anodyne and sudorific effect, followed by gentle sleep.

From A. vincetoxicum (Linn.), 'TamePoison," besides the glucoside Asclepiadin said closely to resemble emetine in its physiological properties, the glucoside Vincetoxir has been isolated. The root of this species sometimes occurs in commercial Senega Root (Polygala Senega).

An infusion of its root was formerly recommended in dropsical cases and disorders peculiar to women, as well as for promoting perspiration in fevers, measles and other eruptive complaints, but is now much less used.

A. curas-savica (Blood-weed and Redhead) is also called in the West Indies 'Bastard Ipecacuanha."

It is a native of the West Indies, abounding especially in Nevis and St. Kitts.

Both root and expressed juice are emetic, the former in the dose of 20 to 40 grains, the latter in that of a fluid ounce.

They are also cathartic and vermifuge in somewhat smaller doses (Amer. Journ. Ph. XIX, 19). The juice, made into a syrup, is given as a powerful anthelmintic to children in the West Indies. The plant is used by the negroes as an emetic and the root as a purgative.

According to the Kew Bulletin, 1897 this plant has insecticidal properties, being especially obnoxious to fleas. The rooms infected are thoroughly swept with rough brooms made from the weed and the pests are said to disappear. D. St. Cyr commends it in phthisis (Ph. Journ., 1903, 714).

Other Species

A. Pulchra (Ehrh.), by many regarded as a variety of incarnata, from which it is distinguished by its hairiness, the other being nearly smooth, is indiscriminately used under the same names.

A. syrica (Willd.) (A. Cornuti, Decaisne), found abundantly in Syria, cultivated in some parts of Europe.

ASH

Botanical: Fraxinus excelsior (LINN.)
Family: N.O. Oleaceae
Synonyms: Common Ash. Weeping Ash.
Parts Used: Leaves, bark.

Description

The Common Ash (Fraxinus excelsior, Linn.), a tall, handsome tree, common in Britain, is readily distinguished by its light-grey bark (smooth in younger trees, rough and scaly in older specimens) and by its large compound leaves, divided into four to eight pairs of lance-shaped leaflets, tipped by a single one, an arrangement which imparts a light feathery arrangement to the foliage. The leaflets have sharply-toothed margins and are about 3 inches long.

In April or May, according to season, and before the appearance of the leaves, the black flower-buds on the previous year's shoots expand into small dense clusters of a greenish white or purplish color, some of the minute flowers having purple stamens, others pistil only, and some both, but all being devoid of petals and sepals, which, owing to the pollen being wind-borne, are not needed as protection, or as attraction to insect visitors.

After fertilization, the oblong ovary develops into a thick seed-chamber, with a long, strap-shaped wing which is known as an Ash-key (botanically: a samara). The bunches of 'keys' hang from the twigs in great clusters, at first green and then brown as the seeds ripen. They remain attached to the tree until the succeeding spring, when they are blown off and carried away by the wind to considerable distances from the parent tree. They germinate vigorously and grow in almost any soil.

The Common Ash and the Privet are the only representatives in England of the Olive tribe: Oleaceae.

There are about fifty species of the genus Fraxinus, and cultivation has produced and perpetuated a large number of distinct varieties, of which the Weeping Ash and the Curl-leaved Ash are the best known.

As a timber tree, the Ash is exceedingly valuable, not only on account of the quickness of its growth, but for the toughness and elasticity of its wood, in which quality it surpasses every European tree. The wood is heavy strong, stiff and hard and takes a high polish; it shrinks only moderately in seasoning and bends well when seasoned. It is the toughest and most elastic of our timbers (for which purpose it was used in olden days for spears and bows and is still used for otter-spears) and can be used for more purposes than the wood of other trees.

It is known that Ash timber is so elastic that a joist of it will bear more before it breaks than one of any other tree. It matures more rapidly than Oak and as sapling wood is valuable. Ash timber always fetches a good price, being next in value to Oak and surpassing it for some purposes, being in endless demand in railway and other waggon works for carriage building. From axe-handles and spade-trees to hop-poles, ladders and carts, Ash wood is probably in constant handling on every countryside - for agricultural plenishings it cannot be excelled. It makes the best of oars and the toughest of shafts for carriages. In its younger stages, when it is called Ground Ash, it is much used, as well as for hop-poles (for which it is extensively grown), for walking-sticks, hoops, hurdles and crates, and it matures its wood at so early an age that an Ash-pole 3 inches in diameter is as valuable and durable for any purpose to which it can be applied as the timber of the largest tree. Ash also makes excellent logs for burning, giving out no smoke, and the ashes of the wood afford very good potash.

The finest Ash is that grown in the Midlands, but so little first-class Ash has been of late years obtained in England that in I 90 I the Coachbuilders' Association appealed to the President of the Board of Agriculture to try and stimulate landowners to grow more of this valuable timber, as English Ash is better in quality than that imported from other European countries or from America. Any owner of a devastated woodland or other suitable ground may demand a grant of L. 2 (pounds sterling) an acre if he is planting pine, and L. 4 (pounds sterling)if he is planting hard woods, such as Ash. The supply of standing Ash timber is also becoming limited in America.

Ash is the second most important wood used in aeroplanes, and a study of the spacious afforestation scheme now in force over the Crown Lands of the New Forest reveals the fact that especial trouble has been taken to find suitable homes for the Ash. The great bulk of the wood used in aeroplanes is Spruce from the Pacific Coast.

Ash bark is astringent and has been employed for tanning nets.

Both bark and the leaves have medicinal use and fetch prices which should repay the labour of collecting them, especially the bark.

The bark is collected from the trunk and the root, the latter being preferred.

Ash bark occurs in commerce in quills which are grey or greenish-grey externally, with numerous small grey or brownish white warts, the inner surface yellowish or yellowish brown and nearly smooth; fracture smooth, fibrous in the inner layer, odors light; taste bitter and astringent.

Constituents

The bark contains the bitter glucoside Fraxin, the bitter substance Fraxetin, tannin, quercetin, mannite, a little volatile oil, gum, malic acid, free and combined with calcium.

Medicinal Action and Uses

Ash bark has been employed as a bitter tonic and astringent, and is said to be valuable as an antiperiodic. On account of its astringency, it has been used, in decoction, extensively in the treatment of intermittent fever and ague, as a substitute for Peruvian bark. The decoction is odorless, though its taste is fairly bitter. It has been considered useful to remove obstructions of the liver and spleen, and in rheumatism of an arthritic nature.

A ley from the ashes of the bark was used formerly to cure scabby and leprous heads.

The leaves have diuretic, diaphoretic and purgative properties, and are employed in modern herbal medicine for their laxative action, especially in the treatment of gouty and rheumatic complaints, proving a useful substitute for Senna, having a less griping effect. The infusion of the leaves, 1 OZ. to the pint, may be given in frequent doses during the twenty-four hours.

The distilled water of the leaves, taken every morning, was considered good for dropsy and obesity.

A decoction of the leaves in white wine had the reputation of dissolving stone and curing jaundice.

The leaves should be gathered in June, well dried, powdered and kept in well corked bottles.

The leaves have been gathered to mix with tea and in some parts of the country are used to feed cattle, when grass is scarce in autumn, but when cows eat the leaves or shoots, the butter becomes rank.

The fruits of the different species of Ash are regarded as somewhat more active than the bark and leaves. Ash Keys were held in high reputation by the ancient physicians, being employed as a remedy for flatulence. They were also in more recent times preserved with salt and vinegar and sent to table as a pickle. Evelyn tells us: 'Ashen keys have the virtue of capers," and they were often substituted for them in sauces and salads.

The keys will keep all the year round if gathered when ripe.

In Mexico, the bark and leaves of F. nigra (Marsh), the Black Swamp, Water Hoop or Basket Ash, are similarly employed to those of the Common Ash. In Mexico, also, the bark and leaves of F. lanceolata (Borch.), the Green or Blue Ash, are employed as a bitter tonic and the root as a diuretic.

In the United States, the bark of the American White Ash (F. Americana, Linn.) (F. acuminata, Lam.) finds similar employment. It has numerous small circular depressions externally and a slightly laminate structure.

Gerard tell us:

'The leaves and bark of the Ash tree are dry and moderately hot . . . the seed is hot and dry in the second degree. The juice of the leaves or the leaves themselves being applied or taken with wine cure the bitting of vipers, as Dioscorides saith, "The leaves of this tree are of so great virtue against serpents as that they dare not so much as touch the morning and evening shadows of the tree, but shun them afar off as Pliny reports." "

There are many old superstitions concerning the tree. The ancient couplets connecting the flowering precedence of the Oak and Ash with the rainfall of the following summer, 'Oak choke, Ash splash," etc., have no basis on fact.

According to another superstition, if the trunk of a sapling Ash were split and a ruptured child passed through, the sufferer would be cured.

The Ash had the reputation of magically curing warts: each wart must be pricked with a new pin that has been thrust into the tree, the pins are withdrawn and left in the tree, and the following charm is repeated:

'Ashen tree, ashen tree,
Pray buy these warts of me."

And there was another superstition that if a live shrew mouse were buried in a hole bored in an Ash trunk and then plugged up a sprig of this Shrew Ash would cure the paralysis supposed to have been caused by a shrew creeping over the sick person's limbs.

ASH, BITTER

Botanical: Picraena excelsa (SWARTZ)
Family: N.O. Simarubeae
Synonym: Jamaica Quassia.
Habitat: West Indies.

Description

The Bitter Ash (Picraena excelsa, Swartz), a native of the West Indies, a lofty tree somewhat resembling the Ash Tree, the wood of which is the Jamaica Quassia of commerce, is employed in the place of the original Quassia amara of Surinam and Trinidad.

Uses

It abounds in a peculiar extractive substance of great bitterness which, as a drug, is purely tonic, invigorating the digestive organs with little excitement of the circulation or increase of bodily heat.

The wood is generally sold in small chips, yellowish white, about an inch wide and 1 to 4 inches long and 1/8 to 1/12 inch thick. Their taste is extremely bitter, but there is no odor.

Exhausted Quassia chips having hardly any bitterness are sometimes met with in commerce and also chips with greyish markings due to a fungus. Neither of these are, of course, suitable for an infusion.

Sometimes cups turned out of the wood are made. These are sold as Bitter Cups, and water standing in them for a short time acquires the bitterness of the wood.

From Syrup of Quassia, made with molasses, a harmless fly-poison is prepared, with which cloth or filtering-papers are moistened.

Quassia has been used by brewers as a substitute for hops and is in general use by gardeners, mixed with soft soap, for spraying plants affected with green-fly.

Preparations

An infusion of Quassia, 2 oz. in a pint of water, affords a valuable and safe injection for seat-worms.

The dose of the fluid extract is 15 to 30 drops; of the tincture, official in the B.Ph. and U.S.Ph., 1/2 to 1 drachm; of the U.S.Ph. powdered extract the dose is 1 grain. Of the concentrated solution of the B.Ph. the dose is 1/2 drachm. The dose of the solid extract is 1/2 to 2 grains.

ASH, MANNA

Botanical: Fraxinus ornus (LINN.)
Family: N.O. Oleaceae
Synonym: Flake Manna.
Part Used: Concrete exudation.

Description

A foreign species of Ash (Fraxinus ornus, Linn.), the South European Flowering Ash, a small tree indigenous to the coasts of the Mediterranean from Spain to Smyrna, yields from its bark a sugary sap called Manna, used in pharmacy.

The tree blossoms early in summer, producing numerous clusters of whitish flowers; in this country it only attains a height of 15 or 16 feet.

To-day, the Manna of commerce is collected exclusively in Sicily, from cultivated trees, exported from Palermo. The trees are grown in plantations placed about 7 feet apart. When from eight to ten years old, when the trunk is at least 3 inches in diameter, the collection of Manna is begun. In July and August, when the trees have ceased to put forth leaves freely, a vertical series of oblique incisions are made in the bark on alternate sides of the trunk. Dry, warm weather is essential for a good crop of the Manna which exudes. The larger pieces of incrustation that form, and which are collected in September and October, when the heat has begun to moderate, are known as Flake Manna, and this is the best. It is put on the market in long pieces or granulated fragments of a whitish and pale yellow color, irregular on one side and smoother and curved on the other, rarely more than 1 inch broad and 2 to 3 inches or more long.

The pieces adhering to the stem after the finer pieces have been gathered are scraped off and form part of the small Manna of commerce. The pieces that form on the lowest incisions, or the pieces that are collected on tiles placed under the tree, and known as 'gerace," are less crystalline, more glutinous, and are in moist adhesive masses of a dark brown color. These are less esteemed.

Medicinal Action and Uses

Manna has a peculiar odor and a sweetish taste.

It was formerly used in medicine as a gentle laxative, but is now chiefly used as a children's laxative or to disguise other medicines.

It is a nutritive and a gentle tonic, usually operating mildly, but in some cases produces flatulence and pain.

It is still largely consumed in South America and is official in the United States Pharmacopoeia.

It is generally given dissolved in water or some aromatic infusion, but the best Flake Manna may be administered in substance, in doses of a teaspoonful up to 1 or 2 oz.

Usually it is prescribed with other purgatives, particularly senna, rhubarb, magnesia and the neutral salts, the taste of which it conceals while it adds to the purgative effect.

For infants, a piece about the size of a hazel-nut is dissolved in a little warm water and added to the food. To children, 30 to 60 grams may be given dissolved in warm milk or a mixture prepared with syrup, or syrup of senna and dill water.

Syrups of Manna are prepared with or without other purgatives.

Manna is sometimes used as a pill excipient, especially for calomel.

Under the name of Dulcinol, a mixture of Manna and common salt has been recommended by Steinberg in 1906 as a sweetening agent in diabetes, the dose 1/2 to 1 OZ.

The Codex of the British Pharmacopeia contains a Syrup of Manna to be prescribed as a mild laxative for children, in the proportion of 1 part of Manna to 10 of water.

The Compound Syrup of Manna of the B.P. Codex is stronger than the Syrup of Manna and contains Senna and fennel in addition, the dose being 1 to 4 fluid drachms.

Constituents

Manna of the best quality dissolves in about 6 parts of water, forming a clear liquid. It has no bitterness or acridity.

The chief constituent of Manna is a peculiar, crystallizable, sweet principle called Mannite or Manna Sugar, present to the extent of about 70 per cent. It also contains a fluorescent body named Fraxin, which occasionally gives a greenish color to Manna and on which is thought to depend its purgative property. Some true sugar and a small quantity of mucilage are also present.

Mannite is white, in odorous, crystallizable in semi-transparent needles of a sweetish taste, soluble in 5 parts of cold water, scarcely soluble in cold alcohol, but readily dissolved by alcohol when hot and deposited when cool. Unlike sugar, it is incapable of undergoing vinous fermentation.

Definition of Manna in Italy

An Italian Decree-law, dated August 12, 1927, dealing with the repression of fraud and adulteration in the preparation and trade in substances of vegetable origin, states that the name 'Manna' is reserved for the product obtained by incision into the cortex of the flowering or Manna Ash (F. ornus or F. excelsior). It is forbidden to prepare, sell, or expose for sale or introduce into trade Manna containing milk sugar, starchy matter, or containing foreign substances of whatever nature, other than those bodies which are present naturally as impurities in the normal proportions existing in the various types of Manna.

In Italy, Mannite is prepared for sale in the shape of small cones, resembling loaf sugar in shape, and is frequently prescribed in medicine instead of Manna.

The term 'Manna' is extremely old and is applied to the saccharine exudence of a number of plants, e.g. Quercus Vallones and persica (Oak Manna); Alhagi maurorum (Alhagi Manna), Tamarix gallica, var. mannifera (Tamarisk Manna); Larix Europaea (Briancon Manna).

The Manna of the present day appears to have been unknown before the fifteenth century. In the sixteenth century, it was collected in Calabria, but none is now brought into commerce from this part of Italy.

Although the name Manna, at first applied to the Manna of the Scriptures, has (as stated) also been applied to various saccharine substances of different origin, none of these corresponds in any way to the Manna of Scripture, inasmuch as they are saccharine substances and do not become corrupt in a night.

The Manna of the biblical narrative answers otherwise in its description to the Tamarisk Manna, exuded in June and July from the slender branches of Tamarisk gallica, var. mannifera, in the form of honey-like drops, which in the cool temperature of the early morning are found in the solid state. This secretion is caused by the puncture of an insect, Coccus manniparus. In the valleys of the peninsula of Sinai, this Manna is collected by the Arabs and sold by them to the monks of St. Catherine, who dispose of it to the pilgrims visiting the convent, under the name of 'gazangabin," which means 'Tamarisk Honey." It appears to consist of cane sugar, inverted sugar, and dextrin.

A report issued in 1927 by an expedition of entomologists from the Hebrew University of Jerusalem declares that Manna is not an exudation from the Tamarisk tree, as is popularly supposed, but an excretion from the bodies of the coccid insects themselves. Clear, syrup-like drops (the report states) come from the abdomen of the insects and fall to the ground, where they form grains of sugar, ranging from the size of a pinhead to that of a pea. The amount varies with the abundance or scarcity of the winter rains and the Bedouins assert that during a good season a man can collect nearly 3 1/2 lb. in a day. The expedition, which was led by Dr. Fritz Bodenheimer of the Zionist experimental agricultural station, observed Manna deposits throughout the long stretch of country which was covered by its journey. The report goes on to state that 'modern science, it seems, was equally ignorant of the true nature of manna till now, and it has been revealed by descendants of those wanderers in the wilderness."

The only substance which in all respects seems to agree with the Manna of the Israelites is that described a few years ago by Mr. A. J. Swann, in his book on Fighting the Slave Driver in Central Africa. The Manna which he saw on the plateaux between the lakes Tanganyika and Nyasa occupied by the Ananbwi tribe Mr. Swann describes as possessing all the characters of the Manna which is said to have fallen for the benefit of the Israelites. In appearance it resembled coriander seed, was white in color like hoar-frost and sweet to taste, melted in the sun, and if kept overnight was full of worms in the morning. It required to be baked to keep it any length of time. A cake of this Manna was baked and sent to England, but no one seemed able to identify it, though there can be little doubt that it is a small fungus. The baking process would, of course, destroy its structure, and it is evident that to determine its nature, some of the Manna should be sent home in formaldehyde or corrosive sublimate, when it would be quite possible to make out its structure and classification and to describe it, if new. It does not appear to be regular in its occurrence, as travellers have reported its appearance only at long intervals.

ASH, MOUNTAIN

Botanical: Pyrus Aucuparia (GAERTN.), Sorbus Aucuparia (LINN.)
Family: N.O. Rosaceae
Synonym: Rowan Tree.
Parts Used: Bark, fruit.

Description

The Mountain Ash (Pyrus Aucuparia, Gaertn.) is not related to the true Ashes, but has derived its name from the similarity of the leaves.

In comparison to the true Ash, it is but a small tree, rarely more than 30 feet high. It belongs to the order Rosacece and is distinguished from its immediate relations the Pear, Crab Apple, White Beam and Wild Service Tree by its regularly pinnate, Ash-like leaves. It is generally distributed over the country in its wild state, but is also much cultivated as an ornamental tree.

All parts of the tree are astringent and may be used in tanning and dyeing black. When cut, the Mountain Ash yields poles and hoops for barrels.

Both the bark and fruit have medicinal properties.

The fruit is rather globose, with teeth at the apex and two to three seeded cells. They are used medicinally in either the fresh or the dried state.

Constituents

The fruit contains tartaric acid before, citric and malic acids after ripening; two sugars, sorbin and sorbit, the latter after fermentation; parasorbic acid, which is aromatic and is converted into isomeric sorbic acid by heating under pressure with potassa; bitter, acrid and coloring matters. A crystalline saccharine principle, Sorbitol, which does not undergo the vinous fermentation, has also been found in the fruit.

The seeds contain 22 per cent. of fixed oil. It has been claimed that these seeds killed a child, apparently by prussic acid poisoning.

The bark has a soft, spongy, yellowishgrey outer layer and an inner thicker portion, with many layers of a light brown color. It has a bitterish taste, but is odourless.

It is astringent and also yields amygdalin.

Medicinal Action and Uses

In herbal medicine, a decoction of the bark is given for diarrhea and used as a vaginal injection in leucorrhoea, etc.

The ripe berries furnish an acidulous and astringent gargle for sore throats and inflamed tonsils. For their anti-scorbutic properties, they have been used in scurvy. The astringent infusion is used as a remedy in hemorrhoids and strangury.

The fruit is a favorite food of birds. A delicious jelly is made from the berries, which is excellent with cold game or wild fowl, and a wholesome kind of perry or cider can also be made from them.

In Northern Europe they are dried for flour, and when fermented yield a strong spirit. The Welsh used to brew an ale from the berries, the secret of which is now lost .

AMERICAN MOUNTAIN ASH

Pyrus Americana (D.C.)

American Mountain Ash bark is derived from Pyrus Americana (D.C.), which has many local names.

It has similar properties to the bark of the European species and was formerly used as a tonic in fevers of supposed malarial type, where it was often substituted for cinchona bark.

No analysis of the bark of the American species has been made, though the fruit has been found to yield 4.92 to 6.6 of malic acid.

ASH, PRICKLY

Botanical: Xanthoxylum Americanum (MILL.)
Family: N.O. Rutacea
Synonyms: Toothache Tree. Yellow Wood. Suterberry.
Parts Used: Root-bark, berries.

Description

The Prickly Ash (Xanthoxylum Americanum, Mill., X. fraxineum Willd.; X. Carolinianum, Lamb.) is a small North American tree growing in the open air in this country. It has pinnate leaves and alternate branches, which are covered with sharp and strong prickles: the common footstalk is also sometimes prickly, and also the bark.

It belongs to the Yellow Wood family (Rutaceae), which all possess aromatic and pungent properties.

The berries, growing in clusters on the top of the branches, are black or deep blue and enclosed in a grey shell.

The leaves and berries have an aromatic odor similar to that of oil of Lemons, and the berries and bark have a hot, acrid taste.

The root-bark and berries are used medicinally, being official in the United States Pharmacopoeia.

Constituents

The barks of numerous species of Xanthoxylum and the allied genus Fagara have been used medicinally. There are two principal varieties of Prickly Ash in commerce: X. Americanum (Northern Prickly Ash) and Fagara Clava-Herculis (Southern Prickly Ashj, which is supposed to be more active. Although not absolutely identical, the two Prickly Ash barks are very similar in their active constituents. Both contain small amounts of volatile oil, fat, sugar, gum, acrid resin, a bitter alkaloid, believed to be Berberine and a colorless, tasteless, inert, crystalline body, Xanthoxylin, slightly different in the two barks. Both yield a large amount of Ash: 12 per cent. or more. The name Xanthoxylin is also applied to a resinous extractive prepared by pouring a tincture of the drug into water.

The fruits of both the species are used similarly to the barks. Their constituents have not been investigated, but they apparently agree in a general way with those of the bark.

The drug is practically never adulterated. The Northern bark occurs in commerce in curved or quilled fragments about 1/24 inch thick, externally brownish grey, with whitish patches, faintly furrowed, with some linearbased, two-edged spines about 1/4 inch long. The fracture is short, green in the outer, and yellow in the inner part. The Southern bark, which is more frequently sold, is 1/12 inch thick and has conical, corky spines, sometimes 4/5, inch in height.

Xanthoxcylin is included in the United States Pharmacopeia for the preparation of a fluid extract, the dose of which is 1/2 to 1 drachm.

Medicinal Action and Uses

It acts as a stimulant - resembling guaiacum resin and mezereon bark in its remedial action and is greatly recommended in the United States for chronic rheumatism, typhoid and skin diseases and impurity of the blood, administered either in the form of fluid extract or in doses of 10 grains to 1/2 drachm in the powdered form, three times daily.

The following formula has also become popular in herbal medicine: Take 1/2 oz. each of Prickly Ash Bark, Guaiacum Raspings and Buckbean Herb, with 6 Cayenne Pods. Boil in 1 1/2 pint of water down to 1 pint . Dose: a wine glassful three or four times daily.

On account of the energetic stimulant properties of the bark, it produces when swallowed a sense of heat in the stomach, with more or less general arterial excitement and tendency to perspiration and is a useful tonic in debilitated conditions of the stomach and digestive organs, and is used in colic, cramp and colera, in fever, ague, lethargy, for cold hands and feet and complaints arising from a bad circulation.

A decoction made by boiling an ounce in 3 pints of water down to a quarter may be given in the quantity of a pint, in divided doses, during the twenty-four hours. As a counter-irritant, the decoction may be applied on compresses. It has also been used as an emmenagogue.

The powdered bark forms an excellent application to indolent ulcers and old wounds for cleansing, stimulating, drying up and healing the wounds. The pulverized bark is also used for paralytic affections and nervous headaches and as a topical irritant the bark, either in powdered form, or chewed, has been a very popular remedy for toothache in America, hence the origin of a common name of the tree in the States: Toothache Tree.

The berries are considered even more active than the bark, being carminative and antispasmodic, and are used as an aperient and for dyspepsia and indigestion; a fluid extract of the berries being given, in doses of 10 to 30 drops.

Xanthoxylin. Dose, 1 to 2 grains.

Both berries and bark are used to make a good bitter.

The name Prickly Ash has also been given to Aralia spinosa (Linn.), the Prickly Elder, or Angelica Tree, the bark, roots and berries of which are used as alteratives.

ASH, WAFER

Botanical: Ptelea trifoliata (LINN.)

Family: N.O. Rutaceae
Synonyms: Swamp Dogwood. Shrubby Trefoil. Wingseed. Hop Tree.
Part Used: Root-bark.

Description

The Wafer Ash is a shrub growing 6 to 8 feet high, a native of North America, but cultivated here, having been introduced in 1714. In America it is also called the Swamp Dogwood, Wingseed, and Hop Tree.

The root-bark is employed medicinally, both in herbal medicine and in homeopathy, but it has never been an official drug, though formerly it was employed to a certain extent by physicians in the western United States.

It has a peculiar, somewhat aromatic odor and a bitter, persistently pungent and slightly acrid, but not disagreeable taste.

Constituents

The bark contains at least three active constituents, a powerful volatile oil, a salt, acrid resin, and an alkaloid: Berberine. The alkaloid Arginine is also stated to be present in the root.

Medicinal Action and Uses

The bark has tonic, antiperiodic and stomachic properties, and has been employed in dyspepsia and debility, and also in febrile diseases, especially in those requiring a mild, non-irritating bitter tonic, as it has a soothing influence upon the mucous membrane and promotes appetite, being tolerated when other tonics cannot be retained.

It is also useful in chronic rheumatism.

The dose of the powdered bark is 10 to 30 grains. The infusion of the bark is taken in tablespoonful doses three or four times daily.

The bark occurs in commerce in quilled or curved pieces, 1 1/2 to 3 inches long and 1 to inch in diameter, 1/8 to 3/4 inch thick, transversely wrinkled, with a whitish brown surface of thin, papery layers, the inner surface being smooth, with faintly projecting medullary layers. It breaks with a short fracture, yellowish white, the papery layer pale buff.

ASPARAGUS

Botanical: Asparagus officinalis
Family: N.O. Liliaceae

Medicinal Action and Uses

This well-known table delicacy may be found wild on the sea-coast in the South-west of England, especially near the Lizard, in the Isle of Anglesea, otherwise it is a rare native. In the southern parts of Russia and Poland the waste steppes are covered with this plant, which is there eaten by horses and cattle as grass. It is also common in Greece, and was formerly much esteemed as a vegetable by the Greeks and Romans. It appears to have been cultivated in the time of Cato the Elder, 200 years B.C., and Pliny mentions a species that grew near Ravenna, of which three heads would weigh a pound.

Asparagus is noticed by Gerard in 1597, and in 1670 forced Asparagus was supplied to the London market.

Medicinal Action and Uses

The virtues of Asparagus are well known as a diuretic and laxative; and for those of sedentary habits who suffer from symptoms of gravel, it has been found very beneficial, as well as in cases of dropsy. The fresh expressed juice is taken medicinally in tablespoonful doses.

Prussian Asparagus, which is brought to some English markets, is not a species of Asparagus at all, but consists of the spikes of Ornithogalum pyrenaicum, which grows abundantly in hedges and pastures (especially in the locality of Bath).

Culpepper tells us 'The decoction of the roots (Asparagus) boiled in wine, and taken is good to clear the sight, and being held in the mouth easeth the toothache." He also tells us it helps those sinews that 'are shrunk by cramps and convulsions, and helpeth the sciatica ."

ASPHODEL

Botanical: Asphodelus Ramosus
Family: N.O. Liliaceae
Synonyms: White Asphodel. Asphodele Rameux. Royal Staff. Branched Asphodel. King's Spear.
Part Used: The roots.
Habitat: Middle Europe. The shores of the Mediterranean.

Description

The plant is about 3 feet high, with large, white, terminal flowers, and radical, long, numerous leaves. It is only cultivated in botanical and ornamental gardens, though it easily grows from seeds or division of roots.

The roots must be gathered at the end of the first year.

The ancients planted the flowers near tombs, regarding them as the form of food preferred by the dead, and many poems refer to this custom. The name is derived from a Greek word meaning sceptre.

The roots, dried and boiled in water, yield a mucilaginous matter that in some countries is mixed with grain or potato to make Asphodel bread. In Spain and other countries they are used as cattle fodder, especially for sheep. In Barbary the wild boars eat them greedily.

In Persia, glue is made with the bulbs, which are first dried and then pulverized. When mixed with cold water, the powder swells and forms a strong glue.

Hippocrates, Dioscorides, and Pliny said the roots were cooked in ashes and eaten. The Greeks and Romans used them in several diseases, but they are not employed in modern medicine.

Constituents

An acrid principle separated or destroyed by boiling water, and a matter resembling inuline have been found. An alcohol of excellent flavor has been obtained from plants growing abundantly in Algeria.

Medicinal Action and Uses

Acrid, heating, and diuretic. Said to be useful in menstrual obstructions and as an antispasmodic. The bruised root has been recommended for rapidly dissolving scrofulous swellings.

Other Species

A. luteus, or Yellow Asphodel, Jacob'sStaff, is a native of Sicily.

A. fistulosus, or Onion-leaved Asphodel, of Southern France and Crete, is also employed.

BOG OR LACASHIRE ASPHODEL is a common name of Narthecium ossifragum. The name of 'bone-breaker' was unfortunately given, because, as It grows on wet moors and mountains, sheep pasturing there frequently suffered from foot rot, and this was attributed to their browsing on the plants.

FALSE ASPHODEL is an American name for Tofieldia.

SCOTCH ASPHODEL is a common name of Tofieldia palustris.

AVENS

Botanical: Geum urbanum (LINN.)
Family: N.O. Rosaceae
Synonyms: Colewort. Herb Bennet. City Avens. Wild Rye. Way Bennet. Goldy Star. Clove Root.
Parts Used: Herb, root.

Habitat

The Avens (Geum urbanum, Linn.), belonging to the order Rosacece, its genus being nearly related to the Potentilla genus, is a common wayside plant in Great Britain, abundant in woods and hedges in England, Ireland and southern Scotland, though becoming scarcer in the north. It is common in the greater part of Europe, Russia and Central Asia.

Description

It has thin, nearly upright, wiry stems, slightly branched, from 1 to 2 feet in height, of a reddish brown on one side. Its leaves vary considerably in form, according to their position. The radical leaves are borne on long, channelled foot-stalks, and are interruptedly pinnate, as in the Silverweed the large terminal leaflet being wedge-shaped and the intermediate pairs of leaflets being very small. The upper leaves on the stem are made up of three long, narrow leaflets: those lower on the stems have the three leaflets round and full. The stem-leaves are placed alternately and have at their base two stipules (leaf-like members that in many plants occur at the junction of the base of the leaf with the stem). Those of the Avens are very large, about an inch broad and long, rounded in form and coarsely toothed and lobed. All the leaves are of a deep green color, more or less covered with spreading hairs, their margins toothed.

The rhizomes are 1 to 2 inches long terminating abruptly, hard and rough with many light brown fibrous roots. The flowers, rather small for the size of the plant, are on solitary, terminal stalks. The corolla is composed of five roundish, spreading, yellow petals, the calyx cleft into ten segments - five large and five small - as in the Silverweed. The flowers, which are in bloom all the summer and autumn, often as late as December, are less conspicuous than the round fruitheads, which succeed them, which are formed of a mass of dark crimson achenes, each terminating in an awn, the end of which is curved into a hook.

History

The plant derives its name of Avens from the Latin Avencia, Mediaeval Latin, avantia or avence, a word of obscure origin and which in varieties of spelling has been applied to the plant from very early times.

The botanical name, Geum, originated from the Greek geno, to yield an agreeable fragrance, because, when freshly dug up, the root has a clove-like aroma. This gives rise to another name, Radix caryophylata, or Clove Root, and its corruption, Gariophilata.

Avens had many names in the fourteenth century, such as Assarabaccara, Pesleporis, or Harefoot, and Minarta.

It was called 'the Blessed Herb' (Herba benedicta), of which a common name still extant - Herb Bennet - is a corruption, because in former times it was believed that it had the power to ward off evil spirits and venomous beasts. It was worn as an amulet. The Ortus Sanitatis, printed in 1491, states: 'Where the root is in the house, Satan can do nothing and flies from it, wherefore it is blessed before all other herbs, and if a man carries the root about him no venomous beast can harm him." Dr. Prior (Popular Names of English Plants) considers the original name to have probably been " St . Benedict's Herb," that name being assigned to such as were supposed to be antidotes, in allusion to a legend respecting the saint. It is said that on one occasion a monk presented him with a goblet of poisoned wine, but when the saint blessed it, the poison, being a sort of devil, flew out of it with such force that the glass was shivered to atoms, the crime of the monk being thus exposed. Hemlock is also known as Herb Bennet, probably for the same reason.

Goldy Star of the Earth, City Avens, Wild Rye and Way Bennet are other local names for the plant.

In mediaeval days, the graceful trefoiled leaf and the five golden petals of the blossoms symbolized the Holy Trinity and the five wounds of Our Lord, and towards the end of the thirteenth century the plant frequently occurs as an architectural decoration in the carved leafage on the capitals of columns and in wall patterns.

The roots should be dug up in spring; some of the old physicians were so particular on this point that the 25th March was fixed for procuring the root (and it was specified that the soil should be dry). At this time the root was said to be most fragrant. It loses much of its odor in drying, so must be dried with great care, and gradually, then sliced and powdered as required, as they are less likely to lose their properties in this form than when kept in slices.

Externally, the rhizome, when dried, is of a brownish to a brownish-yellow color. The fracture is short. Internally, it is of a light purplish-brown when dried. In transverse section, it shows a large pith, a narrow woody ring, with thin bark. The taste of the drug is astringent, slightly bitter and clove-like.

Constituents

The principal constituent is a volatile oil, which is mainly composed of Eugenol, and a glucoside, Gein, geum-bitter, tannic acid, gum and resin. It imparts its qualities to water and alcohol, which it tinges red. Distilled with water, it yields 0.04 per cent. of thick, greenish, volatile oil.

The root has been found by Milandi and Moretti to contain one-eleventh of its weight of tannin.

Medicinal Action and Uses

Astringent, Styptic, febrifuge, sudorific, stomachic, antiseptic, tonic and aromatic.

In earlier days the roots were not only used medicinally, as at present, but to flavor ale, and to put among linen to preserve from moths and to impart a pleasant odor.

The Augsburg Ale is said to owe its peculiar flavor to the addition of a small bag of Avens in each cask. The fresh root imparts a pleasant clove-like flavor to the liquor, preserves it from turning sour, and adds to its wholesome properties.

A cordial against the plague was made by boiling the roots in wine. Gerard recommends a 'decoction made in wine against stomach ills and bites of venomous beasts." On account of its stomachic properties, chewing of the root was recommended for foul breath.

Culpepper says:

'It is governed by Jupiter and that gives hopes of a wholesome healthful herb. It is good for the diseases of the chest or breath, for pains and stitches in the sides, it dissolveth inward congealed blood occasioned by falls and bruises and the spitting of blood, if the roots either green or dried be boiled in wine and drunk. The root in the spring-time steeped in wine doth give it a delicate flavor and taste and being drunk fasting every morning comforteth the heart and is a good preservative against the plague or any other poison. It is very safe and is fit to be kept in every body's house."

In modern herbal medicine Avens is considered useful in diarrhea, dysenteries, leucorrhoea, sore throat, ague, chills, freshcatarrh, intermittent fevers, chronic and passive hemorrhages, gastric irritation and headache.

The infusion or decoction is made from 1/2 oz. of the powdered root or herb to 1 pint of boiling water, strained and taken cold. The infusion is the most grateful, but the decoction may be made much stronger by boiling it down to half.

The simple tincture is made by pouring a pint of proof spirit on an ounce of the bruised root and macerating it for fourteen days and then filtering through paper. Two or three teaspoonsful of this tincture in any watery vehicle, or in a glass of wine, are a sufficient dose.

An excellent compound tincture may be made as follows: Take of Avens root 1 1/2 OZ.; Angelica root, bruised, and Tormentil root bruised, of each 1 OZ.; Raisins, stoned, 2 OZ.; French brandy, 2 pints. Macerate for a month in a warm place. Filter then through paper. Dose, 1/2 oz.

The same ingredients infused in a quart of wine will form an excellent vinous tincture.

The infusion is considered an excellent cordial sudorific at the commencement of chills and catarrh, cutting short the paroxysm, and the continued use of it has restorative power in weakness, debility, etc.

Its astringency makes it useful in diarrhea, sore throat, etc. It is taken, strained and cold, in wine glassful doses, three or four times a day.

The infusion is also used in some skin affections. When used externally as a wash, it will remove spots, freckles or eruptions from the face.

Taken as decoction in the spring, Avens acts as a purifier and removes obstructions of the liver.

The powdered root has been used both in America and Europe as a substitute for Peruvian bark and has frequently been found to cure agues when the latter has failed, a drachm of powder being given every two hours.

The dose of the fluid extract of the herb is 1 drachm, of the fluid extract of the root, 1/2 to 1 drachm. As a tonic, the usual dose of the powdered herb or root is 15 to 30 grains.

As Arnica adulterant, the rhizome is sometimes present in the imported drug.

AVENS, MOUNTAIN

Botanical: Dryas octopetala (LINN,)
Family: N.O. Rosaceae

Description

The Mountain Avens (Dryas octopetala, Linn.) is a small plant, 2 to 3 inches high, distinguished from all other plants of the order Rosaceae by its oblong deeply-cut leaves, which are white with a woolly down beneath, and by its large, handsome, anemone-like, white flowers, which have eight petals. It blooms in the spring. It is not uncommon in the mountainous parts of the British Isles, especially on limestone.

When cultivated, it likes a sunny spot, not too dry, and prefers a little lime in the soil. It is propagated by layers or seeds, layers being the easiest method.

Although our native species are not striking enough to be made use of by the horticulturist, there are many garden varieties of Geum which are easily grown in fairly rich, loamy soil and are mostly propagated by dividing the roots in early autumn or in spring as growth commences. Seeds can be sown in the spring, either in the open or in well-drained pots or shallow boxes in cold frames.

The favorite varieties are the Scarlet Avens of Chile, Geum coccineum, the red G. sylvaticum, and the yellow-flowered G. montanum and G. elatum of the Himalayas, and G. reptans of the Alps.

AVENS, WATER

Botanical: Geum rivale (LINN.)
Family: N.O. Rosaceae
Synonyms: Nodding Avens. Drooping Avens. Cure All. Water Flower. Indian Chocolate.
Part Used: Root.

Habitat

The Water Avens (Geum rivale, Linn.) flourishes freely in the northern parts of Europe, in Canada and Siberia, and in Britain is more common in the northern counties and in Scotland than in the southern counties.

It is a lover of moist situations, found chiefly in damp woods and in ditches and among the coarse herbage fringing canals.

Description

It is a much stouter plant than the Common Avens, the stem 1 foot high or more, scarcely branching and with few leaves, of a simpler form. The lower part of the stem is clothed with bent-back hairs and is very downy above. The radical leaves, in the form of a rosette, as in the Common Avens, are long-stalked, lobed, the terminal leaflet larger, with more numerous segments than in Geum urbanum.

The flowers are larger than those of the Common Avens, fewer in number, not a widely-spreading star, but drooping, the petals forming together a compact and belllike corolla, of a dull purplish hue with darker veins, the calyces brownish, deeply tinged with purple. The awns feathery, not hooked.

Medicinal Action and Uses

The Water Avens has similar properties to those of the Common Avens and is employed in the same way, the root having tonic and powerfully astringent action and being beneficial in passive hemorrhage and diarrhea.

In the eastern states of North America (where it is called Indian Chocolate, Cure All and Water Flower) it is much used as a popular remedy in pulmonary consumption, simple dyspepsia and diseases of the bowels consequent on disorders of the stomach, and is valued as a febrifuge and tonic.

AZADIRACHTA

Botanical: Melia Azadirachta
Family: N.O. Meliaceae
Synonyms: Bead Tree. Pride of China. Nim. Margosa. Neem. Holy Tree. Indiar. Lilac Tree.
Parts Used: The bark of the root and trunk; the seed.
Habitat: Widely distributed through Tropics.

Description

Under the name of Neem it grows luxuriantly in Bengal, where it was known to the author. It grows from 30 to 50 feet high, leaves bipinnate, large bunches of lilac flowers agreeably perfumed. In Southern France and Spain it is found growing in avenues. It is said to be a native of China. The bark should be new and is a rusty grey color, inside yellow and foliated, coarsely fibrous, no odor, powerfully bitter and less astringent than the outer coarser bark, if taken from old roots the outer crust must be taken off.

Constituents

Margosin, a crystalline principle, and tannic acid.

Medicinal Action and Uses

The oil obtained from the fruit is used for burning, that from the bark is used medicinally and is anthelmintic and emetic; it is applied externally for rheumatism. The decoction of Azadirachta is said to be cathartic and in large doses slightly narcotic; it is also supposed to have febrifuge properties, it is used as a remedy for hysteria. The Hindu considers it a stomachic and taps it for toddy. The name Bead Tree is derived from the hard nuts which are used for making rosaries. An ointment to destroy lice is made from the pulp and is also used for scald head and other skin diseases. The oil from the nuts is useful for cramps, obstinate ulcers, etc.

Dosages and Preparations

The decoction is made from 2 OZ. of bark to 1 pint of water boiled down to 1/2 pint, one tablespoonful every two or three hours for a dose. This, or 20 grains of the powdered bark, is an effective dose for worms if followed by a purgative.

Poisons

The name Azadarach implies a poisonous plant and the fruit is considered to be so.

B

BAEL

Botanical: Aegle Marmelos (CORREA)
Family: N.O. Rutaceae
Synonyms: Belae Fructus. Bel. Indian Bael.
Part Used: Unripe fruit.
Habitat: India.

Description

Fruit 2 1/2 to 3 1/4 inches in diameter, globular or ovoid in shape, color greyish brown, outside surface hard and nearly smooth. Rind about 1/8 inch thick and adherent to a light red pulp, in which are ten to fifteen cells, each containing several woolly seeds. It has a faint aromatic odor and mucilagenous taste.

Constituents

The chief constituents appear to be mucilage and pectin contained in the pulp of the unripe fruit; the ripe fruit differs in yielding a tannin reaction and possessing a distinct aroma.

Medicinal Action and Uses

Fresh half-ripe Bael fruit is mildly astringent and is used in India for dysentery and diarrhea; the pulp may be eaten or the decoction administered. The dried fruit does not contain the constituents requisite for the preparation of the decoction. It is said to cure without creating any tendency to constipation.

Dosages and Preparations

Decoction Belae, B.P.C., 1 in 2 1/2: dose, 1/2 to 2 OZ. Fluid extract, 1/2 to 2 drachms.

Other Species

Mangosteen Fruit (Garania Mangostana) is sometimes substituted for it, also another species of the order Rutacece, Wood Apple or Elephant Apple (Feronia Elephantum), but neither are as effective as the fruit of the Bael Tree.

BALM

Botanical: Melissa officinalis (LINN.)
Family: N.O. Labiatae
Synonyms: Sweet Balm. Lemon Balm.
Part Used: Herb.

Habitat

A native of South Europe, especially in mountainous situations, but is naturalized in the south of England, and was introduced into our gardens at a very early period.

Description

The root-stock is short, the stem square and branching, grows 1 to 2 feet high, and has at each joint pairs of broadly ovate or heart-shaped, crenate or toothed leaves which emit a fragrant lemon odor when bruised. They also have a distinct lemon taste. The flowers, white or yellowish, are in loose, small bunches from the axils of the leaves and bloom from June to October. The plant dies down in winter, but the root is perennial.

The genus Melissa is widely diffused, having representatives in Europe, Middle Asia and North America. The name is from the Greek word signifying 'bee," indicative of the attraction the flowers have for those insects, on account of the honey they produce.

History

The word Balm is an abbreviation of Balsam, the chief of sweet-smelling oils. It is so called from its honeyed sweetness It was highly esteemed by Paracelsus, who believed it would completely revivify a man. It was formerly esteemed of great use in all complaints supposed to proceed from a disordered state of the nervous system. The London Dispensary (1696) says: 'An essence of Balm, given in Canary wine, every morning will renew youth, strengthen the brain, relieve languishing nature and prevent baldness." John Evelyn wrote: 'Balm is sovereign for the brain, strengthening the memory and powerfully chasing away melancholy." Balm steeped in wine we are told again, 'comforts the heart and driveth away melancholy and sadness." Formerly a spirit of Balm, combined with lemon-peel, nutmeg and angelica root, enjoyed a great reputation under the name of Carmelite water, being deemed highly useful against nervous headache and neuralgic affections.

Many virtues were formerly ascribed to this plant. Gerard says: 'It is profitably planted where bees are kept. The hives of bees being rubbed with the leaves of bawme, causeth the bees to keep together, and causeth others to come with them." And again quoting Pliny, 'When they are strayed away, they do find their way home by it." Pliny says: 'It is of so great virtue that though it be but tied to his sword that hath given the wound it staunchеth the blood." Gerard also tells us: 'The juice of Balm glueth together greene wounds," and gives the opinion of Pliny and Dioscorides that 'Balm, being leaves steeped in wine, and the wine drunk, and the leaves applied externally, were considered to be a certain cure for the bites of venomous beasts and the stings of scorpions. It is now recognized as a scientific fact that the balsamic oils of aromatic plants make excellent surgical dressings: they give off ozone and thus exercise anti-putrescent effects. Being chemical hydrocarbons, they contain so little oxygen that in wounds dressed with the fixed balsamic herbal oils, the atomic germs of disease are starved out, and the resinous parts of these balsamic oils, as they dry upon the sore or wound, seal it up and effectually exclude all noxious air.

Cultivation

Balm grows freely in any soil and can be propagated by seeds, cuttings or division of roots in spring or autumn. If in autumn, preferably not later than October, so that the offsets may be established before the frosts come on. The roots may be divided into small pieces, with three or four buds to each, and planted 2 feet apart in ordinary garden soil. The only culture required is to keep them clean from weeds and to cut off the decayed stalks in autumn, and then to stir the ground between the roots.

Medicinal Action and Uses

Carminative, diaphoretic and febrifuge. It induces a mild perspiration and makes a pleasant and cooling tea for feverish patients in cases of catarrh and influenza. To make the tea, pour 1 pint of boiling water upon 1 oz. of herb, infuse 15 minutes, allow to cool, then strain and drink freely. If sugar and a little lemon peel or juice be added it makes a refreshing summer drink.

Balm is a useful herb, either alone or in combination with others. It is excellent in colds attended with fever, as it promotes perspiration .

Used with salt, it was formerly applied for the purpose of taking away wens, and had the reputation of cleansing sores and easing the pains of gout.

John Hussey, of Sydenham, who lived to the age of 116, breakfasted for fifty years on Balm tea sweetened with honey, and herb teas were the usual breakfasts of Llewelyn Prince of Glamorgan, who died in his 108th year. Carmelite water, of which Balm was the chief ingredient, was drunk daily by the Emperor Charles V.

Commercial oil of Balm is not a pure distillate, but is probably oil of Lemon distilled over Balm. The oil is used in perfumery.

Balm is frequently used as one of the ingredients of pot-pourri. Mrs. Bardswell, in The Herb Garden, mentions Balm as one of the bushy herbs that are invaluable for the permanence of their leaf-odors, which,

'though ready when sought, do not force themselves upon us, but have to be coaxed out by touching, bruising or pressing. Balm with its delicious lemon scent, is by common consent one of the most sweetly smelling of all the herbs in the garden. Balm-wine was made of it and a tea which is good for feverish colds. The fresh leaves make better tea than the dry."

Refreshing Drink in Fever

'Put two sprigs of Balm, and a little woodsorrel, into a stone-jug, having first washed and dried them; peel thin a small lemon, and clear from the white; slice it and put a bit of peel in, then pour in 3 pints of boiling water, sweeten and cover it close."

Claret Cup

One bottle of claret, one pint bottle of German Seltzer-water, a small bunch of Balm, ditto of burrage, one orange cut in slices, half a cucumber sliced thick, a liqueurglass of Cognac, and one ounce of bruised sugar-candy.

'Process: Place these ingredients in a covered jug well immersed in rough ice, stir all together with a silver spoon, and when the cup has been iced for about an hour, strain or decanter it off free from the herbs, etc." (Francatelli's Cook's Guide.)

A bunch of Balm improves nearly all cups.

BALMONY

Botanical: Chelone Glabra (LINN.)
Family: N.O. Scrophulariaceae
Synonyms: Chelone. Snake-head. Turtle-head. Turtle-bloom. Shellflower. Salt-rheum Weed. Bitter Herb. Chelone Obliqua. Glatte. White Chelone. The Hummingbird Tree.
Part Used: The whole fresh herb.
Habitat: Eastern United States and Canada.

Description

This erect little plant, from 2 to 4 feet high, grows sparingly on the margins of swamps, wet woods, and rivers. It is a perennial, smooth herb, bearing opposite, oblong leaves, and short, dense, terminal spikes of two-lipped, white or purplish, cream or rose flowers, the lower lip bearded in the throat and the heart-shaped anthers and filaments woolly. The leaves have a slight somewhat tea-like odor and a markedly bitter taste. They should be planted in pots to prevent the roots from creeping too far.

The name of the genus Chelone comes from the Greek word meaning a tortoise, from the resemblance of the corolla to a tortoise-head. The whole, fresh plant is chopped, pounded to a pulp, and weighed, and a tincture is prepared with alcohol. The decoction is made with 2 oz. of the fresh herb to a pint.

Constituents

The bitter leaves communicate their properties to both water and alcohol. Chelonin is an eclectic medicine prepared from Chelone, and is a brown, bitter powder given as a tonic laxative.

Medicinal Action and Uses

The leaves have anti-bilious, anthelmintic, tonic and detergent properties, with a peculiar action on the liver, and are used largely in consumption, dyspepsia, debility and jaundice, in diseases of the liver, and for worms in children for which the powder or decoction may be used internally or in injection. As an ointment it is recommended for inflamed tumors, irritable ulcers, inflamed breasts, piles, etc.

For long it has been a favorite tonic, laxative and purgative among the aborigines of North America, though their doses render its tonic value doubtful.

Dosages

Of decoction, 1 to 2 fluid ounces. Of fluid extract, 1/2 to 1 drachm. Of the powder, 1 drachm. Of the tincture, 1 to 2 fluid drachms. Of Chelonin, 1 to 2 grains.

BALSAM OF GILEAD

Botanical: Commiphora Opobalsamum
Family: N.O. Burseraceae
Synonyms: Balsamum Meccae var. Judiacum. Balsamum Gileadense. Baume de la Mecque. Balsamodendrum Opobalsamum. Balessan. Bechan. Balsam Tree. Amyris Gileadensis. Amyris Opobalsamum. Balsumodendron Gileadensis. Protium Gileadense. Dossémo.
Part Used: The resinous juice.
Habitat: The countries on both sides of the Red Sea.

Description

This small tree, the source of the genuine Balm of Gilead around which so many mystical associations have gathered stands from 10 to 12 feet high, with wandlike, spreading branches. The bark is of a rich brown color, the leaves, trifoliate, are small and scanty, the flowers unisexual small, and reddish in color, while the seeds are solitary, yellow, and grooved down one side. It is both rare, and difficult to rear, and is so much valued by the Turks that its importation is prohibited. They have grown the trees in guarded gardens at Matarie, near Cairo, from the days of Prosper Alpin, who wrote the Dialogue of Balm, and the balsam is valued as a cosmetic by the royal ladies. In the Bible, and in the works of Bruce Theophrastes, Galen, and Dioscorides, it is lauded.

History

Balm, Baulm or Bawm, contracted from Balsam, may be derived from the Hebrew bot smin, 'chief of oils," or bâsâm, 'balm," and besem, 'a sweet smell." Opobalsamum is used by Dioscorides to mean 'the juice flowing from the balsam-tree."

Pliny states that the tree was first brought to Rome by the generals of Vespasian, while Josephus relates that it was taken from Arabia to Judea by the Queen of Sheba as a present to Solomon. There, being cultivated for its juice, particularly on Mount Gilead, it acquired its popular name. Later, it was called Opobalsamum, its dried twigs Xylobalsamum, and its dried fruit Carpobalsamum.

Its rarity, combined with the magic of its name, have caused the latter to be adopted for several other species.

Abd-Allatif, a Damascan physician of the twelfth century, noted that it had two barks the outer reddish and thin, the inner green and thick, and a very aromatic odor.

The juice exudes spontaneously during the heat of summer, in resinous drops, the process being helped by incisions in the bark. The more humid the air, the greater the quantity collected. When the oil is separated, it is prepared with great secrecy, and taken to the stores of the ruler, where it is carefully guarded. The quantity of oil obtained is roughly one-tenth the amount of juice. It is probable that an inferior kind of oil is obtained after boiling the leaves and wood with water.

The wood is found in small pieces, several kinds being known commercially, but it rapidly loses its odor.

The fruit is reddish grey, and the size of a small pea, with an agreeable and aromatic taste.

In Europe and America it is so seldom found in a pure state that its use is entirely discontinued .

Constituents

The liquid balm is turbid whitish, thick, grey and odorous, and becomes solid by exposure. It contains a resin soluble in alcohol, and a principle resembling Bassorin.

Medicinal Action and Uses

It has been used in diseases of the urinary tracts, but is said to possess no medicinal properties not found in other balsams.

Other Species

Abies Balsamea, Balm of Gilead Fir, orAmerican Silver Fir. The name is applied to this Canadian species, in Europe, because of the supposed resemblance of its product, an oleoresinous fluid obtained from punctured blisters in the bark, which is really a true turpentine, known as Canada Balsam or Canada Turpentine. Its odor distinguishes it from Strassburg Turpentine, which is sometimes substituted for it. It is diuretic, and stimulates mucous tissues in small doses. In large doses it is purgative, and may cause nausea.

Populus Candicans is called Balm of Gilead in America. The buds are used, and called Balm of Gilead Buds, as are those of P. Nigra and P. balsamifera, the product of the last being imported into Europe under the name of Tacomahaca. They are covered with a fragrant, resinous matter, which may be separated in boiling water, the odor being like incense, and the taste bitter and rather unpleasant. They are stimulant, tonic, diuretic, and antiscorbutic. A tincture of them is useful for complaints of the chest, stomach, and kidneys, and for rheumatism and scurvy. With lard or oil they are useful as an external application in bruises, swellings, and some cutaneous diseases. In ointments they are a little inferior to paraffin as a preventive of rancidity.

The bark of P. balsamifera is tonic and cathartic.

Dosages

Of solid extract, 5 to 10 grains. Of tincture, 1 to 4 fluid drachms. Of fluid extract, 1 to 2 drachms. Of extract of the bark, 5 to 15 grains.

Dracocephalum Canariense or Cedronella Triphylla is known as a garden plant something like Salvia, and called Balm of Gilead for no better reason than that its leaves are fragrant. It is a native of America and the Canaries.

BALSAM OF PERU

Botanical: Myroxylon Pereiræ (KLOTSCH)
Family: N.O. Leguminosae
Synonyms: Toluifera Pereira. Myrosperum Pereira.
Part Used: Oleoresinous liquid.
Habitat: Central America in the forests of San Salvado.

Description

A large and beautiful tree with a valuable wood like mahogany, and a straight smooth trunk; the last is coarse grey, compact, heavy granulated and a pale straw color, containing a resin which changes from citron to dark brown; smell and taste balsamic and aromatic. Leaves alternately, abruptly pinnate, leaflets two pairs mostly opposite, ovate, lanceolate with the end blunt emarginate; every part of the tree including the leaves abounds in a resinous juice. The mesocarp of the fruit is fibrous, and the balsamic juice which is abundant is contained in two distinct receptacles, one on each side. The beans contain Coumarin, the husks an extremely acrid bitter resin, and a volatile oil; a gum resin, quite distinct from the proper balsam, exudes from the trunk of the tree and contains gum resin and a volatile oil; the tree commences to be productive after five or six years, and continues to yield for thirty years; the flower has a fragrance which can be smelt a hundred yards away.

The process of extraction produces three grades of balsam; the title 'Balsam of Peru' is derived from the fact of its being shipped from Peru. There are several fictitious Peruvian balsams found in commerce, but they do not contain the same properties. A white balsam is made from the fruit of Myroxylon Peruviatta or Pereiræ, which has a peculiar resinous body and none of the chemical constituents of Balsam of Peru; this is termed Myroxocarpin. Another substance obtained from the same tree and much used in Central America is termed Balsamito, it is an alcoholic extract of the young fruit. This is used as a stimulant, diuretic, anthelmintic and external application to gangrenous ulcers and to remove freckles. Balsam of Peru is warm and aromatic, much hotter and more stimulating than Balsam of Copaiba and is used for similar complaints. It is specially useful for rheumatic pains and chronic coughs.

Constituents

A colorless, aromatic, oily liquid, termed cinnamein, dark resin peruviol, small quantity of vanillin and cinnamic acid.

Medicinal Action and Uses

Stimulant, expectorant, parasiticide. Used in scabies and skin diseases; it destroys the itch acarus and its eggs, and is much to be preferred to sulphur ointment, also of value in prurigo, pruritis and in later stages of acute eczema. It is a good antiseptic expectorant and a stimulant to the heart, increasing blood pressure; its action resembles benzoic acid. It is applied externally to sore nipples and discharges from the ear. Given internally, it lessens mucous secretions, and is of value in bronchorrhoea gleet, leucorrhoea and chronic bronchitis, and asthma. It is also used in soap manufacturing, for its fragrance, and because it makes a soft creamy lather, useful for chapped hands. Balsam of Peru can be applied alone or as an ointment made by melting it with an equal weight of tallow.

Dose

10 to 30 drops, best given in syrup, with the yolk of an egg added, or with gumarabic.

Adulterations

Castor oil, Copaiba, Canada turpentine, etc.

Other Species

MYROXYLON FRUTESCENS

Habitat: Trinidad.

The pod is used in the island as a carminative, and externally in the form of a tincture. As a lotion for rheumatic pains, the stems yield a balsamic juice.

GUINA-GUINA

Habitat: Paraguay.

This bark is used in powder and in decoction for wounds and ulcers, and the dried concrete juice of the trunk of the tree IS very similar to Balsam of Peru.

BALSAM OF TOLU

Botanical: Myrospermum Toluiferum
Family: N.O. Leguminosae
Synonyms: Balsamum Tolutanum. Tolutanischer Balsam. Balsamum Americanum.
Part Used: Exudation.

History

There is still some obscurity about the origin of the different South American balsam-yielding trees. The appearance of the above variety is said to differ but slightly from the Peruvian, but the method of gathering the balsam is quite different. V-shaped cuts are made in the tree, and the liquid is received into calabash cups placed at an angle; these are emptied into flasks of raw hide, conveyed by donkeys to the depôts, and finally shipped in tin or earthen vessels, which occasionally contain large pieces of red brick. On arrival the balsam is soft and sticky, but exposure to the air makes it hard and brittle, more like resin, with a crystalline appearance. In color it is pale, yellowish red or brown. It has a sweet, aromatic, resinous taste - becoming soft again when chewed - with an odor resembling vanilla or benzoin, especially fragrant when the balsam is burned, but completely changing and resembling the clove-pink if dissolved in a minute portion of liquor potassa.

As the balsam solidifies, its odor becomes more feeble, but the quantity of cinnamic acid increases, and it thus becomes valuable to perfumers as a fixative, an ounce added to a pound of volatile perfume making it much more permanent.

Tolu Balsam is frequently adulterated with turpentines, styrax, colophony, etc., and may be tested by heating it in sulphuric acid. If pure, it will yield a cherry-red liquid, and will dissolve without any appearance of sulphurous acid.

Constituents

About 80 per cent amorphous resin, with cinnamic acid, a volatile oil, and a little vanillin, benzyl benzoate and benzyl cinnamate. It is freely soluble in chloroform, glacial acetic acid, acetone, ether, alcohol and liquor potassa, scarcely soluble in petroleum-benzine and benzol.

To distinguish it from Balsam of Peru it can be tested with sulphuric acid and water, yielding a grey mass instead of the lovely violet color of the genuine Peruvian Balsam.

Medicinal Action and Uses

Stimulant and expectorant, much used as the basis of cough mixtures. The vapor from the balsam dissolved in ether when inhaled, is beneficial in chronic catarrh and other noninflammatory chest complaints. The best form is that of an emulsion, made by titurating the balsam with mucilage and loaf sugar, and adding water.

Two parts of Tolu, 3 of Almond oil, 4 of gum-arabic, and 16 of Rose-water, make an excellent liniment for excoriated nipples.

Preparations

Tincture, B.P. and U.S.P., 1/2 to 1 drachm. Syrup, B.P. and U.S.P., 1/2 to 1 drachm. Lozenges, incense and pastilles are also prepared.

BALSAM, WHITE

Botanical: Gnaphalium polycephalum
Family: N.O. Asteraceae
Synonyms: Indian Posy. Sweet-scented Life Everlasting. Old Field Balsam. Gnaphalium Obtusifolium or Blunt-leaved Everlasting. Gnaphalium Connoideum. Fragrant Everlasting. None-so-Pretty.

Catsfoot. Silver Leaf.
Parts Used: Herb, leaves, flowers.
Habitat: Virginia, Pennsylvania and New England.

Description

Leaves lanceolate; stalk tomentose, panicled; flowers tubular, yellow, glomerate, conical, terminating; stems single, 9 inches high. Corollas yellow, flowering July to August. Leaves have a pleasant aromatic smell and an aromatic, slightly bitter, astringent, agreeable taste. The Antennaria Margaritacea or Gnaphalium Margaritacea, or Pearl-flowered Life Everlasting, has the same properties as White Balsam.

Medicinal Action and Uses

Astringent. Beneficial for ulcerations of the throat and mouth; warm infusions used to produce diaphoresis; also of service in quinsy, pulmonary complaints, leucorrhoea. Can be used internally and as a local application, likewise used as fomentations to bruises, indolent tumors. An infusion given in diseases of the bowels - hemorrhages etc. The fresh juice is reputed anti-venereal and anti-aphrodisiac; the cold infusion vermifugal; the dried flowers are used as a sedative filling for the pillows of consumptives. A tincture is made from whole plant.

BAMBOO BRIER

Botanical: Aralia nudicaulis (LINN.)
Family: N.O. Araliaceae
Synonyms: Wild Sarsaparilla. Shot Bush. Wild Liquorice.
Part Used: The root.
Habitat: United States.

Description

An indigenous perennial in shady rocky woods, very common in rich soil, rhizome horizontal, creeping several feet in length and more or less twisted; of a yellowish-brown color externally and about 1/4 inch in diameter, has a fragrant odor and a warm, aromatic, sweetish taste.

Constituents

Contains 3.05 per cent of resin, 0.33 per cent of oil tannin, an acid albumen, mucilage and cellulose.

Medicinal Action and Uses and Dosage

As Sarsaparilla.

BANEBERRY

POISON
Botanical: Actaea spicata (LINN.)
Family: N.O. Ranunculacea
Synonyms: Herb Christopher. Bugbane. Toadroot.
Part Used: Root.

Habitat

It is to be found in copses on limestone in Yorkshire and the Lake District, but is so uncommon as to be regarded by some botanists as almost a doubtful native.

The Baneberry, or Herb Christopher, is a rather rare British plant belonging (like the Paeony) to the Buttercup order, but distinguished from all other species in the order by its berry-like fruit. It is considered to have similar anti-spasmodic properties to the Paeony.

Description

The black, creeping root-stock is perennial, sending up each year erect stems, growing 1 to 2 feet high, which are triangular and either not branched, or very sparingly so. The foot-stalks of the leaves are long and arise from the root. These divide into three smaller foot-stalks, and are so divided or re-divided that each leaf is composed of eighteen, or even twenty-seven, lobes or leaflets.

The flower-stem arises from the roots and has leaves of the same form, but smaller. The flowers grow in spikes and are of a pure white.

The whole plant is dark green and glabrous (without hairs), or only very slightly downy. It flowers in June and in autumn ripens its fruits, which are egg-shaped berries, 1/2 inch long, black and shining, many-seeded and very poisonous, well justifying the popular name of Baneberry.

The plant is of an acrid, poisonous nature throughout, and though the root has been used in some nervous cases, and is said to be a remedy for catarrh, it must be administered with great caution.

Medicinal Action and Uses

Antispasmodic. The juice of the berries, mixed with alum, yields a black dye.

There are two varieties of this species, one of British origin, only distinguished from the rest of the species by its berries being red, instead of black and the other an American plant (Actaea alba, or White Cohosh) with white berries. Both varieties grow in the writer's garden.

The American species is considered by the natives a valuable remedy against snake-bite, especially of the rattlesnake, hence it is - with several other plants - sometimes known as one of the 'Rattlesnake herbs."

It is said the name 'Herb Christopher' was also formerly applied to the flowering fern, Osmunda regalis.

The name of the genus is from the Greek acte, the elder, which these plants resemble as regards the leaves and berries.

Toads seem to be attracted by the smell of the Baneberry, which causes it also to be termed Toadroot, the name arising possibly also from its preference for the damp shady situations in which the toad is found.

It is also called Bugbane, because of its offensive smell, which is said to drive away vermin.

Closely allied to this plant, and at one time assigned to the same genus, is the plant known as Black Cohosh.

BARBERRY, COMMON

Botanical: Berberis vulgaris (LINN.)
Family: N.O. Berberidaceae
Synonyms: Berbery. Pipperidge Bush. Berberis Dumetorum.
Parts Used: Bark, root-bark.

Habitat

The Common Barberry, a well-known, bushy shrub, with pale-green deciduous leaves, is found in copses and hedges in some parts of England, though a doubtful native in Scotland and Ireland. It is generally distributed over the greater part of Europe, Northern Africa and temperate Asia. As an ornamental shrub, it is fairly common in gardens.

Description

The stems are woody, 8 to 10 feet high, upright and branched, smooth, slightly grooved, brittle, with a white pith and covered with an ash-coloured bark.

The leaves of the barren shoots of the year are alternate, 1 to 1 1/2 inch long, shortly petioled, presenting various gradations from leaves into spines, into which they become transformed in the succeeding year. The primary leaves on the woody shoots are reduced to three-forked spines, with an enlarged base. The secondary leaves are in fascicles from the axil of these spines and are simple, oval, tapering at the base into a short foot-stalk, the margins finely serrate, with the teeth terminating in small spines.

The flowers are small, pale yellow, arranged in pendulous racemes, produced from the fascicles of leaves, towards the ends of the branches. Their scent is not altogether agreeable when near, but by no means offensive at a distance. Their stamens show remarkable sensibility when touched springing and taking a position closely applied to the pistil. Insects of various kinds are exceedingly fond of the Barberry flower. Linnaeus observed that when bees in search of honey touch the filaments, they spring from the petal and strike the anther against the stigma, thereby exploding the pollen. In the original position of the stamens, Iying in the concavity of the petals, they are sheltered from rain, and there remain till some insect unavoidably touches them. As it is chiefly in fine, sunny weather that insects are on the wing, the pollen is also in such weather most fit for the purpose of impregnation, hence this curious contrivance of nature for fertilizing the seeds at the most suitable moment.

The berries are about 1/2 inch long, oblong and slightly curved; when ripe, of a fine, red color and pleasantly acidulous.

The leaves are also acid, and have sometimes been employed for the same purposes as the fruit. Gerard recommends the leaves 'to season meat with and instead of a salad."

Cows, sheep and goats are said to eat the shrub, horses and swine to refuse it, and birds, also, seldom touch the fruit, on account of its acidity; in this respect it approaches the tamarind.

History

In many parts of Europe, farmers have asserted that wheat planted within three or four hundred yards of a Barberry bush became infected with rust or mildew, but this belief has not been substantiated by recent observations.

Professor Henslow (Floral Rambles in Highways and Byways) writes:

'It was thought by farmers in the middle of the last century that the Barberry blighted wheat if it grew near the hedge. Botanists then ridiculed the idea; but in a sense the farmers were right! What they observed was that if a Barberry bush grew, say, at the corner of a wheatfield the leaves of the wheat became "rusty," i.e. they were streaked with a red color when close to the bush; and that this "red rust" extended steadily across the field till the whole was rusted. The interpretation was at that time unknown. A fungus attacks the leaves of the Barberry, making orange-coloured spots. It throws off minute spores which do attack the wheat. These develop parasitic threads within the leaf, from which arise the red rust-spores: subsequently dark brown or black spores, consisting of two cells, called wheat-mildew, appear. After a time these throw off red, onecelled spores which attack the Barbarry; and so a cycle is completed. Though it was not really the bush which blighted the wheat, the latter suffered through its agency as the primary host plant."

Uses

The Barberry used to be cultivated for the sake of the fruit, which was pickled and used for garnishing dishes. The ripe berries can be made into an agreeable, refreshing jelly by boiling them with an equal weight of fine sugar to a proper consistence and then straining it. They were formerly used as a sweetmeat, and in sugar-plums, or comfits. It is from these berries that the delicious confitures d'epine vinette, for which Rouen is famous, are commonly prepared.

The roots boiled in Iye, will dye wool yellow, and in Poland they dye leather of a beautiful yellow color with the bark of the root. The inner bark of the stems will also dye linen of a fine yellow, with the assistance of alum.

Provincially, the plant is also termed Pipperidge Bush, from 'pepon," a pip, and 'rouge," red, as descriptive of the scarlet, juiceless fruit.

Berberis is the Arabic name of the fruit, signifying a shell, and many authors believe the name is derived from this word, because the leaves are glossy, like the inside of an oyster-shell.

Among the Italians, the Barberry bears the name of Holy Thorn, because it is thought to have formed part of the crown of thorns made for our Saviour.

Cultivation

It is generally propagated by suckers, which are put out in plenty from the roots, but these plants are subject to send out suckers in greater plenty than those which are propagated by layers, therefore the latter method should be preferred.

The best time for laying down the branches is in autumn (October), and the young shoots of the same year are the best- these will be well rooted by the next autumn, when they may be taken off and planted where they are designed to remain.

Barberry may also be propagated by ripened cuttings, taken also in autumn and planted in sandy soil, in a cold frame, or by seeds, sown in spring, or preferably in autumn, 1 inch deep in a sheltered border when, if fresh from the pulp, or berry, they will germinate in the open in the following spring.

Parts Used

Stem-bark and root-bark. The stem-bark is collected by shaving and is dried spread out in trays in the sun, or on shelves in a well-ventilated greenhouse or in an airy attic or loft, warmed either by sun or by the artificial heat of a stove, the door and window being left open by day to ensure a warm current of air. The bark may be also strung on threads and hung across the room.

When dried, the pieces of bark are in small irregular portions, about 2 inches long and 1/2 inch wide, and of a dark-yellowish grey color externally, and marked with shallow longitudinal furrows. It frequently bears the minute, black 'fruits' of lichen. The bark is dark yellowish brown on the inner surface separating in layers of bast fibres.

The bark has a slight odor and a bitter taste, and colors the saliva yellow when chewed.

The root-bark is greyish brown externally and is dried in a similar manner after being peeled off. When dry, it breaks with a short fracture. It contains the same constituents as the stem-bark and possesses similar qualities.

Constituents

The chief constituent of Barberry bark is Berberine, a yellow crystalline, bitter alkaloid, one of the few that occurs in plants belonging to several different natural orders. Other constituents are oxyacanthine, berbamine, other alkaloidal matter, a little tannin, also wax, resin, fat, albumin, gum and starch.

Medicinal Action and Uses

Tonic, purgative, antiseptic. It is used in the form of a liquid extract, given as decoction, infusion or tincture, but generally a salt of the alkaloid Berberine is preferred.

As a bitter stomachic tonic, it proves an excellent remedy for dyspepsia and functional derangement of the liver, regulating the digestive powers, and if given in larger doses, acting as a mild purgative and removing constipation.

It is used in all cases of jaundice, general debility and biliousness, and for diarrhea.

Preparations

Powdered bark, 1/4 teaspoonful several times daily. Fluid extract, 1/2 to 1 drachm. Solid extract, 5 to 10 grains.

It possesses febrifuge powers and is used as a remedy for intermittent fevers. It also forms an excellent gargle for a sore mouth.

A good lotion for application to cutaneous eruptions has also been made from it.

The berries contain citric and malic acids, and possess astringent and anti-scorbutic properties. They are useful in inflammatory fevers, especially typhus, also in bilious disorders and scurvy, and in the form of a jelly are very refreshing in irritable sore throat, for which also a syrup of Barberries made with water, proves an excellent astringent gargle.

The Egyptians are said still to employ a diluted juice of the berries in pestilential fevers, and Simon Paulli relates that he was cured of a malignant fever by drinking an infusion of the berries sweetened with sugar and syrup of roses.

Recipes

Barberry Drops

The black tops must be cut off; then roast the fruit before the fire till soft enough to pulp with a silver spoon through a sieve into a china basin; then set the basin in a sauce pan of water, the top of which will just fitit, or on a hot hearth, and stir it till it grows thick. When cold, put to every pint 1 1/2 lb. of sugar, the finest double-refined, pounded and sifted through a lawn sieve, which must be covered with a fine linen to prevent its wasting while sifting. Beat the sugar and juice together 3 1/2 hours if a large quantity, but 2 1/2 for less; then drop it on sheets of white, thick paper, the size of the drops sold in the shops. Some fruit is not so sour and then less sugar is necessary. To know if there be enough, mix till well incorporated and then drop; if it runs, there is not enough sugar, and if there is too much it will be rough. A dry room will suffice to dry them. No metal must touch the juice but the point of a knife, just to take the drop off the end of the wooden spoon, and then as little as possible.

To prepare Barberries for Tartlets

Pick Barberries that have no stones, from the stalks, and to every pound weigh 3/4 lb. of lump sugar; put the fruit into a stone jar, and either set it on a hot hearth or in a saucepan of water, and let them simmer very slowly till soft; put them and the sugar into a preserving-pan, and boil them gently 15 minutes. Use no metal but silver.

Barberries in Bunches

Have ready bits of flat white wood, 3 inches long and 1/4 inch wide. Tie the stalks of the fruit on the stick from within an inch of one end to beyond the other, so as to make them look handsome. Simmer them in some syrup two successive days, covering them each time with it when cold. When they look clear they are simmered enough. The third day do them like other candy fruit.

BARBERRY, NEPAL

Botanical: Berberis aristata
Family: N.O. Berberidaceae
Synonyms: Ophthalmic Barberry. Darlahad.
Part Used: Dried stems.
Habitat: A shrub indigenous to India and Ceylon.

It is known as 'Darlahad," under which names are included the dried stems of Berberis Iycium and B. asiatica, but only the stem of B. aristata is official in the Indian and Colonial Addendum for use in India and the Eastern Colonies, in intermittent fevers.

Medicinal Action and Uses

A bitter tonic antiperiodic and diaphoretic. The chief constituents are those of common Berberiabark, the bitter principle being the alkaloid Berberine, which is present in considerable quantity, together with tannin, resin, gum, starch and other alkaloidal matter. When dried, it occurs in undulating, cylindrical pieces, 1 to 2 inches in diameter. The drug has a faint odor and a bitter taste.

BARBERRY (INDIAN)

Botanical: Berberis asiatica
Family: N.O. Berberiaceae
Part Used: Root-bark.

The root-bark is light coloured, corky, almost inodorous, with a bitter, mucilaginous taste. It contains much Berberine, and a dark-brown extract is made from it employed in India under the name of 'Rusot." This extract is sometimes prepared from the wood or roots of different species of Barberry. It has the consistency of opium and a bitter, astringent taste.

BARLEY

Botanical: Hordeum distichon (LINN.)
Family: N.O. Graminaceae
Synonyms: Pearl Barley. Perlatum.
Part Used: Decorticated seeds.
Habitat: Britain.

Description

Pearl Barley is the grain without its skin; rounded and polished; this is the official variety. Taste and odor farinaceous. The Scotch, milled, or pot barley isthe grain with husks only partly removed. Patent Barley is the ground decorticated grain.

Constituents

Pearl Barley contains about 80 per cent of starch and about 6 per cent of proteins, cellulose, etc.

Medicinal Action and Uses

Pearl Barley is used for the preparation of a decoction which is a nutritive and demulcent drink in febrile conditions and in catarrhal affections of the respiratory and urinary organs: barley water is used to dilute cows' milk for young infants, it prevents the formation of hard masses of curd in the stomach. Malt is produced from barley by a process of steeping and drying which develop a ferment 'diatase' needed for the production of alcoholic malt liquors, but in the form of Malt Extract it is largely used in medicine. Vinegar is an acid liquid produced by oxidation of fermented malt wort. Malt vinegar is the only vinegar that should be used medicinally.

Dosage and Preparation

Barley water. Pearl Barley washed 10 parts, water to 100 parts, boil for 20 minutes, strain. Dose, 1 to 4 oz.

Adulterants

Pearl Barley is sometimes treated with french chalk and starch to whiten it and increase the weight.

BARTSIA, RED

Botanical: Bartsia odontites
Family: N.O. Scrophulariaceae
Part Used: Herb

This common little plant, which has no old popular name, is an abundant weed in cornfields and by the roadside. It is not very attractive in appearance, its narrow, tapering leaves being of a dingy purplish green and the flowers of a dull rose color, small and in onesided spikes, which usually droop at the ends.

A less common species, Bartsia viscosa, is found in marshes and damp places- the flowers are yellow, and might be mistaken for Yellow Rattle, from which it may be easily distinguished by its solitary, unspiked, yellowflowers, and by being covered with clammy down. It grows to a height of 6 to 12 inches, and is very common in many parts of Devon and Cornwall, where it sometimes grows 2 feet high.

Botanical: Bartisa Latifolia
Family: N.O. Scrophulariaceae
Synonyms: Red Nettle

A small annual with reddish stems, leaves and flowers; partly parasitic on the roots of grasses.

BASIL, BUSH

Botanical: Ocymum minumum
Family: N.O. Labiatae
Part Used: Leafy tops.

Bush Basil (Ocymum minumum) is a low, bushy plant, seldom above 6 inches in height, much smaller than Sweet Basil.

The leaves are ovate, quite entire, the white flowers in whorls towards the top of the branches, smaller than those of Sweet Basil, and seldom succeeded by ripe seeds in England.

There are two varieties, one with black-purple leaves and the other with variable leaves.

Both Bush and Garden Basil are natives of India, from whence it was introduced in 1573. Bush Basil may occasionally live through the winter in this country, though Sweet Basil never does.

Both varieties flower in July and August.

The leafy tops of Bush Basil are used in the same manner as the Sweet Basil for seasoning and in salads. t

The leaves of O. viride, a native of Western Africa, possess febrifugal properties; and at Sierra Leone, where it bears the name of 'Fever-plant," a decoction of them, drunk as tea, is used as a remedy for the fevers so prevalent there.

The leaves of O. canum, and O. gratissimum in India, and of O. crispum in Japan, all sweet-scented varieties, are prescribed as a remedy for colds.

O. teniflorum is regarded as an aromatic stimulant in Java; and 0. guineense is much employed by the negroes as a medicine in cases of bilious fever.

These plants are all free of any deleterious secretions; for the most part they are fragrant and aromatic, and hence they have not only been used as tonics, but are also valuable as kitchen herbs.

In Persia and Malaysia Basil is planted on graves, and in Egypt women scatter the flowers on the resting-places of those belonging to them.

These observances are entirely at variance with the idea prevailing among the ancient Greeks that it represented hate and misfortune. They painted poverty as a ragged woman with a Basil at her side, and thought the plant would not grow unless railing and abuse were poured forth at the time of sowing. The

Romans, in like manner, believed that the more it was abused, the better it would prosper.

The physicians of old were quite unable to agree as to its medicinal value, some declaring that it was a poison, and others a precious simple. Culpepper tells us:

'Galen and Dioscorides hold it is not fitting to be taken inwardly and Chrysippusrails at it. Pliny and the Arabians defend it. Something is the matter, this herb and rue will not grow together, no, nor near one another, and we know rue is as great an enemy to poison as any that grows."

But it was said to cause sympathy between human beings and a tradition in Moldavia still exists that a youth will love any maiden from whose hand he accepts a sprig of this plant. In Crete it symbolizes 'love washed with tears," and in some parts of Italy it is a love-token.

Boccaccio's story of Isabella and the Pot of Basil, immortalized by Keats, keeps the plant in our memory, though it is now rarely cultivated in this country. It was formerly grown in English herb gardens. Tusser includes it among the Strewing herbs and Drayton places it first in his poem Polyolbion.

'With Basil then I will begin
Whose scent is wondrous pleasing."

In Tudor days, little pots of Basil were often given as graceful compliments by farmers' wives to visitors. Parkinson says:

'The ordinary Basill is in a manner wholly spent to make sweete or washing waters among other sweet herbs, yet sometimes it is put into nosegays. The Physicall properties are to procure a cheerfull and merry hearte whereunto the seeds is chiefly used in powder."

Cultivation

Basil dies down every year in this country, so that the seeds have to be sown annually. If in a very warm sheltered spot, seeds may be sown in the open, about the last week in April, but they are a long time coming up, and it is preferable to sow in a hot bed, about the end of March, and remove to a warm border in May, planting 10 inches to a foot apart.

Basil flourishes best in a rich soil.

Part Used Medicinally

The whole herb, both fresh and dried, gathered in July.

Medicinal Action and Uses

Aromatic and carminative. Though generally employed in cooking as a flavoring, Basil has been occasionally used for mild nervous disorders and for the alleviation of wandering rheumatic pains- the dried leaves, in the form of snuff, are said to be a cure for nervous headaches.

An infusion of the green herb in boiling water is good for all obstructions of the internal organs, arrests vomiting and allays nausea.

The seeds have been reckoned efficacious against the poison of serpents, both taken internally and laid upon the wound. They are also said to cure warts.

In common with other labiates, Basil, both the wild and the sweet, furnishes an aromatic, volatile, camphoraceous oil, and on this account is much employed in France for flavoring soups, especially turtle soup. They also use it in ragoûts and sauces. The leafy tops are a great improvement to salads and cups.

Although it is now comparatively little used in England for culinary purposes, this herb was one of our favorite pot-herbs in older days, and gave the distinctive flavor that once made Fetter Lane sausages famous.

Recipes

A Recipe for Aromatic Seasoning

'Take of nutmegs and mace one ounce each, of cloves and peppercorns two ounces of each, one ounce of dried bay-leaves, three ounces of basil, the same of marjoram, two ounces of winter savory, and three ounces of thyme, half an ounce of cayenne-pepper, the same of grated lemon-peel, and two cloves of garlic; all these ingredients must be well pulverized in a mortar and sifted through a fine wire sieve, and put away in dry corked bottles for use." (Francatelli's Cook's Guide.)

O. Americanum. First recorded in 1789 as found in the West Indies.

The name 'Ocymum' is said by Mathiolus to be derived from the Greek word 'To smell," because of the powerful aromatic and pungent scent characterizing most of the plants of this genus. Decoctions made from 0. Americanum are used in cases of chest trouble and dysentery; and an essential oil is also extracted from the plant.

Closely akin to the above-named is the O. gratissimum cultivated in China as a culinary herb.

O. canum is used as a tincture made from the leaves in homeopathy.

BASIL, SWEET

Botanical: Ocymum basilium (LINN.)
Family: N.O. Labiatae
Part Used: Herb.

Description

Common or Sweet Basil which is used in medicine and also for culinary purposes, especially in France, is a hairy, labiate plant, growing about 3 feet high. The stem is obtusely quadrangular, the labiate flowers are white, in whorls in the axils of the leaves, the calyx with the upper lobe rounded and spreading. The leaves, greyish-green beneath and dotted with dark oil cells, are opposite, 1 inch long and 1/3 inch broad, stalked and peculiarly smooth, soft and cool to the touch, and if slightly bruised exale a delightful scent of cloves.

There are several varieties, differing in the size, shape, odor and color of the leaves. The Common Basil has very dark green leaves, the curled-leaved has short spikes of flowers, the narrow-leaved smells like Fennel, another has a scent of citron and another a tarragon scent, one species has leaves of three colors, and another 'studded' leaves.

History

The derivation of the name Basil is uncertain. Some authorities say it comes from the Greek basileus, a king, because, as Parkinson says, 'the smell thereof is so excellent that it is fit for a king's house," or it may have been termed royal, because it was used in some regal unguent or medicine. One rather unlikely theory is that it is shortened from basilisk, a fabulous creature that could kill with a look. This theory may be based on a strange old superstition that connected the plant with scorpions. Parkinson tells us that 'being gently handled it gave a pleasant smell but being hardly wrung and bruised would breed scorpions. It is also observed that scorpions doe much rest and abide under these pots and vessells wherein Basil is planted." It was generally believed that if a sprig of Basil were left under a pot it would in time turn to a scorpion. Superstition went so far as to affirm that even smelling the plant might bring a scorpion into the brain.

Culpepper says:

'Being applied to the place bitten by venomous beasts, or stung by a wasp or hornet, it speedily draws the poison to it. - Every like draws its like. Mizaldus affirms, that being laid to rot in horse-dung, it will breed venomous beasts. Hilarius, a French physician, affirms upon his own knowledge, that an acquaintance of his, by common smelling to it, had a scorpion breed in his brain."

In India the Basil plant is sacred to both Krishna and Vishnu, and is cherished in every Hindu house. Probably on account of its virtues, in disinfecting, and vivifying malarious air, it first became inseparable from Hindu houses in India as the protecting spirit of the family.

The strong aromatic scent of the leaves is very much like cloves.

Every good Hindu goes to his rest with a Basil leaf on his breast. This is his passport to Paradise.

BASIL, WILD

Botanical: Calamintha Clinopodium
Family: N.O. Labiatae
Synonyms: Hedge Basil. Hedge Calamint.

Habitat

The plant is widely distributed throughout the North Temperate Zone, and is common in England and Scotland in dry hedges and the borders of copses, mostly in high situations. In Ireland it is somewhat rare.

The Wild Basil, or Hedge Basil (Calamintha Clinopodium) (sometimes called Hedge Calamint), is a straggling plant with somewhat weak-looking, though erect stems, rising to a height of a foot or 18 inches, and thickly covered with soft hairs.

Description

The shortly - stalked, egg shaped leaves, 1 to 2 inches long, are placedopposite to one another on the four-angled stem, the pairs being some distance apart. They are only slightly toothed at their edges and like the stem are downy with soft hairs.

The flowers, with tubular, lipped corollas of a pinkish color, are arranged on the stem in several crowded, bristly rings or whorls, at the points from which the leaf-stalks spring, and are in bloom from July to September.

The whole herb is aromatic and fragrant, with a faint Thyme-like odor, and like Calamint has been used to make an infusion for similar complaints.

The name of the species, Clinopodium, signifies 'bedfoot." An old writer says 'the tufts of the plant are like the knobs at the feet of a bed," but the comparison is not very obvious. By some botanists the plant has been described under the name of C. vulgare, but it is now assigned to the genus, Calamintha.

BAYBERRY

Botanical: Myrica cerifera (LINN.)
Family: N.O. Myricaceae
Synonyms: Wax Myrtle. Myrica. Candle Berry. Arbre à suif. Myricae Cortex. Tallow Shrub. Wachsgagle.
Parts Used: The dried bark of the root. The wax.
Habitat: Eastern North America.

Description

The only species of a useful family that is regarded as official, Myrica cerifera grows in thickets near swamps and marshes in the sand-belt near the Atlantic coast and on the shores of Lake Erie. Its height is from 3 to 8 feet, its leaves lanceolate, shining or resinous, dotted on both sides, its flowers unisexual without calyx or corolla, and its fruit small groups of globular berries, having numerous black grains crusted with greenish-white wax. These are persistent for two or three years. The leaves are very fragrant when rubbed.

The bark as found in commerce is in curved pieces from 1 to 7 inches long, covered with a thin, mottled layer, the cork beneath being smooth and red-brown. The fracture is reddish, granular, and slightly fibrous. The odor is aromatic, and the taste astringent, bitter, and very acrid. It should be separated from the fresh root by pounding, in late autumn, thoroughly dried, and when powdered, kept in darkened, well-closed vessels.

The wax was first introduced into medicinal use by Alexandre in 1722. It is removed from the berries by boiling them in water, on the top of which it floats. It melts at 47 to 49 C. (116.6 to 120.2 F.). It is harder and more brittle than beeswax. Candles made from it are aromatic, smokeless after snuffing, and very brittle. It makes a useful body for surgeon's soap plasters, and an aromatic and softening shaving lather. It has also been used for making sealing-wax. Four-fifths of this wax is soluble in hot alcohol, and boiling ether dissolves more than a quarter of its weight. Four pounds of berries yield about one pound of wax.

Constituents

There has been found in the bark of stem and root volatile oil, starch, lignin, gum, albumen, extractive, tannic and gallic acids, acrid and astringent resins, a red coloring substance, and an acid resembling saponin.

The wax (Myrtle Wax) consists of glycerides of stearic, palmitic and myristic acids, and a small quantity of oleaic acid.

Medicinal Action and Uses

Astringent and stimulant. In large doses emetic. It is useful in diarrhea, jaundice, scrofula, etc. Externally, the powdered bark is used as a stimulant to indolent ulcers, though in poultices it should be combined with elm. The decoction is good as a gargle and injection in chronic inflammation of the throat, leucorrhoea, uterine hemorrhage, etc. It is an excellent wash for the gums.

The powder is strongly sternutatory and excites coughing. Water in which the wax has been 'tried," when boiled to an extract, is regarded as a certain cure for dysentery, and the wax itself, being astringent and slightly narcotic, is valuable in severe dysentery and internal ulcerations.

Dosages

Of powder, 20 to 30 grains. Of decoction, 1 to 2 fluid ounces. Of alcoholic extract, or Myricin, 5 grains.

Other Species

MURICA GALE, SWEET GALE, ENGLISEI BOGMYRTLE, or DUTCH MYRTLE, the badge of the Campbells. The leaves of this species have been used in France as an emmenagogue and abortifacient, being formerly official under the name of Herba Myrti Rabantini, and containing a poisonous, volatile oil. The plant is bitter and astringent, and has been employed in the northern counties as a substitute for hops, and also mingled with bark for tanning, and dyeing wool yellow. The dried berries are put in broth and used as spices. Formerly it was much used in cottage practice, its properties being similar to those of M. cerifera. It is covered with a golden, aromatic dust, and is thus used to drive away insects. The leaves are infused like tea, especially in China, as a stomachic and cordial. See GALE (SWEET).

M. nagi. A glucoside, Myricitrin, resembling quercitrin, has been separated from the yellow coloring matter, or myricetin.

M. cordifolia, of the Cape of Good Hope, yields a wax which is said to be eaten by Hottentots.

M. Pensylvanica has roots with emetic properties.

A Brazilian species yields a waxy-resinous product called Tabocas combicurdo, which is used as a 'pick-me-up."

BAYBERRY is a synonym for the Wild Cinnamon or Pimenta acris of the West Indies and South America, which yields Bay Rum and oil of Bayberry.

BEAN, KIDNEY

Botanical: Phaceolus vulgaris
Family: N.O. Leguminaceae
Part Used: Dried ripe seeds.
Habitat: Native of Indies; cultivated all over Europe; also said to be found in ancient tombs in Peru.

History

This well-known plant has been cultivated from remote times. Because of the seeds close resemblance to the male testicle, the Egyptians made it an object of sacred worship and forbad its use as food. In Italy at the present day beans are distributed among the poor, on the anniversary of a death. The Jewish high priest is forbidden to eat beans on the day of Atonement.

Constituents

Starch and starchy fibrous matter, phaseoline, extractive albumen mucilage, pectic acid, legumin fatty matter, earthy salts, uncrystallizable sugar, inosite, sulphur.

Medicinal Action and Uses

When bruised and boiled with garlic Beans have cured otherwise uncurable coughs. If eaten raw they cause painful severe frontal headache, soreness and itching of the eyeball and pains in the epigastrium. The roots are dangerously narcotic.

BEARBERRY

Botanical: Arctostaphylos Uva-Ursi
Family: N.O. Ericaceae
Synonyms: Arbutus Uva-Ursi. Uva-Ursi.
Part Used: Leaves.

Habitat

The Bearberry (Arctostaphylos Uva-Ursi, Sprengel), a small shrub, with decumbent, much branched, irregular stems and evergreen leaves, is distributed over the greater part of the Northern Hemisphere, being found in the northern latitudes and high mountains of Europe, Asia and America. In the British Isles, it is common in Scotland, on heaths and barren places in hilly districts, especially in the Highlands, and extends south as far as Yorkshire; it grows also on the hills of the north-west of Ireland. In America it is distributed throughout Canada and the United States as far south as New Jersey and Wisconsin.

It is very nearly related to the Arbutus, and was formerly assigned to the same genus - in Green's Universal Herbal, 1832, it will be found under the name Arbutus Uva- Ursi - but it differs from Arbutus in having a smooth berry with five one-seeded stones, whereas the Arbutus has a rough fruit, each cell of the ovary being four to five seeded.

The only other British species assigned to the genus, Arctostaphylos, the Black Bearberry (A. alpina), with black berries, found on barren mountains in northern Scotland, and not at all in England, is the badge of the clan of Ross.

The generic name, derived from the Greek, and the Latin specific name, UvaUrsi, mean the same: the Bear's grape, and may have been given to the plant, either from the notion that bears eat the fruit with relish, or from its very rough, unpleasant flavor, which might have been considered only fit for bears.

Description

The much-branched trailing stems are short and woody, covered with a pale brown bark, scaling off in patches, and form thick masses, 1 to 2 feet long. The long shoots rise obliquely upward from the stems for a few inches and are covered with soft hairs

The evergreen leaves are of a leathery texture, from 1/2 inch to an inch long, like a spatula in form, being rounded at the apex and tapering gradually towards the base to a very short stalk or petiole. The margin is entire and slightly rolled back and the young leaves fringed with short hairs. The upper surface of the leaf is dark, shining green, the veins deeply impressed, the lower side is of a paler green, with the veins prominent and forming a coarse network. The leaves have no distinctive odor, but they have a very astringent and somewhat bitter taste.

The pretty waxy-looking flowers are in small, closely-crowded, drooping clusters, three to fifteen flowers together, at the ends of the branches of the preceding year, appearing in early summer, May - June, before the young leaves. The corolla, about two-thirds inch across, is urn-shaped, reddish white or white with a red lip, transparent at the base, contracted at the mouth, which is divided into four to five short reflexed, blunt teeth, which are hairy within. There are ten stamens, with chocolate-brown, awned anthers. The berry, which ripens in autumn, is about the size of a small currant, very bright red, smooth and glossy, with a tough skin enclosing an insipid mealy pulp, with five one-seeded stones.

Parts Used Medicinally

The dried leaves are the only part of the plant used in medicine. The British Pharmacopeia directs that the leaves should be obtained only from indigenous plants. They should be collected in September and October, only green leaves being selected and dried by exposure to gentle heat.

Leaves must be gathered only in fine weather, in the morning, after the dew has dried, any stained and insect-eaten leaves being rejected. Drying may be done in warm, sunny weather out-of-doors, but in half-shade, as leaves dried in the shade retain their color better than those dried in direct sun. They may be placed on wire sieves, or frames covered with wire or garden netting, at a height of 3 or 4 feet from the ground to ensure a current of air, and must be taken indoors to a dry room, or shed, before there is any risk of damp from dew or showers. The leaves should be spread in a single layer, preferably not touching, and may be turned during drying.

Failing sun, which in the case of leaves collected like the Bearberry in September and October cannot be relied on, any ordinary shed, fitted with racks and shelves can be used, provided it is ventilated near the roof and has a warm current of air, caused by a coke or anthracite stove. Empty glasshouses can readily be adapted into dryingsheds, especially if heated by pipes and the glass is shaded; ventilation is essential, and there must be no open tank in the house to cause steaming. For drying indoors, a warm sunny attic or loft may be employed, the window being left open by day, so that there is a current of air and the moist, hot air may escape: the door may also be left open. The leaves can be placed on coarse butter-cloth stented, i.e. if hooks are placed beneath the window and on the opposite wall, the buttercloth can be attached by rings sewn on each side of it, and hooked on so that it is stretched taut. The drying temperature should be from 70 to 100 degrees F.

All dried leaves should be packed away at once in wooden or tin boxes, in a dry place as otherwise they re-absorb moisture from the air.

Dried Bearberry leaves are usually quite smooth, and entirely free from the hairs that are present on the margins of the growing leaves and on the foot-stalks, which drop off during the drying process.

The commercial drug frequently consists of the entire plants, and therefore contains a large quantity of stems, but the latter should not be present, according to the official definition of the United States Pharmacopoeia, in greater amount than 5 per cent.

The leaves of other plants have been mistaken for Bearberry leaves, notably those of the Cowberry (Vaccinium Vitis-idaea) and of the Box (Buxus sempervirens), and have occasionally been used to adulterate the drug, but Bearberry leaves are readily distinguished by the characteristics given, viz. the spatulate outline, entire margin and rounded apex. Those of the Box have a notch cut out at the apex (emarginate) and have the epidermis loose and separable on the under surface of the leaf, and are, moreover, quite devoid of astringency. The leaves of the Cowberry may be distinguished by the glandular brown dots scattered over their under surface and the minute teeth on their margins. They have only a very slight astringent taste.

Constituents

The chief constituent of Bearberry leaves is a crystallizable glucoside named Arbutin. Other constituents are methyl-arbutin, ericolin (an ill-defined glucoside), ursone (a crystalline substance of resinous character), gallic acid, ellagic acid, a yellow coloring principle resembling quercetin, and probably also myricetin. Tannin is present to the extent of 6 to 7 per cent. On incineration, the leaves yield about 3 per cent. of ash.

Medicinal Action and Uses

In consequence of the powerful astringency of theleaves, Uva-Ursi has a place not only in all the old herbals, but also in the modern Pharmacopoeias. There are records that it was used in the thirteenth century by the Welsh 'Physicians of Myddfai." It was described by Clusius in 1601, and recommended for medicinal use in 1763 by Gerhard of Berlin and others. It had a place in the London Pharmacopoeia for the first time in 1788, though was probably in use long before. It is official in nearly all Pharmacopceias, some of which use the name Arbutus.

The usual form of administration is in the form of an infusion, which has a soothing as well as an astringent effect and marked diuretic action. Of great value in diseases of the bladder and kidneys, strengthening and imparting tone to the urinary passages. The diuretic action is due to the glucoside Arbutin, which is largely absorbed unchanged and is excreted by the kidneys. During its excretion, Arbutin exercises an antiseptic effect on the urinary mucous membrane: Bearberry leaves are, therefore, used in inflammatory diseases of the urinary tract, urethritis, cystisis, etc.

Besides the simple infusion (1 OZ. of the leaves

to 1 pint of boiling water), the combination of 1/2 oz. each of Uva-Ursi, Poplar Bark and Marshmallow root, infused in 1 pint of water for 20 minutes is used with advantage.

The tannin in the leaves is so abundant that they have been used for tanning leather in Sweden and Russia.

An ash-coloured dye is said to be obtained from the plant in Scandinavian countries.

The berries are only of use as food for grouse. Cattle, however, avoid the plant.

Allied Species

Manzanita, the leaves of A. glauca from California, are employed like Uva-Ursi.

The leaves of A. polifolia from Mexico and A. tomentosa (madrona) are also used in medicine.

BEARSFOOT (AMERICAN)

Botanical: Polymnia uvedalia (LINN.)
Family: N.O. Compositae
Synonyms: Uvedalia. Leaf Cup. Yellow Leaf Cup.
Part Used: Root.
Habitat: New York to Missouri and southward.

Description

A tall branching plant found growing in very rich soil the root is greyish brown in color and furrowed, bark thin, brittle and easily scales off, odourless, taste salty and slightly bitter.

Medicinal Action and Uses

Anodyne laxative and stimulant, valuable in malarial enlargements of the spleen, swollen glands and dyspepsia caused by the spleen. Of great use applied externally in stimulating the growth of the hair, and is an ingredient of many American hair ointments and lotions.

Dosage and Preparation

Fluid extract, dose, 15 to 60 minims.

BEDSTRAW, LADY'S

Botanical: Galium verum (LINN.)
Family: N.O. Rubiaceae
Synonyms: Our Lady's Bedstraw. Yellow Bedstraw. Maid's Hair. Petty Mugget. Cheese Renning. Cheese Rennet.

Habitat

Yellow Bedstraw is abundant on dry banks, chiefly near the sea. Its small, bright yellow flowers are closely clustered together in dense panicles at the tops of the wiry, square, upright stems, which are I to 3 feet high, and bear numerous very narrow, almost thread-like leaves, placed six to eight together in whorls. The flowers are in bloom in July and August.

The plant is scentless, but has an astringent, acidulous and bitterish taste.

The common English name of this plant, 'Our Lady's Bedstraw," is derived from its use in former days, even by ladies of rank, for stuffing beds.

Dr. Fernie tells us that because of its bright yellow blossoms, this herb is also named 'Maid's Hair," for in Henry VIII's reign 'maydens did wear silken callis to keep in order their hayre made yellow with dye." It has also been known as 'Petty Mugget," from the French petit muguet, a little dandy.

The plant has the property of curdling milk, hence another of its popular names " Cheese Rennet." It was called " Cheese Renning' in the sixteenth century, and Gerard says (quoting from Matthiolus, a famous commentator of Dioscorides), 'the people of Thuscane do use it to turne their milks and the cheese, which they make of sheepes and goates milke, might be the sweeter and more pleasant to taste. The people in Cheshire especially about Nantwich, where the best cheese is made, do use it in their rennet, esteeming greatly of that cheese above other made without it." The rich color of this cheese was probably originally derived from this plant, though it is now obtained from annatto.

The Highlanders also made special use of Yellow Bedstraw to curdle milk and color their cheese, and it has been used in Gloucestershire for the same purpose, either alone or with the juice of the stinging-nettle.

The name of this genus, Galium, from the Greek word gala, milk, is supposed to have been given from this property of the plants which is shared more or less by most of the group.

Medicinal Action and Uses

Galium verum contains the same chemical principles as G. aparine.

It is still used to a limited degree as a popular remedy in gravel, stone and urinary diseases.

It was formerly highly esteemed as a remedy in epilepsy and hysteria, and was applied externally in cutaneous eruptions, in the form either of the recently expressed juice, or of a decoction from the fresh plant.

'An ointment," says Gerard, 'is prepared which is good for anointing the weary traveller."

Culpepper recommends the decoction to stop inward bleeding and bleeding at the nose, and to heal all inward wounds generally.

The flowering tips, distilled with water, are stated to yield an acid liquor which forms a pleasant summer drink.

The flowers of this species and still more those of G. elatum, an allied non-British species, are considered in France a remedy for epilepsy.

The Yellow Bedstraw can furnish a red dye, like its ally, the Madder of the Continent, Rubia tinctorum. It has been cultivated for the purpose, but with little or no profit, as the roots are too small, though it has been used in the Hebrides for dyeing woollen stuffs red. When attempts have been made to cultivate it, the produce per acre has occasionally exceeded 12 cwt., which is considered an average crop for Madder, but the roots do not yield as much in proportion, and its cultivation has never been undertaken on a very large scale, the crops having been found too small to pay under ordinary circumstances. The same cultivation is necessary as for Madder, the plant requiring a deep, light, but rich loam to succeed well, and the land must be well trenched an manured before planting. The running roots are to be planted, though it may be raised from seed, a plan that has also sometimes been adopted with Madder.

The stem and leaves of this Galium yield good yellow dye, which has been used to great extent in Ireland.

Several other species of this genus have roots capable of yielding red or yellow dye but none of them have been practical applied, their produce being too small to admit of their successful cultivation as dyed plants.

BEECH

Botanical: Fagus sylvatica
Family: N.O. Corylaceae
Synonyms: Buche. Buke. Boke. Bog. Bok. Buk.
Hetre. Faggio. Faya. Haya. Fagos.
Part Used: The oil of the nuts.
Habitat: Europe, including Britain. (Indigenous only in England.) Armenia, Palestine, Asia Minor Tanan.

History

The common name of the Beech tree, found in varying forms throughout the Teutonic dialects, means, with difference of gender, either 'a book' or 'a beech," the Runic tablets, or early books, having been made of this wood. Fagus is from a Greek word meaning 'to eat," referring to the edible character of the Beechmast.

The Beech is one of the largest British trees, especially on chalky and sandy soil. In England it may grow to 140 feet in height, or spread to 130 feet in diameter, with a trunk 21 feet in girth. As the wood is brittle and short-grained, it is not well suited for purposes where strength and durability are required. One of the principal objections to it is that it is liable to be perforated by a small beetle. Its chief uses are for panels for carriages, carpenter's planes, stonemason's mallets wooden bowls, granary shovels, boot-lasts, sabots, and for chair-making, small articles in turnery, also for making charcoal for color manufacturers, and gunpowder. On the Continent Beech is used for parquet flooring, wood pavement and bent-wood furniture, and very extensively as fuel for domestic heating, as its heating power surpasses that of most other timber.

Owing to the capacity of its root system for assisting in the circulation of air throughout the soil, and by the amount of potash in the leaves, Beech trees conserve the productive capacity of the soil better than any other kind of tree, and improve the growth of other trees when planted with them.

Fences of young Beech trees may be employed with advantage in flower gardens, as their leaves generally remain on the branches during the winter and screen the young plants .

The nuts of Beech, called 'mast," are chiefly used in England as food for park deer. In other countries they are valued for feeding farm animals: in France for feeding swine and fattening domestic poultry, especially turkeys, and pigs which are turned into Beech woods to utilize the fallen mast. Beech mast has even been used as human food in time of distress or famine. Horses, however, should not be fed on it.

Well-ripened mast yields from 17 to 20 per cent. of a non-drying oil - similar to hazel and Cotton-seed oils - and is used in European countries for cooking, as well as for burning, and in Silesia as a substitute for butter. The cake left when the oil has been pressed out may be used as a cattle food.

During the War an attempt was made in Germany to use Beech leaves as a substitute for tobacco, and a mixture was served to the army, but proved a failure.

Constituents

The wood ash of the Beech affords a large proportion of potash. The oil of the nuts occupies a position in the fixed oils between the vegetable non-drying and the true drying oils. Like the Cotton-seed oils, it forms more or less elaidin on treatment with nitrous acid or mercuric nitrate, but does not become wholly solidified. Beech tar is completely soluble in 95 per cent. acetic acid. Turpentine oil, chloroform and absolute ether do not entirely dissolve it. The petroleum ether is not coloured by copper acetate solution. Choline is present in the seeds.

Medicinal Uses

The tar is stimulating and antiseptic, used internally as a stimulating expectorant in chronic bronchitis, or externally as an application in various skin diseases.

The oil is used in the same ways as the other fixed oils of its class.

Other Species

BEECH DROPS (OROBANCHE VIRGINIANA,EPIFAGUS VIRGINIANA, BROOM RAPE, CANCER ROOT), a parasite on Beech tree roots, has a bitter, nauseous, astringent taste, diminished by drying. It is given internally in bowel affections, and is reputed to cure cancer, though this is doubtful As a local application to wounds or ulcers it will arrest gangrene. It appears to act upon the capillary system like the tincture of muriate of iron.

ALBANY BEECH DROPS (Pterospora Andromeda) is a rare plant of North America valuable as a sedative diaphoretic in typhus, pleurisy and erysipelas

COPPER-BEECH (F. sylvatica var. purpurea). The leaves of this species may be used like those of the Red-leaved Hazel for the extraction of anthocyan pigment.

BEETROOTS

Family: N.O. Chenopodiaceae
Synonyms: Spinach Beet. Sea Beet. Garden Beet. White Beet. Mangel Wurzel.
Parts Used: Leaves, root.

Description

Beta vulgaris (Linn.) is a native of South Europe,

extensively cultivated as an article of food and especially for the production of sugar, and presents many varieties.

It is derived from the Sea Beet (B. maritima, Linn.), which grows wild on the coasts of Europe, North Africa and Asia, as far as India, and is found in muddy maritime marshes in many parts of England, a tall, succulent plant, about 2 feet high, with large, fleshy, glossy leaves, angular stems and numerous leafy spikes of green flowers, much like those of the Stinking Goosefoot.

The lower leaves, when boiled, are quite equal in taste to Spinach, and the leaf-stalks and midrib of a cultivated form, the Spinach Beet (B. vulgaris, var. cicla), are sometimes stewed, under the name of Swiss Chard (being the Poirée à Carde of the French, with whom it is served as Sea Kale or Asparagus). This white-rooted Beet is also cultivated for its leaves, which are put into soups, or used as spinach, and in France are often mixed with sorrel, to lessen its acidity. It is also largely used as a decorative plant for its large handsome leaves, blood red or variegated in color. Its root, thoughcontaining almost as much sugar as the red Garden Beet, neither looks so appetizing nor tastes so well.

The Mangel Wurzel, or Mangold, also a variety of the Beet, too coarse for table use, is good for cattle, who thrive excellently upon this diet, both its leaves and roots affording an abundance of valuable and nutritious food.

In its uncultivated form, the root of the Sea Beet is coarse and unfit for food, nor has any use been made of the plant medicinally, but the Garden Beet has been cultivated from very remote times as a salad plant and for general use as a vegetable. It was so appreciated by the ancients, that it is recorded that it was offered on silver to Apollo in his temple at Delphi.

Constituents

The root contains about a tenth portion of pure sugar, which is one of the glucoses or fruit sugars and is very wholesome. It is softer than cane sugar and does not crystallize as well as the latter. There is a treacle principle in it, but this renders it all the more nutritious. Canesugar has to be converted by the digestive juices into fruit sugar, before the body can absorb it, but the sugar present in the Beetroot is already in the more easily assimilated form, thus making the Beet a valuable food. Its sugar is a force-giver and an energy creator, a source of vitality to the human body. Besides its tenth portion of pure sugar, Beetroot has as much as a third of its weight in starch and gum.

The Beet makes an appetizing vegetable, plain boiled, stewed, or baked and a good pickle, and in Russia forms an appetizing soup - called Bortsch - the red root in this case being made to exude all its juice into a rich, white stock.

A pleasant wine can be made from the roots and an equally good domestic ale has also been brewed from Mangolds. A considerable amount of alcohol can be obtained by distillation.

Although modern medicine disregards the Beet, of old it was considered to have distinct remedial properties.

Medicinal Action and Uses

The juice of the White Beet was stated to be 'of a cleansing, digestive quality," to open obstructions of the liver and spleen, and, says Culpepper, 'good for the headache and swimmings therein and all affections of the brain." Also,

'effectual against all venomous creatures and applied upon the temples, it stayeth inflammations in the eyes, it helpeth burnings, being used without oil and with a little alum put to it is good for St. Anthonys Fire. It is good for all weals, pushes, blisters and blains in the skin: the decoction in water and vinegar healeth the itch if bathed therewith and cleanseth the head of dandriff, scurf and dry scabs and relieves running sores and ulcers and is much commended against baldness and shedding the hair."

The juice of the Red Beetroot was recommended 'to stay the bloody flux' and 'to help the yellow jaundice," also the juice 'put into the nostrils, purgeth the head, helpeth the noise in the ears and the toothache."

The Sugar Beet, or White Beet, is a selected form of the ordinary red-rooted Garden Beet and is now the chief source of our sugar; as food for animals, it has been preferred to turnips and carrots.

About 1760, the Berlin apothecary Marggraff obtained in his laboratory by means of alcohol, 6.2 per cent. of sugar from a white variety of Beet and 4.5 per cent. from a red variety. At the present day, as a result of careful study of many years, improvement of cultivation, careful selection of seed and suitable manuring, especially with nitrate of soda, the average Beet worked up contains 7 per cent. of fibre and 92 per cent. of juice. The average yield of its weight in sugar was stated in 1910 to be 12.79 per cent. in Germany and 11.6 per cent. in France.

In Great Britain, the cultivation of Beet for sugar was first seriously undertaken in Essex in 1910, as the result of careful consideration during several years and since the War. The Beet Sugar Industry, aided by Government subsidy, can now be regarded as on a permanent basis. In 1926-7, no less than fourteen factories were handling the Beet crops, mostly in Norfolk, Cambridgeshire, Lincolnshire and Nottinghamshire, producing large quantities of white refined sugar.

BENNE

Botanical: Sesamum Indicum (LINN.)
Family: N.O. Pedaliaccac
Synonyms: Gingilly, Teel.
Parts Used: Leaves, seeds.
Habitat: America, Southern States, and India. Cultivated in Africa and Asia.

Description

An annual plant with branching stem 4 or 5 feet high, leaves opposite, petiolate, shape varies; flower reddish white, single, on short peduncles in axils of leaves; fruit an oblong capsule with small oval yellowish seeds. The genus Sesamum comprises ten or twelve species. In India two species occur wild, it is cultivated in the U.S.A. and in the West Indies; it grows as far north as Philadelphia.

Constituents

The seeds by expression yield a fixed oil consisting essentially of the glycerides of oleic and linoleic acids with small preparations of stearin, palmitin and myristin. Sesamin, another constituent of the oil, may be obtained in long crystalline needles melting at 118 degrees F., insoluble in water, light petroleum, ether alkaloids and mineral acids, easily soluble in chloroform, benzine, and glacial acetic acid. Liquid fatty acids are present to about 70 per cent., solid fatty acids 12 to 14 per cent.

Medicinal Action and Uses

Sesame oil is used in the preparation of Iodinol and Brominol, which are employed for external internal or subcutaneous use. The best qualities of the oil are largely used in the manufacture of margarine. Sesame oil may be used as a substitute for Olive oil in making the official liniments, ointments and plasters in India and the African, Eastern, and North America Colonies. The negroes use the seed as food, boiling them for broth and making them into puddings and other dishes. The leaves which abound in gummy matter when mixed with water form a rich bland mucilage used in infantile cholera, diarrhea, dysentery, catarrh and bladder troubles, acute cystitis and strangury. The oil is said to be laxative and to promote menstruation.

Dosage

1 or 2 full-sized leaves stirred in 1/2 pint of cold water, or in hot water if the dried leaves are used.

BENZOIN

Botanical: Styrax benzoin (DRY.)
Family: N.O. Styraceae
Synonyms: Gum Benzoin. Gun Benjamin. Siam Benzoin. Sumatra Benzoin.
Part Used: Resin.
Habitat: Siam, Sumatra and Java.

Description

Benzoin is a balsamic resin. Normally the trees do not produce it or any substance analogous to it, but the infliction of a wound sufficiently severe to injure the cambium results in the formation of numerous oleoresin ducts in which the secretion is produced, it is, therefore, a pathological product. The trunk of the tree is hacked with an axe, and after a time the liquid Benzoin either accumulates beneath the bark or exudes from the incisions. When it has sufficiently hardened it is collected and exported, either in the form of loose pieces (tears) or in masses packed in oblong boxes or in tins; several varieties are known, but Siam and Sumatra Benzoins are the most important. The incisions are made when the tree is seven years old, and in Sumatra each tree yields about 3 lb. annually for ten or twelve years. The first three years' collections give the finest Benzoin; after that the runnings are known as the 'belly," and finally the tree is cut down and the resin scraped out, this being termed the 'foot." Siam Benzoin externally is reddish yellow, internally milky white, has an agreeable odor, recalling vanilla, contains benzoic acid but not cinnamic acid. Sumatra Benzoin is always in blocks of a dull reddish or greyish-brown color. Fine qualities have a strong storax-like odor, quite distinct from the vanilla odor of the Siamese variety. Sumatra Benzoin contains cinnamic acid.

Constituents

The chief constituent of Siam Benzoin is benzoic acid (up to 38 per cent.), partly free and partly combined with benzoresinol and siaresinotannol; it also contains vanillin and an oily aromatic liquid. When quite pure it should be entirely soluble in alcohol and yield only traces of ash. Sumatra benzoin contains 18 per cent. or more of benzoic acid and about 20 per cent. of cinnamic acid the latter partly free and partly combined with benzoresinol and sumarisinotannol; it also contains 1 per cent. of vanillin, styrol, styracin, phenyl-prophyl cinnamate and benzaldehyde, all of which combine to produce its characteristic odor.

Medicinal Action and Uses

It is used externally in the form of a tincture, diluted with water as a mild stimulant and antiseptic in irritable conditions of the skin. It acts as a carminative when taken internally is rapidly absorbed, and mildly expectorant diuretic and antiseptic to the urinary passages. In the form of Compound Tincture of Benzoin, it is used as an inhalant with steam in laryngitis and bronchitis. It is a preservative of fats, and is used for that purpose in Adips Benzoatus.

Dosages and Preparations

Benzoic Acid B.P., 5 to 15 grains. Compound Tincture of Benzoin, B.P. and U.S.P., 1/2 to 1 drachm. Compound Tincture of Camphor, B.P. (paregoric) poison, 1/2 to 1 drachm. Tincture of Benzoin, B.P.C. 1/2 to 1 drachm. Tincture of Benzoin, U.S.P., 15 minims.

BERGAMOT

Botanical: Monarda didyma
Family: N.O. Rustaceae
Synonyms: Scarlet Monarda. Oswego Tea. Bee Balm.

So far, Monarda punctata is considered the only plant indigenous to North America which can be looked upon as a fruitful source of Thymol, though another American swamp plant, closely allied to it, M. didyma, the Scarlet Monarda, is said to yield an oil of similar composition, though not to the same degree.

Description

This species, on account of its aromatic odor, has become a favorite in our gardens. It has showy, scarlet flowers in large heads or whorls at the top of the stem, supported by leafy bracts, the leaflets of which are of a pale-green color tinged with red. Its square, grooved and hard stems rise about 2 feet high, and the leaves which it bears in pairs are rather rough on both surfaces.

The whole plant is strongly impregnated with a delightful fragrance; even after the darkly-coloured leaves have died away, the surface rootlets give off the pleasant smell by which the plant has earned its common name 'Bergamot," it being reminiscent of the aroma of the Bergamot Orange.

It is known in America as 'Oswego Tea," because an infusion of its young leaves used to form a common beverage in many parts of the United States.

It is also sometimes called 'Bee Balm," as bees are fond of its blossoms, which secrete much nectar.

It delights in a moist, light soil, and in a situation where the plants have only the morning sun, where they will continue in flower longer than those which are exposed to the full sun. It is a very ornamental plant and readily propagated by its creeping roots and by slips or cuttings, which, if planted in a shady corner in May, will take root in the same manner as the other Mints.

BETEL

Botanical: Piper betel (LINN.)
Family: N.O. Peperaceae
Synonyms: Chavica Betel. Artanthe Hixagona.
Part Used: The leaves.
Habitat: India, Malaya and Java.

Description

The Betel plant is indigenous throughout the Indian Malay region and also cultivated in Madagascar, Bourbon and the West Indies. It is a climbing shrub and is trained on poles or trellis in a hot but shady situation. The leaves are pressed together and dried, sometimes being sewn up together in packets for commerce.

Constituents

The chief constituent of the leaves is a volatile oil varying in the leaves from different countries and known as Betel oil. It contains two phenols, betelphenol (chavibetol) and chavicol. Cadinene has also been found. The best oil is a clear yellow color obtained from the fresh leaves. The Indians use the leaves as a masticatory (the taste being warm, aromatic and bitter), together with scraped areca nut and lime.

Medicinal Action and Uses

The leaves are stimulant antiseptic and sialogogue; the oil is an active local stimulant used in the treatment of respiratory catarrhs as a local application or gargle, also as an inhalant in diphtheria. In India the leaves are used as a counter-irritant to suppress the secretion of milk in mammary abscesses. The juice of 4 leaves is equivalent in power to one drop of the oil.

Dosage

Betel oil, 1 to 2 minims.

BETHROOT

Botanical: Trillium pendulum (WILLD.)
Trillium erectum (LINN.)
Family: N.O. Liliaceae
Synonyms: Indian Shamrock. Birthroot. Lamb's Quarters. Wake-Robin. Indian Balm. Ground Lily.
Parts Used: The dried root and rhizome. The leaves.
Habitat: Middle and Western United States.

Description

All the seventeen species of the genus are North American plants, distinguished by their possession of three green, persistent sepals and three larger withering petals, of varying color.

Trillium erectum or T. pendulum, perennial, smooth herb, has an erect stem of from 10 to 15 inches in height, bearing three leaves, broad, almost rhomboid, and drooping white flowers, terminal and solitary. Grows in the rich soil of damp and shady woodlands, flowering in May and June.

The official description of the rhizome is 'oblique, globular, oblong or obconical, truncate below., terminated by a small bud surrounded by a sheath of scarious leaf bases annulated by leaf scars and fissured by stem scars. It is from 0.6 to 5 cm. in length, and from 0.6 to 3.5 cm. in width, more or less compressed laterally, rootlet scars in several concentrie rows on the underside in the upper portions. Externally yellowish to reddish brown; internally of a pale yellow; fracture somewhat uneven with a more or less spongy appearance. Odor distinct; taste bitter and acrid, with a sensation of warmth in the throat, and when chewed causing an increased flow of saliva. Trillium yields not more than 5 per cent. of ash."

The drug is one of those prepared by the Shakers.

Constituents

There have been found in it volatile and fixed oils, tannic acid, saponin, a glucoside resembling convallamarin, an acid crystalline principle coloured brown tinged with purple by sulphuric acid, and light green with sulphuric acid and potassium dichromate, gum, resin, and much starch.

The fluid extract is an ingredient in Compound Elixir of Viburnum Opulus.

Professor E. S. Wayne isolated the active principle, calling it Trilline, but the preparation sold under that name has no medicinal value, while the Trilline of Professor Wayne has not been used.

Medicinal Action and Uses

Is said to have been in use among the aborigines and early settlers of North America. It is antiseptic, astringent and tonic expectorant, being used principally in hemorrhages, to promote parturition, and externally, usually in the form of a poultice, as a local irritant in skin diseases, or to restrain gangrene.

The leaves, boiled in lard, are sometimes applied to ulcers and tumors.

The roots may be boiled in milk, when they are helpful in diarrhea and dysentery.

Dosages

Of powdered root, a drachm three times a day. Of fluid extract, 30 minims, as astringent and tonic expectorant. Trilline, 2 to 4 grains.

Other Species

Most of the genus Trillium have medicinal properties, especially T. erythrocarpum, T. grandiflorum, T. sessile, and T. nivale.

The acrid species are useful in fevers and chronic affections of the air-passages. Merely smelling the freshly-exposed surface of the red Beth roots will check bleeding from the nose.

BETONY, WOOD

Botanical: Stachys Betonica (BENTH.), Betonica officinalis (LINN.)
Family N.O. Labiatae
Synonym: Bishopswort.
Part Used: Herb.

Habitat

It is a pretty woodland plant, met with frequently throughout England, but by no means common in Scotland. Though generally growing in woods and copses, it is occasionally to be found in more open situations, and amongst the tangled growths on heaths and moors.

There are five species of Stachys growing wild in this country - the once much-valued Betony (S. Betonica); the Marsh Stachys, or Clown's Woundwort (S. palustris); the true Woundwort (S. Germanica), a doubtful native, occurring occasionally on limestone soils in England, but very common on the Continent, where the dense covering of its leaves was at one time in rustic surgery employed in the place of lint for dressing wounds, the low-creeping Field Stachys (S. arvensis); and the Hedge Stachys, or Hedge Woundwort (S. sylvatica), perhaps the commonest of them all.

History

The Wood Betony (S. Betonica according to present-day nomenclature, though nemed Betonica officinalis, by Linnaeus) was held in high repute not only in the Middle Ages, but also by the Greeks who extolled its qualities. An old Italian proverb, " Sell your coat and buy Betony," and 'He has as many virtues as Betony," a saying of the Spaniards, show what value was placed on its remedial properties. Antonius Musa, chief physician to the Emperor Augustus, wrote a long treatise, showing it was a certain cure for no less than fortyseven diseases.

Throughout the centuries, faith in its virtues as a panacea for all ills was thoroughly ingrained in the popular estimation. It was largely cultivated in the physic gardens, both of the apothecaries and the monasteries, and may still be found growing about the sites of these ancient buildings. Robert Turner, a physician writing in the latter half of the seventeenth century, recounts nearly thirty complaints for which Betony was considered efficacious, and adds, 'I shall conclude with the words I have found in an old manuscript under the virtues of it: "More than all this have been proved of Betony." "

In addition to its medicinal virtues, Betony was endowed with power against evil spirits. On this account, it was carefully planted in churchyards and hung about the neck as an amulet or charm, sanctifying, as Erasmus tells us, 'those that carried it about them," and being also 'good against fearful visions' and an efficacious means of 'driving away devils and despair." An old writer, Apelius, says:

'It is good whether for the man's soul or for his body; it shields him against visions and dreams, and the wort is very wholesome, and thus thou shalt gather it, in the month of August without the use of iron; and when thou hast gathered it, shake the mold till nought of it cleave thereon, and then dry it in the shade very thoroughly, and with its root altogether reduce it to dust: then use it and take of it when thou needst."

Many extravagant superstitions grew up round Betony, one, of very ancient date, was that serpents would fight and kill each other if placed within a ring composed of it; and others declared that even wild beasts recognized its efficacy and used it if wounded, and that stags, if wounded with a dart, would search out Betony, and, eating it, be cured.

Description

It comes up year after year from a thickish, woody root. The stems rise to a height of from 1 to 2 feet, and are slender, square and furrowed. They bear at wide intervals a few pairs of oblong, stalkless leaves, 2 to 3 inches long, and about 3/4 to 1 inch broad, with roughly indented margins in other plants of this group, the pairs of leaves arise on alternate sides of the stem. The majority of the leaves, however, spring from the root and these are larger, on long stalks and of a drawn-out, heart shape. All the leaves are rough to the touch and are also fringed with short, fine hairs; their whole surface is dotted with glands containing a bitter, aromatic oil.

At the top of the stem are the two-lipped flowers of a very rich purplish-red, arranged in dense rings or whorls, which together form short spikes. Then there is a break and a piece of bare stem, with two or four oblong, stalkless leaves and then more flowers, the whole forming what is termed an interrupted spike, a characteristic peculiarity by which Wood Betony is known from all other labiate flowers. The cup or calyx of each flower is crowned by five sharp points, each representing a sepal. The corolla is a long tube ending in two lips, the upper lip slightly arched, the lower one flat, of three equal lobes. The four stamens lie in two pairs within the arch of the upper lip, one pair longer than the other, and shed their pollen on to the back of bee visitors who come to drink the honey in the tube, and thus unconsciously effect the fertilization of the next flower they visit, by carrying to it this pollen that has been dusted upon them. After fertilization, four brown, smooth three-cornered nutlets are developed. The flowers are in bloom during July and August.

The common name of this plant is said by Pliny to have been first Vettonica, from the Vettones a people of Spain, but modern authors resolve the word into the primitive or Celtic form of bew (a head) and ton (good), it being good for complaints in the head. It has sometimes, also, been called Bishopswort, the reason for which is not evident. The name of the genus, Stachys, is a Greek word, signifying a spike, from the mode of flowering.

Part Used Medicinally

The whole herb, collected from wild plants in July, when at their best, and dried.

Collect only on a fine day, in the morning, but after the dew has been dried by the sun, Cut off the stems shortly above the root (which is no longer used, as in olden days); strip off all discoloured or insect-eaten leaves, and as the stems are fairly firm, tie them up in bunches of about six stalks together, spread out fanwise, so that the air can penetrate to them all, and hang them over strings to dry, either in half-shade, in the open air, or in the drying room. The bunches should be of uniform sizes to facilitate packing when dry. If dried out-of-doors, take in before there is any risk of becoming damp from dew or showers. For drying indoors, a warm, sunny attic or loft may be employed, the window being left open by day, so that there is a current of air, and the moist, hot air may escape: the door may also be left open. The temperature should be from 70 to 100 degrees F. Failing sun any ordinary shed, fitted with racks and shelves, can be used as a drying room, provided it is ventilated near the roof and has a warm current of air, caused by an ordinary coke or anthracite stove. The important point in drying is rapidity and the avoidance of steaming: the quicker the process of drying, the more even the color obtained, making the product more saleable.

All dried leaves and herbs should be packed away at once in wooden boxes or tins in a dry place, as otherwise they re-absorb about 12 per cent. of moisture from the air, and are liable to become mouldy. The herbs should not be pressed down heavily when packing, or they will tend to crumble.

Medicinal Action and Uses

Betony was once the sovereign remedy for all maladies of the head, and its properties as a nervine and tonic are still acknowledged, though it is more frequently employed in combination with other nervines than alone. It is useful in hysteria, palpitations pain in the head and face, neuralgia and all nervous affections. In the Medicina Britannica (1666) we read: 'I have known the most obstinate headaches cured by daily breakfasting for a month or six weeks on a decoction of Betony made with new milk and strained."

As an aromatic, it has also astringent and alterative action, and combined with other remedies is used as a tonic in dyspepsia and as an alterative in rheumatism, scrofula and impurities of the blood.

The weak infusion forms a very acceptable substitute for tea, and in this way is extensively used in many localities. It has somewhat the taste of tea and all the good qualities of it, without the bad ones. To make Betony tea, pour a pint of boiling water on an ounce of the dried herb. A wine glassful of this decoction three times a dayproves a benefit against languid nervous headaches.

The dried herb may also be smoked as tobacco, combined with Eyebright and Coltsfoot, for relieving headache.

A pinch of the powdered herb will provoke violent sneezing. The dried leaves formed an ingredient in Rowley's British Herb Snuff, which was at one time quite famous for headaches.

The fresh leaves are said to have an intoxicating effect. They have been used to dye wool a fine yellow.

Gerard tells us, among other uses, that Betony,

'preserveth the lives and bodies of men from the danger of epidemical diseases. It helpeth those that loathe and cannot digest their food. It is used either dry or green either the root or herb - or the flowers, drunk in broth or meat or made into conserve syrup, water, electuary or powder - as everyone may best frame themselves, or as time or season requires."

He proceeds to say that the herb cures the jaundice, falling sickness, palsy, convulsions, gout, dropsy and head troubles, and that 'the powder mixed with honey is no less available for all sorts of colds or cough, wheezing, of shortness of breath and consumption," also that 'the decoction made with mead and Pennyroyal is good for putrid agues," and made in wine is good as a vermifuge, 'and also removes obstructions of the spleen and liver." Again,

'the decoction with wine gargled in the mouth easeth the toothache.... It is a cure for the bites of mad dogs.... A dram of the powder taken with a little honey in some vinegar is good for refreshing those that are wearied by travel. It stayeth bleeding at the nose and mouth, and helpeth those that spit blood, and is good for those that have a rupture and are bruised. The green herb bruised, or the juice, applied to any inward hurt, or outward wound in body or head will quickly heal and close it up. It will draw forth any broken bone or splinter, thorn or other thing gotten into the flesh, also healeth old sores or ulcers and boils. The root is displeasing both to taste and stomach, whereas the leaves and flowers by their sweet and spicy taste, comfort both in meat and medicine."

BILBERRY

Botanical: Vaccinium myrtillus (LINN.)
Family: N.O. Vacciniaceae
Synonyms: Whortleberry. Black Whortles. Whinberry. Trackleberry. Huckleberry. Hurts. Bleaberry. Hurtleberry. Airelle. Vaccinium Frondosum. Blueberries.
Parts Used: The ripe fruit. The leaves.
Habitat: Europe, including Britain, Siberia and Barbary.

Description

V. myrtillus grows abundantly in our heathy and mountainous districts, a small branched shrub, with wiry angular branches, rarely over a foot high, bearing globular wax-like flowers and black berries, which are covered when quite ripe with a delicate grey bloom, hence its name in Scotland, 'Blea-berry," from an old North Countryword, 'blae," meaning livid or bluish. The name Bilberry (by some old writers 'Bulberry') is derived from the Danish 'bollebar," meaning dark berry. There is a variety with white fruits.

The leathery leaves (in form somewhat like those of the myrtle, hence its specific name) are at first rosy, then yellowish-green, and in autumn turn red and are very ornamental. They have been utilized to adulterate tea.

Bilberries flourish best on high grounds, being therefore more abundant in the north and west than in the south and east of England: they are absent from the low-lying Cambridgeshire and Suffolk, but on the Surrey hills, where they are called 'Hurts," cover the ground for miles.

The fruit is globular, with a flat top, about the size of a black currant. When eaten raw, they have a slightly acid flavor. When cooked, however, with sugar, they make an excellent preserve. Gerard tells us that 'the people of Cheshire do eate the black whortles in creame and milke as in these southern parts we eate strawberries." On the Continent, they are often employed for coloring wine.

Stewed with a little sugar and lemon peel in an open tart, Bilberries make a very enjoyable dish. Before the War, immense quantities of them were imported annually from Holland, Germany and Scandinavia. They were used mainly by pastrycooks and restaurant-keepers.

Owing to its rich juice, the Bilberry can be used with the least quantity of sugar in making jam: half a pound of sugar to the pound of berries is sufficient if the preserve is to be eaten soon. The minuteness of the seeds makes them more suitable for jam than currants.

Constituents

Quinic acid is found in the leaves, and a little tannin. Triturated with water they yield a liquid which, filtered and assayed with sulphate of iron, becomes a beautiful green, first of all transparent, then giving a green precipitate.

The fruits contain sugar, etc.

Medicinal Action and Uses

The leaves can be used in the same way as those of UvaUrsi. The fruits are astringent, and are especially valuable in diarrhea and dysentery, in the form of syrup. The ancients used them largely, and Dioscorides spoke highly of them. They are also used for discharges, and as antigalactagogues. A decoction of the leaves or bark of the root may be used as a local application to ulcers, and in ulceration of the mouth and throat.

The fruit is helpful in scurvy and urinary complaints, and when bruised with the roots and steeped in gin has diuretic properties valuable in dropsy and gravel. A tea made of the leaves is also a remedy for diabetes if taken for a prolonged period.

Dosages

Of powder of the berries, 4 grammes. Of syrup, 60 grammes to a litre of water. Of fluid extract, 1/2 to

2 drachms.

Other Species

V. arboreum, or Farkleberry. This is the most astringent variety, and both berries and root-bark may be used internally for diarrhea, chronic dysentery, etc. The infusion is valuable as a local application in sore throat, chronic ophthalmia, leucorrhoea, etc.

V. resinosum, V. damusum, and V. gorymbosum have properties resembling those of V. myrtillus.

The Bog Bilberry (V. uliginosum) is a smaller, less erect plant, with round stems and untoothed leaves, greyish green beneath. Both flowers and berries are smaller than those of the common Bilberry. This kind is quite absent in the south and only to be found in mountain bogs and moist copses, in Scotland, Durham and Westmorland.

The berries of both species are a favorite food of birds.

The 'Huckleberry' of North America, so widely appreciated there, is our Bilberry - the name being an obvious corruption of 'Whortleberry."

Recipe

Recipe for Bilberry Jam

Put 3 lb. of clean, fresh fruit in a preserving pan with 1 1/2 lb. of sugar and about 1 cupful of water and bring to the boil. Then boil rapidly for 40 minutes. Apple juice made from windfalls and peelings, instead of the water, improves this jam. To make apple juice, cover the apples with water, stew down, and strain the juice through thick muslin. Blackberries may also be added to this mixture.

If the jam is to be kept long it must be bottled hot in screw-top jars, or, if tied down in the ordinary way, more sugar must be added.

Bilberry juice yields a clear, dark-blue or purple dye that has been much used in the dyeing of wool and the picking of berries for this purpose, as well as for food, constitutes a summer industry in the 'Hurts' districts. Owing to the shortage of the aniline dyestuffs formerly imported from Germany, Bilberries were eagerly bought up at high prices by dye manufacturers during the War, so that in 1917 and 1918 a large proportion of the Bilberry crop was not available for jam-making, as the dyers were scouring the country for the little blue-black berries.

BINDWEEDS

Family: N.O. Convolvulaciae

Uses

All the Convolvulus family have purgative properties in a greater or less degree. Convolvulus Scammonia is used in homeopathy. A tincture is made from the gum resin. The drugs known as Jalap and Scammony are produced from the Jalap Bindweed and the C. Scammonia.

There are three kinds of Convolvulus or Bindweed in our native flora: the Field, Hedge, and the Sea Convolvulus. We have also many southern species growing in our gardens, chief among which are the handsome Morning Glory (Ipomea purpurea Linn.), C. purpureus, a native of Asia and America, with large purple flowers, and the pretty little annual, C. minor, a native of southern Europe, its cheerful flowers a combination of blue, yellow and white.

BINDWEED, GREATER

Botanical: Convolvulus sepium

Synonyms: Hedge Convolvulus. Old Man's Night Cap. Hooded Bindweed. Bearbind.

Habitat

The Greater Bindweed, or Hedge Convolvulus (C. sepium), is a hedge plant found abundantly throughout England and Scotland, but only of local occurrence in Scotland. Like the Field Convolvulus, it is, in spite of the beauty of its flowers, regarded as a pest by both the farmer and the gardener, its roots being long and penetrating in a dense mass that exhausts the soil, and its twining stems extending in masses over all other plants near, and strangling them to a still greater degree than its smaller relative

Description

The leaves of this Bindweed are arrow-shaped and large, somewhat thin and delicate in texture. They are arranged singly on alternate sides of the stem, as is the case with all species of Convolvulus and from their axils spring the flower-stalks, which are square and in every case bear only one large blossom, conspicuous for its snowy whiteness. The flowers are among the largest which this country produces. The calyx is entirely hidden by the two large bracts that enclose it, and which completely hide the flower while in bud, a feature that has gained it also the name of 'Hooded Bindweed," and has led some botanists to place it in a different genus, Calystegia, the name being derived from two Greek words signifying 'beautiful covering." The specific name, sepium, is derived from the Latin sepes, a hedge, andrefers to its place of growth.

The flowers are in bloom from July to September, and like all the other species expand during sunshine and remain closed during dull weather. They do not, however, like those of the Field Convolvulus, close during a shower.

Anne Pratt (Flowers and their Associations) notices the fact that while some twining plants follow the apparent course of the sun and turn round the supporting stem from left to right, others, like the large White Bindweed or Convolvulus, twine contrary to the sun, from right to left, and never otherwise; even if the gardener turn it in another direction, the plant, if unable to disengage itself and assume its natural bias, will eventually perish.

BINDWEED, JALAP

Botanical: Convolvulus Jalapa (LINN.)
Synonym: Ipomea purga

Habitat

The Jalap Bindweed (C. Jalapa, Linn.), but more often called Ipomea Jalapa or purga, is a native of South America and Mexico. It derives its name from Xalapa, in Mexico, where it is very abundant. It is freely grown out of doors, however, in the southern countries of Europe, and plants have been grown here in the garden of the Society of Apothecaries and also in Norfolk and Hampshire.

Description

It is a handsome climbing convolvulaceous plant with crimson flowers and a tuberous root, which is of officinal value. The tubers, varying in size from a walnut to an orange, are dark, umber-brown in color and much wrinkled. They are imported either whole or sliced.

Medicinal Action and Uses

The drug Jalap is prepared from a resin which abounds in the roots. It has a slight smoky odor and the taste is unpleasant, followed by pungent acridity. It has strong cathartic and purgative action, and is used in constipation, pain and colic in the bowels and general intestinal torpor, being combined, in compound powder, with other laxatives, and with carminatives such as ginger, cloves, etc. It accelerates the action of rhubarb.

Jalap forms a safe purge for children, being given in sugar or jam to disguise the taste, and has been used thus with calomel or wormwood as a vermifuge. It proves an excellent purge in rheumatism.

Preparations

Powdered root, 3 to 20 grains. Tincture, B.P., 1/2 to 1 drachm. Powdered resin, 2 to 5 grains. Compound powder, B.P., 1 to 2 drachms. Jalapin, 1 to 3 grains.

Other members of this Convolvulus family have economic uses. C. dissectus, an American species abounds in prussic acid, the liquor known as Noyau being prepared from it with the aid of alcohol, and the oil of Rodium, which is so attractive to rats as to cause them to swarm to it without fear, even if held in the hand of a rat-catcher, is the produce of another Convolvulus, known as C. Rhodorhiza.

One of the most important members of the order economically is C. Batatas, the tuberous-rooted Bindweed, or SWEET POTATO, the roots of which abound in starch and sugar and form a nourishing food, very valuable in the tropics, where it is largely cultivated. The roots are somewhat in shape like an oblong and ugly potato, often club-shaped, and are of a reddish color. When cooked, they are excessively sweet, not unlike liquorice, and not attractive in appearance. They are usually of greater size and weight than ordinary potatoes.

Before the introduction of the Potato into Europe, the Sweet Potato was regularly imported as a wholesome article of diet, and was grown in Spain and Portugal, to which it had been brought from the West Indies. The Potato which Shakespeare mentions twice - in the Merry Wives of Windsor and in Troilus and Cressida - is the Sweet Potato, and not the more familiar tuber of our days.

BINDWEED, SEA

Botanical: Convolvulus Soldanella

Habitat

The Sea Bindweed (C. Soldanella) is a very beautiful species growing only on sandy sea-shores, decorating the sloping sides of sand-hills with its large, pale rosecoloured flowers striped with red.

Description

Its stems are not climbing being usually buried beneath the sand, the flowers and leaves merely rising above the surface. The leaves are fleshy, roundish or kidney-shaped, about the size of the Lesser Celandine, placed singly on alternate sides of the stem on long foot-stalks. The flowers are produced singly at each side of the stem, on four-sided, winged stalks, and blossom in July, being succeeded by round capsules. The bracts are large, egg-shaped and close to the flower, which is nearly as large as the Great Bindweed, and expands in the morning and in bright weather, closing before night. This species is also frequently assigned to the genus Calystegia.

BINDWEED, SYRIAN

Botanical: Convolvulus Scammonia
Synonym: Scammony.

Habitat

The Syrian Bindweed, or Scammony (C. Scammonia), can be grown here and will thrive well on dry soil, but we import from Smyrna and Aleppo what is needed for medicinal purposes.

Description

It has flowers of a very delicate tint of sulphur yellow and leaves of a similar shape to our native species.

The roots are 3 to 4 feet long and from 9 to 12 inches in circumference; tapering, covered with a light grey bark and containing a milky juice. Scammony is a gummy resin, obtained from this milky juice of the root by clearing away the earth from the upper part of the root and cutting off the top obliquely, about 2 inches below where the stalks spring. Then a vessel is fixed in such a position as to receive the exuding juice, which gradually hardens and becomes the Scammony of commerce. The best Scammony is black, resinous and shining when in the lump, but of a whitish-ash color when powdered, with a strong cheesy smell and a somewhat acrid taste, turning milky when touched by the tongue. It occurs in commerce in irregular pieces 1 to 2 inches or more in diameter.

Medicinal Action and Uses

Scammony is a drastic cathartic, closely allied in its operation to Jalap; though not so nauseous, it is more active and irritating, and in inflammatory conditions of the alimentary canal should not be used.

The root itself is seldom used: the resin prepared from it is generally combined with other cathartics to diminish its action and prevent griping.

Preparations

Powdered root, 3 to 12 grains. Powdered resin, B.P., 3 to 8 grains. Compound Powder, B.P., 10 to 20 grains.

It appears to have been well known to the Greek and Arabian physicians, who used it for various other purposes as well as for a purgative. The dose is generally from 3 to 12 grains. Seven grains of Scammony resin gradually rubbed well up with 3 oz. milk forms a safe purgative, to which a taste of ginger can be added. It is used as a smart purge for children, especially for those with worms, on account of the smallness of the dose necessary to produce its effect, the slight taste and the energy of its operation.

It is useful as a hydragogue in dropsies. Meyrick considered it a rough and powerful, but very useful purgative of great service in rheumatic and other chronic disorders, reaching the seat of many sources of trouble that an ordinary purge does not affect.

The leaves of the Sea Bindweed abound with a milky juice which has been employed as a purge - in 1/2 oz. doses. Applied externally, the leaves are reputed to diminish dropsical swelling of the feet. The whole plant used to be gathered fresh, when about to Hower, and boiled in ale, with nutmegs and cloves, and the decoction given as a strong purge, which was said to be best adapted to robust constitutions, being very violent in its action. The juice oozing from the stalks and root of the Sea Bindweed hardens into a kind of resin, which is also used as a purge in the same way as Scammony - a closelyrelated plant of foreign origin, which is much imported for this purpose.

Both the preceding species of Convolvulus also possess the virtues of Scammony. The smallness of their roots prevents the juice being collected in the same way as the foreign species, but an extract made from the expressed juice of the roots or any preparation of them has the same purgative quality, only in less degree. Meyrick states that the root of C. arvensis is a rough purgative, and to such constitutions as can bear it, will prove serviceable in jaundice, dropsy and other disorders arising from obstructions of the viscera, the best method of administering it being to bruise the roots and give their expressed juice in strong beer. The juice of theGreater Bindweed, taken in doses of 20 to 30 grains is also a powerful drastic purge, and country people often boil its freshly-gathered roots in ale in the same manner as the Field Bindweed. Though for those of a strong constitution there is no better purge, on account of the nausea which it tends to produce, it is not considered fit for the delicate.

Botanical: Convolvulus Duartinus
Common: MORNING GLORY
Synonyms: Ipomoea. Vona-nox.

A tincture of the flowers is used for headaches, rheumatism and inflamed eyes.

BIRCH, COMMON

Botanical: Betula alba (LINN.)
Family: N.O. Betulaceae
Synonyms: White Birch. Bouleau. Berke. Bereza. Monoecia triandria. B. pubescens. B. verrucosa.
Parts Used: The bark and the leaves.
Habitat: Europe, from Sicily to Iceland. Northern Asia.

History

The name is a very ancient one, probably derived from the Sanscrit bhurga, 'a tree whose bark is used for writing upon." From its uses in boat-building and roofing it is also connected with the A.S. beorgan, 'to protect or shelter."

Coleridge speaks of it as the 'Lady of the Woods." It is remarkable for its lightness, grace, and elegance, and after rain it has a fragrant odor.

The young branches are of a rich red brown or orange brown, and the trunks usually white, especially in the second species of B. alba, B. verrucosa. B. pubescens is darker, and has downy instead of warted twigs.

The wood is soft and not very durable, but being cheap, and the tree being able to thrive in any situation and soil, growing all over Europe, is used for many humble purposes, such as bobbins for thread mills, herring-barrel staves, broom handles, and various fancy articles. In country districts the Birch has very many uses, the lighter twigs being employed for thatching and wattles. The twigs are also used in broom making and in the manufacture of cloth. The tree has also been one of the sources from which asphyxiating gases have been manufactured, and its charcoal is much used for gunpowder.

The white epidermis of the bark is separable into thin layers, which may be employed as a substitute for oiled paper and applied to various economical uses. It yields oil of Birch Tar, and the peculiar, well-known odor of russia leather is due to the use of this oil in the process of dressing. It likewise imparts durability to leather, and it isowing to its presence that books bound in russia leather are not liable to become mouldy. The production of Birch Tar oil is a Russian industry of considerable importance. It is also distilled in Holland and Germany, but these oils are appreciably different from the Russian oil. It has the property of keeping away insects and preventing gnatbites when smeared on the hands. It is likewise employed in photography.

When the stem of the tree is wounded, a saccharine juice flows out which is susceptible, with yeast, of vinous fermentation. A beer, wine, spirit and vinegar are prepared from it in some parts of Europe. Birch Wine, concocted from this thin, sugary sap of the tree, collected from incisions made in the trees in March, honey, cloves and lemon peel being added and then the whole fermented with yeast, makes a very pleasant cordial, formerly much appreciated. From 16 to 18 gallons of sap may be drawn from one large tree, and a moderate tapping does no harm.

Constituents

Birch bark only contains about 3 per cent. of tannic acid, but is extensively used for tanning, wherever there are large birch forests, throughout Northern Europe. As it gives a pale color to the skin, it is used for the preliminary and the final stages of tanning. It contains betulin and betuls camphor.

The leaves contain betulorentic acid.

By destructive distillation, the white epidermis of the bark yields an empyreumatic oil, known variously in commerce as oil of Birch Tar, Oleum Rusci, Oleum Betulinum or Dagget. This is a thick, bituminous, brownish-black liquid, with a pungent, balsamic odor. It contains a high percentage of methylsalicylate, and also creosol and guaiacol. The Rectified Oil (Oleum Rusci Rectificatum) is sometimes substituted for oil of Cade.

Birch Tar oil is almost identical with Wintergreen oil. It is not completely soluble in 95 per cent. acetic acid, nor in aniline, but Turpentine oil dissolves it completely.

Medicinal Action and Uses

Various parts of the tree have been applied to medicinal uses. The young shoots and leaves secrete a resinous substance having acid properties, which, combined with alkalies, is said to be a tonic laxative. The leaves have a peculiar, aromatic, agreeable odor and a bitter taste, and have been employed in the form of infusion (Birch Tea) in gout, rheumatism and dropsy, and recommended as a reliable solvent of stone in the kidneys. With the bark they resolve and resist putrefaction. A decoction of them is good for bathing skin eruptions, and is serviceable in dropsy.

The oil is astringent, and is mainly employed for its curative effects in skin affections, especially eczema, but is also used for some Internal maladies.

The inner bark is bitter and astringent, and has been used in intermittent fevers.

The vernal sap is diuretic.

Moxa is made from the yellow, fungous excrescences of the wood, which sometimes swell out from the fissures.

Dosage

Of alcoholic extract of the leaves, 25 to 30 grains daily.

Other Species

B. benta (Cherry Birch, Black Birch, Sweet Birch, Mahogany Birch, or Mountain Mahogany) is an American variety, with richlymarked wood suitable for the use of cabinet and pianoforte makers. The liquor is used in Kamschatka without previous fermentation. The cambium, or the layer between the wood and the bast, is eaten in the spring, cut into strips like vermicelli, and the bark is stimulant, diaphoretic, and astringent, in a warm infusion. In decoction or syrup it forms an excellent tonic for dysentery, and is said to be useful in gravel and female obstructions.

B. trophylla is a syn. of Rhus Aromatica, or Fragrant Sumach.

B. papyracea, or Paper Birch, is largely used for canoe-making in America.

B. nana, or Smooth Dwarf Birch, rarely grows above 3 feet in height. The leaves are said to dye a better yellow than the Common Birch; the seeds are a principal food of ptarmigan in Lapland; Moxa is prepared from it and regarded as an effective remedy in all painful diseases.

BIRTHWORT

Botanical: Aristolochia longa (LINN.)
Family: N.O. Aristolochiaceae
Synonym: Long-rooted Birthwort.
Part Used: The root.
Habitat: Southern Europe and Japan.

Description

There are several species of the Aristolochias used by herbalists in India. The root is spindle-shaped from 5 cm. to 3 dm. in length, about 2 cm. in thickness, fleshy, very brittle, greyish externally, brownish-yellow inside, bitter and of a strong disagreeable odor when fresh.

Constituent

Aristolochine.

Medicinal Action and Uses

Said to be useful as an aromatic stimulant in rheumatism and gout and for removing obstructions, etc., after childbirth. Dose, 1/2 to 1 drachm of the powdered root.

Other Species

Aristolochia, cymbifera from Brazil and Mexico is said to have medicinal properties similar to the official species. Butte affirms it is a depressant to the sensory nerve centres and is useful in neuralgia and pruritis; it was formerly considered alexiteric, antiparalytic, antiperiodic and aphrodisiac.

A. Argentina root is used in that republic as a diuretic and diaphoretic, especially for rheumatism.

A. Indica is used as an emmenagogue, antiarthritic, stomachic, purgative and vermifuge, and in the East Indies is used for similar purposes as the American and European species.

A. Sempervirens is said to be used by the Arabians as a remedy against the poisonous effects of snakebite.

A. Foetida in Mexico is used as a stimulant to foul ulcers.

A. serpentaria used in bilious, typhoid and typhus fevers, smallpox, pneumonia, amenorrhoea and fevers of a septicaemic type. It is often given in combination with Peruvian Bark, rendering it more active and preventing ill effects on the stomach. It is also used in North America, as are several other varieties of the species, as an alexiteric and for the bites of mad dogs.

BISTORT

Botanical: Polygonurn Bistorta (LINN.)
Family: N.O. Polygonaceae
Synonyms: Osterick. Oderwort. Snakeweed. Easter Mangiant. Adderwort. Twice Writhen.
Part Used: The root-stock, gathered in March, when the leaves begin to shoot, and dried.

Habitat

A native of many parts of Northern Europe, occurring in Siberia and in Japan and in Western Asia to the Himalayas. It is common in the north of England and in southern Scotland, growing in moist meadows, though only of local occurrence; in Ireland, it is very rare.

History

In many places, it can only be regarded as an escape from cultivation, its leaves and young shoots having formerly been widely used in the spring as a vegetable, being still, indeed, in the north of England an ingredient in Herb Pudding, under the name of 'Easter-mangiant," the latter word a corruption of mangeant, i.e. a plant to be eaten at Easter, 'Easter

Giant' and 'Easter Ledges' being variations of this name In Lancashire and Cumberland, the leaves and young shoots were eaten as a green vegetable under the name of Patience Dock and Passions. The roots and leaves had also a great reputation as a remedy for wounds, so that the plant was generally cultivated for medicinal use, as well as for employment as a vegetable.

The name Bistort (Latin bis = twice, torta = twisted) bears reference to the twice-twisted character of the root-stock, an old local name, 'Twice-Writhen," being a literal translation of the Latin. Its twisted, creeping nature is also the origin of the names Snakeroot, Adderwort and Snakeweed. It was at one time called Serpentaria, Columbrina, Dracunculus and Serpentary Dragonwort, and has been thought to be the Oxylanathum Britannicum and Limonium of the ancients.

Externally, the root-stock is black, but internally is coloured red and is rich in tannic and gallic acids, which makes it a powerful astringent and has enabled it to be used in tanning leather, when procurable in sufficient quantity.

The root-stock, as it appears in commerce, is about 2 inches long and 3/5 inch broad, twice bent, as in the letter S, more or less annulate, bearing a few slender roots, otherwise smooth, reddish brown internally, dark purplish or blackish brown externally, depressed or channelled on the upper surface, convex and with depressed root-scars below with a thick bark surrounding a ring of small woody wedges, which encloses a pith equal in thickness to the bark.

The drug has an astringent and starchy taste, but no odor.

Besides being one of the strongest vegetable astringents among our native plants, the roots contain much starch, and after being steeped in water and subsequently roasted have been largely consumed in Russia, Siberia and Iceland in time of scarcity and are said after such preparation to be nutritious and a useful article of food, bread having been made of the root-flour of this and another Siberian species of Polygonum.

Where established, the Bistort becomes often a noxious weed in low-lying pastures, frequently forming large patches difficult to extirpate on account of its creeping root-stock.

Description

A number of tuberous roots are produced from the S-shaped root-stock from the upper side of which spring directly large oval leaves, with heart-shaped bases, of a bluish-green color on the upper side and ash-grey, tinged with purple, underneath, both leafstalks and blades being about 6 inches long. The upper part of the leafstalk is winged. The flower-stalk, 12 to 18 inches high, is very erect, slender, unbranched, and bears leaves smaller than the root-leaves and few in number, broader at their base and on very short stalks. The stems terminate in a dense, cylindrical spike of striking flesh-coloured flowers, which consist of five coloured sepals, eight stamens and an ovary with two to three styles. The flowers are grouped in twos, one flower complete, the other with normal stamens, but only a rudimentary ovary. The styles of the complete flower do not mature and become receptive of pollen from visiting insects, till their stamens have shed their pollen and fallen, cross-fertilization thus being ensured. The flowers are produced in May and June and again in September and October. The fruit is three-seeded, the ripe seeds are small, brown and shining. Birds commonly feed upon the seeds, which can be employed to fatten poultry.

Cultivation

The plant may be propagated by division of the root-stock, in early autumn or spring. Bistort is sometimes used to ornament moist parts of the rockery and shady border. When grown in bold masses, it is a handsome and attractive plant.

When it has a corner in the kitchen garden, it is well to pluck it now and then, even when it is not immediately required for culinary purposes, as the plant has a strong tendency to disappear.

Constituents

Bistort root has never been carefully analysed, but it is known to contain about 20 per cent. of tannin and a large amount of starch, as well as some gallic acid and gum. Its virtues are extracted by water and its decoction becomes inky black on the addition of a persalt of iron and with gelatine it forms a precipitate. Red coloring matter is also present.

Medicinal Action and Uses

Bistort root is one of the strongest astringent medicines in the vegetable kingdom and highly styptic and may be used to advantage for all bleedings, whether external or internal and wherever astringency is required. Although its use has greatly been superseded by other astringents of foreign origin, it is of proved excellence in diarrhea, dysentery, cholera and all bowel complaints and in hemorrhages from the lungs and stomach, and is a most effectual remedy for bleeding from the nose and exceedingly useful in dealing with hemorrhoids. It is used - as a medicine, injection and gargle - in mucous discharges, as well as for hemorrhages.

A teaspoonful of the powdered root, in a cupful of boiling water, may be drunk freely as required.

The decoction, often also used, is made from 1 OZ. of the bruised root boiled in 1 pint of water. One tablespoonful of this is given every two hours in passive bleedings and for simple diarrhea. The decoction is also useful as an injection in profuse menstruation and in leucorrhoea and is a useful wash in ulcerated mouth and gums, and as a gargle. It is also used as a lotion to ulcers attended with a discharge.

Bistort is considered valuable for diabetes, given in conjunction with tonics, and has itself tonic action.

The older herbalists considered both the leaves and roots to have 'a powerful faculty to resist poison." Combined with the bitter flag root (calamus), the root was used to cure intermittent fever and ague. Green (Universal Herbal, 1832) cites its frequent use in intermittent fever, both alone and with gentian, 3 drachms daily being administered.

It was used, dried, and powdered on cuts and wounds to stop bleeding. The decoction in wine, made from the powder, was drunk freely 'to stay internal bleedings and fluxes," and was considered 'available against ruptures, burstings and bluises from falls and blows'- also to 'help jaundice, expel the venom of the plague, smallpox, measles or other infectious disease, driving it out by sweating." A distilled water of the leaves and roots was used to wash any part stung or bitten by a venomous creature, or to wash running sores or ulcers; also as a gargle in sore throat and to harden spongy gums, attended with looseness of teeth and soreness of the mouth. Gerard stated that the root would have this effect, 'being holden in the mouth for a certaine space and at sundry times." He also states that 'the juice of Bistort put into the nose prevaileth much against the disease called Polybus."

The root was also employed externally as a poultice.

The powdered leaves were employed to kill worms in children.

In Salmon's Herbal the following preparations are given, with their uses:

1. A liquid juice of the whole plant.

2. A distilled water of the roots and leaves.

3. A powder of the leaves (good to killworms and for other things.)

4. A powder of the root. (Prevails against malignity of measles and small-pox and expels the poyson of the Plague or Pestilence or of any other infectious disease, driving it out by sweating.)

5. A compound powder of the root (made of equal quantities of Bistort, Pellitory of Spain and burnt Alum made into a paste with a little honey and put in hollow of a tooth or at the side, eases their pain and stops the defluxion of rheum on the part cleanses the head and brain and causes evacuation of abundance of rheumatic matter.

6. A decoction of the root in wine or water.

7. A decoction compound of the root. (6 oz. Bistort root, 4 oz. Angelica, 4 oz. of Zedoary, 1 oz. of Winter's Cinnamon, all being bruised, infuse in red port wine or Canary, 5 quarts, for 6 hours, then giving it 2 or 3 boils, take it from the fire, strain out the wine from the ingredients, which let settle, then decant the clear from the rest sweeten with syrup of lemons or syrup of vinegar. This is a notable medicament against Measles, Small-Pox Calenture, Spotted Fever and even the Plague. It also prevails against any vegetable poison, which is taken inwardly, if timely given.)

8. The diet drink, made of the roots, leaves and seeds.

9. The spiritous tincture.

10. The acid tincture.

11. The oily tincture.

12. The saline tincture.

13. The fixed salt (resists putrefaction).

14. The essence.

Dosage

The root is generally administered in powder, the dose being from 1/4 to 1/2drachm in water.

A fluid extract is also prepared from the root, the dose being 1/2 to 1 drachm.

A decoction is also much employed.

Recipes for Ailments

Infants' Diarrhea Syrup

1 OZ. Bistort root, 1/4 oz. Cloves, 1/2 oz. Marshmallow root, 1/4 oz. Angelica powder, 1/4 oz. best Ginger powder.

Bruise the root and cloves small. Add 1 1/2 pint boiling water and simmer down to a pint. Then pour boiling mixture upon the powder, mix well and let it simmer for 10 minutes. Allow to get cold, strain and add lump sugar, sufficient to form a syrup, boil up again, skim, and when cold bottle for use.

This may be given to children in a little Raspberry Leaf Tea, 3 to 6 teaspoonfuls daily, according to age of child. If bleeding from bowels, or flux, a tea of Cranesbill is recommended instead of Raspberry Tea.

Hemorrhoids

1/2 OZ. Marshmallow root powder, 1/2 oz. Bistort root powder, 1/2 oz. Cranesbill root powder.

Mix the powders thoroughly and then form into a stiff paste with treacle. Preserve in a jar and take a small quantity (about the size of a bean) three times a day. When constipation is present, 1/4 oz. Turkey rhubarb powder may be added to the other powdered roots. For the blind piles, 1/2 oz. Barberry bark should be added.

Pile Ointment should be applied at the same time, made as follows: 1/2 oz. Bistort root, 1/2 oz. Cranesbill herb, cut up fine.

Simmer gently for an hour with 2 OZ. lard and 2 OZ. mutton suet. Strain through a coarse cloth and squeeze out as much strength as possible. Add 1 OZ. Olive oil and mix well. Allow to cool gradually. This is equally good for Chapped Hands, Sore Lips, etc.

Decoction for Piles

1 OZ. Marshmallow root, 1 oz. Bistort root, 1 oz. Comfrey root, 1 OZ. White Poplar bark, 1 OZ. Cranesbill, 1 OZ. Yarrow, drachms each Cloves and Cinnamon.

Bruise the roots, add 2 quarts of water and boil 20 minutes, then add the herbs, Cloves and Cinnamon and boil 10 minutes longer. Strain and sweeten with brown sugar.

Dose, a wine glassful four times a day. Also use Celandine (Pilewort) Ointment. (Medical Herbalist.)

Gargle for Ulcerated Tonsils

2 drachms Tincture of Bistort root, 2 drachms Tincture of Bloodroot. Add 2 tablespoonsful of warm water.

Use as gargle, or spray the throat.

Compound Bistort Wash

1 drachm Tincture of Bistort, 1/2 oz. Bayberry powder.

Infuse the powder in 8 oz. of boiling water let it remain until cold, strain the liquid off clear, add the tincture and use freely morning, noon and night.

In inflamed mucous discharges from the ears, nose, vagina, urethra or any other part, this wash is exceedingly useful. (National Botanic Pharmacopoeia.)

For Diabetes

Fluid Extract Bistort, Jambul Seed, Pinus Can, Rhus Aromat., Potentilla Tormentilla of each 2 drachms. The same quantity of Tincture of Hydrastis.

Put the whole into a 12-OZ, bottle and fill with distilled water. Dose, 1 tablespoonful every four hours after meals. (Medical Herbalist.)

Recipes for Culinary Use

Recipe for Bistort Pudding

The Herb Pudding still eaten in Cumberland and Westmorland, where Bistort is common in moist meadows and is also cultivated, is a very wholesome dish and very suitable in May, when ordinary green vegetables used to be scarce.

The chief constituents are Bistort shoots and Nettles, and the younger and fresher these greens are the more satisfactory is the resultant food. Allow about 1 1/2 lb. of Bistort to 1 lb. of Nettles. A few leaves of Black Currant and Yellow Dock may be added and a sprig of Parsley. Wash the vegetables thoroughly (in salt and water in the last rinsing), then chop them fairly fine. Place them in a bowl and mix in about a teacupful of barley (washed and soaked), half a teacupful of oatmeal, salt and pepper to flavor, and if liked, a bunch of chives mixed. Boil the whole in a bag for about 2 1/2 hours, to allow the barley to get thoroughly cooked. The bag should be tied firmly, for while the greens shrink, the barley swells. Turn out into a very hot bowl, add a lump of butter and a beaten egg: the heat of the turned-out pudding is sufficient to cook the egg.

Other Species

About forty species of Polygonum are recorded as having been medicinally employed. A number of species yield blue or yellow dyestuffs.

BITTER ROOT

Botanical: Apocynum androsaemifolium (LINN.)
Family: N.O. Apocynacae
Synonyms: Milkweed. Dogsbane. Fly-Trap.
Parts Used: The dried rhizome, roots.
Habitat: North America.

Description

The genus Apocynum contains only four species, two of which Apocynum androsaemifolium and A. cannabinum, or Black Indian Hemp, resemble each other very closely, the roots being distinguished by the thick-walled stone cells, which in the former are found in an interrupted circle near the middle of the bark, and in the latter are absent.

A. androsaemifolium is a perennial herb, 5 or 6 feet in height, branching, and, in common with the other three members of the genus, yielding on incision a milky juice resembling indiarubber when dry.

The leaves are dark green above, paler and downy beneath, ovate, and from 2 to 3 inches long. The flowers are white, tinged with red, having five scales in the throat of the corolla which secrete a sweet liquid, attractive to flies. These scales are very sensitive, and when touched bend inward, imprisoning the insects.

The tough, fibrous bark of all four species is used by the Indians of California as a substitute for hemp, in making twine, bags, fishing-nets and lines, and linen.

The milky root is found in commerce in cylindrical, branched pieces, about a quarter of an inch thick, reddish or greyish brown outside, longitudinally wrinkled, and having a short fracture and small pith. There is scarcely any odor, and the taste is starchy, afterwards bitter and acrid.

Constituents

The nature of the active principle is uncertain. A glucoside, Apocynamarin, was separated, but the activity is thought to be due not to the glucoside, but to an intensely bitter principle, Cymarin.

Medicinal Action and Uses

One of the digitalis group of cardiac tonics, apocynum, is the most powerful in slowing the pulse, and its action on the vaso-motor system is also very strong. Being rather irritant to mucous membranes, it may cause nausea and catharsis, so that some cannot tolerate it. It is a powerful hydragogue, helpful in dropsies due to heart-failure, and in the ascites of hepatic cirrhosts has been called the 'vegetable trocar."

It is used as an alterative in rheumatism, syphilis and scrofula.

Dosage

5 to 15 grains.

Poisons and Antidotes

The absorption in the gastro-intestinal tract being very irregular, the dosage and patient must be carefully watched and guarded.

Other Species

A. cannabinum, or Black Indian Hemp, Canadian Hemp, American Hemp, Amyroot, Bowman's Root, Indian Physic Bitter Root, Rheumatism Weed, Milkweed, Wild Cotton, Choctaw Root, is diuretic, expectorant, diaphoretic, emetic, and cathartic. It should not be substituted for A. androsaemifolium or vice versa.

It is not the Indian Hemp (Cannabis Indica) which yields 'hashish."

A. hypericifolium bears some resemblance to the above.

A. venetum contains an alkaloid, Apocynteine, said to be a cardiac sedative.

BITTER ROOT is also a common name of Gentiana lutea, or Yellow Gentian, the wellknown bitter, and of Lewisia rediviva or Spathulum, with a starchy, edible root.

MILKWEED is also a common name of Asclepias.

DOG'S BANE is also a common name of Aconitum Cynoctonum.

BLACKBERRY

Botanical: Rubus fructicosus
Family: N.O. Rosacea
Synonyms: Bramble. Bumble-Kite. Bramble-Kite. Bly. Brummel. Brameberry. Scaldhead. Bramble-berry.
Parts Used: Root, leaves.

Habitat

In Australia, the Blackberry grows more luxuriantly than in any other part of the world, though it is common everywhere.

The Blackberry, or Bramble, growing in every English hedge-row, is too well known to need description. Its blossoms, as well as its fruits, both green and ripe, may be seen on the bush: at the same time, a somewhat unusual feature, not often met with in other plants.

History

The name of the bush is derived from brambel, or brymbyl, signifying prickly. We read of it as far back as the days of Jonathan, when he upbraided the men of Shechem for their ingratitude to his father's house, relating to them the parable of the trees choosing a king, the humble bramble being finally elected, after the olive, fig-tree and vine had refused the dignity. The ancient Greeks knew Blackberries well, and considered them a remedy for gout.

Opinions differ as to whether there is one true Blackberry with many aberrant forms; or many distinct types. Professor Babington divides the British Rubi into forty-one species, or more.

Rubus rhamnifolius and R. coryfolius furnish the Blackberries of the hedges, in which the calyx of the fruit is reflexed; has also a reflexed calyx, but the leaves are hoary underneath. R. coesius furnishes Dewberries, distinguished by the large size of the grains, which are covered with bloom and few in number, the whole being closely clasped by the calyx. R. saxatilis, the Roebuck-berry, and the badge of the McNabs, is an herbaceous species found in mountainous places in the North, and distinguished by its ternate leaves and fruit of few red large grains.

R. chamaenorus, the Cloudberry, and badge of the McFarlanes, is also herbaceous, with an erect stem, 6 to 8 inches high, lobed leaves and a single flower which is succeeded by a large orange-red fruit of an agreeable flavor. The double-flowering Rubus of gardens is a variety of R. fructicosus. R. lancinatus, of which the native country is unknown, is a rampant species with deeplycut leaves and large black fruit, which are highly ornamental in autumn.

R. odoratus, the American Bramble, is an erect, unbranched shrub, with large fivelobed leaves and rose-coloured flowers.

R. occidentalis, the Virginian raspberry, has pinnate and ternate leaves, white flowers and black fruit. It is well known that the barren shoots of most of our British Rubi from being too flexile to keep upright, bend downwards even from the hedges and thickets, and root their ends in the soil, thus following that mode of increase which in the strawberry is effected by the scion. The loop thus formed was formerly an object of occasional search, being reputed in some counties (and we have known it so in Gloucestershire) as capable of curing hernia or rupture when used aright, to which end the afflicted child is passed backwards and forwards through the arching bramble. The origin of this custom is difficult to trace; but quoting from Notes and Queries, the passing of children through holes in the earth, rocks, and trees, once an established rite, is still practised in various parts of Cornwall. Children affected with hernia are still passed through a slit in an ash sapling before sunrise, fasting; after which the slit portions are bound up, and as they unite so the malady is cured.

It would appear that in Cornwall the bramble-cure is only employed for boils, the sufferer being either dragged or made to crawl beneath the rooted shoot. We have heard of cows that were said to be 'mouse-crope," or to have been walked over by a shrew-mouse (an ancient way of accounting for paralysis), being dragged through the bramble-loop, in which case, if the creature could wait the time of finding a loop large enough, and suffer the dragging process at the end, we should say the case would not be so hopeless as that of our friend's fat pig, who, when she was ailing, 'had a mind to kill her to make sure on her!" (LINDLEY S Treasury of Botany.)

The Blackberry is known in some parts of the country as 'Scaldhead," either from producing the eruption known as scaldhead in children who eat the fruit to excess - the over-ripe fruit being indigestible - or from the curative effects of the leaves and berries in this malady of the scalp, or from the remedial effects of the leaves, when applied externally to scalds. The leaves are said to be still in use in England as a remedy for burns and scalds; formerly their operation was helped by a spoken charm. Creeping under a Bramble-bush was itself a charm against rheumatism, boils, blackheads, etc. Blackberries were in olden days supposed to give protection against all 'evil runes," if gathered at the right time of the moon. The whole plant had once a considerable popular reputation both as a medicine and as a charm for various disorders. The flowers and fruit were from very ancient times used to remedy venomous bites; the young shoots, eaten as a salad, were thought - though Gerard cautiously suggests the addition of a little alum - to fasten loose teeth. Gerard and other herbalists regard the bramble as a valuable astringent, whether eaten or applied: its leaves 'heal the eies that hang out," and are a most useful application for piles, its fruit stops looseness of the bowels and is good for stone, and for soreness in mouth and throat.

Medicinal Action and Uses

The bark of the root and the leaves contain much tannin, and have long been esteemed as a capital astringent and tonic, proving a valuable remedy for dysentery and diarrhea, etc. The root is the more astringent.

Preparations

Fluid extract, 1/2 to 1 drachm. Fluid extract, root, U.S.P., 15 drops. Syrup, U.S.P., 1 drachm.

The fruit contains malic and citric acids, pectin and albumen. If desiccated in a moderately hot oven and then reduced to a powder, it is a reliable remedy for dysentery.

The root-bark, as used medicinally, should appear in thin tough, flexible bands, inodorous, strongly astringent and somewhat bitter. It should be peeled off the root and dried by artificial heat or in strong sun. One ounce, boiled in 1 1/2 pint water or milk down to a pint, makes a good decoction. Half a teacupful should be taken every hour or two for diarrhea. One ounce of the bruised root, likewise boiled in water, may also be used, the dose being larger, however. The same decoction is said to be useful against whooping-cough in the spasmodic stage.

The leaves are also employed for the same purpose. One ounce of the dried leaves, infused in one pint of boiling water, and the infusion taken cold, a teacupful at a time, makes a serviceable remedy for dysentery, etc.

Recipes

Blackberry Wine

Blackberry jelly has been used with good effects in cases of dropsy caused by feeble, ineffective circulation, and the London Pharmacopoeia (1696) declared the ripe berries of the bramble to be a great cordial, and to contain a notable restorative spirit. Blackberry wine is made by crushing the fruit and adding one quart of boiling water to each gallon of the fruit, allowing to stand for 24 hours, stirring occasionally, and then straining off the liquid. 2 lb. of white sugar are then added to every gallon, and it is kept in a tightly corked cask till the following October. This makes a trustworthy cordial astringent, used in looseness of the bowels. Another delicious cordial is made from pressing out the juice from the ripe Blackberries, adding 2 lb. of sugar to each quart and 1/2 oz. of nutmegs and cloves. Boil all together for a short time, allow to get cold and then add a little brandy.

In Crusoe's Treasury of Easy Medicines (1771) a decoction of Blackberry leaves is recommended as a fomentation for longstanding ulcers. There is also a popular country notion that the young shoots, eaten as a salad, will fasten loose teeth. A noted hair-dye has been made by boiling the leaves in strong lye, which imparts to the hair a permanent soft black color.

Blackberry Vinegar

is a wholesome drink that is easily made and can with advantage have its place in the store cupboard for use in winter, being a fine cordial for a feverish cold.

Gather the berries on a fine day, stalk them, put into an earthenware vessel and cover with malt vinegar. Let them stand three days to draw out the juice. Strain through a sieve, drain thoroughly, leaving them to drip through all day. Measure the juice and allow a pound of sugar to each pint. Put into a preserving pan, boil gently for 5 minutes, removing scum as it rises, set aside to cool, and when cold, bottle and cork well.

A teaspoonful of this, mixed with water will often quench thirst when other beverages fail and makes a delicious drink in fever.

BLACKBERRY, AMERICAN

Botanical: Rubus villosus (AIT.)
Family: N.O. Rosaceae
Synonyms: Brombeere. Bramble, or Fingerberry. Or. Nigrobaccus, and R. Cuneifolius.
Parts Used: Leaves, root, bark.
Habitat: Cultivated in United States of America from a Eurobean species.

Description

It is prepared in thin tough flexible bands, outer surface blackish or blackish grey, inner surface, pale brownish, sometimes striped, with whitish tasteless wood adhering. It is inodorous, very astringent (root more so than the leaves) and rather bitter.

Constituents

Tannic acid is abundant in it up to 10 per cent, and can be extracted readily by boiling water or dilute alcohol.

Medicinal Action and Uses

An astringent tonic for diarrhea, dysentery, etc. It is very similar in action to the wild English Blackberry.

Preparations

Fluid extract of dried bark of root Rubus, U.S.P., 15 minims.

Syrup of Rubus, U.S.P., 1 fluid drachm.

Other Species

Of the genus Rubus a large number are indigenous in the United States, where they are called Blackberry, Dewberry, Cloudberry. Most of them are shrubby or suffruticose briers, with astringent roots and edible berries, some have annual stems without prickles, these are called Raspberries.

BLACK ROOT

Botanical: Leptandra Virginica (NUTT.)
Family: N.O. Scrophulariaceae
Synonyms: Veronica Virginica. Veronica purpurea. Paederota Virginica. Eustachya purpurea and Eustachya alba. Culveris Root. Culver's Physic. Physic Root. Leptandra-Wurzel.
Parts Used: The dried rhizome, roots.
Habitat: Eastern United States.

Description

This tall, herbaceous perennial was included by Linnaeus in the genus Veronica, but was later assigned by Nuttall to the genus Leptandra, a nomenclature followed by present-day botanists. It has a simple, erect stem, 3 or 4 feet high or more, smooth and downy, furnished with leaves in whorls and terminating in a long spike of white flowers, 6 to 10 inches long. The leaves, of which there are from four to seven in each whorl, are lanceolate, pointed and minutely serrate, and stand on short footstalks. A variety with purple flowers has been described as a distinct species under the name of Leptandra purpurea. The plant flowers in July and August. It grows throughout the United States, in the south mostly in mountain meadows - in the north in rich woods, and is not unfrequently cultivated. It will grow readily in Britain. The rhizome and roots are nearly odourless, the taste bitter and rather acrid, and are generally used dried. The rhizome is of horizontal growth, nearly cylindrical, somewhat branched, externally dark brown to purplish brown, smooth and faintly longitudinally wrinkled, and showing stem bases at intervals of 1/2 to 1 1/2 inch. The rootlets, rising from the under portion, are wiry and brittle when dry.

Constituents

The roots contain volatile oil, extractive, tannic acid, gum, resin, a crystalline principle, a saccharine principle resembling mannite, and a glucoside resembling senegin. Both the crystalline principle and the impure resin obtained by precipitating with water a tincture of the root have been called Leptandrin and is said to be the active principle. The properties are extracted by both water and alcohol.

An ester of p-methoxycinnamic acid, a phytosterol verosterol, and some dimethoxycinnamic acid are also obtained.

Medicinal Action and Uses

The fresh root is a violent cathartic and may also be emetic. The dried root is milder and less certain. Leptandrin excites the liver gently and promotes the secretion of bile without irritating the bowels or purging. As it is also a tonic for the stomach, it is very useful in diarrhea, chronic dysentery, cholera infantum, and torpidity of the liver.

The accounts of its use are conflicting, perhaps owing to the difference in the action of the root in its dry and fresh states. There appears to be a risk of the fresh root producing bloody stools and possibly abortion, though a decoction may be useful in intermittent fever. It has been stated that the dried root has been employed with success in leprosy and cachetic diseases, and in combination with cream of tartar, in dropsy.

Dosages

15 to 60 grains. Of the impure resin, 2 to 4 grains. Of the powdered extract, U.S.P., 4 grains. Of the fluid extract, 15 minims as a laxative. Leptandrin, 1/4 to 2 grains.

BLADDERWRACK

Botanical: Fucus vesiculosis (LINN.)
Family: N.O. Fucaceae
Synonyms: Fucus. Sea-Wrack. Kelp-Ware. Black-Tang. Quercus marina. Cutweed. Bladder Fucus. Fucus (Varech) vesiculeux. Blasentang. Seetang. Meeriche.
Parts Used: The dried mass of root, stem and leaves. (The thallus.)
Habitat: North Atlantic Ocean.

Description

Almost all the more solid Algae were formerly described by the name of Fucus, but now it is applied to one genus of Fucaceae, most of the species of which are found only in the northern seas, many being more or less exposed at low water. Fucus vesiculosis is found on submerged rocks on both coasts of North America, and in Europe north of the Mediterranean, where it drifts in from time to time through the Strait of Gibraltar.

The perennial frond or thallus is coarse, light yellow or brownish-green in color, erect, and from 2 to 3 feet in height. It attaches itself to the rocks by branched, rootlike, discoid, woody extremities, developed from the base of the stalk. The frond is almost fan-shaped, narrow and strap-shaped at the base, the rest flat and leaf-like in form, wavy, many times divided into two with erect divisions having a very strong, broad, compressed midrib running to the apex. The margin is entire, the texture tough and leathery, mainly olive brown in color, the younger portion yellower, shining. Air vesicles developed in the substance of the frond, usually in pairs, one on either side of the midrib and often one at the fork of the divisions, broadly oval, or spherical, attaining when fully grown half an inch in diameter, are the characteristics of this species which have suggested both the English and Latin names.

The fructification is contained in small globose conceptacles with a firm wall lined with numerous jointed hairs and sunk in the surface of large ovoid-oblong or narrower pointed or blunt, swollen receptacles, filled with a transparent mucous. These attain an inch in length and are situated at the ends of the divisions of the fronds.

The entire living plant is gathered from the rocks about the end of June and dried rapidly in the sun, when it becomes brittle and may be easily reduced to a coarse powder. Care should be taken to turn it frequently, to avoid the development of a putrid odor. If dried by artificial heat, it retains its hygroscopic qualities and does not become brittle. It is in perfect condition only during early and middle summer, and should not be collected when too fully matured, as it quickly undergoes decomposition. When thrown up on the shore by the sea, the seaweed is not suitable for medicinal purposes, as the soaking of the detached plants in sea-water causes the loss of important constituents by diffusion from cells containing protoplasm which has lost its vitality.

As found in commerce, the drug Fucus is hard and brittle, forming a much wrinkled mass, blackish or with more or less of a whitish efflorescence or incrustation, but it acquires a cartilaginous consistency when slightly moistened. It has a strong, sea-weed-like odor and a nauseous, saline and mucilaginous taste. Occasionally, from some unexplained cause, it is very astringent. The powder is reddish brown, with numerous fragments of epidermal tissue, with polygonal cells from 0.012 to 0.025 mm. in length.

Bladderwrack is a valuable manure for potatoes and other crops and is gathered for this purpose all along the British coast. It is largely used in the Channel Islands, where it is called Vraic, the early potatoes from Jersey being grown by seaweed manure. Fresh seaweed contains 20 to 40 lb. of potash to the ton, and dried seaweed 60 to 230, so that its collection and use were strongly recommended to farmers while the War caused a shortage of artificial fertilizers. It may be spread on the land and left for some time before ploughing in, but should not be left in heaps, as rotting liberates the potash which may be wasted. The seaweed may be dried and burnt to ashes, then sprinkled on the ground as Kelp.

The early broccoli from Cornwall is fertilized with wrack, and on the west coast of Ireland, driftweed is almost the only manure used for raising potatoes. In the Channel Islands it is used for producing the smoke for drying bacon and fish, while in the Hebrides, cheeses while drying are covered with the salty ashes, and horses, cattle and sheep have been fed with it.

During the War the French Ministry of War experimented with regard to the value of seaweed as food for horses. A batch of twenty fed on the usual ration of oats and fodder gained eleven kilogrammes less in two months than a similar number fed on the same weight of seaweed. Another trial resulted in the cure of some sick horses fed on seaweed, while others fed on oats remained out of health.

In Denmark, a few years ago, the possibility of making paper from seaweed was mooted, but the cost of collecting probably proved too serious an obstacle.

It is also possible that considerable quantities of alcohol might be obtained from various species.

Many attempts have been made to make kelp-burning successful by finding a use for by-products from destructive distillation in retorts, but the cost of collection, drying and fuel prevents such experiments being financially profitable. There were at one time flourishing kelp industries in the Hebrides, and Lord Leverhulme, the owner of Lewis Isle, sent experts to report on the possibilities, but his death and lack of official support caused the matter to be dropped.

Kelp is prepared from several species of Fucus (including Black Wrack, F. serratus and Knobbed Wrack, F. nodosus, and on the coast of France about a dozen other species) and from the deep-sea tangle, Laminaria species, especially L. digitata. The latter yield 'drift-wood kelp," obtainable only when cast up on the shore by gales or other causes. These contain ten times as much iodine as the Fuci and are practically now the only kelps used in making iodine. The species of Fucus growing within the tidal range and cut at low water are called 'cut-weeds."

F. vesiculosis is the badge of the M'Neills.

Constituents

Bladderwrack contains about 0.1 per cent. of a volatile oil, cellulose, mucilage, mannite, coloring and bitter principles, soda and iodine, and bromine compounds of sodium and potassium. These saline ingredients constitute 14 to 20 per cent. of its ashes, which the dry plant yields in the proportion of 2.5 to 4 per cent., and also remain in the charcoal resulting from its exposure to heat in closed vessels. The proportions, especially of iodine, vary according to both locality and season. They are most abundant at the end of June. It has been stated that 0.8 per cent. of a sugar named Fucose exists in dried seaweed, and that this yields an alcohol, Fucitol. The air in the vesicles consists of a considerably higher percentage of Oxygen and a lower percentage of Nitrogen than in the outer atmosphere. Its value as a fertilizer is due to its potash.

One hundred pounds of red wrack, dried to a moisture content of 10 per cent., when heated for a short time with weak sulphuric acid and the acidity still further reduced after cooling, may be fermented with brewers' yeast and is then capable of yielding about 6 litres of alcohol on distillation. It is alleged that under industrial conditions this amount might be increased.

Kelp, or dried seaweed, was the original source of iodine, being discovered as such by Courtois in 1812, when investigating the products obtained from the mother-liquors prepared by lixiviating burnt seaweed. Iodine does not occur in nature in the uncombined condition, but is widely, though sparingly distributed in the form of iodides and iodates, chiefly of sodium and potassium, in seawater, some seaweeds, and various mineral and medicinal springs.

Kelp-burning as a source of iodine is a dead industry, owing to a cheaper process of obtaining it from the mother-liquors obtained in the purification of Chile saltpetre, and the use of kelp - an impure carbonate of soda, containing sulphate and chloride of sodium and a little charcoal - as a source of alkalies for soap and glass manufacture has been rendered obsolete by the modern process of obtaining carbonate of soda cheaply from common salt. Unless very recently discontinued, however, the preparation of iodine from kelp is still carried on at Glasgow.

Several methods were employed: (1) the weeds being dried in the sun, burned until formed into a confused mass, and sprinkled with water to break it up into pieces which were treated at chemical works; or (2) the seaweed was heated in large retorts, whereby tarry and ammoniacal liquors pass over and a very porous residue of kelp remained; or (3) the weeds were boiled with sodium carbonate, the liquid filtered and hydrochloric acid added to the filtrate, when alginic acid is precipitated; this is filtered off, the filtrate neutralized by caustic soda and the whole evaporated to dryness and carbonized.

The resulting kelp was then lixiviated with water, which extracts the soluble salts, and the liquid concentrated to crystallize the less soluble salts for removal. The addition of sulphuric acid set chemical processes in action, which finally liberated the iodine from its compounds.

Three tons of Tangle (Laminaria) give a ton of kelp, or 20 tons of cut-weed, or Fucus.

Good drift may yield as much as 10 to 15 lb. of iodine per ton, and cut-weed kelp only 3 to 4 lb. Other constituents vary from 2 to 10 per cent. in different samples.

Medicinal Action and Uses

Bladderwrack is not largely used at present, any virtues it may have being due to the iodine contained in it. It has alterative properties, has been used in scrofula, and is thought by some authorities to reduce obesity through stimulating the thyroid gland.

The charcoal derived from Kelp has been used in the treatment of goitre and scrofulous swellings under the name of Æthiops vegetabilis or vegetable ethiops, introduced by Dr. Russell in 1750, who also used a jelly for similar purposes, both internally and externally. He was also successful in dispersing scrofulous tumors by rubbing in the mucus of the vesicles of Bladderwrack, afterwards washing the parts with sea-water. The charcoal was also helpful in goitre. The iodine from other sources led to the neglect of kelp products.

In 1862 Dr. Duchesne-Duparc found while experimenting in cases of chronic psoriasis, that weight was reduced without injuring health, and used the drug with success for the latter purpose. Dr. Godfroy experimented on himself, losing five and a quarter pounds in a week after taking before three meals a day an extract made into pills containing 25 grams (3.75 grains). The bromine and iodine stimulated the absorbent glands to increased activity, without causing an atrophied wasting of the glands. Later experiments of Hunt and Seidell indicated that the result is brought about by stimulation of the thyroid gland.

Sea-pod liniment, is the expressed juice and decoction of fresh seaweed as dispensed by sea-side chemists for rheumatism, and the extract, taken continuously in pills or fluid form is reputed to relieve rheumatic pains as well as to diminish fat without harm.

Sea-pod essence is good for rubbing into sprains and bruises, or for applying on wet lint under oiled silk, as a compress, changed as often as hot or dry. It may be preceded by fomentations of the hot decoction.

Embrocation for strengthening the limbs of rickety children can be made from the glutinous substance of the vesicles, bottled in rum.

Fucus or Seaweed wine, from grapes and dried Fucus, has been praised as a remedy in diseases of the hip and other joints and bones in children.

For external application to enlarged or hardened glands, the bruised weed may be applied as a cold poultice.

Dosage

Of charcoal, 10 grains to 2 drachms.

Of extract, 3 to 10 grains, in pills, massed with powdered Liquorice or Marshmallow roots, to reduce swelling and obesity.

Of liquid extract, 1 to 2 fluid drachms. It is the basis of many advertised nostrums. Sodium and potassium iodides are often added to supplement the small proportion of iodine. It is used in mixture form, generally with alkali iodides and sometimes in combination with Liquor Thyroidei.

Of decoction, 2 fluid ounces, three times daily.

Of infusion, 1 wine glassful.

Solid extract may be dissolved in diluted alcohol and mixed with syrup.

(All doses for combating obesity are gradually increased.)

Of fluid extract, 10 minims.

The Alginic acid obtained from seaweed is used to form an organic compound with iron, which is sold under the trade name of Algiron or Alginoid Iron. It contains about 11 per cent. of iron and is given in doses of 2 to 10 decigrams (3 to 15 grains).

Fucol is a trade name for a cod-liver oil substitute, said to be obtained from roasted Bladderwrack with a bland oil. It is green in color, and resembles coffee in odor and taste.

Fucusin tablets are recommended in obesity.

Other Species

F. nodosus the Knobbed Wrack, has anarrower thallus, without a midrib and single vesicles.

F. serratus, the Black Wrack, has a veined and serrate frond, without vesicles . Both contain the same constituents as Bladderwrack.

F. serratus has been much used in Norway for feeding cattle, being called there 'cowweed." Linnaeus stated that in Gothland the inhabitants boiled it with water, mixed it with a little coarse meal or flour, and fed their hogs with it, for which reason they called the plant 'Swine-tang." In Sweden the poor people covered their cottages with it and sometimes used it for fuel.

F. siliquosus has a very narrow frond, with short branches and articulated vesicles of a pod-like appearance.

This and the two preceding species are permitted by the French Codex to be employed in the place of F. vesiculosis.

F. natans (Sargassum bacciferum) is the Gulfweed of the Atlantic Ocean and is often found in immense masses floating in the sea.

The frond is terrate and has linear and serrate branches and globular vesicles of the size of a pea.

F. vesiculosis was reputed to be the Antipolyscarcique nostrum of Count Mattei.

F. canaliculatus is remarkable for its amphibious habits, growing on large boulders and recovering after being baked by the sun into hard brown masses.

F. amylaceus, or Ceylon Moss, abounding in starch and vegetable jelly, is used like carrageen, or Irish moss.

F. Helminthocorton (Corsican Moss or Gigartina Helminthocorton) is regarded in Europe as an anthelmintic and febrifuge. It is an ingredient in the trade mixture called Corsican Moss, used in decoction of from 4 to 6 drachms to a pint, the dose being 1 wine glassful three times a day.

Another seaweed, Agar-agar, of the East Indies, is sent to China in large quantities for making jellies and for a size used in stiffening silks. An aperient medicine is known by its name. (American.)

Laminaria digitata, sea-girdles or tangles, of Scotland, gives a good substance for bougies. The stems are strong and tenacious, from 2 to 12 inches long and an inch or more wide, drying easily with much shrinkage and becoming firm, only slightly softer than horn, and yet elastic. It may be kept thus for years, and will absorb moisture at any time and swell to the original size, thus being valuable for dilating bougies and tents.

The Laminariaceae species are very remarkable in many ways. L. digitata, L. stenophylla, and L. saccharina are the principal ones associated with the kelp industry.

F. crispus is a name of Chondrus crispus or Gigartina mamillosa (Irish Moss or Carrageen) of European coasts, well known as a demulcent. Dosage, 4 drachms.

BLITES

Family: N.O. Chenopodiaceae

Habitat

They grow only on seashores, or in saline plains and other places where the soil is impregnated with salt, and are almost exclusively confined to the temperate and tropical regions of the Northern Hemisphere, very few being found in the Southern.

The Sea-blites are members of the genus Suaeda, the name derived from the Greek word for soda, in which the plants abound.

They are smooth or downy herbaceous, or more frequently shrubby, plants, with alternate, somewhat tapering, fleshy, stalkless leaves, bearing solitary or clustered stalkless or short-stalked, usually perfect flowers in their axils. Their fruits, utricles, are enclosed in the slightly enlarged or inflated berry- like calyx, but do not adhere to it.

BLITE, SEA

Botanical: Sueada fruticosa
Synonym: Shrubby Sea Blite

The Shrubby Sea-Blite is one of our rarer British species. It grows on sandy and shingly beaches, mostly on the east coast, but it is very common in the warmer parts of Europe and also in Northern Africa and Western Asia.

It is a shrubby, erect, branching, evergreen, perennial plant, 2 to 5 feet high, with thick and succulent, semi-cylindrical, bluntish, pale-green leaves, and small stalkless flowers, either solitary, or two or three together.

It is one of the plants burned in Southern Europe for the manufacture of barilla.

BLITE, ANNUAL SEA

Botanical: Suaeda maritima

Suaeda maritima (Linn.), the Annual Sea-Blite, is our other British species and is common on muddy seashores. It is a low straggling plant, smooth, glaucous and reddish in winter, with slender branches rising 1 to 2 feet; acute, semi-cylindrical, short fleshy leaves; flowers, 1 to 5 together, styles two. It is in flower from July to October.

Culpepper tells us there are

'two sorts, the white and the red. The white hath leaves somewhat like unto beets but smaller, rounder and of a whitish-green color. The red is in all things like the white, but that its leaves and tufted heads are exceedingly red at first and after turn more purplish.... They are all of them cooling, drying and binding and useful in fluxes of blood, especially the red."

He also mentions

'another sort of wild Blites, like the other wild kinds, but having long and spiky heads of greenish seeds, seeming by the thick setting together to be all seed. This sort fishes are delighted with, and it is a good and usual bait, for fishes will bite fast enough at them, if you have but wit enough to catch them when they bite."

The name Blite has also been applied to several of the Chenopodiums.

BLITE, STRAWBERRY

Botanical: Amaranthus blitus
Synonyms: Strawberry Spinach. Berry-bearing Orache.

The Strawberry Blite belongs to the closely allied order Amaranthacece, and is not strictly a native of Britain, only occasionally appearing on rubbish heaps. It is an inconspicuous weed, and to the casual observer would be regarded as an Orache or Goosefoot. Its trailing stems are a foot or so in length, bearing more or less oval leaves and numerous green flowers clustered in the leaf axils. The flowers are unisexual and without petals, both kinds of flowers being borne, however, on the same plant. The female flower develops into a juicy crimson capsule, full of purple juice, having somewhat the appearance of a Wood Strawberry, hence the popular name of the plant. Was formerly much used for coloring in cookery. It flowers in August.

BLOODROOT

POISON
Botanical: Sanguinaria Candensis (LINN.)
Family: N.O. Papaveraceae
Synonyms: Indian Paint. Tetterwort. Red Pucoon. Red Root. Paucon. Coon Root. Snakebite. Sweet Slumber.
Parts Used: Root, whole plant.

Habitat

United States of America and Canada, found in rich open woods from Canada, south to Florida and west to Arkansas. and Nebraska.

Description

A perennial plant, one of the earliest and most beautiful spring flowers. In England it will grow freely if cultivated carefully, it has even grown in the open in gravelly dry soil in the author's garden. It has a lovely white flower and produces only a single leaf and a flowering scape about 6 inches high. When the leaf first appears it is wrapped round the flower bud and is a greyish-green color covered with a downy bloom - Leaves palmate five to nine lobed, 6 to 10 inches long. After flowering the leaves increase in size, the underside paler showing prominent veins. The white flower is wax-like with golden stamens. The seed is an oblong narrow pod about 1 inch long. The rootstock is thick, round and fleshy, slightly curved at ends, and contains an orange-red juice, and is about 1 to 4 inches long, with orange-red rootlets. When dried it breaks with a short sharp fracture, little smell, taste bitter acrid and persistent, powdered root causes sneezing and irritation of the nose. The root is collected in the autumn, after leaves die down; it must be stored in a dry place or it quickly deteriorates.

Constituents

Alkaloids Sanguinarine, Chelerythrine, Protopine and B. homochelidonine; Sanguinarine forms colorless crystals. Chelerythrine is also colorless and crystalline. Protopine (also found in opium) is one of the most widely diffused of the opium alkaloids. The rhizome also contains red resin and an abundance of starch.

Medicinal Action and Uses

Emetic cathartic expectorant and emmenagogue, and of great value in atonic dyspepsia, asthma, bronchitis and croup. (The taste is so nauseating, that it may cause expectorant action.) Of value in pulmonary consumption, nervous irritation and helpful in lowering high pulse, and in heart disease and weakness and palpitation of heart of great use. For ringworm apply the fluid extract. Also good for torpid liver, scrofula, dysentery. It is applied to fungoid growths, ulcers fleshy excrescences, cancerous affections and as an escharotic. Sanguinaria root is chiefly used as an expectorant for chronic bronchitis and as a local application in chronic eczema, specially when secondary to varicose ulcers. In toxic doses, it causes burning in the stomach, intense thirst, vomiting, faintness vertigo, intense prostration with dimness of eyesight.

The root has long been used by the American Indians as a dye for their bodies and clothes and has been used successfully by American and French dyers.

Preparations and Dosages

Fluid extract of Sanguinaria, U.S.P., dose 1 1/2 minims. Tincture of Sanguinaria, U.S.P., 15 minims. Powdered root, 10 to 30 grains. Sanguinarin, 1/4 to 1 grain. Fluid extract, 10 to 30 drops .

BLUEBELL

Botanical: Scilla nutans (S. M.)
Hyacinthus nonscriptus (LINN.)
Synonyms: Calverkeys. Culverkeys. Auld Man's Bell. Ring-o'-Bells. Jacinth. Wood Bells. Agraphis nutans, Link.
Part Used: Bulb, dried and powdered.

Habitat

Abundant in Britain, Western Europe to Spain, eastward to Central France, along the Mediterranean to Italy.

Description

From the midst of very long, narrow leaves, rising from the small bulb, and overtopping them, rises the flower-stem, bearing the pendulous, bell-shaped blossoms, arranged in a long curving line. Each flower has two small bracts at the base of the short flower-stalk. The perianth is bluish-purple and composed of six leaflets.

The Wild Hyacinth is in flower from early in April till the end of May, and being a perennial and spreading rapidly, is found year after year in the same spot, forming a mass of rich color in the woods where it grows. The long leaves remain above ground until late in the autumn.

Linnaeus first called it Hyacinthus, tradition associating the flower with the Hyacinth of the Ancients, the flower of grief and mourning. Hyacinthus was a charming youth whom both Apollo and Zephyrus loved, but Hyacinthus preferred the Sun-God to the God of the West Wind, who sought to be revenged, and one day when Apollo was playing quoits with the youth, a quoit (blown by Zephyrus out of its proper course) killed Hyacinthus. Apollo, stricken with grief, raised from his blood a purple flower, on which the letters Ai, Ai were traced, so that his cry of woe might for evermore have existence upon earth. As our native variety of Hyacinth had no trace of these mystic letters our older botanists called it Hyacinthus nonscriptus, or 'not written on." A later generic name, Agraphis, is of similar meaning, being a compound of two Greek words, meaning 'not to mark."

It is the 'fair-hair'd hyacinth' of Ben Jonson, a name alluding to the old myth. We also find it called Jacinth in Elizabethan times. In Walton's Angler it is mentioned as Culverkeys.

Constituents

The bulbs contain inulin, but are characterized by the absence of starch (which in many other monoeotyledons is found in company with inulin). Even if fed on cane-sugar, Bluebell bulbs will not form starch. They also contain a very large quantity of mucilage.

Medicinal Action and Uses

Though little used in modern medicine, the bulb has diuretic and styptic properties.

Dried and powdered it has been used as a styptic for leucorrhoea; 'There is hardly a more powerful remedy," wrote Sir John Hill (1716-75), warning at the same time that the dose should not exceed 3 grains. He also informs us that a decoction of the bulb operates by urine.

Tennyson speaks of Bluebell juice being used to cure snake-bite.

The flowers have a slight, starch-like scent, but no medicinal uses have been ascribed to them.

The bulbs are poisonous in the fresh state. The viscid juice so abundantly contained in them and existing in every part of the plant has been used as a substitute for starch, and in the days when stiff ruffs were worn was much in request. From its gummy character, it was also employed as bookbinders' gum.

Gerard informs us that it was also used for setting feathers upon arrows. De Candolle (1778-1841) suggested that the abundant mucilage might be put to some economic purpose.

Dosage

3 grains.

Substitutes

any other bulbous plants related to Scilla (Hyacinthus, Muscari Gagea, etc.) have been used as diuretics, and probably contain related, if not identical substances.

BOGBEAN

Botanical: Menyanthes trifoliata (TOURNEF.)
Family: N.O. Gentianaceae
Synonyms: Buckbean. Marsh Trefoil. Water Trefoil. Marsh Clover.
(Dutch) Bocks. Boonan.
(German) Bocksbohne or Scharbocks-Klee.
Part Used: Herb.

Habitat

The Buckbean, or Bogbean, grows in spongy bogs, marshes and shallow water throughout Europe, being rather scarce in the south of England, though common in the north and in Scotland.

Description

It is a green, glabrous plant, with creeping rootstock and procumbent stem, varying in length according to situation, covered by the sheaths of the leaves, which are on long, fleshy, striated petioles and three-partite, the leaflets being entire and about 2 inches long and 1 broad. It blossoms from May to July, the flowers being borne on long stalks, 6 to 18 inches high, longer than the leaves and clustered together in a thick short spike, rendering them very conspicuous. The corollas, 3/4 inch across, are outwardly rose-coloured and inwardly white and hairy, with reddish stamens. The Buckbean is one of the prettiest of our wild flowers deserving of cultivation in the garden, where it grows and thrives well, if planted in peat with water constantly round the roots.

History

The plant was held to be of great value as a remedy against the once-dreaded scurvy. Scharbock, its German name, is a corruption of the Latin scorbutus, the old medical name for the disease.

'Bean' is probably an affix from the resemblance of the foliage to that of the beans grown in cottage gardens. Gerard says that the leaves are 'like to those of the garden beane."

Its specific name, trifoliata, carries the same reference to the form of its leaves.

The generic name, Menyanthes, is from two Greek words signifying month and flower. It was a name bestowed by Linnaeus, and it has been suggested that the plant was so called because it remains in flower for a month; but it is actually often in bloom during May, June and July!

One of the older writers describes its inflorescence as a 'bush of feather-like floures of a white color, dasht ouer slightly with a wash of light carnation."

Buckbean has a reputation for preserving sheep from rot, but it is doubtful whether they really touch it, on account of its extreme bitterness.

Constituents

The chief constituents are a small quantity of volatile oil and a bitter principle, a glucoside called Menyanthin. The bitterness is imparted to both alcohol and water.

Medicinal Action and Uses

Tonic, cathartic, deobstruent and febrifuge. An extract is made from the leaves, which possesses strong tonic properties, and which renders great service in rheumatism, scurvy, and skin diseases. An infusion of 1 OZ. of the dried leaves to 1 pint of boiling water is taken in wine glassful doses, frequently repeated. It has also been recommended as an external application for dissolving glandular swellings. Finely powdered Buckbean leaves have been employed as a remedy for ague, being said to effect a cure when other means fail. In large doses, the powder is also purgative. It is used also as a herb tobacco.

The juice of the fresh leaves has proved efficacious in dropsical cases, and mixed with whey has been known to cure gout.

In Halliwell's Popular Rhymes and Nursery Tales this rhyme occurs:

'Buckee, Buckee, biddy Bene,
Is the way now fair and clean?
Is the goose ygone to nest,
And the fox ygone to rest?
Shall I come away?"

These curious lines are said by Devonshire children when they go through any passages in the dark, and are said to be addressed to Puck or Robin Goodfellow. Biddy bene= Anglo-Saxon biddan, to ask or pray; bén, a supplication or entreaty. Buckee is perhaps a corruption of Puck.

Buckbean tea, taken alone or mixed with wormwood, centaury or sage, is said to cure dyspepsia and a torpid liver.

Preparation

Fluid extract, 10 to 40 drops.

BOLDO

Botanical: Peumus Boldus (MOLINA)
Family: N.O. Monimiaceae
Synonyms: Boldu. Boldus. Boldoa Fragrans.
Part Used: The leaves.
Habitat: Chile.

Description

An evergreen shrub growing in the fields of the Andes in Chile, where its yellowish-green fruit is eaten, its bark used for tanning, and its wood utilized in charcoal making.

Leaves are opposite, sessile, about 2 inches long entire, and color when dried red brown, coriaceous, prominent midrib, a number of small glands on their surface. Odor peculiar, when crushed very strongly disagreeable, not unlike oil of Chenopodium (wormseed). The leaves contain about 2 per cent on distillation of an aromatic volatile oil, chemically related to oil of Chenopodium.

A peculiar alkaloid called Boldine has been found in the leaves and when injected hyperdermically, paralyses both motor and sensory nerves, also the muscle fibres. When given internally, in toxic doses, it causes great excitement, exaggerates the reflexes and the respiratory movements, increases diuresis, causes cramp and convulsions ending in death from centric respiratory paralysis, the heart continuing to beat long after respiration ceases. Of late years Boldine has been largely used in veterinary practice for jaundice.

Constituents

Boldo leaves contain about 2 per cent of volatile oil, in which, in addition to terpenes, terpineol has been detected. They also contain the bitter alkaloid Boldine and the glucoside Boldin or Boldoglucin.

Medicinal Action and Uses

Tonic, antiseptic, stimulant. Useful in chronic hepatic torpor. The oil in 5-drop doses has been found useful in genito-urinary inflammation. Has long been recognized in South America as a valuable cure for gonorrhea.

Preparations

Tincture of Boldo, B.P.C., used as a diuretic. Dose, 10 to 40 minims. Fluid extract, 1/4 to 1/2 drachm.

Other Species

The Australian tree Monimia rotundifolia contains an oil rather similar, which may be safely substituted for Boldo.

BONESET

Botanical: Eupatorium perfoliatum (LINN.)
Family: N.O. Compositae
Synonym: Thoroughwort.
Part Used: Herb.

Habitat

Thoroughwort or Boneset is a very common and familiar plant in low meadows and damp ground in North America, extending from Nova Scotia to Florida.

Boneset was a favorite medicine of the North American Indians, who called it by a name that is equivalent to 'Ague-weed," and it has always been a popular remedy in the United States, probably no plant in American domestic practice having more extensive and frequent use; it is also in use to some extent in regular practice, being official in the United States Pharmacopeia, though it is not included in the British Pharmacopoeia.

Constituents

All parts of the plant are active, but the herb only is official, the leaves and tops being gathered after flowering has commenced. They contain a volatile oil, some tannic acid, and Eupatorin, a bitter glucosidal principle, also resin, gum and sugar. The virtues of the plant are yielded both to water and alcohol.

Description

Boneset is a perennial herb, with an erect stout, cylindrical hairy stem, 2 to 4 feet high, branched at the top. The leaves are large, opposite, united at the base, lance-shaped, 4 to 8 inches long (the lower ones being the largest), tapering to a sharp point, the edges finely toothed, the veins prominent, the blades rough above, downy and resinous and dotted beneath. The leaves serve to distinguish the species at the first glance - they may be considered either as perforated by the stem, perfoliate (hence the specific name), or as consisting of two opposite leaves joined at the base, the botanical term for which is connate. The flower-heads are terminal and numerous, large and slightly convex, with from ten to twenty white florets, having a bristly pappus, the hairs of which are arranged in a single row. The odor of the plant is slightly aromatic, the taste astringent and strongly bitter. This species shows considerable variety in size, hairiness, form of leaves and inflorescence. It flowers from July to September.

Medicinal Action and Uses

Stimulant, febrifuge and laxative. It acts slowly and persistently, and its greatest power is manifested upon the stomach, liver, bowels and uterus.

It is regarded as a mild tonic in moderate doses, and is also diaphoretic, more especially when taken as a warm infusion, in which form it is used in attacks of muscular rheumatism and general cold. In large doses it is emetic and purgative.

Many of the earlier works allude to this species as a diuretic, and therefore of use in dropsy, but this is an error, this property being possessed by Eupatorium purpureum, the purple-flowered Boneset, or Gravel Root.

It has been much esteemed as a popular febrifuge, especially in intermittent fever, and has been employed, though less successfully, in typhoid and yellow fevers. It is largely used by the negroes of the Southern United States as a remedy in all cases of fever, as well as for its tonic effects. As a mild tonic it is useful in dyspepsia and general debility, and particularly serviceable in the indigestion of old people. The infusion of 1 OZ of the dried herb to 1 pint of boiling water may be taken in wine glassful doses, hot or cold: for colds and to produce perspiration, it is given hot; as a tonic, cold.

As a remedy in catarrh, more especially in influenza, it has been extensively used and with the best effects, given in doses of a wine glassful, warm every half hour, the patient remaining in bed the whole time; after four or five doses, profuse perspiration is caused and relief is obtained. It is stated that the popular name Boneset is derived from the great value of this remedy in the treatment of a species of influenza which had much prevailed in the United States, and which from the pain attending it was commonly called Break-Bone Fever.

This species of Eupatorium has also been employed in cutaneous diseases, and in the expulsion of tapeworm.

Preparations

Powdered herb. Dose 12 to 20 grains.

Fluid extract, 1/2 to 1 drachm.

Eupatorin. Dose, 1 to 3 grains.

BORAGE

Botanical: Borago officinalis (LINN.)
Family: N.O. Boraginaceae
Synonym: Burrage.
Parts Used: Leaves and flowers.

Habitat

The Common Borage is a hardy annual plant coming originally from Aleppo but now naturalized in most parts of Europe and frequently found in this country, though mostly only on rubbish heaps and near dwellings, and may be regarded as a garden escape. It has long been grown freely in kitchen gardens, both for its uses as a herb and for the sake of its flowers, which yield excellent honey.

Description

The whole plant is rough with white, stiff, prickly hairs. The round stems, about 1 1/2 feet high, are branched, hollow and succulent; the leaves alternate, large, wrinkled, deep green, oval and pointed, 3 inches long or more, and about 1 1/2 inch broad, the lower ones stalked, with stiff, one celled hairs on the upper surfaces and on the veins below, the margins entire, but wavy. The flowers, which terminate the cells, are bright blue and star-shaped, distinguished from those of every plant in this order by their prominent black anthers, which form a cone in the centre and have been described as their beauty spot. The fruit consists of four brownish-black nutlets.

History

In the early part of the nineteenth century, the young tops of Borage were still sometimes boiled as a pot-herb, and the young leaves were formerly considered good in salads.

The fresh herb has a cucumber-like fragrance. When steeped in water, it imparts a coolness to it and a faint cucumber flavor, and compounded with lemon and sugar in wine, and water, it makes a refreshing and restorative summer drink. It was formerly always an ingredient in cool tankards of wine and cider, and is still largely used in claret cup.

Our great grandmothers preserved the flowers and candied them.

Borage was sometimes called Bugloss by the old herbalists, a name that properly belongs to Anchusa officinalis, the Alkanet, the Small Bugloss being Lycopsis arvensis, and Viper's Bugloss being the popular name for Echium vulgare.

Some authorities consider that the Latin name Borago, from which our popular name is taken, is a corruption of corago, from cor, the heart, and ago, I bring, because of its cordial effect.

In all the countries bordering the Mediterranean, where it is plentiful, it is spelt with a double 'r," so the word may be derived from the Italian borra, French bourra, signifying hair or wool, words which in their turn are derived from the Low Latin burra, a flock of wool, in reference to the thick covering of short hairs which clothes the whole plant.

Henslow suggests that the name is derived from barrach, a Celtic word meaning 'a man of courage."

Gerard says:

'Pliny calls it Euphrosinum, because it maketh a man merry and joyfull: which thing also the old verse concerning Borage doth testifie:

Ego Borago - (I, Borage)

Gaudia semper ago. - (Bring alwaies courage.)

Those of our time do use the flowers in sallads to exhilerate and make the mind glad. There be also many things made of these used everywhere for the comfort of the heart, for the driving away of sorrow and increasing the joy of the minde. The leaves and floures of Borage put into wine make men and women glad and merry and drive away all sadnesse, dulnesse and melancholy, as Dios corides and Pliny affirme. Syrup made of the floures of Borage comforteth the heart, purgeth melancholy and quieteth the phrenticke and lunaticke person. The leaves eaten raw ingender good bloud, especially in those that have been lately sicke."

According to Dioscorides and Pliny, Borage was the famous Nepenthe of Homer, which when drunk steeped in wine, brought absolute forgetfulness.

John Evelyn, writing at the close of the seventeenth century tells us: 'Sprigs of Borage are of known virtue to revive the hypochrondriac and cheer the hard student."

Parkinson commends it 'to expel pensiveness and melanchollie." Bacon says that it 'hath an excellent spirit to repress the fuliginous vapor of dusky melancholie." Culpepper finds the plant useful in putrid and pestilential fever, the venom of serpents, jaundice, consumption, sore throat, and rheumatism."

Cultivation

Borage flourishes in ordinary soil. It may be propagated by division of rootstocks in spring and by putting cuttings of shoots in sandy soil in a cold frame in summer and autumn, or from seeds sown in fairly good, light soil, from the middle of March to May, in drills 18 inches apart, the seedlings being thinned out to about 15 inches apart in the rows. If left alone, Borage will seed itself freely and comes up year after year in the same place. Seeds may also be sown in the autumn. Those sown then will flower in May, whereas those sown in the spring will not flower till June.

Part Used Medicinally

The leaves, and to a lesser extent, the flowers. Gather the leaves when the plant is coming into flower. Strip them off singly and reject any that are stained and insect-eaten. Pick only on a fine day, when the sun has dried off the dew.

Constituents

Borage contains potassium and calcium, combined with mineral acids. The fresh juice affords 30 per cent, the dried herb 3 per cent of nitrate of potash. The stems and leaves supply much saline mucilage, which when boiled and cooked likewise deposits nitre and common salt. It is to these saline qualities that the wholesome invigorating properties of Borage are supposed to be due. Owing to the presence of nitrate of potash when burnt, it will emit sparks with a slight explosive sound.

Medicinal Action and Uses

Diuretic, demulcent, emollient. Borage is much usedin France for fevers and pulmonary complaints. By virtue of its saline constituents, it promotes the activity of the kidneys and for this reason is employed to carry off feverish catarrhs. Its demulcent qualities are due to the mucilage contained in the whole plant.

For internal use, an infusion is made of 1 OZ of leaves to 1 pint of boiling water, taken in wine glassful doses.

Externally, it is employed as a poultice for inflammatory swellings.

Preparation

Fluid extract. Dose, 1/2 to 1 drachm.

The flowers, candied and made into a conserve, were deemed useful for persons weakened by long sickness, and for those subject to swoonings; the distilled water was considered as effectual, and also valuable to cure inflammation of the eyes.

The juice in syrup was thought not only to be good in fevers, but to be a remedy for jaundice, itch and ringworm. Culpepper tells us that in his days: 'The dried herb is never used, but the green, yet the ashes thereof boiled in mead or honeyed water, is available in inflammation and ulcers in the mouth or throat, as a gargle."

BOX

Botanical: Buxus sempervirens (LINN.)
Family: N.O. Buxaceae
Synonym: Dudgeon.
Parts Used: Wood and leaves.

Habitat

Chiefly in limestone districts in western and

southern Europe, westward to the Himalayas and Japan, northward to central and western France and in Britain, in some parts of southern and central England.

Description

Box in its familiar dwarfed state is merely a shrub, but when left to grow naturally it will become a small tree 12 to 15 feet in height, rarely exceeding 20 feet, with a trunk about 6 inches in diameter covered with a rugged, greyish bark, that of the branches being yellowish. It belongs to the family Buxacece, a very small family of only six genera and about thirty species, closely related to the Spurge family - Euphorbiaceae. Only this evergreen species has been utilized in medicine.

Its twigs are densely leafy and the leaves are about 1/2 inch in length, ovate, entire, smooth, thick, coriaceous and dark green. They have a peculiar, rather disagreeable odor and a bitter and somewhat astringent taste. The flowers are in heads, a terminal female flower, surrounded by a number of male flowers. The fruit dehisces explosively the inner layer of the pericarp separating from the outer and shooting out the seed by folding into a U-shape.

Constituents

The leaves have been found to contain besides a small amount of tannin and unimportant constituents, a butyraceous volatile oil and three alkaloids: (i) Buxine, the important constituent, chiefly responsible for the bitter taste and now regarded as identical with the Berberine of Nectander bark, (ii) Parabuxine, (iii) Parabuxonidine, which turns turmeric paper deep red. The bark contains chlorophyll, wax, resin, argotized tallow, gum, lignin, sulphates of potassium and lime, carbonates of lime and magnesia, phosphates of lime, iron and silica.

Medicinal Action and Uses

The wood in its native countries is considered diaphoretic, being given in decoction as an alterative for rheumatism and secondary syphilis. Used as a substitute for guaiacum in the treatment of venereal disease when sudorifics are considered to be the correct specifics.

It has been found narcotic and sedative in full doses; emetico-cathartic and convulsant in overdose. The tincture was formerly used as a bitter tonic and antiperiodic and had the reputation of curing leprosy.

A volatile oil distilled from the wood has been prescribed in cases of epilepsy. The oil has been employed for piles and also for toothache.

The leaves, which have a nauseous taste, have sudorific, alterative and cathartic properties being given in powder, in which form they are also an excellent vermifuge.

Various extracts and perfumes were formerly made from the leaves and bark. A decoction was recommended by some writers as an application to promote the growth of the hair. The leaves and sawdust boiled in Iye were used to dye hair an auburn color.

Dried and powdered, the leaves are still given to horses for the purpose of improving their coats. The powder is regarded by carters as highly poisonous, to be given with great care. In Devonshire, farriers still employ the old-fashioned remedy of powdered Box leaves for bot-worm in horses.

In former days, Box was the active ingredient in a once-famous remedy for the bite of a mad dog.

Animals in this country will not touch Box, and though camels are said to readily eat the leaves, they are poisoned by them.

The timber, though small, is valuable on account of its hardness and heaviness, being the hardest and heaviest of all European woods. It is of a delicate yellow color, dense in structure with a fine uniform grain, which gives it unique value for the wood-engraver, the most important use to which it is put being for printing blocks and engraving plates. An edge of this wood stands better than tin or lead, rivalling brass in its wearing power. A large amount is used in the manufacture of measuring rules, various mathematical instruments, flutes and other musical instruments and the wooden parts of tools, for which a perfectly rigid and non-expansive material is required, as well as for toilet boxes, pillrounders and similar articles.

The Boxwood used by cabinet-makers and turners in France is chiefly the root. Gerard tells us:

'The root is likewise yellow and harder than the timber, but of greater beauty and more fit for dagger haftes, boxes and suchlike. Turners and cuttlers do call this wood Dudgeon, wherewith they make Dudgeonhafted daggers."

In France, Boxwood has been used as a substitute for hops and the branches and leaves of Box have been recommended as by far the best manure for the vine, as it is said no plant by its decomposition affords a greater quantity of vegetable manure.

Dosage

As a purgative: dose of the powdered leaves, 1 drachm.

As vermifuge: 10 to 20 grains of the powdered leaves.

As sudorific: 1 to 2 oz. of the wood, in decoction.

Other Species

DWARF BOX (Buxus suffructaca) possesses similar medicinal properties.

The American Boxwood used in herbal medicine as a substitute for Peruvian Bark, being a good tonic, astringent and stimulant, is not this Box but a kind of Dogwood, native to America, Cornus florida.

Adulterant

Box bark which is also bitter and free from tannin, is sometimes substituted for Pomegranate Bark, which is employed as a worm-dispeller.

Box leaves have sometimes been substituted for Bearberry leaves (Uva-Ursi), from which they are distinguished by their notched apex.

Box leaves are also sometimes used as adulteration of senna, but are easily detected by their shape and thickness.

The custom of clipping Dwarf Box in topiary gardening is said to have originated with the Romans, a friend of Julius Caesar having invented it.

BOXWOOD, AMERICAN

Botanical: Cornus florida (LINN.)
Family: N.O. Cornaceae
Synonyms: Bitter Redberry. Cornel. New England Boxwood. Dog-Tree. Flowering Dogwood. American Dogwood. Benthamidia florida. Box Tree. Virginian Dogwood. Cornouiller à grandes fleurs. Mon-ha-can-ni-min-schi. Hat-ta-wa-no-minschi.
Part Used: The dried bark of the root.
Habitat: The United States, from Massachusetts to Florida.

Description

An ornamental little tree introduced into English cultivation about 1740, but still uncommon. It grows from 10 to 30 feet in height, with oval, opposite leaves, dark, clear green above and lighter below. The flowers occur in a small bunch surrounded by four large, white, involucral bracts that give the tree the appearance of bearing large white flowers. The name 'Florida' alludes to this effect, and the name 'Cornus," from cornu, 'a horn," refers to the density of the wood. It flowers so punctually in the third week in May that it sets the time for the Indians' corn-planting. The oval berries are a brilliant red. The bark is blackish, and cut into almost square sections. The inner bark can be utilized to make black ink, half an ounce of bark being mixed with two scruples of sulphate of iron and two scruples of gum-arabic dissolved in sixteen ounces of rainwater. A scarlet pigment can be obtained from the root bark. The wood is heavy and fine-grained, valuable for small articles because it takes an excellent polish. It is cut in autumn and dried before using. The twigs, stripped of their bark, whiten the teeth, and are used as a dentifrice by the Creoles who inhabit Virginia. The juice of the twigs preserves and hardens the gums. A bitter but agreeable drink can be prepared from the fruits infused in eau-de-vie.

In commerce the bark is usually in quilled pieces several inches long and from 1/2 to 2 inches broad, which may be covered with the greyish-red outer bark or may be deprived of it. They are brittle, and the short fracture shows a mottled red and white color. There is a slight odor, and the taste is bitter and a little aromatic; when fresh, almost acrid. The powder is a reddish-grey color.

Constituents

The bark has been found to contain tannic and gallic acids, resin, gum, extractive, oil, wax, red coloring matter, lignin, potassa, lime, magnesia, iron, and a neutral, crystalline glucoside called Cornin. Either water or alcohol extracts the virtues of the bark. The flowers are said to have similar properties, and to be sometimes used as a substitute. It is said that the berries, boiled and pressed, yield a limpid oil.

Medicinal Action and Uses

Before Europeans discovered America, the Red Indianswere using the bark in the same way as Peruvian bark. It is valuable in intermittent fevers, as a weak tonic for the stomach, and antiperiodic, as a stimulant and astringent. As a poultice in anthrax, indolent ulcers, and inflamed erysipelas, it is tonic, stimulant and antiseptic. In the recent state it should be avoided, as it disagrees with stomach and bowels. Cinchona bark or sulphate of quinea often replace it officially. 35 grains of Cornus bark are equal to 30 grains of cinchona bark.

The leaves make good fodder for cattle, and in Italy the oil is used in soups.

The ripe fruit, infused in brandy, is used as a stomachic in domestic practice, and a tincture of the berries restores tone to the stomach in alcoholism. Hippocrates, Dioscorides, and Pliny recommend them in diarrhea.

Dosage

Formerly, 1 to 2 oz. of the powder between paroxysms of intermittent fever.

Of fluid extract, 30 minims as a tonic.

Of cornin, 2 grains.

Other Species

C. circinata, or Round leaved Dogwood, and C. Amomum or C.Sericea (Silky Cornel or Swamp Dogwood), have similar properties and are sometimes used as substitutes.

C. sanguinea or C. stolonifera, a European species, is stated to have cured hydrophobia. A decoction was formerly used for washing mangy dogs, hence its name of Dogberry or Hound's Tree. It also yields an oil that is both edible and good for burning.

A Chilian species has edible berries, with which a drink called Theca is prepared. The juice of the leaves, or Maqui, is administered in angina.

C. caerulea has an astringent bark.

C. mascula, called in Greece akenia, and in Turkey kizziljiek, or redwood, yields the red dye used for the fez, and the astringent fruit is good in bowel complaints, and is used in cholera and for flavoring sherbet. The flowers are used in diarrhea, and the berries were formerly made into tarts called rob de cornis.

The dwarf C. suecica has small red berries which form part of the Esquimaux' winter food-store. In Scotland they have such a reputation as a tonic for the appetite that the tree is called lus-a-chraois, or Plant of Gluttony.

Dogwood is also a popular name of Pisicia Erythrina, which yields a powerful soporific used for toothache. Its chief use is for poisoning birds, fish, or animals, which may be eaten afterwards without ill effect. Fish after eating it may be caught in the hand, stupefied.

BROOKLIME

Botanical: Veronica beccabunga (LINN.)
Family: N.O. Scrophulariaceae
Synonyms: Water Pimpernel. Becky Leaves. Cow Cress. Horse Cress. Housewell. Grass. Limewort.

Brooklembe. Limpwort. Wall-ink. Water-Pumpy. Well-ink.
Part Used: Herb.

Habitat

Brooklime is found in all parts of Great Britain, being very common and generally distributed, occurring as far north as the Shetlands, and in the Highlands ascending up to 2,800 feet. It is found in Ireland and the Channel Islands.

Description

It grows abundantly in shallow streams, ditches, the margins of ponds, etc., flourishing in the same situations as Water Cress and Water Mint, throwing out stout, succulent, hollow stems that root and creep along the ground at the base, giving off roots at intervals, and then ascend, bearing pairs of short, stalked, oval-oblong leaves, smooth, about 1 1/2 inch long, slightly toothed on their margin and thick and leathery in texture. The whole plant is very smooth and shiny in appearance, turning blackish in drying. The flowers are rather numerous, in lax, axillary racemes, 2 to 4 inches long, given off in pairs, whereas in Germander, Speedwell, only one flower stem rises from each pair of leaves. They begin to open in May and continue in succession through the greater part of the summer, though are at their best in May and June. The corollas are bright blue, with darker veins and a white eye, the petals oval and unequal. Occasionally a pink form is found.

The flower is adapted for cross-fertilization in the same manner as Veronica chamaedrys, the stamens and style projecting from the flower and forming an alighting place for insects. The petals are wide open in the sun but only partly expanded in dull weather. The flowers are much visited by insects, especially by a fly, Syritta pipians. The Honey Bee is also a visitor and some other small wild bees. Two species of beetle and the larva of a moth, Athalia annulata, feed on the leaves. The capsule is round, flat notched and swollen and contains winged, smooth seeds.

The specific name of this plant seems to be derived from the German name, Bachbunge bach, signifying a brook, and bunge, a bunch. Another source given for the specific name is from the Flemish beckpunge meaning 'mouth smart," a name suggested by the pungency of its leaves, which were formerly eaten in salads. Dr. Prior tells us that the name Brooklime is in old writers Broklempe or Lympe, from its growing in the lime or mud of brooks, the Anglo-Saxon word lime, coming from the Latin limus, a word that from mud used in the rude buildings of Anglo-Saxon times, has come to be applied to the calcareous stone of which mortar is now made.

Constituents

Tannin and a special bitter principle, a pungent volatile oil and some sulphur.

Medicinal Action and Uses

Alterative, Diuretic. The leaves and young stems were once in favour as an antiscorbutic, and even now the young shoots are sometimes eaten in spring with those of Watercress, the two plants being generally found growing together. As a green vegetable, Brooklime isalso wholesome, but not very palatable.

In earlier days the leaves were applied to wounds, though their styptic qualities appear to be slight. They are sometimes bruised and put on burns.

The juice, with that of scurvy-grass and Seville oranges, formed the 'spring juices' once valued as an antiscorbutic.

The plant has always been a popular simple for scrofulous affections, especially of the skin. An infusion of the leaves is recommended for impurity of the blood, an ounce of them being infused in a pint of boiling water.

In the fourteenth century, Brooklime was used for many complaints, including swellings, gout, etc.

BROOM

Botanical: Cytisus scoparius (LINN.)
Family: N.O. Leguminosae
Synonyms: Spartium scoparium (Linn.). Genista scoparius (Lam.). Sarothamnus scoparius (Koch). Broom Tops. Irish Tops. Basam. Bisom. Bizzom.

Browme. Brum. Breeam. Green Broom.
Part Used: Tops.

Habitat

The densely-growing Broom, a shrub indigenous to England and common in this country, grows wild all over temperate Europe and northern Asia, being found in abundance on sandy pastures and heaths. It is sparingly naturalized in sandy soil in North America.

It is remarkable as the only native medicinal plant used as an official drug that we draw from the important order of the Leguminosae, or pod-bearing tribe. Though now more generally known as Cytisus scoparius (Linn.), it has also been named Spartium scoparium (Linn.), Sarothamnus scoparius (Koch), and Genista scoparius (Lam.).

Its long, slender, erect and tough branches grow in large, close fascicles, thus rendering it available for broom-making, hence its English name. The local names of Basam, Bisom, Bizzom, Breeam, Browme, Brum and Green Broom have all been given it in reference to the habit of making brooms of it, and the name of the genus, Sarothamnus, to which it was formerly assigned, also points out this use of the plant, being formed from the Greek words signifying 'to sweep' and 'a shrub." The specific name, Scoparius, also, is derived from the Latin scopa, a besom. The generic name Cytisus is said to be a corruption of the name of a Greek island, Cythnus, where Broom abounded, though it is probable that the Broom known to the ancients, and mentioned by Pliny and by Virgil under the name of Genista, was another species, the Spanish Broom, Spartium junceum, as the Common Broom is in Greece and not found in Southern and Eastern Europe, being chiefly a native of Western, Northern and Central Europe.

The medicinal use of the brush-like branches of the Broom, under the name Genista, Genesta, or Genestia, is mentioned in the earliest printed herbals, under Passau, 1485, the Hortus Sanitatis, 1491, the Grete Herball, 1516, and others. It is likewise the Genista figured by the German botanists and pharmacologists of the sixteenth century.

Broom was used in ancient Anglo-Saxon medicine and by the Welsh physicians of the early Middle Ages. It had a place in the London Pharmacopeia of 1618 and is included in the British Pharmacopoeia of the present day.

Bartholomew says of Broom:

'Genesta hath that name of bytterness for it is full of bytter to mannes taste. And is a shrub that growyth in a place that is forsaken, stony and untylthed. Presence thereof is witnesse that the ground is bareyne and drye that it groweth in. And hath many braunches knotty and hard. Grene in winter and yelowe floures in somer thyche (the which) wrapped with hevy (heavy) smell and bitter sauer (savour). And ben, netheles, moost of vertue."

Description

It grows to a height of 3 to 5 feet and produces numerous long, straight, slender bright green branches, tough and very flexible, smooth and prominently angled. The leaves are alternate, hairy when young the lower ones shortly stalked, with three small, oblong leaflets, the upper ones, near the tips of the branches, sessile and small, often reduced to a single leaflet. Professor G. Henslow (Floral Rambles in Highways and Byways) says with reference to the 'leaves' of the broom: 'It has generally no leaves, the green stems undertaking their duties instead. If it grows in wet places, it can develop threefoliate leaves." The large bright yellow, papilionaceous, fragrant flowers, in bloom from April to July, are borne on axillary footstalks, either solitary or in pairs, and are succeeded by oblong, flattened pods, about 1 1/2 inch long, hairy on the edges, but smooth on the sides. They are nearly black when mature. They burst with a sharp report when the seeds are ripe flinging them to a distance by the spring-iike twisting of the valves or sides of the pods. The continuous crackling of the bursting seed-vessels on a hot, sunny July day is readily noticeable. The flowers have a great attraction for bees, they contain no honey, but abundance of pollen.

'In flowers without honey, such as the Broom, there is a curious way of "exploding" to expel the pollen. In the Broom the stigma lies in the midst of the five anthers of the longer stamens, and when a bee visits the flower those of the shorter explode and disperse their pollen on the bee pressing upon the closed edges of the keel petal. "The shock is not enough to drive the bee away . . . The split now quickly extends further . . . when a second and more violent explosion occurs." The style was horizontal with a flattened end below the stigma; but when freed from restraint it curls inwards, forming more than a complete spiral turn. It springs up and strikes the back of the bee with its stigma. The bee then gathers pollen with its mouth and legs." (From The Fertilization of Flowers, by Professor H. Mueller, pp. 195-6)

History

As a heraldic device, the Broom was adopted at a very early period as the badge of Brittany. Geoffrey of Anjou thrust it into his helmet at the moment of going into battle, that his troops might see and follow him. As he plucked it from a steep bank which its roots had knit together he is reputed to have said: 'This golden plant, rooted firmly amid rock, yet upholding what is ready to fall, shall be my cognizance. I will maintain it on the field, in the tourney and in the court of justice." Fulke of Anjou bore it as his personal cognizance, and Henry II of England, his grandson, as a claimant of that province, also adopted it, its mediaeval name Planta genista, giving the family name of Plantagenets to his line. It may be seen on the Great Seal of Richard I, this being its first official, heraldic appearance in England. Another origin is claimed for the heraldic use of the Broom in Brittany. A prince of Anjou assassinated his brother there and seized his kingdom, but being overcome by remorse, he made a pilgrimage to the Holy Land, in expiation of his crime. Every night on the journey, he scourged himself with a brush of 'genets," or genista, and adopted this plant as his badge, in perpetual memory of his repentance. St. Louis of France continued the use of this token, founding a special order on the occasion of his marriage in the year 1234. The Colle de Genet, the collar of the order, was composed alternately of the fleur-de-lys of France and the Broomflower, the Broomflower being worn on the coat of his bodyguard of a hundred nobles, with the motto, 'Exaltat humiles," 'He exalteth the lowly." The order was held in great esteem and its bestowal regarded as a high honour. Our Richard II received it, and a Broom plant, with open, empty pods, can be seen ornamenting his tomb in Westminster Abbey. In 1368 Charles V of France bestowed the insignia of the Broom pod on his favorite chamberlain, and in 1389 Charles VI gave the same decoration to his kinsmen.

The Broom is the badge of the Forbes. Thus, according to Sandford, it was the bonny broom which the Scottish clan of Forbes wore in their bonnets when they wished to arouse the heroism of their chieftains, and which in their Gaelic dialect they called bealadh, in token of its beauty.

'This humble shrub," writes Baines, 'was not less distinguished than the Rose herself during the civil wars of the fourteenth century."

Apart from its use in heraldry, the Broom has been associated with several popular traditions. In some parts, it used to be considered a sign of plenty, when it bore many flowers. The flowering tops were used for house decoration at the Whitsuntide festival but it was considered unlucky to employ them for menial purposes when in full bloom.

An old Suffolk tradition runs:

'If you sweep the house with blossomed Broom in May
You are sure to sweep the head of the house away."

And a yet older tradition is extant that when Joseph and Mary were fleeing into Egypt, the plants of the Broom were cursed by the Virgin because the crackling of their ripe pods as they touched them in passing risked drawing the attention of the soldiers of Herod to the fugitives.

The Broom has been put to many uses. When planted on the sides of steep banks, its roots serve to hold the earth together. On some parts of our coast, it is one of the first plants that grow on the sand-dunes after they have been somewhat consolidated on the surface by the interlacing stems of the mat grasses and other sand-binding plants. It will flourish within reach of sea spray, and, like gorse, is a good sheltering plant for sea-side growth.

Broom is grown extensively as a shelter for game, and also in fresh plantations among more important species of shrubs, to protect them from the wind till fully established.

The shrub seldom grows large enough to furnish useful wood, but when its stem acquires sufficient size, it is beautifully veined, and being very hard, furnishes the cabinetmaker with most valuable material for veneering.

The twigs and branches are serviceable not only for making brooms, but are also used for basket-work, especially in the island of Madeira. They are sometimes used in the north of England and Scotland for thatching cottages and cornricks, and as substitutes for reeds in making fences or screens.

The bark of the Common Broom yields an excellent fibre, finer but not so strong as that of the Spanish Broom, which has been employed from very ancient times- it is easily separated by macerating the twigs in water like flax. From the large quantity of fibrous matter contained, the shoots have been used in the manufacture of paper and cloth.

Tannin exists in considerable amount in the bark, which has been used in former times for tanning leather.

Before the introduction of Hops, the tender Freen tops were often used to communicate a bitter flavor to beer, and to render it more intoxicating.

Gerard says of the Broom:

'The common Broom groweth almost everywhere in dry pastures and low woods. It flowers at the end of April or May, and then the young buds of the flowers are to be gathered and laid in pickle or salt, which afterwards being washed or boiled are used for sallads as capers be and be eaten with no less delight."

Broom buds were evidently a favorite delicacy, for they appeared on three separate tables at the Coronation feast of James II. The flowers served the double purpose of an appetizer and a corrective.

Sometimes a bunch of green Broom tied up with coloured ribbons was carried by the guests at rustic weddings instead of rosemary, when that favorite aromatic herb proved scarce.

Withering (Arrangement of Plants) stated that the green tops were a good winter food for sheep, preventing rot and dropsy in them.

The blossoms were used for making an unguent to cure the gout, and Henry VIII used to drink a water made from the flowers against the surfeit.

Dodoens (Herbal, 1606) recommended a decoction of the tops in dropsy and for 'stoppages of the liver."

Gerard tells us: 'The decoction of the twigs and tops of Broom doth cleanse and open the liver, milt and kidnies."

Culpepper considered the decoction of Broom to be good not only for dropsy, but also for black jaundice, ague, gout, sciatica and various pains of the hips and joints.

Some of the old physicians burned the tops to ashes and infused the salts thus extracted in wine. They were known as Salts of Broom (Sal Genistae).

The powdered seeds are likewise administered and sometimes a tincture is employed. Bruised Broom seeds were formerly used infused in rectified spirit, allowed to stand two weeks and then strained. A tablespoonful in a glass of peppermint water was taken daily for liver complaints and ague.

The leaves or young tops yield a green dye.

The seeds have similar properties to the tops, and have also been employed medicinally, though they are not any longer used officially. They have served as a substitute for coffee.

Cultivation

Broom is most easily raised from seed, sown broadcast in the open air, as soon as ripe. Seedlings may be transplanted in autumn or spring to their permanent position. Prune directly after flowering, if the shoots have not been gathered for medicinal use, shortening the old shoots to the base of promising young ones.

As their roots strike down deeply into the ground, the plants can be grown in dry, sandy soil, where others will not grow. They do well on rough banks.

Broom may also be increased by layers. Choice garden varieties are generally increased by cuttings inserted in cold frames in September.

Constituents

Broom contains two principles on which its activity depends. Sparteine, discovered in 1851 by Stenhouse, of which about 0.03 per cent is present, is a transparent, oily liquid, colorless when fresh, turning brown on exposure, of an aniline-like odor and a very bitter taste. It is but slightly soluble in water, but readily soluble in alcohol and ether. Stenhouse stated that the amount of Sparteine in Broom depends much upon external conditions, that grown in the shade yielding less than that produced in sunny places.

Scoparin, the other principal constituent, is a glucoside, occurring in pale-yellow crystals, colorless and tasteless, soluble in alcohol and hot water. It represents most of the direct diuretic activity of Broom.

Volatile oil, tannin, fat, wax, sugar, etc., are also present. Broom contains a very large quantity of alkaline and earthy matter, on incineration yielding about 3 per cent of ash, containing 29 per cent of carbonate of potash.

Sparteine forms certain salts of which the sulphate (official in the British and the United States Pharmacopceias) is most used in medicine. It occurs in colorless crystals, readily soluble in water.

Oxysparteine (formed by the action of acid on Sparteine) is used as a cardiac stimulant.

The flowers contain volatile oil fatty matter, wax, chlorophyll, yellow coloring matter, tannin, a sweet substance, mucilage, albumen and lignin. Scoparin and the alkaloid sparteine have been separated from them.

Part Used Medicinally

The young, herbaceous tips of the flowering branches are collected in early spring, generally in May, as they contain most alkaloid at the close of the winter. They are used officially both in the fresh and dried state.

Broom Juice (Succus Scoparii) is directed to be obtained by pressing out the bruised, fresh tops, adding one-third volume of alcohol and setting aside for seven days, filtering before use.

For the expression of the juice the fresh tops may be gathered in June. Broom Juice is official in the British, French, German and United States Pharmacopoeias.

Infusion of Broom (Infusum Scoparii) is made by infusing the dried tops with boiling water for fifteen minutes and then straining. It was introduced in the British Pharmacopoeia of 1898, in place of the decoction of Broom of the preceding issues.

The Fluid Extract of Broom of the United States Pharmacopeia is prepared from the powdered dried tops.

The drug, as it appears in commerce, consists of very long, much-branched, tough and flexible twigs, which lie parallel with and close to one another and are about 1/25 to 1/12 inch thick, narrowly five-winged, with alternating, slight nodes, dark-green and usually naked; internally, greenish-white.

When fresh, the whole plant has a strong and peculiar odor, especially when bruised, which almost entirely disappears on drying.

The tops are dark green when fresh and dark brownish-green when dried.

The quality of the drug deteriorates with keeping, and this condition can be determined by the partial or complete loss of the slight, peculiar odor of the recently dried drug.

The deep yellow flowers, dried, are considerably employed separately, under the name Flores Genistae, or Flores Scoparii.

Broom Seeds are used sometimes and are as active as the tops. Water and alcohol extract their active properties.

Medicinal Action and Uses

Diuretic and cathartic. Broom tops are used in the form of decoction and infusion, often with squill and ammonium and potassium acetate, as a feeble diuretic, generally in dropsical complaints of cardiac origin. The action is due to the Scoparin contained, whose action on the renal mucous membrane is similar to that of Buchu and Uva-Ursi.

The infusion is made from 1 OZ. of the dried tops to a pint of boiling water, taken in wine glassful doses frequently. When acute renal inflammation is present, it should not be given.

Broom Juice, in large doses, is apt to disturb the stomach and bowels and is therefore more often used as an adjuvant to other diuretics than alone.

A compound decoction of Broom is recommended in herbal medicine as of much benefit in bladder and kidney affections, as well as in chronic dropsy. To make this, 1 OZ. Broomtops and 1/2 oz. of Dandelion Roots are boiled in one pint of water down to half a pint, adding towards the last, 1/2 oz. of bruised Juniper berries. When cold, the decoction is strained and a small quantity of cayenne added. A wine glassful is taken three or four times a day.

The statements of different investigators, both clinical and pharmacological, concerning the effects of the Sparteine in preparations of Broom, have elicited absolutely opposing views on the effect upon the nerves and circulatory system. It is found to produce a transient rise in arterial pressure, followed by a longer period of decreased vascular tension. Small doses slow the heart for a short period of time and then hasten its rate and at the same time increase the volume of the pulse. Those who advocate its employment claim that it is a useful heart tonic and regulator in chronic valvular disease. It has no cumulative action, like Digitalis.

In large doses, Sparteine causes vomiting and purging weakens the heart, depresses the nerve cells and lowers the blood pressure and has a strong resemblance to the action of Conine (Hemlock) on the heart. In extreme cases, death is caused by impairing the activity of the respiratory organs. Shepherds have long been aware of the narcotic properties of Broom, due to Sparteine, having noticed that sheep after eating it become at first excited and then stupefied, but the intoxicating effects soon pass off.

Preparations

Fluid extract, 1/2 to 1 drachm. Juice, B.P., 1 to 2 drachms. Infusion, B.P., 1 to 2 oz.

Substitutes

It is essential that true Broom be carefully distinguished from Spanish Broom (Spartium junceum), since a number of cases of poisoning have occurred from the substitution of the dried flowers of Spartium for those of the true Broom.

BROOM, BUTCHER'S

Botanical: Ruscus aculeatus (LINN.)
Family: N.O. Liliaceae
Synonyms: Kneeholy. Knee Holly. Kneeholm. Jew's Myrtle. Sweet Broom. Pettigree.
Parts Used: Herb and root.

Habitat

Butcher's Broom, a low, shrubby, evergreen plant, which occurs not infrequently in woods and waste and bushy places, especially in the south of England, is sometimes called Knee Holly, though it is in no way allied to the true Holly, being a member of the Lily tribe. It is, however, entirely different in appearance to the bulbous plants we regard as the characteristic representatives of this group, it being, in fact, the only Liliaceous shrub known in this country, and the only representative of its genus among our flora, the other species of the genus, Ruscus, being mostly native to northern Africa.

Description

The name Knee Holly appears to have been given it from its rising to about the height of a man's knee (though occasionally specimens are found growing about 3 feet high), and from its having, like the true Holly, prickly leaves, which are also evergreen.

There is no other British plant exhibiting any similarity to the Butcher's Broom. Its tough, green, erect, striated stems, which are destitute of bark, send out from the upper part many short branches, plentifully furnished with very rigid leaves, which are really a mere expansion of the stem, and terminate each in a single sharp spine. The small greenish-white flowers are solitary growing from the centre of the leaves and blossom in the early spring. They are dioecious, i.e. stamens and pistils are on different plants, as is also mostly the case with the Holly and Mistletoe. The corolla is deeply six-cleft, the stamens, in the one kind of flower, connected at the base, the style, in the fertile flowers, surrounded by a nectary. The fertile flowers are succeeded by scarlet berries as large as cherries, which are ripe in September, and remain attached to the plant all the winter and cause it often to be picked for room decoration.

Another member of the same family is Ruscus racemosus or Alexandrinus, a favorite evergreen shrub with the leaf-like branches unarmed, and the racemes of small flowers terminal. It is the original of the 'poets' laurel' so often seen in classic prints. It, too has red berries - smaller than those of the Butcher's Broom.

Other species are R. androgynous, a native of the Canaries, which bears its flowers along the edges of the so-called leaves; R. Hypophyllum, in which the flowers are borne on the underside of the flattened branches; and R. Hypoglossum, also from southern Europe, in which the flowers are on the upper side under a bract-like branchlet.

The young shoots of Butcher's Broom have often been eaten like those of the Asparagus, a plant to which it is closely allied. The matured branches used to be bound into bundles and sold to butchers for sweeping their blocks, hence the name: Butcher's Broom. It is frequently made into besoms in Italy. One of the names given the plant, 'Jew's Myrtle," points to its use for service during the Feast of Tabernacles. 'Pettigree' is another old popular name, the meaning of which is not clear.

Parkinson tells us that Butcher's Broom was used to preserve 'hanged meate' from being eaten by mice, and also for the making of brooms,

'but the King's Chamber is by revolution of time turned to the Butcher's stall, for that a bundle of the stalkes tied together serveth them to cleanse their stalls and from thence have we our English name of Butcher's broom."

Culpepper says it is

'a plant of Mars, being of a gallant cleansing and opening quality. The decoction of the root drank, and a poultice made of the berries and leaves applied, are effectual-in knitting and consolidating broken bones or parts out of joint. The common way of using it is to boil the root of it, and Parsley and Fennel and Smallage in white wine, and drink the decoction, adding the like quantity of Grassroot to them: The more of the root you boil the stronger will the decoction be; it works no ill effects, yet I hope you have wit enough to give the strongest decoction to the strongest bodies."

Cultivation

Butcher's Broom is very hardy, thriving in almost any soil or situation, and is often planted in shrubberies or edges of woods, on account of its remaining green after the deciduous trees have shed their leaves.

Propagation is generally effected by division of the roots in autumn. The shrub may also be propagated by seed, but quicker results are obtained by the other method. When planted under trees it soon spreads into large clumps.

Part Used

The root or rhizome, collected in autumn. The root is thick, striking deep into the ground. When dry, it is brownish grey, 2 to 4 inches long and 1/3 inch in diameter, having somewhat crowded rings and rounded stem scars on the upper surface and many woody rootlets below. If a transverse section be made, a number of vascular bundles in the central portion are to be seen. The root has no odor, but its taste is sweetish at first and then slightly acrid.

The whole herb is also collected, being dried in the same manner as Holly leaves.

Medicinal Action and Uses

Diaphoretic, diuretic, deobstruent and aperient. Was much recommended by Dioscorides and other ancient physicians as an aperient and diuretic in dropsy, urinary obstructions and nephritic cases.

A decoction of the root is the usual form of administration, and it is still considered of use in jaundice and gravel. One pint of boiling water to 1 OZ. of the twigs, or 1/2 oz. of the bruised fresh root has also been recommended as an infusion, which may be taken as tea.

In scrofulous tumors, advantage has been realized by administering the root in doses of a drachm every morning.

The decoction, sweetened with honey, is said to clear the chest of phlegm and relieve difficult breathing.

The boughs have been employed for flogging chilblains.

BROOM, DYER'S

Botanical: Genista tinctoria (LINN.)
Family: N.O. Leguminosae
Synonyms: Dyer's Greenwood. Dyer's Weed. Woad Waxen.
(French) Genêt des Teinturiers.
(German) Färberginster.
Parts Used: Twigs and leaves.

Habitat

The Dyer's Broom (Genista tinctoria, Linn.) is a small shrubby plant with narrow, pointed leaves and yellow flowers, growing in meadows, pastures and heaths and on the borders of fields, not uncommon in England but rare in Scotland. It is wild throughout Europe and established on barren hills and on roadsides in the eastern states of North America. It is also cultivated in greenhouses in the United States, on account of its profusion of yellow papilionaceous flowers.

Description

The bright green smooth stems, 1 to 2 feet high, are much branched; the branches erect, rather stiff, smooth or only lightly hairy and free from spines. The leaves are spear-shaped, placed alternately on the stem, smooth, with uncut margins, 1/2 to 1 inch in length, very smoothly stalked; the margins fringed with hairs.

The shoots terminate in spikes of brightyellow, pea-like flowers, opening in July. They are 1/2 to 3/4 inch long, on foot-stalks shorter than the calyx. Like those of the Broom, they 'explode' when visited by an insect. The 'claws' of the four lower petals are straight at first, but in a high state of tension, so that the moment they are touched, they curl downwards with a sudden action and the flower bursts open. The flowers are followed by smooth pods, 1 to 1/4 inch long, much compressed laterally, brown when ripe, containing five to ten seeds.

A dwarf kind grows in tufts in meadows in the greater part of England and is said to enrich poor soil.

Cows will sometimes eat the plant, and it communicates an unpleasant bitterness to their milk and even to the cheese and butter made from it.

All parts of the plant, but especially the flowering tops, yield a good yellow dye, and from the earliest times have been used by dyers for producing this color, especially for wool; combined with woad, an excellent green is yielded, the color being fixed with alum, cream of tartar and sulphate of lime. In some parts of England, the plant used to be collected in large quantities by the poor and sold to the dyers.

Tournefort (1708) describes the process of dyeing linen, woollen, cloth or leather by the use of this plant, which he saw in the island of Samos. It is still applied to the same purpose in some of the Grecian islands. The Romans employed it for dyeing, and it is described by several of their writers.

The plant is called in French Genêt des Teinturiers and in German Färberginster. Its English name in the fourteenth century was Wede-wixin, or Woudwix, which later became Woad Waxen. We find it also called Green Weed and Dyer's Weed.

It has diuretic, cathartic and emetic properties and both flower tops and seeds have been used medicinally, though it has never been an official drug.

The powdered seeds operate as a mild purgative, and a decoction of the plant has been used medicinally as a remedy in dropsy and is stated to have proved effective in gout and rheumatism, being taken in wine glassful doses three or four times a day.

The ashes form an alkaline salt, which has also been used as a remedy in dropsy and other diseases.

In the fourteenth century it was used, as well as Broom, to make an ointment called Unguentum geneste, 'goud for alle could goutes," etc. The seed was also used in a plaster for broken limbs.

A decoction of the plant was regarded in the Ukraine as a remedy for hydrophobia, but its virtues in this respect do not seem to rest on very good evidence.

BROOM, SPANISH

Botanical: Spartium junceum (LINN.)
Family: N.O. Leguminosae

Habitat

The Spanish Broom is a small shrub, indigenous in the south of Europe and cultivated as an ornamental plant. The flowers are large, yellow and of an agreeable scent. It is identified with the Spartium of the ancients, which is reputed to have been very violent in action and was said by Gerard and other herbalists 'to cause to vomit with great violence, even as white Hellebor."

Medicinal Action and Uses

The Spanish Broom in its medicinal properties closely resembles the common Broom, but is from five to six times more active. The symptoms produced by overdoses are vomiting and purging, with renal irritation. The seeds have been used to a considerable extent in dropsy, in the form of a tincture. The flowers yield a yellow dye.

The dried flowers of Spanish Broom are readily differentiated, those of the true Broom having a small bell-shaped calyx with two unequal lobes, the upper of which is bi-dentate and the lower minutely tridentate, while in Spartium junceum, the calyx is deeply cleft to the base on one side only.

By macerating the twigs a good fibre is obtained, which is made into thread in Languedoc, and its cord and a coarse sort of cloth in Dalmatia.

The name Spartium is from the Greek word denoting 'cardage," in allusion to the use of the plant.

Coronilla scorpioides (Koch) has been used medicinally as substitute for Broom.

Coronilla is the herbage of various species of the genus of that name, natives of Europe and some naturalized in North America.

The drug, at least that from Coronilla scorpioides (Koch), contains the glucoside Coronillin, a yellow powder. The action and uses of the drug are very similar to those of Broom.

The leaflets are said to produce a dye like indigo by proper fermentation, and are also reported as a laxative.

BROOM-CORN

Botanical: Sorghum vulgare (PERS.)
Family: N.O. Graminacae
Synonyms: Sorghum Seeds. Sorghum Saccharatum (Moench). Guinea Corn.

Part Used: Seeds.

Habitat

Spain. Italy and south of Europe. Cultivated in the United States of America.

Description

Known as Millet or Guinea Corn. Is cultivated in the same way as oats or barley in northern Europe; the seeds are small, round and white, the plant is canelike and similar to Indian Corn, but producing large heads of the small grain. Sorghum is generally classified under two varieties, saccharine and non-saccharine. The saccharine sorghums are not used for producing sugar owing to the difficulty of crystallization.

Medicinal Action and Uses

It yields a very white flour which is used for making bread, and the grain is used for feeding cattle, horses and poultry. The grain is diuretic and demulcent if taken as a decoction. The plant is extensively cultivated in America for the manufacture of brooms and brushes.

The decoction of 2 oz. of seeds to 1 quart of water, boiled down to 1 pint, is used in urinary and kidney complaints.

In the semi-arid districts of western America it is reported that cattle have been poisoned by eating the green sorghum of the second growth; possibly due to hydrocyanic acid in the leaves.

BRYONY, BLACK

POISON
Botanical: Tamus communis (LINN.
Family: N.O. Dioscoreaceae
Synonym: Blackeye Root.
Part Used: Root.

Black Bryony belongs to a family of twining and climbing plants which generally spring from large tubers, some of which are cultivated for food, as the Yam, which forms an important article of food in many tropical countries. Great Britain only furnishes one species of this tribe, Tamus communis, which, from its powerful, acrid and cathartic qualities, ranks as a dangerous irritant poison.

It is a very common plant in woods and hedges, with weak stems twining round anything within reach, and thus ascending or creeping among the trees and bushes to a considerable distance.

Description

The leaves are heart-shaped pointed, smooth and generally shining as if they had been varnished. Late in autumn they turn dark purple or bright yellow, making a very showy appearance. In winter, the stems die down, though the root is perennial.

The flowers are small, greenish-white, in loose bunches and of two kinds, barren and fertile on different plants, the latter being succeeded by berries of a red color when ripe.

The large, fleshy root is black on the outside and exceedingly acrid, and, although an old cathartic medicine, is a most dangerous remedy when taken internally. It is like that of the yam, thick and tuberous and abounding in starch, but too acrid to be used as food in any manner.

The young shoots are said to be good eating when dressed like Asparagus- the Moors eat them boiled with oil and salt, after they have been first soaked in hot water.

Gerard says of this plant:

'The wild black Briony resembleth the white Briony vine, but has not clasping tendrils and is easier to be losed. The root is black without and of a pale yellow color within, like Box. It differs from white Briony only in that the root is of a yellow box color on the inside, and the fruit or berries are black when they come to ripeness."

As to the color of the berries, Gerard is at fault: they are bright red. Other writers have also made the same mistake. The root is nearly cylindrical, 1 to 1 1/2 inch in diameter, 3 to 4 inches long or more, and black.

Medicinal Action and Uses

Rubifacient, diuretic. The expressed juice of the fresh root, mixed with a little white wine, has been used as a remedy for gravel, being a powerful diuretic, but it is not given internally now, and is not included in the British Pharmacopoeia. Death in most painful form is the result of an overdose, while the effect of a small quantity, varying not with the age only, but according to the idiosyncrasies of the patient, leaves little room for determining the limit between safety and destruction. The expressed juice of the root, with honey, has also been used as a remedy for asthmatic complaints, but other remedies that are safer should be preferred.

The berries act as an emetic, and children should be cautioned against eating them.

As an external irritant, Black Bryony has, however, been used with advantage, and it was formerly much employed. The scraped pulp was applied as a stimulating plaster, and in gout, rheumatism and paralysis has been found serviceable in many instances.

A tincture made from the root proves a most useful application to unbroken chilblains, and also the fruits, steeped in gin, are used for the same remedy.

Black Bryony is a popular remedy for removing discoloration caused by bruises and black eyes, etc. The fresh root is scraped to a pulp and applied in the form of a poultice.

For sores, old writers recommend it being made into an ointment with 'hog's grease or wax, or other convenient ointment."

The generic name Tamus is given to the plant from the belief that it is the same as that referred to in the works of Pliny under the name of Uva Taminia.

The Greeks use the young suckers like Asparagus, which they much resemble.

T. cretica is a native of Greece and the Greek Archipelago.

Preparation

Tincture, 1 to 5 drops.

BRYONY, EUROPEAN WHITE

POISON
Botanial: Bryonia alba (LINN.)
Family: N.O. Cucurbitaceae
Synonyms: Black-berried White Bryony. European White Bryony.
Part Used: Root.

The Black-berried White Bryony is a plant very similar in general appearance to Bryonia dioica, having also palmate rough leaves and similar unisexual flowers, which are succeeded, however, by globular black berries.

The root is very similar to that of Bryonia dioica and contains the same substances, but it is stated also to contain a glucoside Brein, which causes the drug to produce a somewhat different physiological effect.

The tincture is used by homoeopathists, and is said to be one of the best diuretics in medicine. It is an excellent remedy in gravel and all other obstructions and disorders of the urinary passages, and has also been used for relieving coughs and colds of a feverish, bronchial nature.

Preparation

Fluid extract, 1/6 to 1 drachm Bryonin, 1/4 to 2 grains.

BRYONY, WHITE

POISON
Botanical: Bryonia dioica (LINN.)
Family: N.O. Cucurbitaceae
Synonyms: English Mandrake. Wild Vine. Wild Hops. Wild Nep. Tamus. Ladies' Seal. Tetterbury. (French) Navet du diable.
Part Used: Root.

Habitat

The Cucumber tribe has a single representative among our wild plants in the Red-berried, common or White Bryony. This is a vine-like plant growing in woods and hedges, and exceedingly common in the south of England, rarer in the Midland counties, and not often found in the north of England. It is of frequent occurrence in central and southern Europe.

Description

The stems climb by means of long tendrils springing from the side of the leaf stalks, and extend among the trees and shrubs often to the length of several yards during the summer, dying away after ripening their fruit. They are angular and brittle, branched mostly at the base, and are, as well as the somewhat vine-shaped leaves very rough to the touch, with short, pricklelike hairs - a general character of the exotic plants of this order.

The leaves are stalked, with the stalk curved, shorter than the blade, which is divided into five lobes, of which the middle one is the longest - all five are slightly angular.

The flowers, which bloom in May, are small, greenish, and produced, generally three or four together, in small bunches springing from the axils of the leaves. Stamens and pistils are never found in the same flower, nor are the flowers which have them individually ever met with on the same plant in this species, whence the name dioica, signifying literally 'two dwellings."The male flowers are in loose, stalked bunches, 3 to 8 flowers in a bunch, or cyme, the stamens having one-celled, yellow anthers. The fertile flowers, easily distinguished from the barren by the presence of an ovary beneath the calyx, are generally either stalkless (sessile) or with very short stalks - two to five together. The corollas in each case consist of five petals, cohering only at the base. The outer green calyx is widely bell-shaped and five-toothed.

The berries, which hang about the bushes after the stem and leaves are withered, are almost the size of peas when ripe, a pale scarlet in color. They are filled with juice of an unpleasant, foetid odor and contain three to six large seeds, greyish-yellow, mottled with black, and are unwholesome to eat.

The whole plant is rather succulent, bright green and somewhat shining.

The name of the genus, Bryonia, derived from the Greek bryo, 1 shoot, or sprout appears to have reference to the vigorous an active growth of its annual stems, which proceed from the perennial roots, and so rapidlycover other shrubs, adhering to them with their tendrils. Bryonia dioica is the only British representative of the genus.

History

Under the name of Wild Nepit was known in the fourteenth century as an antidote to leprosy.

It produces a large, tuberous rootstock which is continuous with a thick, fleshy root which attains an enormous size. Gerard says of it:

'The Queen's chief surgeon, Mr. Wiiliam Godorous, a very curious and learned gentleman, shewed me a root hereof that waied half an hundredweight, and of the bignes of a child of a yeare old."

This large, fleshy, pale-coloured root used often to be seen suspended in herb shops, occasionally trimmed into a rude human form. Green (Universal Herbal, 1832) tells us:

'The roots of Bryony grow to a vast size and have been formerly by imposters brought into a human shape, carried about the country and shown for Mandrakes to the common people. The method which these knaves practised was to open the earth round a young, thriving Bryony plant, being careful not to disturb the lower fibres of the root; to fix a mould, such as is used by those who make plaster figures, close to the root, and then to fill in the earth about the root, leaving it to grow to the shape of the mould, which is effected in one summer."

The plant is still sometimes called Mandrake in Norfolk.

In this fleshy root is found a somewhat milky juice, very nauseous and bitter to the taste. It is of a violently purgative and cathartic nature, and was a favorite medicine with the older herbalists, well known to and much used by the Greeks and Romans prescribed by Galen and Dioscorides, and afterwards by

Gerard, but is now seldom employed by regular practitioners, though sometimes by the homoeopathists, though they mostly use another variety of Bryony that is not indigenous to this country. The French call the root Navet du Diable (Devil's Turnip), from its violent and dangerous action.

Withering says a decoction made by boiling one pound of the fresh root in water is 'the best purge for horned cattle," and it has been considered a sovereign remedy for horse grip.

Gerard declared the root to be profitable for tanners to thicken their hides with.

Bartholomew's Anglicus tells us that Augustus Caesar used to wear a wreath of Bryony during a thunderstorm to protect himself from lightning.

Culpepper says it is a 'furious martial plant," but good for many complaints; among others, 'stiches in the side, palsies, cramps, convulsions " etc.

The acrid and cathartic properties of the root are shared in some measure by all parts of the plant: the berries are emetic and even poisonous. They have been used for dyeing. The young shoots in the spring are considered to be inert, and have sometimes been boiled and eaten as greens without harm resulting. Among animals, goats alone are said to eat this plant.

The extracts made from some exotic species of this tribe, as the Squirting Cucumber (Momordica elaterium) and the Colocynth (Cucumis colocynthis), afford useful medicine.

Part Used

The root is collected in the autumn and used both in the fresh and dry state. When fresh, it is of a dirty yellow or yellowish-white color, externally marked at close intervals with prominent transverse corky ridges, which often extend half round the root and give it the appearance of being circularly wrinkled. Internally, it is whitish, succulent and fleshy, with a nauseous odor - which disappears in great measure on drying - and a bitter, acrid taste. The juice which exudes on cutting the root is milky, owing to the presence of numerous minute starch grains. The root is usually simple, like a carrot or parsnip, but sometimes is forked into two.

When sold dry, Bryony root appears in circular, brittle pieces, 1/4 to 1/3 inch thick about 2 inches in diameter, the thin bark greyish-brown and rough, longitudinally wrinkled, the central portion whitish or greyish, showing numerous round wood bundles arranged in concentric rays, with projecting radiating lines. The taste is disagreeably bitter, but there is no odor.

The large size, tapering shape, transverse corky ridges and nauseously bitter taste of Bryony root are distinctive. Small specimens may resemble Horseradish root, but that is cylindrical and smooth and has a pungent taste.

Medicinal Action and Uses

Irritative, hydragogue, cathartic. Its chief use was as a hydragogue cathartic, but is now superseded by Jalap. Its use as a purgative has been discontinued as dangerous, on account of its powerful and highly irritant nature.

It was formerly given in dropsy and other complaints. It is of so acrid a character that, if applied to the skin, it produces redness and even blisters. It has been used for cataplasms, and praised as a remedy for sciatica, rheumatism and lumbago.

It is still considered useful in small doses for cough, influenza, bronchitis and pneumonia, and has also been recommended for pleurisy and whooping-cough, relieving the pain and allaying the cough.

It has proved of value in cardiac disorders caused by rheumatism and gout, also in malarial and zymotic diseases.

In case of poisoning by Bryony, the stomach must be evacuated and demulcent drinks given. The body temperature must be maintained by the use of blankets and hot bottles.

BUCHU

Botanical: Barosma betulina (BART. and WENDL.)
Family: N.O. Rutaceae
Synonym: Diosma betulina.
Part Used: Leaves.

Habitat

A small shrubby plant chiefly found in the south-west region of Cape Colony.

The standard Buchus of commerce are obtained from three species: Barosma betulina, known as 'shorts'; B. crenulata, known 'ovals' and 'shortbroads," and B. serratifolia, known as 'longs." The leaves of the firstnamed are most valued and constitute the foliea buchu of the British Pharmacopoeia.

The Hottentots use several species, all under the common name of 'Bucku." The leaves have a rue-like smell, and are used by the natives to perfume their bodies.

Buchu leaves are collected while the plant is flowering and fruiting, and are then dried and exported from Cape Town. The bulk of the Buchu exported to London from South Africa eventually finds its way to America, where it is used in certain proprietary medicines.

Description

The leaves of B. betulina (short Buchu) are of a pale green color, 1/2 to 3/4 inch long, 1/2 inch or less wide, leathery and glossy, with a blunt, strongly-curved tip and finely-toothed margin, with round oil glands scattered through the leaf. Frequently the small flowers, with five whitish petals, and the brownish fruits may be found mixed with the drug. The leaves have a strongly aromatic taste and a peppermint-like odor.

Constituents

The principal constituents of Buchu leaves are volatile oil and mucilage, also diosphenol, which has antiseptic properties, and is considered by some to be the most important constituent of Buchu its absence from the variety known as 'Long Buchu' has led to the exclusion of the latter leaves from the British Pharmacopoeia.

The Cape Government exercises strict control over the gathering of Buchu leaves and has lately made the terms and conditions more onerous, in order to prevent the wholesale destruction of the wild plants, no person being permitted to pick or buy Buchu without a licence. Cultivation experiments with Buchu have been made from time to time by private persons, and during the war experiments were conducted at the National Botanic Gardens, Kirstenbosch (near Cape Town), the result of which (given in the South African Journal of Industries, 1919, 2, 748) indicate that, under suitable conditions, the commercial cultivation of Buchu should prove a success, B. betulina, the most valuable kind, being the species alone to be grown. The plant is particularly adapted to dry conditions, and may be cultivated on sunny hillsides where other crops will not succeed.

It is doubtful whether the cultivation of Buehu could be conducted satisfactorily outside South Africa. B. betulina was introduced to this country in 1790, but does not appear to be in eultivation at the present time, except as a greenhouse plant. This and B. serratifolia are grown in Kew Gardens.

Medicinal Action and Uses

In gravel, inflammation and catarrh of the bladder it is specially useful. The infusion (B.P.) of 1 OZ. of leaves to 1 pint of boiling water is taken in wine glassful doses three or four times a day.

Other Preparations

Fluid extract: dose, 1/2 to 1 drachm. Tincture, B.P.: dose, 1/2 to 1 drachm. Solid extract: dose, 5 to 15 grains. Barosmin: dose, 2 to 3 grains.

Buchu has long been known at the Cape as a stimulant tonic and remedy for stomachic troubles, where it is infused in Brandy and known as Buchu Brandy. Its use was learnt from the Hottentots.

It was introdueed into official medicine in Great Britain in 1821 as a remedy for cystitis urethritis, nephritis and catarrh of the bladder.

BUCKTHORNS, COMMON

Family: N.O. Rhamnaceae
Synonyms: Highwaythorn. Waythorn. Hartsthorn. Ramsthorn.
Part Used: Berries.

Three species of the genus Rhamnus (the name derived from the Greek rhamnos, a branch) are possessed of the same medicinal properties in varying degrees.

The Common or Purging Buckthorn, a much-branched shrub, usually about 6 feet high, but sometimes as much as 10 or 12 feet, is indigenous to North Africa, the greater part of Europe and North Asia. Though found throughout England in woods and thickets and near brooks, it is practically confined to a calcareous soil, except in a few counties, such as Bucks., Herts., Oxon. and Wilts. In Scotland it occurs only in a single locality.

Description

The main stem is erect, the bark smooth, of a blackish-brown color, on the twigs ash-coloured. The smaller branches generally terminate in a stout thorn or spine, hence the ordinary name of Buckthorn, and the older names by which the shrub has been known: Highwaythorn and Waythorn. Gerard calls it Ram or Hart's Thorn. The leaves grow in small bunches on footstalks, mostly opposite towards the base of the young shoots, though more generally alternate towards the apex. They are eggshaped and toothed on the edges, the younger ones with a kind of soft down. In the axils of the more closely arranged leaves, developed from the wood of the preceding year, are dense branches of small greenish-yellow flowers, about one-fifth inch across, which are followed by globular berries about the size of a pea, black and shining when ripe, and each containing four hard, dark-brown seeds.

Goats, sheep and horses browse on this shrub, but cows refuse it. Its blossoms are very grateful to bees.

Part Used

The berries are the part used medicinally, collected when ripe and from which an acrid, nauseous, bitter juice is obtained by expression. From this juice, with the addition of sugar and aromatics, syrup of Buckthorn (Succus Rhamni) is prepared.

When freshly gathered in the autumn, the berries are about 1/3 inch in diameter, with the remains of a calyx beneath. The fruit is collected for use chiefly in the counties of Herts., Bucks. and Oxon, and is usually expressed in the locality where it is grown, by the collectors themselves, who sell the juice to the wholesale druggists, generally more or less diluted with water, the admixture being generally about 6 parts water to 1 of juice.

From the dried berries, a series of rich but fugitive colors is obtained; the berries used to be sold under the name of 'French berries' and imported with those of Rhamnus infectorius from the Levant. If gathered before ripe, the berries furnish a yellow dye, used formerly for staining maps or paper. When ripe, if mixed with gum-arabic and limewater, they form the pigment 'Sap or bladder green," so well known to water-color painters. The bark also affords a yellow dye.

Cultivation

Buckthorn is seldom cultivated, the berries being collected from thewild shrubs, but it can be easily raised from seed in autumn, soon after the berries are ripe, usually about September, but if left too late the berries soften and will not bear carriage well. The shrub may also be propagated like any other hardy deciduous tree or shrub by cuttings or layers: if the young shoots be laid in autumn, they will have struck roots by the following autumn, when they may be separated and either planted in a nursery for a year or two, or at once planted in permanent quarters. Buckthorn is not so suitable for hedges as the hawthorn.

Constituents

Buckthorn berry juice contains Rhamnocathartin (which is yellowand uncrystallizable), Rhamnin, a peculiar tannic acid, sugar and gum. The fresh juice is coloured red by acids and yellow by alkalies, and has a bitter taste and nauseous odor. Its specific gravity should be between 1.035 and 1.070, but it is seldom sold pure. The ripe berries yield on expression 40 to 50 percent of juice of a green color, which on keeping turns, however, gradually to a reddish or purplish brown color, on account of the acidification of the saccharine and mucilaginous matter.

Medicinal Action and Uses

Laxative and cathartic.

Buckthorn was well known to the AngloSaxons and is mentioned as Hartsthorn or Waythorn in their medical writings and glossaries dating before the Norman Conquest. The Welsh physicians of the thirteenth century prescribed the juice of the fruit of Buckthorn boiled with honey as an aperient drink.

The medicinal use of the berries was familiar to all the writers on botany and materia medica of the sixteenth century, though Dodoens in his Herbal wrote: 'They be not meat to be administered but to the young and lusty people of the country which do set more store of their money than their lives."

Until late in the nineteenth century, syrup of Buckthorn ranked, however, among favorite rustic remedies as a purgative for children, prepared by boiling the juice with pimento and ginger and adding sugar, but its action was so severe that, as time went on, the medicine was discarded. It first appeared in the London Pharmacopeia of 1650, where, to disguise the bitter taste of the raw juice, it was aromatized by means of aniseed, cinnamon, mastic and nutmeg. It was still official in the British Pharmacopoeia of 1867, but is no longer so, being regarded as a medicine more fit for animals than human beings, and it is now employed almost exclusively in veterinary practice, being commonly prescribed for dogs, with equal parts of castor oil as an occasional purgative.

The flesh of birds eating the berries is stated to be purgative.

There used to be a superstition that the Crown of Thorns was made of Buckthorn.

BUCKTHORN ALDER

Botanical: Rhamnus Frangula (LINN.)
Family: N.O. Rhamnaceae
Synonyms: Black Dogwood. Frangula Bark.
Part Used: Bark.

Habitat

The Alder Buckthorn is a slender shrub, widely distributed over Europe and northern Asia, and found in woods and thickets throughout England, though rare in Scotland.

In place of the violently-acting juice of the berries of the Common Buckthorn, a fluid extract prepared from the bark of the closely allied and milder Alder Buckthorn or Black Alder (Rhamnus Frangula, Linn.) has been proved a very satisfactory substitute. Frangula bark is official both in the United States and the British Pharmacopoeia. Its use has been, however, somewhat neglected and the much advertized Cascara Sagrada (R. purshianus) has greatly taken its place, though itis a less agreeable aperient.

Description

It is generally about the same size as the Common Buckthorn, but is distinguished from it by its less bushy and more tree-like habit, by the absence of thorns on its branches and by its larger and entire, not toothed, feather-veined leaves, which are all arranged alternately on the stem, none opposite to one another. The flowers are produced not only from the wood of the preceding year, but also on the shoots of the current year, and have a five-parted calyx, while that of the Common Buckthorn is four-cleft. They bloom in May and are of an inconspicuous green. Their fruit, which is ripe in September, is not unlike that of the Common Buckthorn, but the berry has only two, or at most three, roundish, angular seeds, instead of four. Bees are likewise constant visitors of the flowers of this species, and goats eat the leaves voraciously.

It grows as a rule in leaf-mould in woods comparatively free from lime.

The bark and leaves of the Alder Buckthorn yield

a yellow dye much used in Russia; when mixed with salts of iron it turns black. The berries, when unripe, afford a good green color, readily taken by woollen stuffs; when ripe, they give various shades of blue and grey.

After removal of the bark from the stem and branches, the wood of this shrub is used for making charcoal, yielding a very light, inflammable kind, and being on that account preferred to that of almost any other tree by gunpowder makers, who name it 'Black Dogwood." In Germany, for the same reason, it is called Pulverholz ('powder-wood').

Cultivation

Frangula bark is usually collected from wild shrubs, but this Buckthorn can readily be cultivated. The seeds should be sown as soon as ripe, not kept till the following spring. The seedlings should be kept free from weeds, and in the autumn planted in the nursery in rows 2 feet asunder and 1 foot distant in the rows. Stock may also be increased by layers and cuttings, though propagation by seedling plants is preferable.

Part Used Medicinally

The dried bark collected from the young trunk and moderately-sized branches in early summer and kept at least one year before being used. It is stripped from the branches and dried either on sunny days, out of doors, in halfshade, or by artificial heat, on shelves or trays, in a warm, well-ventilated room.

The dried bark varies considerably in appearance, according to the age of the branch or stem from which it has been taken. Young bark, which is to be preferred, occurs in narrow, single or double quills and is of papery texture, about 1/25 inch thick. It is of a greyish or blackish-brown color outside, with numerous small, whitish corky warts. When gently scraped, the inner layers are seen to be crimson in color. The inner surface of the bark is smooth, of a pale, yellowish brown and very finely striated. The fracture is short. Older bark is rougher externally, thicker and usually in single quills or channelled pieces.

The bark is nearly inodorous; its taste is pleasant, sweetish and slightly bitter. When masticated, it colors the saliva yellow.

Constituents

The chemical constituents of Frangula Bark, especially those to which the laxative properties are due, are but imperfectly known. A yellow, crystalline glucoside, Frangulin has been isolated from it. Emodin is present in old bark; this principle is also present in rhubarb root; it is allied to Chrysophane, and is said to result from the glucosic fermentation of Frangulin or Frangulic acid, and to its presence the drug owes its purgative action. Possibly other glucosides are also present and contribute to the laxative action, but the evidence in favour of this assumption is not conclusive. Two resins, resinous bitter matter and a little tannic acid are likewise present in the bark.

Medicinal Action and Uses

Tonic, laxative, cathartic.

Dried seasoned bark from one to twoyears old alone should be used, as the freshlystripped bark acts as an irritant poison on the gastro-intestinal canal. The action of the bark becomes gradually less violent when kept for a length of time and more like that of rhubarb.

It is used as a gentle purgative in cases of chronic constipation and is principally given in the form of the fluid extract, in small doses, repeated three or four times daily, a decoction of 1 OZ. of the bark in 1 quart of water boiled down to a pint, may also be taken in tablespoonful doses.

Preparation

Fluid extract, 1/2 to 2 drachms.

This milder English Buckthorn acts likewise as a tonic to the intestine and is especially useful for relieving piles.

Lozenges of the Alder Buckthorn are dispensed under the name of 'Aperient Fruit Lozenges."

The juice of the berries, though little used, is aperient without being irritating.

Country people used to take the bark boiled in ale for jaundice.

BUCKTHORN, CALIFORNIAN

Botanical: Rhamnus purshianus
Family: N.O. Rhamnaceae

The Californian Buckthorn (Rhamnus purshianus), known more commonly as Cascara Sagrada, is a nearly-allied shrub growing in the United States, from northern Idaho westward to the Pacific Ocean. The drug prepared from its bark is now more commonly employed than those prepared from the two previously described species.

The bark is collected in spring and early summer, when it is easily peeled from the wood, and is dried in the shade.

Since, as is the case with R. Frangula, it is considered that the action of the bark becomes milder and less emetic by keeping, matured bark, three years old, is preferred for pharmaceutical purposes.

Description

As imported, the drug mostly occurs in quills or incurved pieces of varying lengths and sizes, smooth or nearly so externally, covered with a greyish-white layer, which is usually easily removed, and frequently marked with spots or patches of adherent lichens. Beneath the surface it is violet-brown, reddish-brown or brownish, and internally a pale yellowish-brown and nearly smooth. It has no marked odor, but a nauseous, bitter taste.

It is frequently also imported in flattened packets, consisting of small pieces of the bark compressed into a more or less compact mass.

The fluid extract is made by maceration and percolation with diluted alcohol and evaporation.

Constituents

The chemical constituents of the bark are but imperfectly known. It has been proved to contain Emodin and an allied substance possibly identical with the Frangula-Emodin of Alder Buckthorn bark. Fat, starch, glucose, a volatile odorous oil, malic and tannic acids are also present. The assertion has been made that the bark contains glucosides which yield on hydrolysis Chrysophanic acid, but the evidence on this point is conflicting.

Medicinal Action and Uses

Cascara Sagrada is a mild laxative, acting principally on the large intestine. It is considered suitable for delicate and elderly persons, and may with advantage be given in chronic constipation, being generally administered in the form of the fluid extract.

It acts also as a stomachic tonic and bitter, in small doses, promoting gastric digestion and appetite.

Preparations

Fluid extract, B.P., 5 drops to 1 drachm.

Fluid extract, U.S.P., 15 drops.

Fluid extract, tasteless, 1/4 to 1 drachm.

Fluid extract, aromatic, U.S.P., 15 drops.

Aromatic syrup, B.P., 1/2 to 2 drachms.

Powder extract, 2 to 10 grains.

Rhamnin, 2 to 6 grains.

In veterinary practice, Cascara Sagrada is also much used and is probably the best mild purgative remedy for dogs with chronic constipation, as the dose does not require to be increased by repetition and the tone of the bowels is improved by the drug.

BUCKTHORN, SEA

Botanical: Hippophae rhamnoides
Family: N.O. Rhamnaceae
Synonym: Sallow Thorn.

The Sea Buckthorn (Hippophae rhamnoides), a

thorny shrub with narrow willowlike leaves growing on sandhills and cliffs on the East Coast, and called also " Sallow Thorn, " is in no way related to these medicinally employed Buckthorns but belongs to a different natural order: Elaeagnaceae. Its fruit, an orange-coloured berry, is made (in Tartary) into a pleasant jelly, because of its acid flavor, and is used in the countries bordering on the Gulf of Bothnia as an ingredient to a fish sauce. The name Hippophae has been variously derived either as meaning 'giving light to a horse," because of a supposed power to cure equine blindness, or as signifying 'shining underneath," an allusion to the silvery underside of the leaf. The stems, roots and foliage are said to impart a yellow dye.

Henslow relates that in some parts of Europe the berries are considered poisonous, and a story is told by Rousseau of a person who saw him eating them, and, though believing them to be poisonous, had too much respect for the great man to caution him against the supposed danger! A decoction of them is said to be useful in cutaneous eruptions. The color may be extracted by hot water and used as a dye for woollen stuffs, but it is not very brilliant when so obtained. This plant runs very much at the root, and by its long suckers often assists in binding loose sandy dunes on which it grows.

Some of the plants of this order (Elaeagnaceae) are said to possess narcotic properties.

BUCKWHEAT

Botanical: Polygonum fagopyrum
Family: N.O. Polygonaceae
Synonyms: Brank. Beechwheat. Le Blé noir. Sarrasin. Buchweizen. Heidekorm. French. Wheat. Saracen Corn.
Part Used: The fruit.

Habitat

A native of Northern or Central Asia. Largely cultivated in the United States.

Description

The Buckwheat is not really a native plant, and when found apparently wild in this country, it is only on cultivated land, where it is grown as food for pheasants, which are very partial to it. One of its local names, 'French Wheat," points to then recognition of the fact that it is a foreign grain.

It is a native of Central Asia, cultivated in China and other Eastern countries as a bread-corn and was first brought to Europe from Asia by the Crusaders, and hence in France is called 'Saracen Corn."

It is a herbaceous plant, with a knotted stem a foot or two in height, round and hollow, generally green, but sometimes tinged with red, lateral branches growing out of the joints, which give off alternately from opposite sides, heart-shaped, or somewhat arrowshaped leaves, and from July to September, spreading panicles of numerous light freshcoloured flowers, which are perfumed. They are dimorphic, i.e. there are two forms of flowers, one with long styles and short stamens, the other with short styles and long stamens and are very attractive to bees. It is frequently cultivated in the Middle United States of Arnerica and also in Brabant as food for bees, and an immense quantity of Buckwheat honey is also collected in Russia. It gives a particularly pleasant flavor to honey.

The nut (so-called 'seed') has a dark brown, tough rind, enclosing the kernel or seed, and is three-sided in form, with sharp angles, resembling the triangular Beech-nut, hence the name of the plant, Buckwheat, a corruption of Boek-weit, the Dutch form of the name, adopted with its culture from the Dutch, meaning 'Beech-wheat' (German Buchweizen), a translation of the Latin name Fagopyrum (Latin fagus, a beech).

By some botanists, the Buckwheat is separated from the Polygonums, receiving the name Fagopyrum esculentum (Moench).

The nut contains a floury endosperm, and though rarely employed in this country as human food is extensively cultivated for that purpose in Northern Europe, North America (where it also goes by the name of Indian Wheat) and in India and the East.

Buckwheat flour is occasionally used for bread, but more frequently employed for cakes, which when baked have an agreeable taste, with a darkish, somewhat violet color and are a national dish throughout America in the winter. They are baked on gridirons and eaten with maple syrup as breakfast cakes. The meal of Buckwheat is also baked into crumpets, which are popular among Dutch children and are said to be nutritious and easily digested.

By the Hindus, Buckwheat, which is extensively cultivated in the Himalayas, is eaten on 'bart' or fast days, being one of the lawful foods for such occasions. Polygonum cymosum (Meism.), the Chinese perennial Buckwheat, and P. Tartaricum Ge.), the Tartary or Rough Buckwheat, also constitute an important source of flour in the East. In Japan, Buckwheat is called Soba, and its flour is prepared in various ways; kneaded with hot water to make a dough, Soba-neri; a kind of macaroni, Soba-kiri; and so on. The grains, steamed and dried, are eaten boiled or made into bread or Manju, a small cake. Its young leaves are eaten as a vegetable and its stalks are used to feed cattle.

In the Russian Army, Buckwheat groats are served out as part of the soldiers' rations and cooked with butter, tallow or hemp-seed oil. In Germany it forms an ingredient in pottage, puddings and other food.

Beer may be brewed from the grain, and by distillation it yields an excellent spirit, in Danzig much used in the preparation of cordial waters.

The blossoms may be used for dyeing a brown color.

Cultivation

It is sown in May or June and ripens rapidly, thriving in the poorest soil. The flowers appear about July and the seeds ripen in October, but so tender are the plants that a single night's frost will destroy a whole crop. As a grian, Buckwheat is chiefly cultivated in England to supply food for pheasants and to feed poultry, which devour the seeds with avidity and thrive on it - hence one of its local names: Fat Hen. Mixed with bran chaff or grain, its seeds are sometimes given to horses, either whole or broken. When used as food for cattle, the hard angular rind must first be removed. The meal is considered specially good for fattening pigs: 8 bushels of Buckwheat have been said to go as far as 12 bushels of barleymeal and a bushel of the seeds to go further than 2 bushels of oats, though all farmers do not quite agree as to the superior food value of Buckwheat. If it is given to pigs at first in too large quantities, they will show symptoms of intoxication. As compared with the principal cereal grains, it is poor in nitrogenous substances and fat, its nutritious properties are greatly inferior to wheat, though as a food it ranks much higher than rice; but the rapidity and the ease with which it can be grown renders it a fit crop for very poor, badly-tilled land which will produce scarcely anything else, its culture, compared with that of other grain, being attended with little expense.

When grown by the preservers of game as a food for pheasants, it is often left standing, as it affords both food and shelter to the birds during the winter. With some farmers it is the practice to sow Buckwheat for the purpose only of ploughing it into the ground as a manure for the land. The best time for ploughing it in is when it is in full blossom, allowing the land to rest till it decomposes.

Whilst green, it serves as food for sheep and oxen, and mixed with other provender it may also with advantage be given to horses. If sown in April, two green crops may be procured during the season.

The best mode of harvesting this grain is said to be by pulling it out of the ground like flax, stripping off the seeds with the hand and collecting these into aprons or cloths tied round the waist.

In the United States, Buckwheat is sown at the end of June or beginning of July, the amount of seed varying from 3 to 5 pecks to the acre. The crop matures rapidly and continues blooming till the frosts set in, so that at harvest, which is usually set to occur just before this period, the grain is in various stages of ripeness. There, after cutting, it is allowed to lie in swaths for a few days and then set up in shocks. Threshing is done on the field in most cases.

It grows so quickly that it will kill off any weeds.

Constituents

The leaves have been found by Schunch to contain a crystalline coloring principle (1 part in a thousand) identical with the Rutin or Rutic acid previously discovered by Weiss in the leaves of the common Rue and probably existing in the leaves of the Holly.

The seeds contain starch, sugar, gum, and various matters soluble in alcohol. A small amount of the glucoside Indican has been found.

Medicinal Action and Uses

Astringent, acrid.

An infusion of the herb has been used in erysipelas, and a poultice made of the flour and buttermilk for restoring the flow of milk in nurses.

The breakfast cakes are very heating, and in many people cause severe itching, felt chiefly after removing the clothing at night, with an eruption of vesicles. The faeces may become so glutinous that expulsion is difficult.

Other Species

The FALSE BUCKWHEAT, or Arrow-leaved Tear Thumb, is Polygonum sagittarum (Linn.), a North American plant that has become naturalized in County Kerry, Ireland.

It is an annual, with a rough stem, 6 inches to 2 feet high, bearing turned-back prickles. The leaves are oblong-ovate to arrow-shaped and the flowers white, in bloom from July to October.

It has been used with success in nephritic colic, relieving the pains caused by gravel.

The CLIMBING BUCKWHEAT, or Black Bindweed, also called Bearbind and Cornbind, is Polygonum Convolvulus (Linn.), a troublesome climbing cornfield weed, which occurs indifferently in all soils.

Its stems are 1 to 3 feet long, angular, twining or trailing, bearing leaves 1 to 3 inches long, from heart-shaped to arrowshaped. The flowers are very small, in loose axillary spikes, about four together, greenish-white, often tinged with red, and are insectpollinated, containing nectar secreted in glands near the base of the stamens. The fruits are three-angled, bearing a resemblance to those of Buckwheat.

It is largely distributed by the seeds being sown with those of the crop among which it has grown. Spraying as for Charlock (with solutions of copper-, iron- or ammonium sulphate) will largely destroy this weed in cereals. It may be injurious to animals, owing to mechanical injury from the seeds when fed with corn, horses are said to have been killed in this way.

BUGLE, COMMON

Botanical: Ajuga reptans (LINN.)
Family: N.O. Labiatae
Synonyms: Carpenter's Herb. Sicklewort. Middle Comfrey.
Part Used: Herb.

Habitat

It is abundantly distributed throughout Britain in damp, shady pastures and woods.

The Bugle and the Self-Heal, nearly related plants (both, with their two-lipped corollas, belonging to the important order Labiatae), for many centuries stood in equally high estimation as valuable vulneraries or wound herbs.

There are three Bugles in the British flora - the common creeping form (Ajuga reptans), the erect Bugle (A. pyramidalis), a rare Highland species, and the Yellow Bugle or Ground Pine (A. Chamaepitys), which likewise has its reputation as a curative herb.

Description

It is a perennial, to be found in flower from the end of April to the beginning of July and well marked by its solitary, tapering flower-stalks, 6 to 9 inches high, and its creeping scions or runners. These are long shoots, sometimes a couple of feet or more long, sent out from the rootstock. At intervals upon them are pairs of leaves, and at the same point rootlets are given off below, which enter the earth. As winter approaches, the runners die, but at every point where the leaf-pairs and the rootlets were formed, there is a dormant plant waiting to develop fully in the spring, a Bugle plant thus being the centre of quite a colony of new young plants, quite independently of setting its seeds, which as a matter of fact do not always ripen, the plant propagating itself more largely by its creeping scions.

The erect flower-stalk sent up from the root-stock is square, pale green, often purplish above, with the leaves opposite in pairs, the lower leaves on stalks, the upper leaves stalkless, oblong and obtuse in form, toothed or almost entire at the margin, having manycelled hairs on both surfaces, the margins also fringed with hairs. The runners are altogether smooth, but the stems are smooth only on two sides and downy on the other two.

The flowers are of a purplish blue, crowded into a spike formed of about six or more rings of whorls, generally six flowers in a whorl. The upper leaves or bracts interspersed between the whorls are also tinged with the same color, so that ordinarily the whole of the upper portion of the plant has a bluish appearance. A white variety is sometimes found, the upper leaves then being of the normal green color.

The flowers are adapted by their lipped formation for cross-fertilization by bees, a little honey being found at the base of the long tube of the corolla. The upper lip is very short and the lower three-cleft. The stamens project. The flowers have practically no scent. After fertilization, small blackish seeds are formed, but many of the ovules do not mature.

The rather singular names of this plant - both popular and botanical - are not very easy to account for. It has been suggested that 'Bugle' is derived from bugulus, a thin, glass pipe used in embroidery, the long, thin tube of the corolla being thought to resemble this bead bugle. It is more likely to be a corruption of the Latin name Ajuga, the generic name which Linnaeus was the first to apply to this plant from a belief that this or some closely-allied species was the one referred to by Pliny and other writers by a very similar name, a name probably corrupted from Abija, in turn derived from the Latin word abigo, to drive away, because the plant was thought to drive away various forms of disease. In former days it was held to possess great curative powers. Prior, writing in the seventeenth century, tells us: 'It is put in drinkes for woundes and that is the cause why some doe commonly say that he that hath Bugle and Sanicle will scarce vouchsafe the chirugeon a bugle." The early writers speak of the plant as the Abija, Ajuga, Abuga and Bugula, and the common English name, Bugle, is clearly a corruption of one or other of these forms.

Part Used Medicinally

The whole herb, gathered in May and early June, when the leaves are at their best, and dried.

Medicinal Action and Uses

Bitter, astringent and aromatic.

In herbal treatment, an infusion of this plant is still considered very useful in arresting hemorrhages and is employed in coughs and spitting of blood in incipient consumption and also in some biliary disorders, a wine glassful of the infusion - made from 1 OZ. of the dried herb to 1 pint of boiling water - being given frequently.

In its action, it rather resembles digitalis, lowering the pulse and lessening its frequency, it allays irritation and cough, and equalizes the circulation and has been termed 'one of the mildest and best narcotics in the world." It has also been considered good for the bad effects of excessive drinking.

Green (Universal Herbal, 1832) gives as his opinion that

'the leaves may be advantageously used in fluxes and disorders of that kind as they do not, like many other plants of the same value, produce costiveness, but rather operate as gentle laxatives."

He states that a decoction of the herb has been employed for quinsy on the Continent, where the herb has been more employed as a remedy than in this country.

The roots have by some authorities been considered more astringent than the rest of the plant.

Culpepper had a great opinion of the value of the Bugle and says,

'if the virtues of it make you fall in love with it (as they will if you be wise) keep a syrup of it to take inwardly, and an ointment and plaster of it to use outwardly, always by you. The decoction of the leaves and flowers in wine dissolveth the congealed blood in those that are bruised inwardly by a fall or otherwise and is very effectual for any inward wounds, thrusts or stabs in the body or bowels; and is an especial help in wound drinks and for those that are liver-grown, as they call it. It is wonderful in curing all ulcers and sores, gangrenes and fistulas, if the leaves, bruised and applied or their juice be used to wash and bathe the place and the same made into lotion and some honey and gum added, cureth the worse sores. Being also taken inwardly or outwardly applied, it helpeth those that have broken any bone or have any member out of joint. An ointment made with the leaves of Bugle, Scabious and Sanicle bruised and boiled in hog's lard until the herbs be dry and then strained into a pot for such occasions as shall require, it is so efficacious for all sorts of hurts in the body that none should be without it."

BUGLE, YELLOW

Botanical: Ajuga chamaepitys (SCHREB.)
Family: N.O. Lahiatae
Synonym: European Ground Pine.
Part Used: Leaves.

Habitat

It is a native of many parts of Europe, the Levant and North Africa, is common in sandy and chalky fields in Kent, Surrey and Essex, but otherwise is a scarce plant in England.

Description

Both in foliage and blossom it is very unlike its near relative, the Common Bugle, forming a bushy, herbaceous plant, 3 to 6 inches high, the four-cornered stem, hairy and viscid, generally purplish red, being much branched and densely leafy. Except the lowermost leaves, which are lanceshaped and almost undivided, each leaf is divided almost to its base into three very long, narrow segments, and the leaves being so closely packed together, the general appearance is not altogether unlike the long, needle-like foliage of the pine, hence the plant has received a second name- Ground Pine. The flowers are placed singly in the axils of leaf-like bracts and have bright yellow corollas, the lower lip spotted with red. They are in bloom during May and June.

The whole plant is very hairy, with stiff hairs, which consist of a few long joints. It has a highly aromatic and turpentiny odor and taste.

Uses

Ground Pine has stimulant, diuretic and emmenagogue action and is considered by herbalists to form a good remedy, combined with other suitable herbs, for gout and rheumatism and also to be useful in female disorders, an infusion of 1 OZ. of the dried herb to 1 pint of boiling water being recommended, taken in tablespoonful doses, frequently repeated.

The herb was formerly regarded almost as a specific in gouty and rheumatic affections, the young tops, dried and reduced to powder being employed. It formed an ingredient of the once famous Portland Powder.

It likewise operates powerfully by urine, removing obstructions and is serviceable in dropsy, jaundice and ague, reputed great cures having been performed by its use, either in infusion, or powder.

BUGLEWEED

Botanical: Lycopus Virginicus (LINN.)
Family: N.O. Labiatae
Synonyms: Water Bugle. Sweet Bugle. Virginian Water Horehound. Gipsyweed.
Part Used: Herb.

Habitat

An American plant. It is a very common weed in North America, growing in low, damp, shady ground and flowering from July to September.

Description

Though a Labiate, it does not actually belong to the same genus as the British Bugles, but has certain points in common. From the perennial, creeping root, the quadrangular, smooth stem rises to a height of from 6 to 24 inches, bearing pairs of opposite leaves on short stalks, those on the upper part being toothed and lance-shaped, the lower ones wedge-shaped and with entire margins. The leaves are destitute of hairs and gland-dotted beneath. The flowers are in clusters in the axils of the leaves; the calyx has four broad, blunt teeth and the corolla is four-lobed, purplish in color, with only two fertile stamens.

Part Used

The whole herb is used. It is slightly aromatic, with a mint-like odor and is used, fresh, when in flower, for the preparation of a tincture and a fluid extract, until recent years official in the United States Pharmacopoeia. It is also used dried for making an infusion.

Constituents

It contains a peculiar bitter principle, insoluble in ether, another soluble in ether, the two forming more than 10 per cent of the whole solid extract, also tannin and a volatile oil.

Medicinal Action and Uses

Sedative, astringent and mildly narcotic. Used in coughs, bleeding from the lungs and consumption. The infusion made from 1 OZ. of the dried herb to 1 pint of boiling water is taken in wine glassful doses, frequently, the fluid extract in doses of 10 to 30 drops, and the dry extract, Lycopin, in doses of 1 to 4 grains.

BUGLOSS, VIPER'S

Botanical: Echium vulgare (LINN.)
Family: N.O. Boraginaceae
Synonym: Blueweed.
Part Used: Herb.

Viper's Bugloss is a showy plant covered with prickly hairs. It grows on walls, old quarries and gravel pits, and is common on calcareous soils. The name Bugloss, which is of Greek origin, signifies an Ox's Tongue, and was applied to it from the roughness and shape of the leaves.

Description

The stems grow from 2 to 3 feet high and are covered with bristly hairs, as are also the leaves, which are 4 or 5 inches long, lanceolate, sessile, quite entire and rough on both sides. The stem is often spotted with red and sometimes the leaves also. The root-leaves form a tuft nearly 18 inches to 2 feet across. They are petioled. The flowers are in curved spikes, numerous, those of each spike pointing one way and closely wedged together. On their first opening they are bright rose-coloured and turn to a brilliant blue. They are in bloom throughout June and July, and are much visited by bees. The corollas are irregularly tubular and funnel-shaped. A variety is occasionally found with white flowers. The fruit consists of four small nutlets. The roots are biennial and descend to a great depth in the loose soil in which the plant generally grows.

Lycopsis arvenis, the Common or Small Bugloss, has small wheel-shaped flowers and wavy toothed leaves, which have also rigid hairs with a bulbous base.

Viper's Bugloss was said of old to be an expellent of poisons and venom, and to cure the bites of a viper, hence its name. Coles tells us in his Art of Simples:

'Viper's Bugloss hath its stalks all to be speckled like a snake or viper, and is a most singular remedy against poyson and the sting of scorpions.

Its seeds are also thought to resemble snake heads, thus specifying it as a cure for the bites of serpents. Its generic name Echium is derived from Echis, a viper.

Parkinson says of it:

'the water distilled in glasses or the roote itself

taken is good against the passions and tremblings of the heart as also against swoonings, sadness and melancholy."

Medicinal Action and Uses

Diuretic, demulcent and pectoral. The leaves, especially those growing near the root, make a good cordial on infusion, which operates by perspiration and alleviates fevers, headaches and nervous complaints, relieving inflammatory pains. The infusion is made of 1 oz. of the dried leaves to a pint of boiling water, and is given in wine glassful to teacupful doses, as required.

A decoction of the seeds in wine, we are told by old writers, 'comforts the heart and drives away melancholy."

BULLACE

Botanical: Prunus insititia (LINN.)
Family: N.O. Rosaceae
Synonyms: Bully-bloom (for the flowers). Bullies, Bolas, Bullions and Wild Damson (for the fruit). (French) Sibarelles.
Parts Used: Fruit, wood and bark.

Habitat

Common in England in thickets, woods and hedges, though more rare in Scotland and probably not wild north of the Forth and Clyde. Common in South-East Europe and in Northern and Central Asia.

Description

A tall shrub, sometimes developing into a small tree about 15 feet high. Resembles the Blackthorn or Sloe (Prunus spinosa), but is less thorny and has straight, not crooked branches, covered by brown, not black bark, only a few of the old ones terminating in spines, the younger ones downy. It has also larger leaves than the Blackthorn, downy underneath, alternate, finely-toothed, on short, downy foot-stalks, and flowers, white like those of the Blackthorn, but larger, with broader petals, borne in less crowded clusters and not on the naked branches, but expanding just after the leaves have begun to unfold.

The globular, fleshy fruit, marked with a faint suture, has generally a black skin, covered with a thin bluish bloom, and is similar to the Sloe, but larger, often an inch across, and drooping from its weight, not erect as the Sloe. Occasionally yellow varieties are found.

Constituents

The volatile oil expressed from the seeds contains benzaldehyde and hydrocyanic acid. These substances are also present in the young leaves and flowers.

Medicinal Action and Uses

The bark of the root and branches is considerably styptic. An infusion of the flowers, sweetened with sugar, has been used as a mild purgative for children.

The wood, branches, fruit and entire plant are used throughout France for the same properties as those of the Sloe, the bark of which is used as a febrifuge and the gin, prepared from the fruit on account of its astringency, as a good remedy in cases of diarrhea.

In this country, the fruit is gathered for 'Bullace Wine," and is also made into excellent pies and puddings and a good preserve is made by mixing the pulp with three times its weight of sugar.

There are several varieties of the Bullace in cultivation, and they frequently appear on the market as 'Damsons." Both Bullace and Damson originate from the same source P. domestica, the only difference being that the former is round and the latter oval. All cultivated Bullaces are immense bearers; the following are the best known:

ROYAL BULLACE. Fruit large, 1 1/4 inch in diameter. Skin bright grass-green, mottled with red on the side next to the sun and becoming yellowish-green as it ripens, with a thin, grey bloom on the surface. Flesh green, separating from the stone, briskly flavoured with sufficient sweetness to make it an agreeable late fruit. Ripe in early October.

WHITE BULLACE. Fruit small, round. Skin pale yellowish-white, mottled with red next the sun. Flesh firm, juicy, sub-acid, adhering to the stone, becoming sweetish when quite ripe in end of October and beginning of November. Often sold in London as 'White Damsons ."

ESSEX BULLACE. Skin green, becoming yellowish as it ripens. Flesh juicy and not so acid as the common Bullace. Ripens end of October and beginning of November. Fruit an inch or more in diameter, larger than the common White Bullace.

BURDOCK

Botanical: Arctium lappa (LINN.)
Family: N.O. Compositae
Synonyms: Lappa. Fox's Clote. Thorny Burr. Beggar's Buttons. Cockle Buttons. Love Leaves. Philanthropium. Personata. Happy Major. Clot-Bur.
Parts Used: Root, herb and seeds (fruits).

Habitat

It grows freely throughout England (though rarely in Scotland) on waste ground and about old buildings, by roadsides and in fairly damp places.

The Burdock, the only British member of its genus, belongs to the Thistle group of the great order, Compositae.

Description

A stout handsome plant, with large, wavy leaves and round heads of purple flowers. It is enclosed in a globular involucre of long stiff scales with hooked tips, the scales being also often interwoven with a white, cottony substance.

The whole plant is a dull, pale green, the stem about 3 to 4 feet and branched, rising from a biennial root. The lower leaves are very large, on long, solid foot-stalks, furrowed above, frequently more than a foot long heart-shaped and of a grey color on their under surfaces from the mass of fine down with which they are covered. The upper leaves are much smaller, more egg-shaped in form and not so densely clothed beneath with the grey down.

The plant varies considerably in appearance, and by some botanists various subspecies, or even separate species, have been described, the variations being according to the size of the flower-heads and of the whole plant, the abundance of the whitish cottonlike substance that is sometimes found on the involucres, or the absence of it, the length of the flower-stalks, etc.

The flower-heads are found expanded during the latter part of the summer and well into the autumn: all the florets are tubular, the stamens dark purple and the styles whitish. The plant owes its dissemination greatly to the little hooked prickles of its involucre, which adhere to everything with which they come in contact, and by attaching themselves to coats of animals are often carried to a distance.

'They are Burs, I can tell you, they'll stick where they are thrown,"

Shakespeare makes Pandarus say in Troilus and Cressida, and in King Lear we have another direct reference to this plant:

'Crown'd with rank Fumiter and Furrow-weeds,

With Burdocks, Hemlocks, Nettles, Cuckoo-flowers."

Also in As You Like It:

ROSALIND. How full of briers is this working-day world!

CELIA. They are but burs, cousin, thrown upon thee in holiday foolery. If we walk not in the trodden paths, our very petticoats will catch them.

The name of the genus, Arctium, is derived from the Greek arktos, a bear, in allusion to the roughness of the burs, lappa, the specific name, being derived from a word meaning 'to seize."

Another source derives the word lappa from the Celtic llap, a hand, on account of its prehensile properties.

The plant gets its name of 'Dock' from its large leaves; the 'Bur' is supposed to be a contraction of the French bourre, from the Latin burra, a lock of wool, such is often found entangled with it when sheep have passed by the growing plants.

An old English name for the Burdock was 'Herrif," 'Aireve," or 'Airup," from the Anglo-Saxon hoeg, a hedge, and reafe, a robber - or from the Anglo-Saxon verb reafian, to seize. Culpepper gives as popular names in his time: Personata, Happy Major and Clot-Bur.

Though growing in its wild state hardly any animal except the ass will browse on this plant, the stalks, cut before the flower is open and stripped of their rind, form a delicate vegetable when boiled, similar in flavor to Asparagus, and also make a pleasant salad, eaten raw with oil and vinegar. Formerly they were sometimes candied with sugar, as Angelica is now. They are slightly laxative, but perfectly wholesome.

Cultivation

As the Burdock grows freely in waste places and hedgerows, it can be collected in the wild state, and is seldom worth cultivating.

It will grow in almost any soil, but the roots are formed best in a light well-drained soil. The seeds germinate readily and may be sown directly in the field, either in autumn or early spring, in drills 18 inches to 3 feet apart, sowing 1 inch deep in autumn, but less in spring. The young plants when well up are thinned out to 6 inches apart in the row.

Yields at the rate of 1,500 to 2,000 lb. of dry roots per acre have been obtained from plantations of Burdock.

Parts Used Medicinally

The dried root from plants of the first year's growth forms the official drug, but the leaves and fruits (commonly, though erroneously, called seeds) are also used.

The roots are dug in July, and should be lifted with a beet-lifter or a deep-running plough. As a rule they are 12 inches or more in length and about 1 inch thick, sometimes, however, they extend 2 to 3 feet, making it necessary to dig by hand. They are fleshy, wrinkled, crowned with a tuft of whitish, soft, hairy leaf-stalks, grey-brown externally, whitish internally, with a somewhat thick bark, about a quarter of the diameter of the root, and soft wood tissues, with a radiate structure.

Burdock root has a sweetish and mucilaginous taste.

Burdock leaves, which are less used than the root, are collected in July. For drying, follow the drying of Coltsfoot leaves. They have a somewhat bitter taste.

The seeds (or fruits) are collected when ripe. They are brownish-grey, wrinkled, about 1/4 inch long and 1/16 inch in diameter. They are shaken out of the head and dried by spreading them out on paper in the sun.

Constituents

Inulin, mucilage, sugar, a bitter, crystalline glucoside - Lappin-a little resin, fixed and volatile oils, and some tannic acid.

The roots contain starch, and the ashes of the plant, burnt when green, yield carbonate of potash abundantly, and also some nitre.

Medicinal Action and Uses

Alterative, diuretic and diaphoretic. One of the best blood purifiers. In all skin diseases, it is a certain remedy and has effected a cure in many cases of eczema, either taken alone or combined with other remedies, such as Yellow Dock and Sarsaparilla.

The root is principally employed, but the leaves and seeds are equally valuable. Both root and seeds may be taken as a decoction of 1 OZ. to 1 1/2 pint of water, boiled down to a pint, in doses of a wine glassful, three or four times a day.

The anti-scorbutic properties of the root make the decoction very useful for boils, scurvy and rheumatic affections, and by many it is considered superior to Sarsaparilla, on account of its mucilaginous, demulcent nature; it has in addition been recommended for external use as a wash for ulcers and scaly skin disorders.

An infusion of the leaves is useful to impart strength and tone to the stomach, for some forms of long-standing indigestion.

When applied externally as a poultice, the leaves are highly resolvent for tumors and gouty swellings, and relieve bruises and inflamed surfaces generally. The bruised leaves have been applied by the peasantry in many countries as cataplasms to the feet and as a remedy for hysterical disorders.

From the seeds, both a medicinal tincture and a fluid extract are prepared, of benefit in chronic skin diseases. Americans use the seeds only, considering them more efficacious and prompt in their action than the other parts of the plant. They are relaxant and demulcent, with a limited amount of tonic property. Their influence upon the skin is due largely to their being of such an oily nature: they affect both the sebaceous and sudoriferous glands, and probably owing to their oily nature restore that smoothness to the skin which is a sign of normal healthy action.

The infusion or decoction of the seeds is employed in dropsical complaints, more especially in cases where there is co-existing derangement of the nervous system, and is considered by many to be a specific for all affections of the kidneys, for which it may with advantage be taken several times a day, before meals.

Preparations

Fluid extract, root, 1/2 to 2 drachms. Solid extract, 5 to 15 grains. Fluid extract, seed, 10 to 30 drops.

Culpepper gives the following uses for the Burdock:

'The Burdock leaves are cooling and moderately drying, wherby good for old ulcers and sores.... The leaves applied to the places troubled with the shrinking in the sinews or arteries give much ease: a juice of the leaves or rather the roots themselves given to drink with old wine, doth wonderfully help the biting of any serpents- the root beaten with a little salt and laid on the place suddenly easeth the pain thereof, and helpeth those that are bit by a mad dog:... the seed being drunk in wine 40 days together doth wonderfully help the sciatica: the leaves bruised with the white of an egg and applied to any place burnt with fire, taketh out the fire, gives sudden ease and heals it up afterwards.... The root may be preserved with sugar for consumption, stone and the lax. The seed is much commended to break the stone, and is often used with other seeds and things for that purpose."

It was regarded as a valuable remedy for stone in the Middle Ages, and called Bardona. As a rule, the recipes for stone contained some seeds or 'fruits' of a 'stony' character, as gromel seed, ivy berries, and nearly always saxifrage, i.e. 'stone-breaker." Even date-stones had to be pounded and taken; the idea being that what is naturally 'stony' would cure it; that 'like cures like' (Henslow).

BURNET, GREAT

Botanical: Sanguisorba Officinalis (LINN.)
Synonyms: Garden Burnet. Common Burnet.
Parts Used: Herb, root.

Habitat

Grows in moist meadows and shady places, chiefly in mountainous districts, almost all over Europe. In Britain it is not uncommon, but is rare in Ireland.

Closely related to the Alchemillas, belonging to the same subdivision, Sanguisorbidae, of the order Rosaceae and having similar medicinal properties to Alchemilla vulgaris, are the Burnets, Sanguisorba officinalis and Poterium sanguisorba.

It is a tall and not inelegant plant, with pinnate leaves on long stalks, bearing thirteen sharply serrate leaflets and branched stems, 2 feet high or more, sparsely clothed with leaves, and oblong heads of deep purple-brown flowers, which have four-toothed, coloured, membraneous calyces. The root is black and long. The plant has no odor.

It is cultivated to a considerable extent in Germany for fodder, and has been grown here with that view, but is not in esteem among English farmers. It will grow tolerably on very poor land, but is not a very valuable fodder plant.

An Italian proverb says: 'The salad is neither good nor good-looking when there is no pimpernel." This pimpernel is our Common Burnet and must not be confused with the plant known by that name which has poisonous properties. The roots are perennial and should be divided in early spring. It likes a dry and chalky soil.

Parts Used Medicinally

The herb and root, the herb gathered in July, and the root dug in autumn.

Culpepper says of 'The Great Wild Burnet':

'This is an herb the Sun challenges dominion over, and is a most precious herb, little inferior to Betony- the continual use of it preserves the body in health and the spirits in vigour, for if the Sun be the preserver of life under God, his herbs are the best in the world to do it by.... Two or three of the stalks, with leaves put into a cup of wine, especially claret, are known to quicken the spirits, refresh and cheer the heart, and drive away melancholy: It is a special help to defend the heart from noisome vapors, and from infection of the pestilence, the juice thereof being taken in some drink, and the party laid to sweat thereupon."

He also recommends it for wounds, both inwardly and outwardly applied.

Cultivation

Burnet may be cultivated. It prefers a light soil. Sow seeds in March and thin out to 9 inches apart. Propagation may also be effected by division of roots, in the autumn, that they may be well-established before the dry summer weather sets in. The flowers should be picked off when they appear, the stem and leaves only of the herb being used.

Medicinal Action and Uses

Astringent and tonic. Great Burnet was formerly in high repute as a vulnerary, hence its generic name, from sanguis, blood, and sorbeo, to staunch. Both herb and root are administered internally in all abnormal discharges: in diarrhea, dysentery, leucorrhoea, it is of the utmost service; dried and powdered, it has been used to stop purgings.

The whole plant has astringent qualities, but the root possesses the most astringency. A decoction of the whole herb has, however, been found useful in hemorrhage and is a tonic cordial and sudorific; the herb is also largely used in Herb Beer.

BURNET, LESSER

Botanical: Pimpinella saxifraga (LINN.)
Family: N.O. Umbelliferae
Synonyms: Salad Burnet. Burnet Saxifrage. Pimpinella sanguisorba.
Parts Used: Root, herb.

Habitat

The Salad Burnet is common in dry pastures and by the wayside, especially on chalk and limestone, but is rarer in Scotland and Ireland than in England.

The Lesser or Salad Burnet is not unlike the Great Burnet in habit, but it is much smaller and more slender. It was known by older writers as Pimpinella sanguisorba, Pimpinella being a corruption of bipennula, from the two pinnate leaves. Pimpinella is now reserved for the name of a genus belonging to the order Umbelliferae, and the Salad Burnet is assigned to the genus Poterium, which name is derived from the Greek poterion, a drinking-cup, from the use to which the leaves of the Salad Burnet were applied in the preparation of the numerous beverages with which the poterion was filled in ancient times. The leaves when bruised smell like cucumber and taste somewhat like it, and it was used to cool tankards in the same manner as Borage, and was also added to salads and cups.

Hooker places both the Great Burnet and the Salad or Lesser Burnet in the same genus, Poterium, rejecting the generic name of Sanguisorba, assigned to the former by Linnaeus.

Description

Its leaflets are more numerous, five to ten pairs, and shorter than thoseof the Great Burnet. The flowers in each head bear crimson tufted stigmas, the lower ones thirty to forty stamens, with very long, drooping filaments. Both the flower and leafstalks are a deep-crimson color.

Turner (Newe Herball, 1551), in his description of the plant, tells us that

'it has two little leives like unto the wings of birdes, standing out as the bird setteth her wings out when she intendeth to flye. Ye Dutchmen call it Hergottes berdlen, that is God's little berde, because of the color that it hath in the topp."

The great Burnet and the Salad Burnet both flower in June and July.

The Salad Burnet forms much of the turf on some of the chalk downs in the southern counties. It is extremely nutritious to sheep and cattle, and was formerly extensively cultivated as a fodder plant on calcareous soils but is now little grown in that way. Cattle do not seem to like it as well as clover when full grown, but when kept closely cropped sheep are fond of it. It has the advantage of keeping green all the winter in dry barren pastures, affording food for sheep when other green crops are scarce. The results of cultivation have, however, not been very satisfactory, except on poor soil, although it contains a larger amount of nutritive matter than many grasses.

In the herb gardens of older days, Salad Burnet always had its place. Bacon recommends it to be set in alleys together with wild thyme and water mint, 'to perfume the air most delightfully, being trodden on and crushed."

Cultivation

It is easily propagated by seeds, sown in autumn, soon after they are ripe. If the seeds be permitted to scatter, the plants will come up plentifully, and can be transplanted into an ordinary or rather poor soil, at about a foot distant each way. If kept clear from weeds, they will continue some years without further care, especially if the soil be dry. Propagation may also be effected by division of roots in spring or autumn.

When used for salad, the flower-stalks should be cut down if not required for seed. The leaves, for salad use, should be cut young, or may be tough.

Part Used Medicinally

The whole herb, as in the Great Burnet, gathered in July and dried in the same manner.

Medicinal Action and Uses

The older herbalists held this plant in greater repute than it enjoys at the present day. Pliny recommended a decoction of the plant beaten up with honey for divers complaints.

Dodoens recommended it as a healer of wounds,

'made into powder and dronke with wine, wherin iron hath bene often quenched, and so doth the herbe alone, being but only holden in a man's hande as some have written. The leaves stiped in wine and dronken, doth comfort and rejoice the hart and are good against the trembling and shaking of the same."

Parkinson grew Burnet in his garden and the early settlers in America introduced it from the Mother Country.

'It gives a grace in the drynkynge," says Gerard, referring to this use of it in cool tankards. We are also told that it affords protection against infection,

'a speciall helpe to defend the heart from noysome vapors and from the infection of the Plague or Pestilence, and all other contagious diseases for which purpose it is of great effect, the juice thereof being taken in some drink."

and that

'it is a capital wound herb for all sorts of wounds, both of the head and body, either inward or outward, used either in juice or decoction of the herb, or by the powder of the herb or root, or the water of the distilled herb, or made into an ointment by itself or with other things to be kept."

It is still regarded as a styptic, an infusion of the whole herb being employed as an astringent. It is also a cordial and promotes perspiration.

Turner advised the use of the herb, infused in wine or beer, for the cure of gout and rheumatism.

BURNING BUSH

Botanical: Dictamnus albus
Family: N.O. Rutaceae
Synonyms: Fraxinella. Bastard. False or White Dittany.
Part Used: The root.
Habitat: Germany. France. Alsace. Spain. Austria. Italy. Asia Minor.

Description

The members of this small genus are plants about 2 feet high, bearing flowers in a long, pyramidal, loose spike, varying in color from pale purple to white. It prefers to grow in woods in warm places. The whole plant, especially when rubbed, gives out an odor like lemon-peel, and when bruised this grows more like that of a fine balsam, strongest in the pedicels of the flowers. It is due to an essential oil, which gives off an inflammable vapor in heat or in dry, cloudy weather, which also congeals as resinous wax, exuding from rusty-red glands in the flowers. This accounts for the fact that the atmosphere surrounding it will often take fire if approached by a lighted candle, without injuring the plant.

The fragrant leaves and handsome flowers cause it to be frequently cultivated in gardens.

The prepared root-bark is whitish, almost odourless, and rolled in pieces from 1 to 2 inches long.

Constituents

The acrid and resinous principles have not been analysed.

Medicinal Action and Uses

The drug is very little used to-day, though it is an ingredient in 'Orvieton' 'Solomon's Opiate," 'Guttète Powder," 'Balm of Fioraventi," 'Eau generale," 'Hyacinth Mixture," etc. It is recommended in nervous complaints and intermittent fevers, and used to be given in scrofulous and scorbutic diseases. It is a cordial and stomachic. The distilled water is used as a cosmetic. An infusion of the leaves is regarded as a substitute for tea. The powder is combined with that of peppermint for use in epilepsy.

Dosage

Of powdered root, 4 to 8 grammes, or double the quantity in infusion.

Other Species

Several drugs bear the name of Dictamnus,such as Dictamnus of Barbados, or Arrowroot des tilles.

The leaves of a plant growing in Crete and Candy were used by the Ancients for wounds, and it is still known as Dictamnus or Dittany of Crete, being Origanum Dictamnus of the Labiatae family.

BUTTERBUR

Botanical: Petasites vulgaris (DESF.)
Family: N.O. Compositae
Synonyms: Langwort. Umbrella Plant. Bog Rhubarb. Flapperdock. Blatterdock. Capdockin. Bogshorns. Butter-Dock.
Part Used: Root.

The Butterbur, a plant nearly allied to the Coltsfoot - being the Tussilago petasites of Linnaeus - is found in wet ground, lowlying, marshy meadows and by riversides, but is usually local.

Description

It has a fleshy, stout root-stock, extensively creeping, which, like the Coltsfoot, sends up the flowers before the leaves appear. The flower-heads are, however, not produced singly, on separate stalks, but in crowned clusters in a dense spike, with many bracts interspersed, at the summit of a round, thick flower-stalk, 4 inches to a little over a foot in height, which first appears at the end of February or beginning of

March, and is generally of a purplish hue.

There are two kinds of flowers - the male or stamen-bearing and the female or seedproducing - as a rule on different spikes, the female flowers being in denser, longer spikes than the male flowers, which are in shorter, loose clusters. Occasionally a few female flowers are found on the male spikes, and a few male flowers on the female spikes. The corollas are pale reddish purple or fleshcoloured, bell-shaped in the male flowers, and containing abundant nectar, but only threadlike in the female flowers, which contain no nectar, and are succeeded by the white feathery pappus, which crowns the seeds.

In April, as the flowers begin to decay, the leaves appear. They are on stout hollowed channelled footstalks, and when full grown very large - the largest leaves of any plant in Great Britain - the blade sometimes attaining 3 feet in diameter. It is roundish, heartshaped at the base, scalloped at the edges, with the portion between the projections finely toothed. The leaves are white and cobwebby with down both above and below when young, but when mature, most of the covering disappears from the upper surface though the leaves still remain grey and more or less downy beneath.

The name of the genus, Petasites, is derived from petasos, the Greek word for the felt hats worn by shepherds, and familiar to us in representations of Mercury, in reference to the large size of the leaves, which could be used as a head-covering. No other vegetation can live where these leaves grow, for they exclude light and air from all beneath, and where the plant abounds, it has been described as 'the most pernicious of all the weeds which this country produces."

The name Butterbur is supposed to have been given it because formerly these large leaves were used to wrap butter in during hot weather. 'Lagwort' is an old name we sometimes find for it, in reference to the leaves delaying their appearance till after the flowers have faded, though once the leaf-shoots make a start, they grow with almost tropical luxuriance.

'The early flowering of this rank weed,'Hooker writes, 'induces the Swedish farmers to plant it near their beehives. Thus we see in our gardens the bees assembled on its affinities, P. alba and P. fragrans, at a season when scarcely any other flowers are expanded."

In Germany an old name for the plant was Pestilenzenwurt, but one finds really very little either of evil or good assigned by the older writers to the Butterbur as compared with most other herbs. The old German name was given it, not as suggesting the plant was provocative of pestilence, but as an indication of its value as a remedy in time of such calamity (Henslow).

Anne Pratt says the former name of this plant was the 'plague-flower," as it gained a successful reputation among the few remedies during the time of that malady. Lyte, in his Herbal, 1578, calls it 'a soveraigne medicine against the plague', and remarks of its leaves that 'one of them is large enough to cover a small table, as with a carpet," and they are often 2 feet in width. Under its ample foliage, the poultry in farm meadows, shelter themselves from the rain, or find a cool retreat from the noonday sun. The Swedish farmers plant it in great quantities near their bechives, as bees are attracted by its flowers.

The seeds in some parts of the country have been used for love divination.

'The seeds of butterdock must be sowed by a young unmarried woman half an hour before sunrise on a Friday morning, in a lonesome place. She must strew the seeds gradually on the grass, saying these words:

I sow, I sow!
Then, my own dear,
Come here, come here,
And mow and mow!

The seed being scattered, she will see her future husband mowing with a scythe at a short distance from her. She must not be frightened, for if she says, "Have mercy on me," he will immediately vanish! This method is said to be infallible, but it is looked upon as a bold, desperate, and presumptuous undertaking!"

Part Used

The rhizome, or root-stock which is blackish on the outside and whitish internally, and has a bitter and unpleasant taste, due to the resinous, bitter juice it contains.

Medicinal Action and Uses

Butterbur root is medicinally employed as a heart stimulant, acting both as a cardiac tonic and also as a diuretic. It has been in use as a remedy in fevers, asthma, colds and urinary complaints, a decoction being taken warm in wine glassful doses, frequently repeated.

Both Butterbur and Coltsfoot are specific homeopathic remedies for severe and obstinate neuralgia in the small of the back and the loins, a medicinal tincture being prepared in each case.

Gerard writes of the Butterbur:

'The roots dried and beaten to powder and drunke in wine is a soveraigne medicine against the plague and pestilent fevers, because it provoketh sweat and driveth from the heart all venim and evill heate; it killeth worms. The powder of the roots cureth all naughty filthy ulcers, if it be strewed therein."

Culpepper says:

'It is a great strengthener of the heart and cheerer of the vital spirits: . . . if the powder thereof be taken in wine, it also resisteth the force of any other poison . . . the decoction of the root in wine is singularly good for those that wheeze much or are shortwinded.... The powder of the root taketh away all spots and blemishes of the skin."

Another species known as the Winter Heliotrope, or Sweet-scented Coltsfoot (P. fragrans), flourishes in warm districts like South Devon, where it is abundant. It is even more spreading and luxuriant in growth than our native Coltsfoot, but as it flowers in the poorest soil and clothes waste land with its handsome foliage, it is certainly welcome outside the garden, and is even frequently planted in shrubberies. The fragrant flowers, which have the scent of vanilla and are like Butterbur in appearance, are freely borne in the depth of winter. The leaves appear in the spring and in favourable situations remain green till the young leaves appear in the succeeding season.

BUTTERCUP, BULBOUS

Botanical: Ranunculus bulbosus (LINN.)
Family: N.O. Ranunculaceae
Parts used: Juice and Herb.
Synonyms: St. Anthony's Turnip. Crowfoot. Frogs-foot. Goldcup.
(French) Jaunet.

The Bulbous Buttercup or Crowfoot is perhaps the commonest of the Ranunculus family, covering the meadows in May with dazzling yellow, being one of the earliest of the varieties to flower, owing to the nourishment stored up in the bulbs.

The specific name bulbosus refers to the bulb-like swelling at the base of the stem, roundish and white, flattened a little both at the top and bottom, somewhat resembling a small turnip - hence one of the popular names for this plant: St. Anthony's Turnip. It is however, not a true bulb, only 'bulb-like."

This is the 'Cuckow buds of yellow hue' of Shakespeare, and in France it is called the jaunet from the brilliance of its blossoms. Frogs-foot (from the form of its leaves) and Goldcup, from the shape and color of its flowers, are other English names it bears.

The Bulbous Buttercup has some superficial resemblance to the Upright Crowfoot and the Creeping Crowfoot, but is distinguished not only by its bulb and by the fact that it never throws out runners, but by the fact that its sepals are turned back in the fully expanded blossom, so as to touch the stemthat supports the flower.

The stems are furrowed slightly, not merely round, as in Ranunculus acris. The upper leaves are composed of long, narrow segments, the lower ones broadened out into very distinct masses.

When once established it is not easily eradicated.

Medicinal Action and Uses

Like most of the Crowfoots, the Bulbous Buttercup possesses the property of inflaming and blistering the skin, particularly the roots, which are said to raise blisters with less pain and greater safety than Spanish Fly, and have been applied for that purpose, especially to the joints, in gout. The juice, if applied to the nostrils, provokes sneezing and cures certain cases of headache. The leaves have been used to produce blisters on the wrists in rheumatism, and when infused in boiling water, as a poultice, at the pit of the stomach.

A tincture made with spirits of wine will cure shingles very expeditiously, it is stated, both the outbreak of the small pimples and the accompanying sharp pains between the ribs, 6 to 8 drops being given three or four times daily. For sciatica, the tincture has been employed with good effect.

The roots on being kept lose their stimulating quality, and are even eatable when boiled. Pigs are remarkably fond of them, and will go long distances to get them.

The herb is too acrid to be eaten alone by cattle, but possibly mixed with grasses it may act as a stimulus.

It is recorded that two obstinate cases of nursing soremouth have been cured with an infusion made by adding 2 drachms of the recent root, cut into small pieces, to 1 pint of hot water, when cold, a tablespoonful was given three or four times a day, and the mouth was frequently washed with a much stronger infusion.

Its action as a counter-irritant is both uncertain and violent, and may cause obstinate ulcers. The beggars of Europe sometimes use it to keep open sores for the purpose of exciting sympathy.

BUTTERNUT

Botanical: Juglans cinerea (LINN.)
Family: N.O. Juglandaceae
Synonyms: White Walnut. Oilnut.
Part Used: Bark of the root.
Habitat: New Brunswick and mountains of Georgia.

Description

The leaves possess much the same properties as the Black Walnut. The inner bark of the root is the best for medicinal use and should be collected in May or June; it is generally found in quills, curved strips or chips from 1/8 to 1/2 inch thick, deep brown in color all through, outer surface smooth and a little warty, inner surface smooth and striate with fragments and thin stringy fibre, short fracture, weak and fibrous, odor slightly aromatic, taste bitter (astringent and acrid). The powdered drug is dark brown.

Constituents

A bitter extractive, a large proportion of oily matter, a volatilizable acid and juglandic acid.

Medicinal Action and Uses

Butternut is a mild cathartic like rhubarb; it does not constipate and is often used as a habitual laxative, also for dysentery and hypatic congestions. It has been employed as a vermifuge and is recommended for syphilis and old ulcers. The expressed oil of the fruit removes tapeworm. The fruit when halfgrown is made into pickles and when matured is a valuable article of diet. The bark is used for dyeing wool a dark brown color but is inferior to that of the black walnut for this purpose. It is said to be rubefacient when applied to the skin.

Preparations

Fluid extract, 1 to 2 drachms. Solid extract, 5 to 10 grains Juglandin, 2 to 5 grains.

C

CABBAGE TREE

POISON
Botanical: Andira inermis
Family: N.O. Leguminosae
Synonyms: Vouacapoua inermis. Bastard Cabbage Tree. Worm Bark. Yellow Cabbage Tree. Jamaica Cabbage Tree.
Part Used: Bark.
Habitat: Jamaica and other West Indian Islands. Senegambi.

Description

A leguminous tree, growing very tall and branching towards the top called Cabbage Tree because it forms a head in growing; it has a smooth grey bark which, cut into long pieces, is the part utilized for medicine. It is thick, fibrous, scaly, and of an ashy brownish color externally, covered with lichens - the inside bark is yellow and contains a bitter sweet mucilage, with an unpleasant smell. In Europe the bark of another species, Avouacouapa retusa, has been utilized. It grows in Surinam, is a more powerful vermifuge than Vouacapoua inermus and does not as a rule produce such injurious after-effects. In the dried state it is without odor, but has a very bitter taste; when powdered it has the color of cinnamon.

Constituents

Jamaicine-Andirin aglucoside, an inodorous, bitter, acrid resin.

Medicinal Action and Uses

Narcotic vermifuge. Cabbage Tree bark used in large doses may cause vomiting, fever and delirium, especially if cold water is drunk just before or after taking it. In the West Indies it is largely employed as a vermifuge to expel worm - ascaris lumbrecoides - but if used incautiously death has been known to occur. The powder purges like jalap.

Dosages

Usually given in decoction, though the powder, syrup and extract are all used. Dose of powder, 20 to 30 grains. Fluid extract, 1/4 to 1 drachm.

Antidote

Lime-juice or Castor oil.

Other Species

Andira retusa, a Brazilian species, has purple flowers, the odor of oranges and a slight aroma. The fruit is said to smell like tonka beans.

CACAO

Botanical: Theobroma cacao (LINN.)
Family: N.O. Sterculiaceae
Synonyms: Cocoa. Chocolate Tree.
Part Used: The seeds.
Habitat: Topical America. Cultivated in Ceylon. Java. etc.

Description and History

Cacao was named Theobroma by Linnaeus, the word meaning 'food of the gods," so called from the goodness of its seeds. Mexicans named the pounded seeds 'Chocolate." The tree is handsome, 12 to 16 feet high; trunk about 5 feet long; wood light and white coloured; bark brown; Ieaves lanceolate, bright green, entire; flowers small reddish, almost odourless; fruit yellowy red, smooth; rind fleshcoloured; pulp white; when seeds are ripe they rattle in the capsule when shaken; each capsule contains about twenty-five seeds; if separated from the capsule they soon become infertile, but if kept therein they retain their fertility for a long time. The tree bears its leaves, flowers and fruit (like the orange tree) all the year round, but the usual season for gathering the fruit is June and December. In Mexico during the time of the Aztec kings the small seeds were utilized as coins twelve approximating to the value of 1d., the smallest actual coin in use then being worth about 6d. The seeds were necessary for small transactions. The method is still in use in some parts of Mexico. The tree is generally cultivated on large estates under the shade of other trees, such as the banana and develops the pods continuously. When ripe they are cut open and the beans or nuts surrounded by their sweetish acid pulp are allowed to ferment so that they may be more easily separated from the shell. The beans are then usually dried in the sun, though sometimes in a steam drying shed.

Constituents

The seeds contain about 2 per cent. of theobromine and 40 to 60 per cent of solid fat. The shells contain about 1 per cent of theobromine, together with mucilage, etc.

Medicinal Action and Uses

Cocoa is prepared by grinding the beans into a paste between hot rollers and mixing it with sugar and starch, part of the fat being removed. Chocolate is prepared in much the same way, but the fat is retained. Oil of Theobroma or cacao butter is a yellowish white solid, with an odor resembling that of cocoa, taste bland and agreeable; generally extracted by expression. It is used as an ingredient in cosmetic ointments and in pharmacy for coating pills and preparing suppositories. It has excellent emollient properties and is used to soften and protect chapped hands and lips. Theobromine, the alkaloid contained in the beans, resembles caffeine in its action, but its effect on the central nervous system is less powerful. Its action on muscle, the kidneys and the heart is more pronounced. It is used principally for its diuretic effect due to stimulation of the renal epithelium; it is especially useful when there is an accumulation of fluid in the body resulting from cardiac failure, when it is often given with digitalis to relieve dilatation. It is also employed in high blood pressure as it dilates the blood-vessels. It is best administered in powders or cachets.

Dosage

Theobromine, 5 to 10 grains.

CAJUPUT

Botanical: Melaleuca leucadendron (LINN.)
Family: N.O. Myrtaceae
Synonyms: Cajeput. White Tea Tree. Swamp Tea Tree. White Wood.
Part Used: The oil.

Habitat

East Indies, Tropical Australia. Imported from Macassar, Batavia, Singapore, Queensland and N.S. Wales.

Description

The tree has a long flexible trunk with irregular ascending branches, covered with a pale thick, lamellated bark it is soft and spongy and from time to time throws off its outer layer in flakes; leaves entire, linear, lanceolate, ash color, alternate on short foot-stalks; flowers sessile, white, on a long spike. The leaves have a very aromatic odor and the oil is distilled from the fresh leaves and twigs, and is volatile and stimulating with an aroma like camphor, rosemary, or cardamom seeds; taste bitter, aromatic and camphoraceous. Traces of copper have been found in it, hence the greenish tint; it should be stored in dark or amber-coloured bottles in a cool place. Cajuput oil is obtained from Melaleuca leucadendron, Roxburgh, and the minor Smith, but several other species of Melaleuca leucadendron are utilized such as M. hypericifolia, M. veridifolia, M. lalifolia, and others. The Australian species M. Decussata and M. Erucifolia are also used. The oil is fluid, clear, inflammable, burns without residue, highly volatile. The trace of copper found may be due to the vessels in which the oil is prepared, but it is doubtless sometimes added in commerce to produce the normal green tinge when other species have been used which do not impart it naturally.

Constituents

The principal constituent of oil is cineol, which should average 45 to 55 per cent. Solid terpineol is also present and several aldehydes such as valeric, butyric and benzoic.

Medicinal Action and Uses

Antispasmodic, diaphoretic, stimulant, antiseptic, anthelmintic. Highly stimulant, producing a sensation of warmth when taken internally, increasing the fullness and rapidity of the pulse and sometimes producing profuse perspiration. Used as a stimulating expectorant in chronic laryngitis and bronchitis, as an antiseptic in cystisis and as an anthelmintic for round worms, also used in chronic rheumatism. Applied externally, it is stimulant and mildly counter-irritant and is usually applied diluted with 2 parts of olive oil or turpentine ointment. Used externally for psoriasis and other skin affections.

Adulterants

The oils of Rosemary and Turpentine, impregnated with Camphor and coloured, are said to be used. Spirit of Cajeput, B.P., 5 to 20 minims. Oil U S P., 3 to 10 minims. Oil, B.P., 1/2 to 3 minims.

CALABAR BEAN

POISON
Botanical: Physostigma venenosum (EALF.)
Family: N.O. Leguminosae
Synonyms: Ordeal Bean. Chop Nut.
Part Used: The seeds.
Habitat: West Africa, Old Calabar. Has been introduced into India and Brazil.

Description

The plant came into notice in 1846 and was planted in the Edinburgh Botanical Gardens, where it grew into a strong perennial creeper. It is a great twining climber, pinnately trifoliate leaves, pendulous racemes of purplish bean-like flowers; seeds are two or three together in dark brown pods about 6 inches long and kidney-shaped thick, about 1 inch long, rounded ends, roughish but a little polished, and have a long scar on the edge where adherent to the placenta. The seeds ripen at all seasons, but are best and most abundant during the rainy season in Africa, June till September. The natives of Africa employ the bean as an ordeal owing to its very poisonous qualities. They call it esere, and it is given to an accused person to eat. If the prisoner vomits within half an hour he is accounted innocent, but if he succumbs he is found guilty. A draught of the pounded seeds infused in water is said to have been fatal to a man within an hour.

Constituents

The chief constituent is the alkaloid physostigmine (eserine), with which are calabarines, eseridine, and eseramine. Eseridine is not employed medicinally.

Medicinal Action and Uses

Chiefly used for diseases of the eye; it causes rapid contraction of the pupil and disturbed vision. Also used as a stimulant to the unstriped muscles of the intestines in chronic constipation. Its action on the circulation is to slow the pulse and raise blood-pressure; it depresses the central nervous system, causing muscular weakness; it has been employed internally for its depressant action in epilepsy, cholera, etc., and given hypodermically in acute tetanus. Physostigmine Salicylas is preferred for the preparation of eyedrops.

Preparation of Doses

Extract of Calabar Bean, B.P.: dose, 1/4 to 1 grain. Extract of Physostigma, U.S.P.: dose, 1/8 grain. Tincture of Calabar Bean, B.P.C.: dose, 5 to 15 minims. Tincture of Physostigma, U.S.P.: dose, 15 minims. Physostigmine Eyedrops, B.P.C. Physostigmine eye ointment, B.P.C. Fluid extract, 1 to 3 drops.

Poisons and Antidotes

In case of poisoning by the beans the stomach should be evacuated and atropine injected until the pulse quickens. With poisoning by physostigmine the stomach should be washed out with 0.2 per cent of potassium permanganate and atropine and strychnine administered hypodermically.

CALAMINT

Botanical: Calamintha officinalis (MOENCH)
Family: N.O. Labiatae
Synonyms: Mill Mountain. Mountain Balm. Basil Thyme. Mountain Mint.
Part Used: Herb.

Description

Calamint belongs to a genus closely related to both the Thymes and to Catnep and Ground Ivy.

It is an erect, bushy plant with square stems, rarely more than a foot high, bearing pairs of opposite leaves, which, like the stems, are downy with soft hairs. The flowers bloom in July and August, and are somewhat inconspicuous, drooping gracefully before expansion: the corollas are of a light purple color.

The plant grows by waysides and in hedges, and is not uncommon, especially in dry places. It may be cultivated as a hardy perennial, propagated by seeds sown outdoors in April, by cuttings of side shoots in cold frames in spring, or by division of roots in October and April.

Constituents

It contains a camphoraceous, volatile, stimulating oil in commonwith the other mints. This is distilled by water, but its virtues are better extracted by rectified spirit.

Medicinal Actions and Uses

Diaphoretic, expectorant, aromatic. The whole herb has a sweet, aromatic odor and an infusion of the dried leaves, collected about July, when in their best condition and dried in the same way as Catmint tops, makes a pleasant cordial tea, which was formerly much taken for weaknesses of the stomach and flatulent colic. It is useful in hysterical complaints, and a conserve made of the young fresh tops has been used, for this purpose.

Culpepper says that it 'is very efficacious in all afflictions of the brain," that it 'relieves convulsions and cramps, shortness of breath or choleric pains in the stomach or bowels," and that 'it cures the yellow jaundice." He also recommends it, taken with salt and honey, for killing worms:

'It relieves those who have the leprosy, taken inwardly, drinking whey after it, or the green herb outwardly applied, and that it taketh away black and blue marks in the face, and maketh black scars become well coloured, if the green herb (not the dry) be boiled in wine and laid to the place or the place washed therewith."

He also considers it 'helpful to them that have a tertian ague," and beneficial in all disorders of the gall and spleen.

Gerard says, 'the seede cureth the infirmities of the hart, taketh away sorrowfulnesse which commeth of melancholie, and maketh a man merrie and glad."

THE LESSER CALAMINT

(Calamintha nepeta) is a variety of the herb possessing almost superior virtues, with a stronger odor, resembling that of Pennyroyal, and a moderately pungent taste somewhat like Spearmint, but warmer. It is scarcely distinct from C. officinalis, and by some botanists is considered a sub-species. The leaves are more strongly toothed, and it bears its flowers on longer stalks. Both this and the Common Calamint seem to have been used indifferently in the old practice of medicine under the name of Calamint.

The name of the genus, Calamintha, is derived from the Greek Kalos (excellent because of the ancient belief in its power to drive away serpents and the dreaded basilisk - the fabled king of the serpents, whose very glance was fatal.

CALISAYA

Botanical: Cinchona calisaya (WEDD.)
Family: N.O. Rubiaceae
Synonyms: Jesuit's Powder. Yellow Cinchona.
Part Used: Bark.
Habitat: Tropical valleys of the Andes. Bolivia and Southern Peru.

Description

Cinchona is an important genus and comprises a large number of evergreen trees and shrubs, flowers white and pinkish arranged in panicles, very fragrant. Not all the species yield cinchona or Peruvian bark. The most important is called Calisaya or yellow bark. Its great value as a tonic and febrifuge depends on an alkaloid, quina (Quinine). This substance chiefly exists in the cellular tissue outside the liber in combination with kinic and tannic acids. Calisaya yields the largest amount of this alkaloid of any of the species - often 70 to 80 per cent of the total alkaloids contained in the bark which is not collected from trees growing wild, but from those cultivated in plantations. The bark for commerce is classified under two headings: the druggist's bark, and the manufacturer's at a low price. The great bulk of the trade is in Amsterdam, and the bark sold there mainly comes from

Java. That sold in London from India, Ceylon and South America. Mature Calisaya bark has a scaly appearance, which denotes maturity and high quality. It is very bitter, astringent and odourless.

Constituents

The bark should yield between 5 and 6 per cent of total alkaloids, of which not less than half should consist of quinine and cinchonidin. Other constituents are cinchonine, quinidine, hydrocinchonidine, quinamine, homokinchonidine, hydroquinine; quinic and cinchotannic acids, a bitter amorphous glucocide, starch and calcium-oxalate.

Medicinal Action and Uses

Febrifuge, tonic and astringent; valuable for influenza, neuralgia and debility. Large and too constant doses must be avoided, as they produce headache, giddiness and deafness. The liquid extract is useful as a cure for drunkenness. The powdered bark is often used in tooth-powders, owing to its astringency, but not much used internally (except as a bitter wine); it creates a sensation of warmth, but sometimes causes gastric intestinal irritation. Cinchona in decoction is a useful gargle and a good throat astringent.

Preparations and Dosages

Decoction of Cinchona, B.P., 1/2 to 2 fluid ounces. Elixir of Cinchona or Elixir of Calisaya, B.P.C., 1/2 to 1 fluid drachm. Tincture of Cinchona, B.P.C., 1/2 to 1 fluid drachm. Cinchona wine, B.P.C., 1/2 to 1 fluid ounce.

CALOTROPIS

POISON
Botanical: Calotropis procera (R. BR.) and gigantea
Family: N.O. Asclepiadaceae
Synonyms: Mudar Yercum.
Parts Used: Bark, root-bark.

Habitat

Native of Hindustan, but widely naturalized in the East and West Indies and Ceylon.

Description

The dried root freed from its outer cork layer and called Mudar. It occurs in commerce in short quilled pieces about 1/5 to 1/10 of an inch thick and not over 1 1/2 inch wide. Deeply furrowed and reticulated, color greyish buff, easily separated from periderm. Fracture short and mealy, taste bitter, nauseous, acrid; it has a peculiar smell and is mucilaginous; official in India and the Colonial addendum for the preparation of a tincture.

Constituents

A yellow bitter resin; a black acid resin; Madaralbum, a crystalline colorless substance; Madarfluavil, an ambercoloured viscid substance; and caoutchouc, and a peculiar principle which gelatinizes on being heated, called Mudarine. Lewin found a neutral principle, Calatropin, a very active poison of the digitalis type. In India the author's husband experimented with it for paper-making, the inner bark yielding a fibre stronger than Russian hemp. The acrid juice hardens into a substance like gutta-percha. It has long been used in India for abortive and suicidal purposes. Mudar root-bark is very largely used there as a treatment for elephantiasis and leprosy, and is efficacious in cases of chronic eczema, also for diarrhea and dysentery.

Preparations

Tincture of Calatropis, 1/2 to 1 fluid drachm. Powder, 3 to 12 grains.

Antidotes

As an antidote to poisoning atropine may be administered. In severe cases the stomach pump may be used and chloral or chloroform administered. Amyl nitrite may also be useful.

CALUMBA

Botanical: Jateorhiza calumba (MIERS)
Family: N.O. Menispermaceae
Synonyms: Cocculus Palmatus. Colombo.
Part Used: The dried root sliced transversely.

Habitat

Forests of Eastern Africa. Indigenous to Mozambique, where it is abundant in the forests.

Description

A dioecious climbing plant with a perennial root, consisting of several tuberous portions, flowers small and inconspicuous, the root is dug in dry weather, in March, but only the fusiform offsets are used; the old root is rejected and the brightest, least worm-eaten and well-shaped pieces are preferred. The root and powder, if kept any length of time, are liable to be attacked by worms; the color of the freshly prepared powder is greenish, later on it turns brown and when moistened very dark; it quickly absorbs moisture from the air and is apt to decompose, so only a small quantity should be prepared at a time. Odor aromatic, taste very bitter, rind more so than the central pith, which is somewhat mucilaginous. It is rarely adulterated since the price has been lowered.

Constituents

Columbamine, Jateorhizine and Palmatine, three yellow crystalline alkaloids closely allied to berberine; also a colorless crystalline principle, Columbine, and an abundance of starch and mucilage.

Medicinal Action and Uses

A bitter tonic without astringency, does not produce nausea, headache, sickness or feverishness as other remedies of the same class. It is best given as a cold infusion; it is a most valuable agent for weakness of the digestive organs. In pulmonary consumption it is useful, as it never debilitates or purges the bowels. The natives of Mozambique use it for dysentery It allays the sickness of pregnancy and gastric irritation. In Africa and the East Indies it is cultivated for dyeing purposes.

Preparations

Calumba is generally combined with other tonics. For flatulence, 1/2 oz. of Calumba, 1/2 oz. of ginger 1 drachm of senna, added to 1 pint of boiling water, is taken three times daily in wine glassful doses.

Calumba can be safely combined with salts of iron and alkalies, as it does not contain tannic or gallic acid. The powdered root, 10 to 15 grains. The solid extract, 2 grains. The powdered extract, 2 grains. The fluid extract, 10 to 30 minims. The infusion, B.P., 1/2 to 1 drachm. The tincture, B.P. and U.S.P., 1/2 to 1 drachm. The concentrated solution, B.P. 1/2 to 1 drachm.

CAMPHOR

Botanical: Cinnamonum camphora (T. NEES and EBERM.)
Family: N.O. Lauraceae
Synonyms: Laurel Camphor. Gum Camphor.
Part Used: Gum.

Habitat

China, Japan, and adjacent parts of East Asia. Formosa official in the U.S.P. Dryobalanops aromatica is indigenous to Borneo and Sumatra.

Description

Camphor is a white crystalline substance, obtained from the tree Cinnamonum camphora, but the name has been given to various concrete odorous volatile products, found in different aromatic plants. The commercial Camphor comes only from C. camphora and Dryobalanops camphora (fam. Dipterocarpacaea). The first gives our official Camphor, the latter the Borneo Camphor, which is much valued in the East, but unknown in Europe and America. C. camphora is an evergreen tree looking not unlike our linden; it grows to a great size, is manybranched, flowers white, small and clustered, fruit a red berry much like cinnamon. While the tree grows in China, etc., it can be cultivated successfully in sub-tropical countries, such as India and Ceylon, and it will thrive in Egypt, Formosa, Madagascar, Canary Islands and southern parts of Europe, California, Florida, and also in Argentina. It grows so slowly that the return financially is a long investment. Some growers think that Camphor cannot be taken from the trees till they are fifty years old. In Japan and Formosa the drug comes from the root, trunk and branches of the tree by sublimation, but there is less injury done to the tree in the American plantations, as it is taken there from the leaves and twigs of the oldest trees. A Camphor oil exudes in the process of extracting

Camphor, which is valued by the Chinese, used for medicinal purposes. Two substances are found in commerce under the name of oil of Camphor: one is the produce of C. cinnamonum, and is known as Formosa or Japanese oil of Camphor; the other as East Indian oil of Camphor, from the D. aromatica but this oil is not found in European or American trade. It is less volatile than the other, and has a distinctive odor; it is highly prized by the Chinese, who use it for embalming purposes and to scent soap. The Chinese attribute many virtues to it. It is mentioned by Marco Polo in the thirteenth century and Camoens in 1571, who called it the 'balsam of disease." During the last few years large quantities have come into the American and European markets as Japanese oil; it varies in quality and color from a thin watery oil to a thick black one. It is imported in tin cans and varies greatly in the amount of Camphor it contains, some cans having had all the solid principle extracted before importation. The odor is peculiar, like sassafras and distinctly camphoraceous; this oil is said to be used in Japan for burning, making varnish and for Chinese inks, as a diluent for artists' colors; it has a capacity for dissolving resins that oil of Turps has not. The properties in the oil are much the same as in Camphor, but it is more stimulant and very useful in complaints of stomach and bowels, in spasmodic cholera and flatulent colic. It is also used as a rubefacient and sedative liniment, and if diluted with Olive oil or soap is excellent for local rheumatism, sprains, bruises, and neuralgia dose, 2 or 3 minims. There is an erroneous idea that Camphor acts as a preventive to infectious diseases. It is very acrid and in large doses very poisonous, and should be used cautiously in certain heart cases. It is a well-known preventive of moths and other insects, such as worms in wood; natural history cabinets are often made of it, the wood of the tree being occasionally imported to make cabinets for entomologists. The Dryobalanops oil of Camphor is said to be found in trees too young to produce Camphor, and is said to be the first stage of the development of Camphor, as it is found in the cavities of the trunk, which later on become filled with Camphor. Its chief constituent is an oil called Borneene. The D. aromatica tree, found in Sumatra and Borneo, grows to an enormous height, often over 100 feet, and trunk 6 or 7 feet in diameter. The Camphor of the older trees exists in concrete masses, in longitudinal cavities, in the heart of the tree, 1 1/2 feet long at certain distances apart. The only way of finding out if Camphor has formed in the tree is by incision. This Camphor is chiefly used for funeral rites, and any that is exported is bought by the Chinese at a high price, as they use it for embalming, it being less volatile than ordinary Camphor. Another Camphor called N'gai, obtained from the Blumea Balcamferi (Compositae), differs chemically from the Borneo species, being levogyrate, and is converted by boiling nitric acid, to a substance considered identical with stearoptene of Chrysanthemum parthenium. This plant grows freely in the author's garden, and is known in Great Britain as Double-flowered Bush Fever-Few.

Medicinal Action and Uses

Camphor has a strong, penetrating, fragrant odor, a bitter, pungent taste, and is slightly cold to the touch like menthol leaves; locally it is an irritant, numbs the peripheral sensory nerves, and is slightly antiseptic; it is not readily absorbed by the mucous membrane, but is easily absorbed by the subcutaneous tissue- it combines in the body with glucuronic acid, and in this condition is voided by the urine. Experiments on frogs show a depressant action to the spinal column, no motor disturbance, but a slow increasing paralysis; in mankind it causes convulsions, from the effect it has on the motor tract of the brain; it stimulates the intellectual centres and prevents narcotic drugs taking effect, but in cases of nervous excitement it has a soothing and quieting result. Authorities vary as to its effect on blood pressure; some think it raises it, others take an opposite view; but it has been proved valuable as an excitant in cases of heart failure, whether due to diseases or as a result of infectious fevers, such as typhoid and pneumonia, not only in the latter case as a stimulant to circulation, but as preventing the growth of pneumococci. Camphor is used in medicine internally for its calming influence in hysteria, nervousness and neuralgia, and for serious diarrhea, and externally as a counter-irritant in rheumatisms, sprains bronchitis, and in inflammatory conditions, and sometimes in conjunction with menthol and phenol for heart failure; it is often given hypodermically, 3 to 5 grains dissolved in 20 to 30 minims of sterile Olive oil - the effect will last about two hours. In nervous diseases it may be given in substance or in capsules or in spirit; dose 2 to 5 grains. Its great value is in colds, chills, and in all inflammatory complaints; it relieves irritation of the sexual organs.

Preparations and Dosages

Spirit of Camphor, B.P., 5 to 20 drops. Tincture of Camphor Comp., B.P. (Paregoric), 1/2 to 1 drachm. Camphor water, B.P., 1 to 2 OZ. Liniment of Aconite, B.P. Liniment of Belladonna, B.P. Liniment of Camphor Comp., B.P. Liniment of Opium, B.P. Liniment of Soap, B.P. Liniment of Mustard, B.P. Liniment of Turpentine, B.P. Liniment of Turpentine and Acetic Acid, B.P. Spirit of Camphor, B.P., 5 to 20 drops. Tincture of Camphor Comp., B.P.

CANDYTUFT, BITTER

Botanical: Iberis amara
Family: N.O. Cruciferae
Parts Used: Leaves, stem, root, seeds.

Habitat

Found in various parts of Europe and in English and Scotch cornfields, specially in limestone districts.

Description

This plant is an erect, rather stiff, very bitter annual, 6 to 12 inches high; flowers milky white, forming a terminal flat corymb; leaves oblong, lanceolate, acute, toothed; pod nearly orbicular, the long style projecting from notch at top; it flowers with the corns.

Medicinal Action and Uses

A tincture made from the ripe seeds is much used in homeopathy, but the plant is more generally used by American herbalists. All parts of the plant are used, leaves, stem, root and seeds, more particularly the latter. It has always been used for gout, rheumatism and kindred ailments, and is now usually combined with other plants for the same diseases in their acute form, and as a simple to allay excited action of the heart, especially when it is enlarged. For asthma, bronchitis and dropsy it is considered very useful.

Dosage

1 to 3 grains of the powdered seeds. In overdoses or too large ones it is said to produce giddiness, nausea and diarrhea.

CARAWAY

Botanical: Carum Carvi (LINN.)
Family: N.O. Umbelliferae
Synonym: Caraway Seed.
Part Used: Fruit.

Habitat

The plant is distributed throughout the northern and central parts of Europe and Asia, though where it occurs in this country it is only considered a naturalized species, having apparently escaped from cultivation.

Caraway is another member of the group of aromatic, umbelliferous plants characterized by carminative properties, like Anise, Cumin, Dill and Fennel. It is grown, however, less for the medicinal properties of the fruits, or so-called 'seeds," than for their use as a flavoring in cookery, confectionery and liqueurs.

Description

It is a biennial, with smooth, furrowed stems growing 1 1/2 to 2 feet high, hearing finely cut leaves, and umbels of white flowers which blossom in June. The fruitswhich are popularly and incorrectly called seeds - and which correspond in general character to those of the other plants of this large family, are laterally compressed, somewhat horny and translucent, slightly curved, and marked with five distinct, pale ridges. They evolve a pleasant, aromatic odor when bruised, and have an agreeable taste.

The leaves possess similar properties and afford an oil identical with that of the fruit. The tender leaves in spring have been boiled in soup, to give it an aromatic flavor.

History

The roots are thick and tapering, like a parsnip,

though much smaller and are edible. Parkinson declared them, when young, to be superior in flavor to Parsnips. Mixed with milk and made into bread, they are said to have formed the 'Chara' of Julius Ceasar, eaten by the soldiers of Valerius.

Caraway was well known in classic days, and it is believed that its use originated with the ancient Arabs, who called the 'seeds' Karawya, a name they still bear in the East, and clearly the origin of our word Caraway and the Latin name Carvi, although Pliny would have us believe that the name Carvi was derived from Caria, in Asia Minor, where according to him the plant was originally found. In old Spanish the name occurs as Alcaravea.

Caraway is frequently mentioned by the old writers. Dioscorides advised the oil to be taken by pale-faced girls. In the Middle Ages and in Shakespeare's times it was very popular.

'The seed," says Parkinson, 'is much used to be put among baked fruit, or into bread, cakes, etc., to give them a rellish. It is also made into comfites and taken for cold or wind in the body, which also are served to the table with fruit."

In Henry IV, Squire Shallow invites Falstaff to 'a pippin and a dish of caraways."The custom of serving roast apples with a little saucerful of Caraway is still kept up at Trinity College, Cambridge, and at some of the old-fashioned London Livery Dinners, just as in Shakespeare's days - and in Scotland to this day a saucerful is put down at tea to dip the buttered side of bread into and called 'salt water jelly."

The scattering of the seed over cakes has long been practised, and Caraway-seed cake was formerly a standing institution at the feasts given by farmers to their labourers at the end of the wheat-sowing. The little Caraway comfits consist of the seeds encrusted with white sugar. In Germany, the peasants flavor their cheese, cabbage, soups, and household bread with Caraway, and in Norway and Sweden, polenta-like, black, Caraway bread is largely eaten in country districts.

The oil extracted from the fruits is used as an ingredient of alcoholic liquors: both the Russians and the Germans make from Caraway a liqueur, 'Kummel," and Caraway enters into the composition of l'huile de Venus and other cordials.

A curious superstition was held in olden times about the Caraway. It was deemed to confer the gift of retention, preventing the theft of any object which contained it, and holding the thief in custody within the invaded house. In like manner it was thought to keep lovers from proving fickle (forming an ingredient of love potions), and also to prevent fowls and pigeons from straying. It is an undoubted fact that tame pigeons, who are particularly fond of the seeds, will never stray if they are given a piece of baked Caraway dough in their cote.

Cultivation - Preparation for Market

Caraway does best when the seeds are sown inthe autumn, as soon as ripe, though they may be sown in March. Sow in drills, 1 foot apart, the plants when strong enough, being thinned out to about 8 inches in the rows. The ground will require an occasional hoeing to keep it clean and assist the growth of the plants. From an autumn-sown crop, seeds will be produced in the following summer, ripening about August.

When the fruit ripens, the plant is cut and the Caraways are separated by threshing. They can be dried either on trays in the sun, or by very gentle heat over a stove, shaking occasionally.

There are several varieties, the English, the Dutch and the German (obtained from plants extensively cultivated in Moravia and Prussia), and other varieties imported from Norway, Finland, Russia and the Morocco ports.

Habitat

One marked peculiarity about Caraway is that it is indigenous to all parts of Europe, Siberia, Turkey in Asia, Persia, India and North Africa, and yet it is cultivated only in a few comparatively restricted areas. It grows wild in many parts of Canada and the United States, but is nowhere grown there as a field or garden crop. Its cultivation is restricted to relatively small areas in England, Holland, Germany, Finland, Russia, Norway and Morocco, where it constitutes one of the chief agricultural industries within its narrow confines. It has so far received comparatively little attention in England, where it is grown only in Essex, Kent and Suffolk, upon old grassland broken up for the purpose. Holland cultivates the main crop, producing and exporting far larger quantities than any other country. It is cultivated most extensively there in the provinces of Groningen and North Holland, in which more than half the acreage is found. In the whole country about 20,000 acres are devoted to this crop, each acre yielding about 1,000 lb., whereas while Caraway is grown commercially throughout Germany, Austria, France and parts of Spain, the character and amounts produced are very variable, and the yield per acre varies only from 400 to 700 lb., and these countries do not produce much more than they require for home consumption. Morocco produces a grade of Caraway that comes regularly into the English and American markets, but is somewhat inferior in quality. Dutch Caraway is preferred among consumers in the United States, and the bulk used there comes from Holland.

During the last year or two there has been a scarcity of Caraway, owing partly to the fact that the extensive area of land in Holland usually employed for the cultivation of the plant was devastated by floods towards the close of 1915. Much Dill seed is now being sold in its place. Quite lately, a small grower reported that she had netted L. 5 (pounds sterling) from growing Caraway on a corner of what otherwise would have been waste ground.

Constituents

The seeds contain from 4 to 7 per cent of volatile oil, according to the variety of Caraway fruit from which obtained that distilled from home-grown fruits being considered the best. Caraway grown in more northerly latitudes is richer in essential oil than that grown in southern regions, and if grown in full sun a greater percentage and a richer oil is obtained.

The oil is distilled chiefly from Dutch, Norwegian and Russian fruits. The Dutch are small and dark brown in color. English fruits, of which only a small quantity is produced, are of a brighter tint.

The chief constituent of the oil is a hydrocarbon termed Carvene, also found in oils of Dill and Cumin, and an oxygenated oil Carvol, a mobile liquid (isomeric with the menthol of Spearmint).

From 6 lb. of the unbruised seeds, 4 oz. of the pure essential oil can be expressed.

The exhausted seed, after the distillation of the oil, contains a high percentage of protein and fat, and is used as a cattle food.

Medicinal Action and Uses

Both fruit and oil possess aromatic, stimulant and carminative properties. Caraway was widely employed at one time as a carminative cordial, and was recommended in dyspepsia and symptoms attending hysteria and other disorders. It possesses some tonic property and forms a pleasant stomachic. Its former extensive employment in medicine has much decreased in recent years, and the oil and fruit are now principally employed as adjuncts to other medicines as corrective or flavoring agents, combined with purgatives. For flatulent indigestion, however, from 1 to 4 drops of the essential oil of Caraway given on a lump of sugar, or in a teaspoonful of water, will be found efficacious. Distilled Caraway water is considered a useful remedy in the flatulent colic of infants, and is an excellent vehicle for children's medicine. When sweetened, its flavor is agreeable.

One ounce of the bruised seeds infused for 6 hours in a pint of cold water makes a good Caraway julep for infants, from 1 to 3 teaspoonsful being given for a dose.

The bruised seeds, pounded with the crumb of a hot new loaf and a little spirit to moisten, was an old-fashioned remedy for bad earache. The powder of the seeds, made into a poultice, will also take away bruises.

CARDAMONS

Botanical: Elettaria cardamomum (MATON)
Family: N.O. Zingiberaceae (Scitamineae)
Synonyms: Amomum Cardamomum. Alpinia Cardamomum. Matonia Cardamomum. Cardamomum minus. Amomum repens. Cardamomi Semina. Cardamom Seeds. Malabar Cardamums. Ebil. Kakelah seghar. Capalaga. Gujatatti elachi. Ilachi. Ailum.
Part Used: The dried, ripe seeds.
Habitat: Southern India.

Description

The large perennial herb. yielding Cardamom seeds is known in its own country as 'Elattari' or 'Ilachi," while 'Cardamomum' was the name by which some Indian spice was known in classical times.

It has a large, fleshy rhizome, and the alternate, lanceolate leaves are blades from 1 to 2 1/2 feet long, smooth and dark green above, pale, glaucous green and finely silky beneath. The flowering stems spread horizontally near the ground, from a few inches to 2 feet long, and bear small, loose racemes, the small flowers being usually yellowish, with a violet lip. The fruits are from 2/5 to 4/5 of an inch long, ovoid or oblong, bluntly triangular in section, shortly beaked at the apex, pale yellowish grey in color, plump, and nearly smooth. They are three-celled, and contain in each cell two rows of small seeds of a dark, reddish-brown color. These should be kept in their pericarps and only separated when required for use. Though only the seeds are official, the retention of the pericarp is an obstacle to adulteration, while it contains some oil and forms a good surface for grinding the seeds. The value is estimated by the plumpness and heaviness of the fruits and the soundness and ripeness of the seeds. Unripe seeds are paler and less plump. The unbroken fruits are gathered before they are quite ripe, as the seeds of fruits which have partially opened are less aromatic, and such fruits are less valued. The seeds have a powerful, aromatic odor, and an agreeable, pungent, aromatic taste, but the pericarps are odourless and tasteless.

There is some confusion as to the different kinds, both botanically and commercially, different writers distinguishing them in varied ways.

The official Cardamums in the United States are stated to be only those produced in India, chiefly in Malabar and Mysore, but in Britain the seeds corresponding most closely to the official description are recognized, in spite of their names, as being imported from Ceylon.

The Cardamom is a native of Southern India, and grows abundantly in forests 2,500 to 5,000 feet above sea-level in North Canara Coorgi and Wynaad, where it is also largely cultivated. It flowers in April and May and the fruit-gathering lasts in dry weather for three months, starting in October. The methods of cultivating and preparing vary in different districts.

In the Bombay Presidency the fruits are washed by women with water from special wells and pounded soap nut (a kind of acacia). They are dried on house-roofs, the stalks clipped, and sometimes a starchy paste is sprinkled over them, in addition to the bleaching.

Bombay ships about 250,000 lb. annually to the London market. They were formerly known by their shapes as shorts, short-longs, and long-longs, but the last are now rarely seen. One hundred parts of the fruit yield on an average 74 parts of seeds and 26 of pericarp. The powdered seeds may be distinguished from the powdered fruit by the absence of the tissues of the pericarp.

The seeds are about 1/5 of an inch long, angular, wrinkled, and whitish inside. They should be powdered only when wanted for use, as they lose their aromatic properties.

In Great Britain and the United States Cardamums are employed to a small extent as an ingredient of curry powder, and in Russia, Sweden, Norway, and parts of Germany are largely used for flavoring cakes and in the preparation of liqueurs, etc. In Egypt they are ground and put in coffee, and in the East Indies are used both as a condiment and for chewing with betel. Their use was known to the ancients. In France and America the oil is used in perfumery.

Constituents

The seeds contain volatile oil, fixed oil, salt of potassium, a coloring principle, starch, nitrogenous mucilage, ligneous fibre, an acrid resin, and ash. The volatile oil contains terpenes, terpineol and cineol. Good 'shorts' yield about 4-6 per cent. It is colorless when fresh, but becomes thicker, more yellow, and less aromatic. It is very soluble in alcohol and readily soluble in four volumes of 70 per cent. alcohol, forming a clear solution.

Its specific gravity is 0.924 to 0.927 at 25 degrees C. (77 degrees F.). It is not used medicinally, but solely for pharmaceutical purposes, being employed as a flavoring in the compound spirit and compound elixir of Cardamums, and in other elixirs and mixtures. It is largely adulterated, owing to the high price of the seeds and the small percentage of volatile oil found in them.

Medicinal Action and Uses

Carminative, stimulant, aromatic, but rarely used alone; chiefly useful as an adjuvant or corrective.

The seeds are helpful in indigestion and flatulence, giving a grateful but not fiery warmth. When chewed singly in the mouth the flavor is not unpleasant, and they are said to be good for colic and disorders of the head.

In flavoring they are combined with oils of Orange, Cinnamon, Cloves, and Caraway.

The substitution of glycerine for honey in the 1880 United States' formula for compound tincture increased its stability.

Dosages

15 to 30 grains of the powdered seeds. Of tincture, 1/2 to 1 fluid drachm. Of compound tincture, B.P., 1/2 to 1 fluid drachm. Fluid extract, 5 to 30 drops.

Adulterations

Various unofficial Cardamums are included, the product of otherspecies. Orange seeds and unroasted grains of coffee are also admixed. The oil is said to be no longer distilled from Eiettaria cardamomum. It is often factitious, and composed of oils of Cajuput, Nutmeg, etc.

Other Species

MADRAS CARDAMUMS, exported from Madras and Pondicherry.

ALEPPY CARDAMUMS, exported from Aleppy and Calicut, are also recognized in Britain, the former being paler and 'short-longs' and the latter 'shorts."

CEYLON WILD CARDAMOMS are the fruits of E. cardamomum var. major, imported from Ceylon, and sometimes called Long Wild Natives. They are cultivated in Kandy, and sometimes called in the East, Grains of Paradise, but they are not the product known by that name in Europe and America.

ROUND or SIAM CARDAMUMS are probably those referred to by Dioscorides, and called Amomi uva by Pliny. They are the fruits of A. cardamomum and A. globosum, growing in Java, Siam, and China, etc., and are nearly the size of a cherry. In their natural clusters they are the amomum racemosum or amome en grappe of the French, and in Southern Europe are sometimes used in the same way as the official kinds.

BENGAL CARDAMOMS, from A. subulatum, are sometimes called Winged Bengal Cardamums, Morung elachi, or Buro elachi. They are oblong or oval, and about an inch long.

NEPAL CARDAMUMS, of unknown origin, are like the Bengal species, but usually stalked, and have a long, tubular calyx.

WINGED JAVA CARDAMOMS, from A. maximum, growing in the Malay islands, are about an inch long, and when soaked in water show from 4 to 13 ragged wings on each side. They are feebly aromatic, and are usually sent abroad from the London markets.

KORARIMA CARDAMOMS, from A. kararima, have recently become known.

MADAGASCAR CARDAMUMS, of A. angustifolium, have pointed, ovate flattened capsules. The flavor of the seeds resembles the official variety.

BASTARD CARDAMUMS, from A. Xanthioides looks like the real kind, but is greenish in color, and tastes like crude camphor.

Cardamomum Siberiense (Star Aniseed), Annis de Siberie of the seventeenth century and badiane of the French, is from Illicium verum, the fruit of which is chiefly used in preparing a volatile oil resembling the official oil of Anise.

CAROBA

Botanical: Jacaranda procera (SPRENG.)
Family: N.O. Bignoniacea
Synonyms: Carob Tree. Carobinha. Bignonia Caroba. Jacaranda Caroba. Caaroba.
Part Used: The leaves.
Habitat: South America.

Description

The genus Jacaranda includes several species which are used medicinally in South America, and especially in Brazil. The trees are small, and the leaves thick, tough, and lanceolate, about 2 1/2 inches long, odourless, and slightly bitter in taste.

Constituents

There has been found in the leaves Caroba balsam, caroborelinic acid carobic acid, steocarobic acid, carobon, and crystalline substance, carobin.

Medicinal Actions and Uses

The value of the Jacaranda active principles has been proved in syphilis and venereal diseases, being widely used by the aborigines of Brazil and other South American countries. The leaves have also been tried in epilepsy for their soothing influence.

Dosage

From 15 to 60 grains.

Other Species

CAROB-TREE, or Ceratonia siliqua, is a small tree of the Mediterranean coasts. Beyond its name it has no connexion with Caroba. It furnishes the St. John's Bread which probably corresponds to the husks of the Prodigal Son parable, and the seed which is said to have been the original jewellers' carat weight.

The Spaniards call it Algaroba, and the Arabs Kharoub, hence Carob or Caroub Pods, Beans, or Sugar-pods. It is also called Locust Pods. These pods are much used in the south of Europe for feeding domestic animals and, in times of scarcity, as human food. Being saccharine, they are more heatgiving than nourishing. The seeds or beans were used as fodder for British cavalry horses during the Spanish campaign of 1811-12.

South American varieties are Prosopis dulcis and P. siliquastrum of the Leguminosae family.

CARROT

Botanical: Daucus carota (LINN.)
Family: N.O. Umbelliferae
Synonyms: Philtron (Old Greek). Bird's Neat.
Part Used: Whole herb.

Habitat

A native wild plant common everywhere in the British Islands.

Both the Carrot and Parsnip are striking examples of the effect of cultivation on wild plants. The roots of the wild variety are small and woody, while those of the cultivated kind are fleshy and succulent and grow to a considerable size.

History

The Carrot was well known to the ancients, and is mentioned by Greek and Latin writers under various names, being, however, not always distinguished from the Parsnip and Skirret, closely allied to it. The Greeks - Professor Henslow tells us - had three words: Sisaron, first occurring in the writings of Epicharmus, a comic poet (500 B.C.); Staphylinos, used by Hippocrates (430 B.C.) and Elaphoboscum, used by Dioscorides (first century A.D.), whose description of the plant applies accurately to the modern Carrot. Pliny says:

'There is one kind of wild pastinaca which grows spontaneously; by the Greeks it is known as staphylinos. Another kind is grown either from the root transplanted or else from seed, the ground being dug to a very considerable depth for the purpose. It begins to be fit for eating at the end of the year, but it is still better at the end of two; even then, however, it preserves its strong pungent flavor, which it is found impossible to get rid of."

In speaking of the medical virtue of the first species (which is evidently the Carrot, the second variety presumably the Parsnip), he adds, 'the cultivated has the same as the wild kind, though the latter is more powerful, especially when growing in stony places."

The name Carota for the garden Carrot is found first in the writings of Athenaeus (A.D. 200), and in a book on cookery by Apicius Czclius (A.D. 230). It was Galen (second century A.D.) who added the name Daucus to distinguish the Carrot from the Parsnip, calling it D. pastinaca, and Daucus came to be the official name in the sixteenth century, and was adopted by Linnaeus in the eighteenth century.

From the time of Dioscorides and Pliny to the present day, the Carrot has been in constant use by all nations. It was long cultivated on the Continent before it became known in this country, where it was first generally cultivated in the reign of Queen Elizabeth, being introduced by the Flemings, who took refuge here from the persecutions of Philip II of Spain, and who, finding the soil about Sandwich peculiarly favourable for it, grew it there largely. As vegetables were at that time rather scarce in England, the Carrot was warmly welcomed and became a general favorite, its cultivation spreading over the country. It is mentioned appreciatively by Shakespeare in The Merry Wives of Windsor. In the reign of James I, it became the fashion for ladies to use its feathery leaves in their head-dresses. A very charming, fern-like decoration may be obtained if the thick end of a large carrot be cut off and placed in a saucer of water in a warm place, when the young and delicate leaves soon begin to sprout and form a pretty tuft of verdant green, well worth the slight trouble entailed.

Its root is small and spindle-shaped whitish, slender and hard, with a strong aromatic smell and an acrid, disagreeable taste, very different to the reddish, thick, fleshy, cultivated form, with its pleasant odor and peculiar, sweet, mucilaginous flavor. It penetrates some distance into the ground, having only a few lateral rootlets.

Description

The stems are erect and branched, generally about 2, feet high, tough and furrowed. Both stems and leaves are more or less clothed with stout, coarse hairs. The leaves are very finely divided, the lowest leaves considerably larger than the upper; their arrangement on the stem is alternate, and all the leaves embrace the stem with the sheathing base, which is so characteristic of this group of plants, the Umbelliferae, to which the Carrot belongs. The blossoms are densely clustered together in terminal umbels, or flattened heads, in which the flower-bearing stalks of the head all arise from one point in rays, like the ribs of an umbrella, each ray again dividing in the case of the Carrot, to form a secondary umbel, or umbellule of white flowers, the outer ones of which are irregular and larger than the others. The wild Carrot is in bloom from June to August, but often continues flowering much longer. The flowers themselves are very small, but from their whiteness and number, they form a conspicuous head, nearly flat while in bloom, or slightly convex, but as the seeds ripen, the umbels contract, the outer rays, which are to begin with 1 to 2 inches long, lengthening and curving inwards, so that the head forms a hollow cup hence one of the old popular names for the plant: Bird's Nest. The fruit is slightly flattened, with numerous bristles arranged in five rows. The ring of finely-divided and leaf-like bracts at the point where the umbel springs is a noticeable feature.

The Carrot is well distinguished from other plants of the same order by having the central flower of the umbel, or sometimes a tiny umbellule, of a bright red or deep purple color, though there is a variety, D. maritimus, frequent on many parts of the sea coast in the south of England, which differs in having somewhat fleshy leaves and in being destitute of the central purple flower. In this case, all the flowers of the head have often a somewhat pinkish tinge. There was a curious superstition that this small purple flower of the Carrot was of benefit in epilepsy.

Parts Used Medicinally

The whole herb, collected in July; the seeds and root. The whole herb is the part now more generally in use.

Medicinal Action and Uses

Diuretic, Stimulant, Deobstruent. An infusion of the whole herb is considered an active and valuable remedy in the treatment of dropsy, chronic kidney diseases and affections of the bladder. The infusion of tea, made from one ounce of the herb in a pint of boiling water, is taken in wine glassful doses. Carrot tea, taken night and morning, and brewed in this manner from the whole plant, is considered excellent for lithic acid or gouty disposition. A strong decoction is very useful in gravel and stone, and is good against flatulence. A fluid extract is also prepared, the dose being from 1/2 to 1 drachm.

The seeds are carminative, stimulant and very useful in flatulence, windy colic, hiccough, dysentery, chronic coughs, etc. The dose of the seeds, bruised, is from one-third to one teaspoonful, repeated as necessary. They were at one time considered a valuable remedy for calculus complaints. They are excellent in obstructions of the viscera, in jaundice (for which they were formerly considered a specific), and in the beginnings of dropsies, and are also of service as an emmenagogue. They have a slight aromatic smell and a warm, pungent taste. They communicate an agreeable flavor to malt liquor, if infused in it while in the vat, and render it a useful drink in scorbutic disorders.

Old writers tell us that a poultice made of the roots has been found to mitigate the pain of cancerous ulcers, and that the leaves, applied with honey, cleanse running sores and ulcers. An infusion of the root was also used as an aperient.

Cultivation

The root of the Carrot consists of Bark and Wood: the bark of theGarden Carrot is the outer red layer, dark and pulpy and sweet to the taste; the wood forms the yellow core, gradually becoming hard, stringy and fibrous. The aim of cultivation, therefore, is to obtain a fleshy root, with the smallest part of wood. This depends on soil and the quality and kind of the seed.

For its successful cultivation, Carrot needs a light, warm soil, which has been well manured in the previous season. The most suitable soil is a light one inclining to sand, a somewhat sandy loam or dry, peaty land being the best, but even heavy ground, properly prepared, may be made to produce good Carrots. Formerly the cultivation of the Carrot was almost entirely confined to the light lands of Norfolk and Suffolk.

The ground should be well prepared some months in advance; heavy ground should be lightened by the addition of wood ash, road scrapings, old potting soil and similar materials. It is essential that the soil be in such a state as to allow the roots to penetrate to their full length without interruption. Previous to sowing the seed, the soil should be lightly forked over, and, if possible, be given a dressing of leaf soil or well decayed vegetable matter, but no fresh manure must be dug into the top spit of ground intended for Carrots and Parsnips, as it may cause the roots to become forked. The crops will, however, benefit by about an ounce of superphosphate to the square yard, raked in before sowing, or by a light dressing of soot.

Sowing of the main crop should be done in calm weather about the middle of March or early in April. The seeds frequently adhere to one another by means of the forked hairs which surround them. These hairs can be removed by rubbing through the hands or a fine chaff sieve. The seeds should then be mixed with about twice the bulk of dry earth, sand or sifted ashes (about one bushel of seeds to 4 or 5 lb. of sand). When the ground is thoroughly prepared and has been firmly trodden, draw flat-bottomed drills from north to south, 1/2 inch deep and 3 inches wide. Distribute the seed along the row evenly and thinly and cover lightly. Carrots can hardly be covered too lightly, 1 inch of fine soil is quite enough, and for ordinary use they may be sown in drills one foot apart, but if extra large roots are desired, more room must be given between the rows. As soon as the young plants are large enough to handle they may be thinned to 6 inches or 8 inches apart. The thinning may be at first to a distance of 3 inches, and then a final thinning later, the second thinnings being used as young Carrots for culinary purposes. Frequent dustings of soot will greatly benefit the crop. Light hoeings between the rows to keep the crop free from weeds is all that is necessary during the period of growth. Partial shade from other crops is often found beneficial.

Scarlet Immediate is the best sort for general purposes.

Main-crop Carrots are generally taken up about the last week in October, or early in November, by three-pronged forks, and stored in sand in a dry place, where they can be kept till the following March or April Some of the roots dug in the autumn can be replanted in February, about 2 feet apart, with the crown or head a few inches below the surface. Leaves and flowers will spring from them, and the seeds produced will ripen in the autumn.

By making successional sowings, good crops of small roots will be always available. In gardens, Carrots are grown in succession of crops from the latter part of February to the beginning of August. For early Carrots sow on a warm border in February: such a sowing, if made as soon as the state of ground allows, will assure early Carrots just when fresh and quickly-grown vegetables are most highly prized. They will be off in time to leave the ground ready for other crops.

After a good dressing of soot has been given, Carrots may be sown again, and even then it leaves the room vacant for winter greens or cabbage for use next spring. Sowing as late as July is generally successful in most districts. Main crops are often sown too early, especially on cold soils. Carrots are liable to attacks of grubs and insects, the upper part of the root being also attacked by the grub of a kind of fly, the best remedy being late sowing, to avoid the period at which these insects are evolved from the egg. Dusting with ashes and a little soot or lime wards off both birds and slugs from the young tender growths.

Carrots are a valuable product for the farmer in feeding his cattle, and for this purpose are raised in large quantities. The produce of an acre of Carrots in Suffolk is on an average 350 bushels per acre, but sometimes much more. In the Channel Islands and Brittany, much larger crops of Carrots and Parsnips are obtained than are yielded in England, the soil being deeply trenched by a spade or specially-constructed plough. Far more Carrots are grown in France, Germany and Belgium for fodder than here. Horses are remarkably fond of Carrots, and when mixed with oats, Carrots form a very good food for them; with a small quantity of oats or other corn, a horse may be supported on from 20 to 30 lb. of Carrots daily. In Suffolk, Carrots were formerly given as a specific for preserving and restoring the wind of horses, but they are not considered good for cattle if fed too long on them. They may also with advantage be given both to pigs and poultry, and rabbits are especially fond of them. The kinds grown for farm purposes are generally larger than those in the kitchen garden and are known as Red Carrots, the more delicate Orange Carrot being the variety used in cooking. Some farmers sow the seeds on the top of the drills, which is said to be an improvement over the gardener, who makes his Carrot-bed on the flat in the ordinary way. This ridge system gives good results the Carrots being clean and well-shaped and free from grubs. The farmers reckon about 2 lb. of seed for an acre for drills, and 5 or 6 lb. if sown broadcast. For ordinary garden purposes, one ounce of seed is reckoned to be sufficient for about 600 feet sown in drills.

Chemical Constituents

The juice of the Carrot when expressed contains crystallizable and uncrystallizable sugar, a little starch, extractine gluten, albumen, volatile oil (on which the medicinal properties of the root depend and which is fragrant, aromatic and stimulating), vegetable jelly or pectin, saline matter, malic acid and a peculiar crystallizable, ruby-red neutral principle, without odor or taste, called Carotin.

Carrots contain no less than 89 per cent of water; their most distinguishing dietical substance is sugar, of which they contain about 4.5 per cent.

Owing to the large percentage of carbohydrate material contained by Carrots, rabbits fed for some days on Carrots alone, are found to have an increased amount of glycogen stored in the liver, carbohydrate being converted into glycogen in the body.

Sir Humphry Davy ascertained the nutritive matter of Carrots to amount to 98 parts in 1,000, of which 95 are sugar, and three are starch. Weight for weight, they stand third in nourishing value on the list of roots and tubers, potatoes and parsnips taking first and second places. Carrots containing less water and more nourlshing material than green vegetables, have higher nutritive qualities than turnips, swedes, cabbage, sprouts, cauliflower, onions and leeks. Moreover, the fair proportion of sugar contained in their composition adds to their nourishing value.

In the interesting collection of the Food Collection at Bethnal Green Museum, prepared by Dr. Lankester, we learn that the maximum amount of work produceable by a pound of Carrots is that it will enable a man to raise 64 tons one foot high, so that it would appear to be a very efficient forceproducer. From 1 lb. of Carrots we can obtain 1 OZ. and 11 grains of sugar, while out of the 16 oz. fourteen are water. When we consider that in an average man of 11 stone or 154 lb. weight, about 111 of these are water, we see what a large supply is needful to repair waste and wear and tear.

Medicinal and General Uses

The chief virtues of the Carrot lie in the strong antiseptic qualities they possess, which prevent all putrescent changes within the body.

Carrots were formerly of some medicinal repute as a laxative, vermifuge, poultice, etc., and the seeds have been employed as a substitute for caraways.

At Vichy, where derangements of the liver are specially treated, Carrots in one form or the other are served at every meal whether in soup or as vegetables, and considerable efficacy of cure is attributed to them.

In country districts, raw Carrots are still sometimes given to children for expelling worms, and the boiled roots, mashed to a pulp, are sometimes used as a cataplasm for application to ulcers and cancerous sores.

Carrot sugar, got from the inspissated juice of the roots, may be used at table, and is good for the coughs of consumptive children.

A good British wine may be brewed from the root of the Carrot, and a very tolerable bread prepared from the roots, dried and powdered. The pectic acid contained can be extracted from the root and solidifies into a wholesome, appetizing jelly.

In Germany, a substitute and adulteration for coffee has been made of Carrots chopped into small pieces, partially carbonized by roasting and then ground.

In France and Germany a spirit is distilled from the Carrot, which yields more spirit than the potato. The refuse after making the spirit is good for feeding pigs.

Attempts have also been made to extract sugar from Carrots, but the resulting thick syrup refuses to crystallize, and in competition with either cane sugar or that obtained from the beetroot, it has not proved commercially successful.

Carrots are also used in winter and spring in the dairy, to give color and flavor to butter, and a dye similar to woad has been obtained from the leaves.

Recipes

Carrot Jam

Wash and grate some carrots; boil until reduced to a thick pulp. To 1 Ib. of this pulp add 9 oz. sugar, the juice and grated rind of 2 lemons, and 3 oz. margarine. Boil the mixture well for 45 minutes to 1 hour. The result is a useful and inexpensive jam, which can be made for 6d. to 8d. a lb. (according to the price of the lemons), if all materials have to be bought, and for considerably less by those who have home-grown carrots available.

Preserved Young Carrots

Turn the carrots in their own shape, and as you do so, them turn into hot water; when all are ready, put them in a stewpan with water enough to cover them; add fresh butter in the proportion of an ounce to the pound of carrots, and salt to season; boil the carrots in this till half done, and then arrange them neatly in tin boxes; fill up with their own liquor, solder down, boil for hour, and put them away in the cool.

CARROT, WILD

Botanical: Daucus carota (LINN.)
Family: N.O. Umbelliferae
Synonyms: Birds' Nest and Bees' Nest.
Parts Used: Whole herb, seeds, root.

Habitat

Britain, near the sea in greatest abundance, and in waste places throughout Europe, Russian Asia, America, and is even found in India.

Probably originally a native of the sea-coasts of Southern Europe degenerated into its present wild state, but of very ancient cultivation. The name 'Carrot' is Celtic, and means 'red of color," and Daucus from the Greek dais to burn, signifying its pungent and stimulating qualities.

The Carrot was in ancient times much valued for its medicinal properties; the Wild Carrot, which is found so plentifully in Britain, both in cultivated lands and by waysides, thriving more especially by the sea, is superior, medicinally, to the cultivated kind.

Description

Its root is small and spindle shaped, whitish, slender and hard, witha strong aromatic smell and an acrid, disagreeable taste, very different to the reddish, thick, fleshy, cultivated form, with its pleasant odor and peculiar, sweet, mucilaginous flavor. It penetrates some distance into the ground, having only a few lateral rootlets.

The stems are erect and branched, generally about 2 feet high, tough and furrowed. Both stems and leaves are more or less clothed with stout coarse hairs. The leaves are very finely divided, the lowest leaves considerably larger than the upper; their arrangement on the stem is alternate, and all the leaves embrace the stem with the sheathing base, which is so characteristic of this group of plants, the Umbelliferae, to which the Carrot belongs. The blossoms are densely clustered together in terminal umbels, or flattened heads, in which the flower-bearing stalks of the head all arise from one point in rays, like the ribs of an umbrella, each ray again dividing in the case of the Carrot, in like manner to form a secondary umbel, or umbellule of white flowers, the outer ones of which are irregular and larger than the others. The Wild Carrot is in bloom from June to August, but often continues flowering much longer. The flowers themselves are very small, but from their whiteness and number, they form a conspicuous head nearly flat while in bloom, or slightly convex, but as the seeds ripen, the umbels contract, the outer rays, which are to begin with 1 to 2 inches long, lengthening and curving inwards, so that the head forms a hollow cup hence one of the old popular names for the plant - Birds' Nest. The fruit is slightly flattened, with numerous bristles arranged in five rows. The ring of finely-divided and leaf-like bracts at the point where the umbel springs is a noticeable feature.

The Carrot is well distinguished from other plants of the same order by having the central flower of the umbel, or sometimes a tiny umbellule, of a bright red or deep purple color, though there is a variety, Daucus maritimus, frequent in many parts of the seacoast in the south of England, which differs in having somewhat fleshy leaves and no central purple flower. In this case, all the flowers of the head have usually a somewhat pinkish tinge. There was a curious superstition that this small purple flower of the Carrot was of benefit for mitigating epilepsy.

Constituents

The medicinal properties of the seeds are owing to a volatile oil which is colorless or slightly tinged with yellow; this is procured by distilling with water. They also yield their virtues by infusion to water at 212 degrees F.; boiling dissipates them. No thorough analysis has been made.

Medicinal Action and Uses

Diuretic, stimulant deobstruent. An infusion of the whole herb is considered an active and valuable remedy in the treatment of dropsy, chronic kidney diseases and affections of the bladder. The infusion, made from 1 OZ. of the herb in a pint of boiling water, is taken in wine glassful doses. Carrot tea, taken night and morning, and brewed in this manner from the whole front, is considered excellent for a gouty disposition. A strong decoction is very useful in gravel and stone, and is good against flatulence. A fluid extract is also prepared, the dose being from 1/2 to 1 drachm.

The seeds are carminative, stimulant and very useful in flatulence, windy colic, hiccough, dysentery, chronic coughs, etc. The dose of the seeds, bruised, is from one-third to one teaspoonful, repeated as necessary. They were at one time considered a valuable remedy for calculus complaints. They are excellent in obstructions of the viscera, in jaundice (for which they were formerly considered a specific), and in the beginnings of dropsies, and are also of service as an emmenagogue. They have a slight aromatic smell and a warm, pungent taste. They communicate an agreeable flavor to malt liquor, if infused in it while working in thc vat, and render it a useful drink in scorbutic disorders.

Old writers tell us that a poultice made of the roots has been found to mitigate the pain of cancerous ulcers, and that the leaves, applied with honey, cleanse running sores and ulcers. An infusion of the root was also used as an aperient.

CASCARA, AMARGA

Botanical: Picramnia antidesma (S. W.)
Family: N.O. Simarubacaea
Synonyms: Mountain Damson Bark. Simaruba Honduras Bark.
Parts Used: Bark, root-bark.
Habitat: Jamaica and South Guiana.

Description

A native of the West Indies and yields the drug known as Simaruba bark. The tree grows to a considerable height and thickness and has alternate spreading branches; the bark on the old trees is black and furrowed, on the younger trees smooth grey, in places spotted with big patches of yellow, the wood is hard, white and without any special taste; it has numerous leaves alternately on the branches, each leaf has several pinnae, nearly elliptical, upper side smooth deep green, under side whitish, short foot-stalks, flowers male and female on different trees, color yellow in long panicles. The bark is rough scaly and poor; inside when fresh is a good yellow color, but when dry paler; it has very little smell and taste and though very bitter is not disagreeable. Macerated in water or rectified spirits it gives a yellow tincture; makes a better and stronger infusion in cold water than in boiling water; the decoction is transparent yellow when hot, but when cooled, is turbid and brownish red in color. The bark was brought from Guiana in 1713 as a remedy for dysentery. In France in 1718 to 1825 an epidemic flux was cured by the bark and this established its medicinal use in Europe.

Constituents

A bitter tonic credited with specific alternative properties. It belongs to an undetermined species of picrammia and contains a bitter sweet amorphous alkaloid.

Medicinal Action and Uses

Purgative, tonic, diaphoretic. A very valuable bitter tonic, useful in diarrhea, dysentery, and in some forms of indigestion; in large doses it is said to act as an emetic. It restores tone to the intestines, allays spasmodic motions, promotes a healthy secretion. Big doses cause vomiting and nausea - should not be used in dysentery attended with fever. In dysentery with weak indigestion it is often preferred to chamonilee.

Dosage

The infusion taken in wine glassful doses every four to six hours.

Other Species

Simaruba versicolor, a Brazilian species,has similar properties; the fruits and barks are also used as anthelmintics, and an infusion of the bark is used for snake-bite. The plant is so bitter that insects will not attack it - on which account the powdered bark has been used to kill vermin.

S. alauca, a native of Cuba, gives a glutinous juice which has been found useful in some forms of skin disease.

CASCARILLA

Botanical: Croton Eleuteria (J. BENN.)
Family: N.O. Euphorbiaceae
Synonyms: Sweetwood Bark. Sweet Bark. Bahama Cascarilla. Elutheria. Clutia Eleuteria. Cascarillae Cortex. Cortex Thuris. Aromatic Quinquina. False Quinquina.
Part Used: The dried bark.
Habitat: The Bahama Islands.

History

The name Croton comes from a Greek word meaning 'a tick," and Eleuteria from the name of one of the Bahama Islands, Eleuthera, near Providence Island.

Description

It is a small tree rarely reaching 20 feet in height, with scanty, alternate, ovate-lanceolate leaves, averaging 2 inches long, closely-scaled below, giving a metallic silver-bronze appearance, with scattered, white scales above. The flowers are small, with white petals, and very fragrant, appearing in March and April. The scented bark is fissured, and pale yellowish brown. It is imported from Nassau, in New Providence.

The quills of dried bark average 2 inches in length, and 3/8 inch in thickness. They are often furrowed in both directions, so that they appear to be chequered. The outer, thin, corky layer is white, often covered with a fine lichen (Verrucaria albissima). The second layer is brownish, and sometimes shows through. The bark is hard and compact, breaking with a short, resinous fracture. The taste is nauseating, warm and bitter, and the odor agreeable and aromatic, especially when burned, resembling weak musk, so that it is used in fumigating pastilles, and sometimes mixed with tobacco, though in the latter case some regard it as being liable to cause giddiness and symptoms of intoxication.

The leaves can be infused for a digestive tea, and the bark yields a good, black dye.

Constituents

There have been found in the bark albumen, tannin, cascar illin (a bitter, crystallizable principle, soluble in alcohol, ether, and hot water), red coloring matter, fatty matter with a sickly odor, volatile oil, gum, wax, resin, starch, pectic acid potassium chloride, a salt of calcium, and lignin.

The oil contains an alcohol, two sesquiterpenes, a free acid consisting of liquid cascarillic acid and a mixture of solid palmitic and stearic acids, eugenol, a terpene (differing from pinene), cymene, and possibly some l-limonene. Betaine has also been found.

Medicinal Action and Uses

An aromatic, bitter tonic, with possibly narcotic properties. It is used in dyspepsia, intermittent and low fevers, diarrhea and dysentery. It is a stimulant to mucous membranes, and in chronic bronchitis is used as an expectorant; while it is valuable in atonia dyspepsia, flatulence, chronic diarrhea, nocturnal pollutions, debility and convalescence. Added to cinchona, it will arrest vomiting caused by that drug.

Dosages

Of Cascarilla powdered Bark, 20 to 30 grains. Of Infusum Cascarillae (B.P. 1 OZ. to 1/2 pint), 1 to 2 fluid ounces. Of Tinctura Cascarillae, 1/2 to 2 fluid drachms. Of fluid extract, 1/2 to 1 fluid drachm. Tincture, B.P. 1/2 to 1 drachm.

Other Species

Cascarilla is also the name of Quina morada, the bark of Pogonopus febrifugus, used in the Argentine Republic as a substitute for cinchona bark. An alkaloid, Moradeine, and a blue fluorescent substance, Moradin, have been separated from it.

Croton Cascarilla, the Wild Rosemary of the West Indies, was at first thought to be the source of the Cascarilla of commerce.

C. Pseudo-China, or Copalchi Bark, of Mexico, also known as Copalche Bark or C. niveus, resembles C. Eleuteria so closely that it can be mistaken for it. It is used in the same way. A second variety, more bitter, may be a product of C. suberosus.

It has also been mistaken for a variety of cinchona.

C. micans is thought to have similar properties.

White, red, and black Cascarillas are also found in commerce, differing in form and properties, but these are other names for varieties of quinquina.

CASHEW NUT

Botanical: Anacardium occidentale (LINN.)
Family: N.O. Anacardiaceae
Synonym: Cassavium pomiferum.
Part Used: Nut.
Habitat: Jamaica, West Indies, and other parts of tropical America.

Description

A medium-sized tree, beautiful, and not unlike in appearance the walnut tree, with oval blunt alternate leaves and scented rose-coloured panicles of bloom - the tree produces a fleshy receptacle, commonly called an apple, at the end of which the kidney-shaped nut is borne; the end of it which is attached to the apple, is much bigger than the other. The outer shell is ashy color, very smooth, the kernel is covered with an inner shell, and between the two shells is found a thick inflammable caustic oil, which will raise blisters on the skin and be dangerously painful if the nuts are cracked with the teeth.

Constituents

Two peculiar principles have been found: Anacardic Acid and a yellow oleaginous liquid Cardol.

Medicinal Action and Uses

The oil must be used with great caution, but has been successfully applied to corns, warts, ringworms, cancerous ulcers and even elephantiasis, and has been used in beauty culture to remove the skin of the face in order to grow a new one. The nuts are eaten either fresh or roasted, and contain a milky juice which is used in puddings. The older nuts are roasted and salted and the dried and broken kernels are sometimes imported to mix with old Madeira as they greatly improve its flavor. In roasting great care must be taken not to let the fumes cover the face or hands etc., as they cause acute inflammation an external poisoning. Ground and mixed with cocoa the nuts make a good chocolate. The fruit is a reddy yellow and has a pleasant sub-acid stringent taste, the expressed juice of the fruit makes a good wine, and if distilled, a spirit much better than arrack or rum. The fruit itself is edible, and its juice has been found of service in uterine complaints and dropsy. It is a powerful diuretic. The black juice of the nut and the milky juice from the tree after incision are made into an indelible marking-ink- the stems of the flowers also give a milky juice which when dried is hard and black and is used as a varnish. A gum is also found in the plant having the same qualities as gumarabic; it is imported from South America under the name of Cadjii gum, and used by South American bookbinders, who wash their books with it to keep away moths and ants. The caustic oil found in the layers of the fruit is sometimes rubbed into the floors of houses in India to keep white ants away.

Other Species

The Oriental Anacardium or Cashew Nut (Semecarpus anacardium), a native of India, has similar qualities to the West Indian Cashew, and is said to contain an alkaloid called Chuchunine.

Ammonium anarcadate. This is the Ammonium compound of beta and delta resinous acids of A. occidentale (Cashew Nut), and is used as a hair-dye, but cannot be used with acids, acid salts, or acetate of lead.

CASSIA (CINNAMON)

Botanical: Cinnamomum cassia (BLUME)
Family: N.O. Lauraceae
Synonyms: Bastard Cinnamon. Chinese Cinnamon. Cassia lignea. Cassia Bark. Cassia aromaticum. Canton Cassia.
Part Used: The dried bark.
Habitat: Indigenous to China. Cochin-China and Annam. Also cultivated in Sumatra, Ceylon, Japan, Java, Mexico and South America.

Description

As its name of Bastard Cinnamon implies, the product of this tree is usually regarded as a substitute for that of the Cinnarmomum zeylanicum of Ceylon, which it closely resembles. The cultivated trees are kept as coppices, and numerous shoots, which are not allowed to rise higher than 10 feet, spring from the roots. Their appearance when the flame-coloured leaves and delicate blossoms first appear is very beautiful. The fruit is about the size of a small olive. The leaves are evergreen, ovaloblong blades from 5 to 9 inches long. The trees are at their greatest perfection at the age of ten to twelve years, but they continue to spread and send up new shoots. The bark may be easily distinguished from that of cinnamon, as it is thicker, coarser, darker, and duller, the flavor being more pungent, less sweet and delicate, and slightly bitter. The stronger flavor causes it to be preferred to cinnamon by German and Roman chocolate makers. The fracture is short, and the quills are single, while pieces of the corky layer are often left adhering. The best and most pungent bark is cut from the young shoots when the leaves are red, or from trees which grow in rocky situations. The bark should separate easily from the wood, and be covered inside with a mucilaginous juice though the flavor of the spice is spoiled if this is not carefully removed. The wood without the bark is odourless and is used as fuel. When clean, the bark is a little thicker than parchment, and curls up while drying in the sun. It is imported in bundles of about 12 inches long, tied together with strips of bamboo and weighing about a pound. It is the kind almost universally kept in American shops.

The dried, unripe fruits, or Chinese Cassia Buds, have the odor and taste of the bark, and are rather like small cloves in appearance. They have been known in Europe as a spice since the Middle Ages, being then probably used in preparing a spiced wine called Hippocras. Now they are employed in confectionery and in making Pot-Pourri. The importation of the buds into the U.S.A. in 1916 was 197,156 lb., and of Cassia and Cassia leaves 7,487,156 lb.

Constituents

Cassia bark yields from 1 to 2 per cent of volatile oil, somewhat resembling that of cinnamon. It should be kept from the light in well-stoppered, ambercoloured bottles. It is cheaper and more abundant than the Ceylon variety, and is the only official oil of Cinnamon in the United States Pharmacopoeia and German Pharmacopoeia. It is imported from Canton and Singapore. Its value depends on the percentage of cinnamic aldehyde which it contains. It is heavier, less liquid, and congeals more quickly than the Ceylon oil.

There are also found in it cinnamyl acetate, cinnamic acid, phenylpropyl acetate and orthocumaric aldehyde, tannic acid and starch.

Ceylon cinnamon, if tested with one or two drops of tincture of iodine to a fluid ounce of a decoction of the powder, is but little affected, while with Cassia a deep blueblack color is produced. The cheaper kinds of Cassia can be distinguished by the greater quantity of mucilage, which can be extracted by cold water.

Eighty pounds of the freshly-prepared bark yield about 2.5 oz. of the lighter of the two oils produced, and 5 5 of the heavier.

An oil was formerly obtained by distilling the leaves after maceration in sea water, and this was imported into Great Britain.

Medicinal Action and Uses

Stomachic, carminative, mildly astringent, said

to be emmenagogue and capable of decreasing the secretion of milk. The tincture is useful in uterine hemorrhage and menorrhagia, the doses of 1 drachm being given every 5, 10 or 20 minutes as required. It is chiefly used to assist and flavor other drugs, being helpful in diarrhea, nausea, vomiting, and to relieve flatulence.

The oil is a powerful germicide, but being very irritant is rarely used in medicine for this purpose. It is a strong local stimulant, sometimes prescribed in gastro-dynia, flatulent colic, and gastric debility.

Dosages

Of oil, 1 to 3 minims. Of powder, 10 to 20 grains.

Poisons and Antidotes

It was found that 6 drachms of the oil would kill a moderately sized dog in five hours, and 2 drachms in forty hours, inflammation of the gastro-intestinal mucous membrane being observed.

Other Species, Substitutes and Adulterations

The powder cinnamon is often adulterated with sugar, ground walnut shells, galanga rhizome, etc.

The oil sometimes contains resin, petroleum, or oil of Cloves. Saigon cinnamon was recognized by the United States Pharmacopoeia in 1890. It comes from French Cochin-China, its botanical origin being uncertain. It is also known as Annam Cinnamon, China Cinnamon, and God's Cinnamon.

C. inners gives the Wild Cinnamon of Japan. It is also found in Southern India, where the buds are more mature, and are employed medicinally by the Indians in dysentery, diarrhea and coughs. The bark is used as a condiment.

C. lignea includes several inferior varieties from the Malabar Coast.

C. Sintok comes from Java and Sumatra.

C. obtusifolium, from East Bengal, Assam, Burmah, etc., is perhaps not distinct from C. Zeylanicum.

C. Culilawan and C. rubrum come from the Moluccas, Amboyna, and have a flavor of cloves.

C. Loureirii grows in Cochin-China and Japan.

C. pauciflorum is found from Silhet and Khasya.

C. Burmanni is said to yield Massoi Bark, which is also a product of Massora aromatica.

The bark of C. Tamala as well as the above species gives the inferior Cassia Vera.

C. inserta is slightly known.

C. nitidum has aromatic leaves, which, when dried, are said to have been the 'folia Malabathri."

Martinique and Cayenne contribute three varieties, from trees introduced from Ceylon and Sumatra. Other kinds are known as Black Cinnamon, Isle of France Cinnamon, and Santa Fé Cinnamon.

Oil of Cassia is now recognized in the United States Pharmacopeia under the name of oil of Cinnamon.

CASTOR OIL PLANT

Botanical: Ricinus communis (LINN.)
Family: N.O. Euphorbiaceae
Synonyms: Palma Christi. Castor Oil Bush.
Part Used: Seeds.

Habitat

By cultivation it has been distributed through not only all tropical and subtropical regions, but also in many of the temperate countries of the globe.

The valuable purgative known as Castor Oil is the fixed oil obtained from the seeds of the Castor Oil plant. Besides being used medicinally, the oil is also employed for lubricating purposes, burning and for leather dressing. The Chinese are said to have some mode of depriving it of its medicinal properties so as to render it suitable for culinary purposes.

The Castor Oil plant is a native of India, where it bears several ancient Sanskrit names, the most ancient and most usual being Eranda, which has passed into several other Indian languages.

It is very variable in habit and appearance, the known varieties being very numerous, and having mostly been described as species. In the tropical latitudes most favourable to its growth, it becomes a tree 30 to 40 feet high; in the Azores and the warmer Mediterranean countries - Algeria, Egypt, Greece and the Riviera - it is of more slender growth, attaining an average height of only 10 to 15 feet, and farther north in France, and in this country, where it is cultivated as an ornamental plant on account of its large and beautiful foliage, it is merely a shrubby branched annual herb, rarely more than 4 to 5 feet high, with thick, hollow, herbaceous stems, which are cylindrical, smooth and shiny, with a purplish bloom in the upper part.

Description

The handsome leaves are placed alternately on the stem, on long, curved, purplish foot-stalks, with drooping blades, generally 6 to 8 inches across, sometimes still larger, palmately cut for threefourths of their depth into seven to eleven lance-shaped, pointed, coarsely toothed segments. When fully expanded, they are of a blue-green color, paler beneath and smooth; when young, they are red and shining.

The flowers are male and female on the same plant, and are produced on a clustered, oblong, terminal spike. The male flowers are placed on the under portion of the spike; they have no corolla, only a green calyx, deeply cut into three to five segments, enclosing numerous, much branched, yellow stamens. The female flowers occupy the upper part of the spike and have likewise no corolla. The three narrow segments of the calyx are, however, of a reddish color, and the ovary in their centre is crowned by deeply-divided, carmine-red threads (styles). The fruit is a blunt, greenish, deeply-grooved capsule less than an inch long, covered with soft, yielding prickles in each of which a seed is developed. The seeds of the different cultivated varieties differ much in size and in external markings but average seeds are of an oval, laterally compressed form. The smaller, annual varieties yield small seeds- the tree forms, large seeds. They have a shining, marble-grey and brown, thick, leathery outer coat, within which is a thin, dark-coloured, brittle coat. A large, distinct, leafy embryo lies in the middle of a dense, oily tissue (endosperm). The seeds contain a toxic substance which make them actively poisonous, so much so that three large seeds have been known to kill an adult.

In the South of England the plant ripens its seeds in favourable situations, and it has been known to come to maturity as far north as Christiania in Norway.

History

It was known to Herodotus, who calls it Kiki, and states that it furnishes an oil much used by the Egyptians, in whose ancient tombs seeds of Ricinus are met with. At the period when Herodotus wrote (the fourth century B.C.), it would appear to have been already introduced into Greece, where it is cultivated to the present day under the same ancient name. The Kikajon of the Book of Jonah, rendered by the translators of the English Bible, 'gourd," is believed to be the same plant. Kiki is also mentioned by Strabo as a production of Egypt, the oil from which is used for burning in lamps and for unguents. Theophrastus and Dioscorides, in the first century, describe the plant, Dioscorides giving an account of the process for extracting the oil and saying that it is not fit for food, but is used externally in medicine, and stating that the seeds are extremely purgative. Pliny, about the same time, also speaks of it as a drastic purgative.

We read of it being employed medicinally in Europe during the early Middle Ages: it is recorded that it was cultivated by Albertus Magnus, Bishop of Ratisbon, in the middle of the thirteenth century, but later it fell into disuse, though Gerard (1597) was familiar with it under the name of Ricinus or Kik: the oil, he says, is called Oleum cicinum and used externally in skin diseases. As a garden plant, it was well known in this country in the time of Turner (1551). In the eighteenth century, its cultivation in

Europe as a medicinal plant had, however, practically ceased, and the small supplies of the seeds and oil required for European medicine were obtained from Jamaica. The name 'Castor' was indeed originally applied about this period to the plant in Jamaica, where it seems to have been called 'Agnus Castus," though it bears no resemblance to the South European plant properly so called. The botanical name is from the Latin Ricinus (a dog-tick), from the form and markings of the seed.

Cultivation

The various varieties of Ricinus, which are perennial in their nativecountries, are generally annuals in England, though sometimes they may be preserved through the winter.

Plants are readily grown from seed, which should be sown on a hot bed early in March. When the plants come up, each should be planted in a separate small pot, filled with light soil and plunged into a fresh hot bed. The young plants are kept under glass till early in June, when they are hardened and put out.

Ricinus (Bronze King) and R. Africanus are two good garden varieties for this country, which if given good soil and kept well supplied with water, grow to a large size and make a fine effect in the garden.

Preparation for Market

The seeds are collected when ripe: as the capsules dry, theyopen and discharge the seeds.

The oil is obtained from the seeds by two principal methods - expression and decoction. The latter process is largely used in India, where the oil on account of its cheapness and abundance, is extensively employed for illuminating, as well as for other domestic andmedicinal purposes.

The oil exported from Calcutta to Europe is prepared by shelling and crushing the seed between rollers. The crushed mass is then placed in hempen cloths and pressed in a screw or hydraulic press. The oil which exudes is mixed with water and heated till the water boils and the mucilaginous matter in the oil separates as a scum. It is next strained, then bleached in the sunlight and stored for exportation.

In France, the oil is obtained by macerating the bruised seeds in alcohol, but the process is expensive and the product inferior.

There are two modes of extracting the oil by expression: (1) without heat, when it is termed 'cold drawn Castor Oil," this process being largely carried out in Italy, Marseilles, Belgium, Hull and London; (2) with heat, the process generally adopted in America.

Italian Castor Oil, which is of an excellent quality, is pressed from seeds grown chiefly in the neighborhood of Verona and Legnago. Two varieties of Ricinus are cultivated in these localities, the black-seeded Egyptian and the red-seeded American, the latter yields the larger percentage, but the oil is not so pale in color. All the Castor Oil pressed in Italy, however, is not pressed from Italian seed, but some seeds are imported from India into Italy - as also into this country.

In the north of Italy, the fresh seeds are alone used, and after they have been crushed and the seed coats very carefully removed with a winnowing machine and by hand, the blanched seeds are put into small hempen bags, which are arranged in superposed layers in a powerful hydraulic press, with a sheet of iron heated to 90 degrees F. between each layer, so as to enable the oil to flow readily, they are finally submitted to pressure in a room, which in the winter is heated to a temperature of about 70 degrees. The oil which first flows is of the finest quality, but an inferior oil is subsequently obtained by pressing the mass at a somewhat higher temperature. The peeled seeds yield about 40 per cent. of oil. After expression, the oil is usually bleached by exposure to sunlight or by chemical means.

In America, where the oil is obtained by expression with heat, the manufacture is conducted on an extensive scale in California. There the seeds are submitted to a dry heat in a furnace for an hour or so, by which they are softened and prepared to part easily with their oil. They are then pressed in a large powerful screwpress, and the oily matter which flows out is mixed with an equal proportion of water, and boiled to purify it from mucilaginous and albuminous matter. After boiling about an hour, it is allowed to cool, the water is drawn off and the oil is transferred to zinc tanks or clarifiers capable of holding from 60 to 100 gallons. In these it stands about eight hours, bleaching in the sun, after which it is ready for storing. By this method, 100 lb. of good seeds yield about five gallons of pure oil.

Of these three varieties of extraction, the Italian or cold drawn is considered the best the East Indian, the poorest, as the mode of purifying by heating with water is considered very imperfect. The former owes its freedom from acridity and unpleasant taste partly to the removal of the seed coats before pressing, and partly to the low temperature used during the manufacture.

Constituents

The seeds contain 50 per cent of the fixed oil, which is a viscid fluid, almost colorless when pure, possessing only a slight odor and mild, yet highly nauseous and disagreeable taste. Its specific gravity is high for an oil, being 0.96, a little less than that of water, and it dissolves freely in alcohol, ether and glacial acetic acid. It contains Palmitic and several other fatty acids, among which there is one - Ricinoleic acid - peculiar to itself. This occurs in combination with glycerine, constituting the greater part of the bulk of the oil. The oil is decomposed by the fat-splitting ferments of the intestinal canal liberating this irritant Ricinoleic acid, to which the purgative action is considered in all probablity to be due.

Both the seeds themselves and the cake left after the expression of the oil are violently purgative, a property which is due to the presence of the highly toxic albumin Ricin. The seeds are never employed in this country on account of their violent action. Ricin exhibits its highest toxicity when injected into the blood. It is of interest to note that the work upon which is based the whole science of Serum therapeutics was carried out by Ehrlich with Ricin. He found that by injecting gradually increasing doses, immunity was established, a condition which he attributed to the formation of an antibody and termed Antiricin.

Medicinal Action and Uses

Castor Oil is regarded as one of the most valuable laxatives in medicine. It is of special service in temporary constipation and wherever a mild action is essential, and is extremely useful for children and the aged. It is used in cases of colic and acute diarrhea due to slow digestion, but must not be employed in cases of chronic constipation, which it only aggravates whilst relieving the symptoms. It acts in about five hours, affecting the entire length of the bowel, but not increasing the flow of bile, except in very large doses. The mode of its action is unknown. The oil will purge when rubbed into the skin, or injected. It is also used for expelling worms, after other special remedies have been administered.

The only serious objections to the use of Castor Oil are its flavor and the sickness often produced by it. The nauseous taste may be disguised by administering it covered by Lemon oil, Sassafras oil and other essential oils, or floating on Peppermint or Cinnamon water, or coffee, or shaken up with glycerine, or given in fresh or warmed milk, the dose varying from 1 to 4 teaspoonsful. Probably the best way, however, is to administer it in capsules. Small repeated doses may be given in the intestinal colic of children.

It may also be made into an emulsion with the yolk of an egg or mucilage; or with orange-wine or gin.

Castor Oil forms a clean, light-coloured soap, which dries and hardens well and is free from smell. It has been recommended for medicinal use. The inferior qualities of the oil are frequently employed in India for soap-making.

Externally, the oil has been recommended for various cutaneous complaints, such as ringworm, itch, etc. The fresh leaves are used by nursing mothers in the Canary Islands as an external application, to increase the flow of milk.

The oil varies much in activity - the East Indian is the more active, but the Italian has the least taste.

Castor Oil is an excellent solvent of pure alkaloids and such solutions of Atropine, Cocaine, etc., as are used in ophthalmic surgery. It is also dropped into the eye to remove the after-irritation caused by the removal of foreign bodies.

'Castor Oil is finding increasing uses in the industrial world. It figures largely in the manufacture of the artificial leather used in upholstery; it furnishes a coloring for butter, and from it is produced the so-called 'Turkey-red' oil used in the dyeing of cotton textures. It is an essential component in some artificial rubbers, in various descriptions of celluloid, and in the making of certain waterproof preparations, and one of the largest uses is in the manufacture of transparent soaps. It also furnishes sebacic acid which is employed in the manufacture of candles, and caprylic acid, which enters into the composition of varnishes, especially suitable for the polishing of high-class furniture and carriage bodies. One of its minor uses is in the manufacture of fly-papers." - 'West India Committee Circular." (Quoted in The Chemist and Druggist.)

The Cleaning of Pictures

Lecturing in London, on November 15, on the preservation and restoration of pictures, Professor A. P. Lawrie, while not prepared to give a final opinion as to the safest methods of cleaning, suggested that where alcohol was used Castor Oil should be laid on the surface with a soft brush; and then a mixture of Castor Oil and alcohol dabbed on with a soft brush, and removed by diluting with turpentine and sopping up with a large dry brush. Where alcohol was not a sufficiently powerful solvent, copaiba balsam emulsified with ammonia might be used, a preparation of copaiba balsam thinned with a little turpentine being laid on first." (Chemist and Druggist, November 25, 1922.)

Combined with citron ointment, it is used as a topical application in common leprosy.

CATECHU, BLACK

Botanical: Catechu nigrum, Acacia catechu (WILLD.)
Family: N.O. Leguminosae
Synonym: Cutch.
Habitat: Burma, India.

Pale Catechu is an extract made from the leaves and young shoots of Uncaria Gambier (Roxb.), a member of the order Rubiaceae, not an Acacia. It occurs in commerce in dark or pale-brown cubes with a dull, powdery fracture, or sometimes in lozenge form.

Black Catechu occurs in black, shining pieces or cakes.

Both substances are sold under the name of Catechu.

Medicinal Action and Uses

Both the dark and the pale Catechu are employed in medicine, the former is more astringent, the latter, being sweeter, is less disagreeable.

It depends almost entirely for its virtues upon the tannic acid it contains and is hence employed as an astringent to overcome relaxation of mucous membranes in general.

An infusion can be employed to stop nosebleeding, and is also employed as an injection for uterine hemorrhage, leucorrhoea and gonorrhea.

Externally, it is applied in the form of powder, to boils, ulcers and cutaneous eruptions, and also used for the same purposes mixed with other ingredients, in an ointment.

A small piece, held in the mouth and allowed slowly to dissolve, is an excellent remedy in relaxation of the uvula and simple pharyngitis.

In powder, applied to spongy gums, it often proves of use and has been recommended as a dentifrice with powdered charcoal, myrrh, etc.

The pharmaceutical preparations are: Powdered Catechu, dose 5 to 15 grains; Compound Powder of

Catechu, B.P., dose 10 to 40 grains; Tincture of Catechu, B.P., dose 1/2 to 1 drachm; Comp. Tincture, U.S.P., dose 1 drachm. Catechu Lozenges are also official preparations in both the British and United States Pharmacopoeias.

Like Acacia arabica, the wood-extract of this species has, however, a larger field in the tanning industry than in medicine. The Pale Catechu (Gambier Catechu) is largely used in the arts, for dyeing purposes, yielding a color known as 'Cutch Brown."

Cutch is subject to the most extensive adulteration, though this exists chiefly in the tanning grades. The chief adulterants are Than (an extract obtained by boiling the bark of Buceras oliverii), dried blood, ashes, sand, clay and starch, and their detection is provided for in the official tests.

CATMINT

Botanical: Nepeta cataria (LINN.)
Family: N.O. Labiatae
Synonym: Catnep.
Parts Used: Leaves, herb.

Habitat

Catmint or Catnep, a wild English plant belonging to the large family Labiatae, of which the Mints and Deadnettles are also members, is generally distributed throughout the central and the southern counties of England, in hedgerows, borders of fields, and on dry banks and waste ground, especially in chalky and gravelly soil. It is less common in the north, very local in Scotland and rare in Ireland, but of frequent occurrence in the whole of Europe and temperate Asia, and also common in North Arnerica, where originally. however. it was an introduced species.

Description

The root is perennial and sends up square, erect and branched stems, 2 to 3 feet high, which are very leafy and covered with a mealy down. The heart-shaped, toothed leaves are also covered with a soft, close down, especially on the under sides, which are quite white with it, so that the whole plant has a hoary, greyish appearance, as though it had had dust blown over it.

The flowers grow on short footstalks in dense whorls, which towards the summit of the stem are so close as almost to form a spike. They are in bloom from July to September. The individual flowers are small, the corollas two-lipped, the upper lip straight, of a whitish or pale pink color, dotted with red spots, the anthers a deep red color. The calyx tube has fifteen ribs, a distinguishing feature of the genus Nepeta, to which this species belongs.

History

The plant has an aromatic, characteristic odor, which bears a certain resemblance to that of both Mint and Pennyroyal. It is owing to this scent that it has a strange fascination for cats, who will destroy any plant of it that may happen to be bruised. There is an old saying about this plant:

'If you set it, the cats will eat it,
If you sow it, the cats don't know it."

And it seems to be a fact that plants transplanted are always destroyed by cats unless protected, but they never meddle with the plants raised from seed, being only attracted to it when it is in a withering state, or when the peculiar scent of the plant is excited by being bruised in gathering or transplanting.

In France the leaves and young shoots are used for seasoning, and it is regularly grown amongst kitchen herbs for the purpose. Both there and in this country, it has an old reputation for its value as a medicinal herb. Miss Bardswell, in The Herb Garden, writes of Catmint:

'Before the use of tea from China, our English peasantry were in the habit of brewing Catmint Tea, which they said was quite as pleasant and a good deal more wholesome. Ellen Montgomery in The Wide, Wide World made Catmint Tea for Miss Fortune when she was ill. It is stimulating. The root when chewed is said to make the most gentle person fierce and quarrelsome, and there is a legend of a certain hangman who could never screw up his courage to the point of hanging anybody till he had partaken of it. Rats dislike the plant particularly, and will not approach it even when driven by hunger."

This dislike of rats for Catmint might well be utilized by growing it round other valuable crops as a protective screen.

Closely allied to the Catmint is the Ground Ivy (Nepeta glechoma, Benth.), named Glechoma hederacea by Linnaeus.

Cultivation

Catmint is easily grown in any garden soil, and does not require moisture in the same way as the other Mints. It may be increased by dividing the plants in spring, or by sowing seeds at the same period. Sow in rows, about 20 inches apart, thinning out the seedlings to about the same distance apart as the plants attain a considerable size. They require no attention, and will last for several years if the ground is kept free from weeds. The germinating power of the seeds lasts five years.

Catmint forms a pretty border plant, especially in conjunction with Hyssop, the soft blues blending pleasingly, and it is also a suitable plant for the rock garden.

Part Used Medicinally

The flowering tops are the part utilized in medicine and are harvested when the plant is in full bloom in August.

Medicinal Action and Uses

Carminative, tonic, diaphoretic, refrigerant and slightly emmenagogue, specially antispasmodic, and mildly stimulating.

Producing free perspiration, it is very useful in colds. Catnep Tea is a valuable drink in every case of fever, because of its action in inducing sleep and producing perspiration without increasing the heat of the system. It is good in restlessness, colic, insanity and nervousness, and is used as a mild nervine for children, one of its chief uses being, indeed, in the treatment of children's ailments. The infusion of 1 OZ. to a pint of boiling water may be taken by adults in doses of 2 tablespoonsful, by children in 2 or 3 teaspoonsful frequently, to relieve pain and flatulence. An injection of Catnep Tea is also used for colicky pains.

The herb should always be infused, boiling will spoil it. Its qualities are somewhat volatile, hence when made it should be covered up.

The tea may be drunk freely, but if taken in very large doses when warm, it frequently acts as an emetic.

It has proved efficacious in nervous headaches and as an emmenagogue, though for the latter purpose, it is preferable to use Catnep, not as a warm tea, but to express the juice of the green herb and take it in tablespoonful doses, three times a day.

An injection of the tea also relieves headache and hysteria, by its immediate action upon the sacral plexus. The young tops, made into a conserve, have been found serviceable for nightmare.

Catnep may be combined with other agents of a more decidedly diaphoretic nature. Equal parts of warm Catnep tea and Saffron are excellent in scarlet-fever and small-pox, as well as colds and hysterics. It will relieve painful swellings when applied in the form of a poultice or fomentation.

Old writers recommended a decoction of the herb, sweetened with honey for relieving a cough, and Culpepper tells us also that 'the juice drunk in wine is good for bruises," and that 'the green leaves bruised and made into an ointment is effectual for piles," and that 'the head washed with a decoction taketh away scabs, scurf, etc."

CATSFOOT

Botanical: Antennaria dioca (GAEERTN.)
Family: N.O. Compositae
Synonyms: Life Everlasting. Mountain Everlasting. Gnaphalium dioicum (Linn.). Cudweed.
Part Used: Whole herb.

Habitat

Europe, Asia, America to the Arctic regions, abundant in Great Britain, often to the coast level.

Description

This plant derives its name from the antennae of a butterfly which the pappus hairs of the Staminate florets resemble.

It is the only British species, a small perennial with tufted or creeping leafly stalks and almost simple flowering stems, from 2 to 5 inches high. Lower leaves obovate or oblong, upper ones linear, white underneath or on both sides. Flowers early summer white and pinky, dioecious. In the males, inner bracts of the involucre have broad white petal-like tips, the females inner bracts narrow and white at tips, florets filiform with long protruding pappus to the achenes. Taste astringent odor pleasant and strongest in the female heads, male plant has white membraneous scales and the female rosecoloured. Gerard alludes to it as 'Live for ever," and says:

'When the flower hath long flourished and is waxen old, then comes there in the middest of the floure a certain brown yellow thrumme, such as is in the middest of the daisie, which floure being gathered when it is young may be kept in such manner (I meane in such freshness and well-liking) by the space of a whole year after in your chest or elsewhere, wherefore our English women have called it "Live Long," or "Live-for ever," which name doth aptly answer thiseffects."

Another variety of Cudweed was called 'Herbe Impious' or 'Wicked Cudweed," a variety

'like unto the small Cudweed, but much larger and for the most part those floures which appeare first are the lowest and basest; and they are over topt by other floures, which come on younger branches, and grow higher as children seeking to overgrow or overtop their parents (as many wicked children do) for which cause it hath been called "Herbe Impious." "

Medicinal Action and Uses

Discutient and used for its astringent properties, as a cure for quinsy, and mumps, said to be efficacious for bites of poisonous reptiles, and for looseness of bowels.

Constituents

Resin, volabile oil tanin and a bitter principle.

Doses

For a mouthwash: 1 OZ. Cudweed, 1 OZ. Raspberry Leaves, 1 OZ. Tincture of Myrrh. As an infusion: 1 OZ. herb to pint boiling water is given internally in wine glassful doses and applied externally, as a gargle and as a fomentation. Fluid extract: Dose, 1/2 to 1 drachm.

CAYENNE

Botanical: Capsicum minimum (ROXB.)
Family: N.O. Solanaceae
Synonyms: African Pepper. Chillies. Bird Pepper.
Part Used: Fruit, ripe and dried.
Habitat: Zanzibar - but now grown in most tropical and sub-tropical countries.

Description

Cayenne or Capsicum derives its name from the Greek, 'to bite," in allusion to the hot pungent properties of the fruits and seeds. Cayenne pepper was introduced into Britain from India in 1548, and Gerard mentioned it as being cultivated in his time. The plant was described by Linnaeus under the name of C. frutescens proper. This species appeared in Miller's Garden Dictionary in 1771. It is a shrubby perennial plant 2 to 6 feet high. Branches angular, usually enlarged and slightly purple at the nodes; petioles medium; peduncles slender, often in pairs, and longer than the fruit; calyx cup-shaped, clasping base of fruit which is red, ovate, and long; seeds small and flat, from ten to twenty-nine. The cuticle of the pericarp is uniformly striated and in this particular is distinct from other species. Taste very pungent and smell characteristic. It is difficult to determine the source of true powdered Capsicum, as the color is affected by light, so that it should always be kept in dark receptacles. African pepper is generally light brownish-yellow color and very pungent; its pungency appears to depend on a principle called Capsicin. Cayenne is sometimes adulterated with oxide of red lead, which may be detected by digesting in dilute nitric acid. Other adulterants are coloured sawdust which can be found by the aid of the microscope. The British Pharmacopeia requires that capsicum should yield not more than 6 per cent of ash, and this test detects the presence of most adulterants.

Constituents

Capsaicin, a red coloring matter, oleic, palmitic and stearic acids.

Medicinal Action and Uses

A powerful local stimulant, with no narcotic effect largely used in hot climates as a condiment, and most useful in atony of the intestines and stomach. It should not be used in ordinary gastric catarrh. For persons addicted to drink it seems to be useful possibly by reducing the dilated blood-vessels and thus relieving chronic congestion. It is often added to tonics and is said to be unequalled for warding off diseases. Herbalists use it largely in pill form and powdered. Externally it is a strong rubefacient and acts gently with no danger of vesication; is applied as a cataplasm or as a liniment; it can be mixed with 10 to 20 per cent of cotton-seed oil. The powder or the tincture is beneficial for relaxed uvula. A preparation in use in the West Indies called Mandram, for weak digestion and loss of appetite, is made of thinly sliced and unskinned cucumbers, shallots, chives, or onions, lemon or lime juice, Madeira, and a few pods of bird pepper well mashed up in the liquids. It can be used as a chutney.

Doses

For a gargle: 1/2 drachm of powder to 1 pint of boiling water, or 1/2 fluid ounce of the tincture to 8 fluid ounces of rose water. If the throat is very sensitive it can be given in pill form - generally made with 1 to 10 grains powder. The infusion is made with 2 drachms to 1/2 pint boiling water taken in 1/2 fluid ounce doses. The tincture is used as a paint for chilblains.

CEDAR, YELLOW

Botanical: Thuja occidentalis (LINN.)
Family: N.O. Coniferae
Synonyms: Tree of Life. Arbor Vitae. American Arbor Vitae. Cedrus Lycea. Western Arbor Vitae. False White Cedar. Hackmatack. Thuia du Canada. Lebensbaum.
Part Used: The recently-dried, leafy young twigs.
Habitat: North America, from Pennsylvania northward.

Description

The tallest of this species of Conifer rarely grows above 30 feet high. These trees have regular, graceful conical forms that make them valuable as high-hedge trees, and they also take easily any other shape to which they may be clipped. The leaves are of two kinds on different branchlets, one awl-shaped and the other short and obtuse. Both have a small, flattened gland, containing a thin, fragrant turpentine. They are persistent, and overlap in four rows. The flowers are very small and terminal, and the cones nodding first ovoid and then spreading, with blunt scales arranged in three rows.

The name Thuja is a latinized form of a Greek word meaning 'to fumigate," or thuo ('to sacrifice'), for the fragrant wood was burnt by the ancients with sacrifices. The tree was described as 'arbor vita " by Clusius, who saw it in the royal garden of Fontainebleau after its importation from Canada. It was introduced into Britain about 1566.

In America the wood is much used for fencing and palings, as a light roofing timber, and, as it is both durable and pliable, for the ribs and bottom of bark boats, and also for limekilns, bowls, boxes, cups, and small articles of furniture.

The fresh branches are much used in Canada for besoms, which have a pleasing scent. The odor is pungent and balsamic and the taste bitter, resembling camphor and terebinth.

The trees grow well on the western coast hills of Britain, and the wood is soft, finely grained, and light in texture.

Constituents

The bitter principle, Pinipicrin, and the tannic acid, said to beidentical with Pinitannic acid, occur also in Pinus sylvestris. Thuja also contains volatile oil, sugar, gelatinous matter, wax, resin, and Thujin. The last is a citron-yellow, crystallizable coloring principle, soluble in alcohol. It has an astringent taste, is inflammable, and can be split up into glucose, Thujigenin and Thujetin (probably identical with Quercitin).

The leaves and twigs are said to yield also a camphor-like essential oil, sp. gr. 0.925, boiling point 190-206 degrees C., easily soluble in alcohol and containing pinene, fenchone, thujone, and perhaps carvone.

A yellow-green volatile oil can be distilled from the leaves and used as a vermifuge.

Medicinal Action and Uses

Aromatic, astringent, diuretic. The twigs may produce abortion, like those of savin, by reflex action on the uterus from severe gastrointestinal irritation. Both fenchone and thujone stimulate the heart muscle. The decoction has been used in intermittent fevers, rheumatism, dropsy, coughs, scurvy, and as an emmenagogue. The leaves, made into an ointment with fat, are a helpful local application in rheumatism. An injection of the tincture into venereal warts is said to cause them to disappear. For violent pains the Canadians have used the cones, powdered, with four-fifths of Polypody, made into a poultice with lukewarm water or milk and applied to the body, with a cloth over the skin to prevent scorching.

Dosage

Of fluid extract, 1/4 drachm, three to six times a day, as stimulating expectorant and diuretic. The infusion of 1 OZ. to a pint of boiling water is taken cold in tablespoonful doses.

Poisons

The oil, resembling camphor, may produce convulsions in warmblooded and paralysis in cold-blooded animals. Sixteen drops of the oil, taken by a girl of fifteen, caused unconsciousness, followed by spasms and convulsions, with subsequent stomachic irritation. It causes great flatulence and distension of the stomach.

Other Species

CHINESE ARBOR VITAE (Thuja orientalis or Biota orientalis), a native of China and Japan has the same properties. The young branches yield a yellow dye and the wood withstands conditions of humidity well.

T. articulata, of Northern Africa, yields the resin known as Sandarac, formerly used as a drug, and for ointments and plasters. At present it is used as varnish and incense, and the powder, or Pounce, is used to prevent ink spreading on paper after letters have been scratched out. It is occasionally adulterated with mastic, rosin, etc. A false sandarac consists largely of colophony.

Sandarac is said to be used in India for hemorrhoids and diarrhea and the tincture for friction in cases of low spirits.

The Australian sandarac, from C. robusta, is very similar.

WHITE CEDAR is a common name of Cupressus thujoides.

RED CEDAR OF BRITISH COLUMBIA, the Giant Arbor Vitae, is next to the Douglas Fir in importance in British Columbia, where it attains its greatest height of 100 feet. It is the best wood to use for shingles.

RED CEDAR, or Juniperus virginiana, resembles savin, but is less energetic. Externally it is an irritant, and an ointment prepared from the fresh leaves is used as a substitute for savin cerate in discharge from blisters. The volatile oil has been used for abortion and has caused death, preceded by burning in the stomach, vomiting, convulsions, coma, and gastrointestinal inflammation. It is used in perfumery, and is a principal constituent of extract of white rose.

Small excrescences called cedar apples are sometimes found on the branches, and used as an anthelmintic. Dosage: from 10 to 20 grains three times a day.

To obtain Cedrene camphor the oil must be cooled until coagulated and the crystalline portion separated by expression.

HAITIAN CEDAR yields an oil resembling that of J. virginiana, but having a higher specific gravity.

HACKMATOCK is also the name of Larix americana.

CEDAR OF LEBANON (Cedrus libani) and its two varieties.

INDIAN CEDAR or DEODAR (C. deodara) and AFRICAN CEDAR (C. Atlantica), or satin-wood, yield an oil which, when distilled, is called Libanol. The oil of the last resembles oil of santal, and is good for phthisis, bronchitis, blennorrhagia, and also for eruptions on the skin, in the form of 25 per cent ointment with vaseline. Dosage: capsules up to 45 grains per day.

Cedrela odorata of the West Indies yields a volatile oil that is said to be a powerful insecticide. The wood is used for making cigar boxes. Another cedar of the same family of Cedrelaceae or Meliaceae is AUSTRALIAN RED CEDAR (C. tooma) or Red Cedar of Queensland, yielding Cedar Gum, containing 68 per cent arabin, and 6 per cent metarabin, but no resin.

NEW ZEALAND CEDAR (Libocedrus bidwillii) and also CALIFORNIAN WHITE CEDAR (L. decurrens) possess some of the same properties.

PRICKLY CEDAR (J. oxycedrus) (syn. Large, Brown-fruited Juniper), of the Mediterranean coasts, yields Oil of Cade by destructive distillation of the wood. It has been used from remote ages for the skin diseases of animals, and more recently in medicine for psoriasis and chronic eczema. It is a good parasiticide in psora and favus.

It is also made into ointments and soaps, and a glycerite is prepared.

On the very rare occasions of its internal use, its action resembles oil of tar. Dosage: 1 to 3 minims.

J. phoenicia is used in Europe to adulterate savin.

CEDRON

Botanical: Simaba Cedron (PLANCH.)
Family: N.O. Simarubaceae
Synonym: Cedron seeds.
Part Used: Seeds.
Habitat: Columbia and Central America.

Description

A small tree, a native of New Grenada, remarkable for the properties of its seed. It has large pinnated leaves with over twenty narrow elliptical leaflets and large panicles of flowers, 3 to 4 feet long; the fruit is about the size of a swan's egg, and contains only one fruit, four of the cells being barren. The Cedron of commerce is not unlike a large blanched almond - it is often yellowish, hard and compact, but can be easily cut, it is intensely bitter, not unlike quassia in taste and has no odor. The Cedron of commerce is obtained from the seed. Cedron has always been used in Central America as a remedy for snake-bite, and first came into notice in Britain in 1699.

Medicinal Action and Uses

It has been found of considerable value in New Grenada as a febrifuge in intermittent fever, and is also recommended as an antiperiodic. There is almost a superstitious belief in its efficacy in eradicating poison, and the natives always carry some of the seeds on their person. For snake-bites, a small quantity is scraped off, mixed with water and applied to the wound, and then about 2 grains are put into brandy or into water and taken internally. Every part of the plant, including the seed, is intensely bitter.

Constituents

A crystalline substance called Cedrin was separated by Lowry, but this has been disputed.

Dosages

Of the crude drug, 5 to 15 grains. Of powdered seeds, 1 to 10 grains.

The infusion, which is taken in tablespoonful doses, is made with 1 OZ. of the herb to 1 pint of boiling water. Hyperdermically, Cedrin has been given, 1/15 of a grain.

The powdered bark is used to kill vermin.

Other Species

The Simaruba versicolor has similar properties.

CELANDINE, GREATER

Botanical: Chelidonium majus (LINN.)
Family: N.O. Papaveraceae
Synonyms: Common Celandine. Garden Celandine.
Part Used: Herb.

Habitat

Found by old walls, on waste ground and in hedges, nearly always in the neighborhood of human habitations.

Description

At first glance, the four petals arranged in the form of a cross make it appear a member of the order Ciferce, but it is not related to these plants, belonging to the same family as the Poppies (Papaveraceae) and has, like these flowers, a dense mass of stamens in the centre of its blossoms.

The Celandine is a herbaceous perennial. The root is thick and fleshy. The stem, which is slender, round and slightly hairy, grows from 1 1/2 to 3 feet high and is much branched; at the points where the branches are given off, it is swollen and jointed and breaks very easily.

The whole plant abounds in a bright, orange-coloured juice, which is emitted freely wherever the stems or leaves are broken. This juice stains the hands strongly and has a persistent and nauseous taste and a strong, disagreeable smell. It is acrid and a powerful irritant.

The yellowish-green leaves, which are much paler, almost greyish below, are very thin in texture, drooping immediately on gathering. They are graceful in form and slightly hairy, 6 to 12 inches long, 2 to 3 inches wide, deeply divided as far as the central rib, so as to form usually two pairs of leaflets, placed opposite to one another, with a large terminal leaflet. The margins (i.e. edges) of the leaflets are cut into by rounded teeth.

The flowers drop very quickly when picked. They are arranged at the ends of the stems in loose umbels. They blossom throughout the summer, being succeeded by narrow, long pods, containing blackish seeds.

History

This plant is undoubtedly the true Celandine, having nothing in common with the Lesser Celandine except the color of its flowers. It was a drug plant in the Middle Ages and is mentioned by Pliny, to whom we owe the tradition that it is called Chelidonium from the Greek chelidon (a swallow), because it comes into flower when the swallows arrive and fades at their departure. (The English name Celandine is merely a corruption of the Greek word.) Its acrid juice has been employed successfully in removing films from the cornea of the eye, a property which Pliny tells us was discovered by swallows, this being a double reason why the plant should be named after these birds.

Gerard says:

'the juice of the herbe is good to sharpen the sight, for it cleanseth and consumeth away slimie things that cleave about the ball of the eye and hinder the sight and especially being boiled with honey in a brasen vessell, as Dioscorides teacheth."

It is one of the twenty-four herbs mentioned in Mercer's Herbal.

In the fourteenth century, a drink made with Celandine was supposed to be good for the blood. Clusius, the celebrated Dutch botanist, considered that the juice, dropped into small green wounds, effected rapid cure, and when dropped into the eye would take away specks and stop incipient suffusions. The old alchemists held that it was good to 'superstifle the jaundice," because of its intense yellow color.

Part Used

The whole herb, collected in the wild state, from May to July, when in flower, and dried. Likewise, the fresh juice.

Constituents

The alkaloids Chelidonine and Chelerythrin, the latter narcotic and poisonous, also the two nearly allied alkaloids, Homochelidonine A, and Homocheli donine B. In addition, Protopine and Sanguinarine, and a body named Chelidoxanthin, a neutral bitter principle.

Medicinal Action and Uses

Alterative, diuretic, purgative. It is used in jaundice, eczema, scrofulous diseases, etc., the infusion of 1 OZ. of the dried herb to a pint of boiling water being taken in wine glassful doses. The infusion is a cordial and greatly promotes perspiration. The addition of a few aniseeds in making a decoction of the herb in wine has been held to increase its efficacy in removing obstructions of the liver and gall.

A fluid extract is also prepared, the dose being 1/2 to 1 drachm. Eight to 10 drops of the tincture made from the whole herb, or of the fresh juice, given as a dose three times a day in sweetened water, is considered excellent for overcoming torpid conditions of the liver. In the treatment of the worst forms of scurvy it has been given with benefit.

The orange-coloured, acrid juice is commonly used fresh to cure warts, ringworm and corns, but should not be allowed to come into contact with any other part of the skin.

In milk, it is employed as an eye-lotion, to remove the white, opaque spots on the cornea. Mixed with sulphur, it was formerly used to cure the itch.

An ointment made of the roots and lard boiled together, also of the leaves and flowers, has been used with advantage for piles.

Celandine is a very popular medicine in Russia, where it is said to have proved effective in cases of cancer.

It is still used in Suffolk as a fomentation for toothache.

CELANDINE, LESSER

Botanical: Ranunculus ficaria (LINN.)
Family: N.O. Ranunculaceae
Synonyms: Small Celandine. Figwort. Smallwort. Pilewort.
Part Used: Herb.

Habitat

The Lesser Celandine, one of the very earliest of spring flowers, its cheery, starlike blossoms lighting up our hedges even before winter is quite spent, is distributed throughout Europe, Western Asia, and North Africa, in these islands, growing up the hillsides in Wales to a height of 2,400 feet. It grows in moist corners of fields and places near watersides, but is found also on drier ground, if shady, being one of the few plants that thrive beneath the shade of trees, where its glossy foliage frequently forms a dense carpet.

Wordsworth, whose favorite flower this was (in recognition of which the blossoms are carved on his tomb), fancifully suggests that the painter who first tried to picture the rising sun, must have taken the idea of the spreading pointed rays from the Celandine's 'glittering countenance." The burnishing of the golden petals gives a brilliant effect to the flowers, which burst into bloom about the middle of February, a few days only after their bright, shining leaves. The leaves are on long stalks, arising from a short, prostrate stem, and are very variable, the first being heart-shaped, the later ones bluntly cut into, somewhat like the ivy. They often have dark markings.

The blossoms shut up before rain, and even in fine weather do not open before nine o'clock, and by 5 p.m. have already closed for the night. The Celtic name of the plant, Grian (i.e. the sun), refers to this habit. The petals are green on the underside, and directly the flowers close they become inconspicuous.

Throughout March and April, this cheerful little plant is in full bloom, but as the spring passes into summer, the flowers pale somewhat, and the whole plant looks rather sickly, the warmth of the lengthening days withdrawing from it the needed moisture. By the end of May, no flowers are to be seen, and all the plant above ground withers and dies, the virtue being stored up in the fibres of the root, which swell into the form of tubers. If the plant is dug up, late in the summer or autumn, these tubers are seen hanging in a bunch, a dozen or more together, looking like figs, hence the plant's specific Latin name ficaria, from ficus (a fig). By these tubers, the plant is increased, as they break off readily, each tuber, like a potato, producing a new plant. To eradicate this plant from any ground, it is necessary to remove the roots bodily, for if the plants are dug into the soil, they work their way up to the surface again, the stems branching as they grow upward from the tubers, and at every branch producing fresh tubers.

The early awakening of the plant is due to these fully-stored tubers, which lie quiescent all the summer and autumn, but all necessary materials being at hand, leaves and flowers are quickly pushed upwards directly the depth of the winter has passed.

Although the Lesser Celandine has been placed by some botanists in a distinct genus, when it is called Ficaria verna, it is more generally assigned to the Buttercup or Crowfoot genus, Ranunculus. The name of this genus, first employed by Pliny, alludes to the damp and marshy localities preferred by the plants of the family, Rana, being the Latin for a frog, whose native haunts are those of the majority of this group of plants. The Lesser Celandine is distinguished from the Buttercup by having nine or ten, even sometimes a dozen narrow petals, instead of five, and only three sepals (the outer, generally green leaves of the flower), which fall off on opening, instead of the usual five, which remain after the flower has expanded, in the other species of Ranunculus. The flowers rise singly from the root, on long, slender, leafless stalks and are about 1 inch in diameter. There are a number of stamens. The fruits are not unlike those of the Buttercups being dry and distinct, set together in a globular head, somewhat like a grain of corn and whitish in color, but comparatively few fertile seeds are produced.

The flowers would originally appear to have been designed with the object of attracting insects for their fertilization, the bright coloured, burnished petals having honey sacs at their base, but the flowers can face colder days than the insects can, for whom the honey has been provided, blooming when few of the insects have emerged, with the result that comparatively few become fertilized in this country and not many seeds are produced. The plant, therefore, has recourse to another method of reproduction, independent of all external aid. At the point where the upper leaves join the stem are to be seen little objects like minute round tumors, which grow about the size of a grain of wheat. In the early summer, when the leaves and stems are dying down, these grains become loose and drop to the ground. Each is capable of producing a new plant. A heavy rain will sometimes wash them from the plants in every direction. Kerner, in his Natural History of Plants, tells us that:

'a sudden downpour of rain in a region abundantly overgrown with Lesser Celandine is sufficient to float away numbers of the tubers, and heap them up on the borders of irrigation channels when the rain disperses. In such places the quantity of tubers which have floated together is often so large that one can hardly gather them in one's hands. In this way arose the idea that the tubers had fallen from heaven with the rain and the myth of a rain of potatoes."

This fact probably accounts, also, for the 'rains of wheat' sometimes vouched for by country people in various parts. These bulbils (i.e. little bulbs) are only produced on those plants whose fruits have failed to set.

The root of the Lesser Celandine is perennial.

Seedlings do not flower in their first year, but collect and store up material to start their accustomed course at the end of the ensuing winter.

The whole plant is glabrous.

It is called the Lesser Celandine to distinguish it

from the Greater Celandine, to which it has neither relationship nor similarity, except in the color of its flowers, though the older herbalists applied the name to both plants indiscriminately. The confusion of names existed in Gerard's time, for he published a list of all the plants in cultivation in his garden on Holborn Hill - to wards the close of the sixteenth century and introduced in it, under the same name, both this and the Greater Celandine (Chelidonium majus) which certainly is in bloom when the swallows arrive, and continues to flower the whole summer, and so would have more right to the name Celandine than this species, which blossoms long before they come, and dies down months before they leave our shores.

A figure of the Lesser Celandine - under the name of Erdöpffel - appears in an old German Herbal of 1533, Rhodion's Kreutterbuch, evidence that this plant was well known to the herbalists of the Middle Ages.

It is also called 'Small-wort."

The old English name of Pilewort is due to the fact that it has long been considered a cure for piles, one of the reasons assigned for this resting on the strange doctrine of signatures. We are told by an old writer: 'If you dig up the root of it you will perceive the perfect image of the disease commonly called the piles." Gerard writes of it:

'It presently, as Galen and Dioscorides affirm (though this perhaps refers to the Greater Celandine) exulcerateth or blistereth the skin: it maketh rough and corrupt nails to fall away. The juice of the roots mixed with honie and drawn up into the nosthrils purgeth the head of foul and filthy humours. The later age use the roots and graines for the piles . . . there be also who think that if the berbe be but carried about one that hath the piles, the pain forthwith ceaseth."

Culpepper, writing fifty years later, tells us:

'It is certain by good experience that the decoction of the leaves and roots doth wonderfully help piles and hemorrhoids; also kernels by the ears and throat called the King's Evil, or any other hard wens or tumors."

He had such faith in the virtues of this little plant that he further tells us, with more definite belief than Gerard: 'The very herb borne about one's body next the skin helps in such diseases though it never touch the place grieved."

The young leaves, the substance of which is soft and mucilaginous, have sometimes been boiled and eaten as a vegetable in Sweden, but have not the reputation of being very palatable, either thus treated or raw as a salad.

Linnaeus advised farmers to eradicate the plant from their land on account of it being disliked by cattle (though wood-pigeons eat it with avidity), also for its injurious effect on other herbs in the meadow, but there seems little ground for this assumption, as although the tissues of most plants in this order contain acrid juices to a high degree, the acrimony of the Lesser Celandine is of a very mild character. A dressing of coal or wood ash is said to effectually destroy the whole plant.

Part Used

The whole herb is collected in the wild state, while in flower in March and April, and dried.

Constituents

Nothing is known definitely concerning the constituents of Pilewort the fresh plant, however, prob ably contains traces of an acrid principle resembling or identical with Anemonin.

Medicinal Action and Uses

Astringent This herb is an old remedy for piles, for which it has recently been re-introduced into the British Pharmacopoeia, and is considered almost a specific.

Internally, the infusion of 1 OZ. in a pint of boiling water is taken in wine glassful doses, and will in most cases be sufficient to effect a cure.

It is also used externally as an ointment, made from the bruised herb with fresh lard, applied locally night and morning, or in the form of poultices, fomentations, or in suppositories.

A most excellent ointment has been recommended for external abscesses, etc., made from Pilewort, Elder-buds, House-leek, and leaves of the Broad Plantain, prepared in the early spring, when the Pilewort is in flower.

The roots are highly valued as a medicine in Cochin-China.

Recipes

The following old-time recipes connected with this herb occur in A Plain Plantain (R. G. Alexander):

For a Sore Throat

'Take a pinte of whitewine, A good handful of Sallendine, and boile them well together; put to it A piece of the best Roach Allome, sweeten it with English honey, and use it."

A Marvellous Precious Water

'Take Gallingall (Galingale), Cloves, Cubibs, Ginger, Mellilote, Cardamonia, Maces, Nutmegs, one dram- of the juice of Salendine, 8 drams; mingle all these made in powder with the said juice and a pint of Aquavitae, and 3 pints of Whitewine; putt itt into A Stillitory of Glass; and the next day still it with An easy fire.

'This water is of an excellent Virtue Agst A Consumption or any other Disease that proceeds from Rheume Choller or Fleagnie."

All the species of Ranunculus, except the Water Crowfoot, are acrid, and before the introduction of Cantharides (Spanish Fly), many, especially R. sceleratus, were used as vesicatories. They are said to act with less pain and without any action on the urinary passages, but their action is supposed to be uncertain, and they are accused of frequently leaving ill-conditioned ulcers. Since the introduction of Cantharides, their employment has therefore fallen into disuse. Formerly it was not at all uncommon for beggars to produce sores about their bodies by the medium of various species of Ranunculus, for the sake of getting alms, afterwards curing these sores by applying fresh Mullein leaves to heal them.

Pliny tells us that:

'they raise blisters like those caused by fire, hence the plant is used for the removal of leprous spots. They form an ingredient in all caustic preparations."

CELERY (WILD)

Botanical: Apium graveolens (LINN.)
Family: N.O. Umbelliferae
Synonyms: Smallage. Wild Celery.
Parts Used: Ripe seeds, herb and root.
Habitat: Levant, South Europe, and cultivated in Great Britain, etc.

Description

Odor characteristic and agreeable. Taste, aromatic, warm, and slightly pungent.

Constituents

Celery seed contains two oils - one heavy, the other lighter; it also contains apiol, but not so much as is found in parsley.

Medicinal Action and Uses

Carminative stimulant, diuretic, tonic, nervine, useful in hysteria, promoting restfulness and sleep, and diffusing through the system a mild sustaining influence. Good combined with Scutellaria for nervous cases with loss of tone. On this account it is recommended to eat the cultivated fresh root as well as taking the oil or fluid extract. Is said to be very good for rheumatism, when it is often combined with Coca, Damiana, etc. Dose: fluid extract, 3 to 7 drops every four hours.

CENTAURY

Botanical: Erythraea centaurium (PERS.)
Family: N.O. Gentianaceae
Synonyms: Centaury Gentian. Century. Red Cen-

taury. Filwort. Centory. Christ's Ladder. Feverwort. Parts Used: Herb and leaves.

Habitat

The plant is a native of Europe and North Africa. Though common in this country in dry pastures and on chalky cliffs, it cannot be easily reared in a garden, and for its medicinal use is, therefore, collected in the wild state.

Description

The Red Centaury (Erythraea centaurium, Pers.) is an annual, with a yellowish, fibrous, woody root, the stem stiff, square and erect, 3 to 12 inches in height, often branching considerably at the summit. The leaves are of a pale green color, smooth and shiny, their margins undivided. The lowest leaves are broader than the others, oblong or wedge-shaped, narrowed at the base, blunt at the end and form a spreading tuft at the base of the plant, while the stalkless stem-leaves are pointed and lance-shaped, growing in pairs opposite to one another at somewhat distant intervals on the stalk, which is crowned by flat tufts (corymbs) of rose-coloured, star-like flowers, with five-cleft corollas. The stamens are five in number: the anthers have a curious way of twisting themselves round after they have shed their pollen, this being one of the distinctive points between the plants of this genus and those of the genus Gentiana, with which it has much in common, having by some earlier botanists been assigned to that genus, under the name of Gentiana centaurium, or Centaury Gentian. The flowers open only in fine weather and not after mid-day: Gerard chronicles their love of light, saying that they 'in the day-time and after the sun is up, do open themselves and towards evening do shut up again." A variety is sometimes found with white corollas.

Centaury varies a great deal according to) its situation, and some botanists enumerate several distinct species, namely: E. pulchella (Dwarf Centaury), a minute plant, 2 to 8 inches high, with an exceedingly slender stem and a few stalked flowers (often only one); this is found on the sandy seashore, especially in the West of England, and has been picked at Newquay, Cornwall; E. littoralis (Dwarf Tufted Centaury), a stunted plant, with broad leaves, and flowers crowded into a kind of head; this occurs on turfy sea-cliffs, and E. latifolia (Broadleaved Centaury), which has even broader leaves than the last, and bears its flowers in forked tufts, the main stem being divided into three branches. There are other minute differences, for which the student may consult more scientific works.

Besides the English species, others from the south of Europe, the Azores, etc., with yellow or pink flowers, are occasionally grown in gardens.

History

The name of the genus to which it is at present assigned, Erythraea, is derived from the Greek erythros (red), from the color of the flowers. The genus was formerly called Chironia, from the Centaur Chiron, who was famous in Greek mythology for his skill in medicinal herbs, and is supposed to have cured himself with it from a wound he had accidentally received from an arrow poisoned with the blood of the hydra. The English name Centaury has the same origin. The ancients named the plant Fel Terrae, or Gall of the Earth from its extreme bitterness. The old Engiish name of Felwort is equivalent in meaning to this, and is applied to all the plants of the Gentian family. It is also thought to be the 'Graveolentia Centaurea' of Virgil, to which Lucretius gives the more significant epithet of tristia, in reference to this same intense bitterness. As this bitterness had a healing and tonic effect attributed to it, we sometimes find the Centaury called Febrifuga and Feverwort. It is known popularly also as Christ's Ladder, and the name Centaury has become corrupted in Worcestershire to 'Centre of the Sun."

We find a reference to it in Le Petit Albert. Fifteen magical herbs of the Ancients are given:

'The eleventh hearbe is named of the Chaldees, Isiphon . . . of Englishmen, Centory . . . this herbe hath a marvellous virtue, for if it be joined with the blood of a female lapwing, or black plover, and put with oile in a lamp, all that compass it about shall believe themselves to be witches, so that one shall believe of another that his head is in heaven and his feete on earth; and if the aforesaid thynge be put in the fire when the starres shine it shall appeare yt the sterres runne one agaynste another and fyghte." (English translation, 1619.)

Also in a translation of an old mediaeval Latin poem of the tenth century, by Macer, there is mention of Centaury (with other herbs) as being powerful against 'wykked sperytis."

Of all the bitter appetizing wild herbs which serve as excellent simple tonics, the Centaury is the most efficacious, sharing the antiseptic virtues of the Field Gentian and the Buckbean.

Part Used

The whole herb, collected in July, when just breaking into flower and dried. The plant has a slight odor, which disappears when dried.

The Field Gentian is dried in the same manner.

Constituents

Centaury contains a bitter principle, Erythrocentaurin, which is colorless, crystalline, non-nitrogenous, reddened by sunlight; a bitter glucoside, Erytaurin; Valeric acid, wax, etc.

Medicinal Action and Uses

Aromatic bitter, stomachic and tonic. It acts on the liver and kidneys, purifies the blood, and is an excellent tonic.

The dried herb is given in infusion or powder, or made into an extract. It is used extensively in dyspepsia, for languid digestion with heartburn after food, in an infusion of 1 OZ. of the dried herb to 1 pint of water. When run down and suffering from want of appetite, a wine glassful of this infusion Centaury Tea - taken three or four times daily, half an hour before meals, is found of great benefit. The same infusion may also be taken for muscular rheumatism.

Culpepper tells us that:

'the herbe is so safe that you cannot fail in the using of it, only give it inwardly for inward diseases, use it outwardly for outward diseases. 'Tis very wholesome, but not very toothsome."

He says:

'it helps those that have the dropsy, or the green-sickness, being much used by the Italians in powder for that purpose. It kills worms ... as is found by experience.... A dram of the powder taken in wine, is a wonderful good help against the biting and poison of an adder. The juice of the herb with a little honey put to it, is good to clear the eyes from dimness, mists and clouds that offend or hinder sight. It is singularly good both for green and fresh wounds, as also for old ulcers and sores, to close up the one and cleanse the other, and perfectly to cure them both, although they are hollow or fistulous; the green herb, especially, being bruised and laid thereto. The decoction thereof dropped into the ears, cleanses them from worms . . . and takes away all freckles, spots, and marks in the skin, being washed with it."

The Saxon herbalists prescribed it largely for snake-bites and other poisons, and it was long celebrated for the cure of intermittent fevers, hence its name of Feverwort.

The herb formed the basis of the once famous Portland Powder, which was said to be a specific for gout.

Centaury is given with Barberry Bark for jaundice. It has also been much employed as a vermifuge, and a decoction of the plant is said to destroy body vermin.

The green herb, bruised, is reputed to be good as an application to wounds and sores.

CENTAURY, CHILIAN

Botanical: Erythraea chilensis
Family: N.O. Gentianaceae
Synonym: Canchalagua.
Part Used: The herb.
Habitat: Chile.

Description

A small, herbaceous plant, with branched stems and pink or yellow flowers, widely used in Chile as a mild tonic.

Medicinal Action and Uses

Stimulant bitter, tonic. Useful in dyspepsia and indigestion. An infusion may be made of 1 oz. to 1 pint of boiling water.

Dosage

Of infusion - a wine glassful. Of fluid extract - 1/2 to 1 drachm.

Other Species

Erythraea acaulis, a native of Southern Algeria, has roots that yield a yellow dye.

Sabatia angularis, or American Centaury, is a simple bitter used as a tonic and antiperiodic, in doses of 1 drachm of fluid extract or decoction of the whole plant. It has been found to contain a small proportion of Erythrocentaurin. The root of S. Elliottii is used in a similar manner in the south-eastern United States, and the whole plant of S. campestris in the south-western. S. Elliottii is known as the Quinine Flower, its properties resembling quinine.

CEREUS, NIGHT BLOOMING

Botanical: Cereus grandiflorus (LINN.)
Family: N.O. Cactaceae
Synonyms: Vanilla Cactus. Sweet-scented Cactus. Large-flowered Cactus.
Parts Used: The flowers, young and tender stems.
Habitat: Tropical America, Mexico, West Indies, and Naples.

Description

A fleshy, creeping, rooting shrub, stems cylindrical, with five or six not very prominent angles, branching armed with clusters of small spines, in radiated forms. Flowers, terminal and lateral from the clusters of spines, very large 8 to 12 inches in diameter, expanding in the evening and only lasting for about six hours, exhaling a delicious vanilla-like perfume. Petals are white, spreading, shorter than the sepals, which are linear, lanceolate, outside brown, inside yellow. Fruit ovate, covered with scaly tubercles, fleshy and of a lovely orange-red color, seeds very small and acid. The flower only lasts in bloom about six hours and does not revive- when withered, the ovary enlarges, becomes pulpy and forms an acid juicy fruit, something like a gooseberry. The plant was brought to the notice of the medical profession by Dr. Scheile but it aroused little interest till a homeopathic doctor of Naples, R. Rubini, used it as a specific in heart disease. The flowers and young stems should be collected in July and a tincture made from them whilst fresh. The plant contains a milky acrid juice.

Constituents

No special analysis seems yet to have been made; the chief constituents are resins, the presence of the alleged alkaloid cactine not having been confirmed.

Medicinal Action and Uses

Diuretic Sedative, Cardiac. Cereus has been used as a cardiac stimulant and as a partial substitute for digitalis. In large doses it produces gastric irritation, slight delirium, hallucinations and general mental confusion. It is said to greatly increase the renal secretion. It does not appear to weaken the nervous system. It has a decided action on the heart and frequently gives prompt relief in functional or organic disease. It has been found of some service in haemoptysis, dropsy and incipient apoplexy.

Dosages and Preparations

Liquid extract of Cereus, B.P.C.: dose, 1 to 10 minims. Tincture of Cereus, B.P.C.: dose, 2 to 30 minims.

Other Species

Cactus bomplandi, a cardiac stimulant notnow used. Cereus caespitosus. An alkaloid separated from this variety, called Pectenine, produces tetanus convulsions in animals. C. pilocereus gives an alkaloid which produces central paralysis with great cardiac depression in frogs and death by cardiac arrest in warm-blooded animals.

C. flagelliformis and C. divaricatus are said to have anthelmintic properties.

Opuntias decumana and other species are often

substituted for C. grandiflorus, but are of little use. C. giganteus, the Suwarron or Saguaro of the Mexicans, is the largest, and most striking species of the genus. The fruits are 2 to 3 inches long, oval and green, having a broad scar at the top caused by the flowers falling away when the fruits are ripe. They burst into three or four pieces, which curve back to resemble a flower. Inside they contain small black seeds embedded in a crimson pulp, which the Pimos and Papagos Indians make into an excellent preserve. They also eat the ripe fruit as a food and gather it by means of a forked stick tied to the end of a long pole.

Opuntia vulgaris (Prickly Pear), of the Cactus tribe, is cultivated in the south of Europe, and much esteemed by the Spaniards, who consume large quantities. In homeopathy a tincture is made from the flowers and wood for spleen troubles and diarrhea.

O. cochinellifera, the Cochineal Insect Cactus, is a native of Mexico, but cultivated in the West Indies and other places. There are two kinds of O. grana - finagrana and sylvestre. The substance which envelops the insect is pulverulent in the first species and flocculent in the second. It has not yet been decided whether they are different species of COCCUS or whether the difference is in the plant.

CHAMOMILES

Botanical: N.O. Compositae

Habitat

There are a number of species of Chamomile spread over Europe, North Africa and the temperate region of Asia, but in Great Britain we have four growing wild: the sweet-scented, true Chamomile (Anthemis nobilis); the Fcetid Chamomile or Stinking Mayweed (A. cotula), which has what Gerard calls 'a naughty smell'; the Corn Chamomile (A. arvensis), which flowers rather earlier and is noticeable because its ray florets are empty and wholly for show and possess no sort of ovary or style, and fourthly, the Yellow Chamomile, with yellow instead of white rays, which is found sometimes on ballast heaps, but is not a true native.

CHAMOMILE, COMMON

Botanical: Anthemis nobilis (LINN.)
Family: N.O. Compositae
Synonyms: Manzanilla (Spanish). Maythen (Saxon).
Parts Used: Flowers and herb.

Chamomile is one of the oldest favorites amongst garden herbs and its reputation as a medicinal plant shows little signs of abatement. The Egyptians reverenced it for its virtues, and from their belief in its power to cure ague, dedicated it to their gods. No plant was better known to the country folk of old, it having been grown for centuries in English gardens for its use as a common domestic medicine to such an extent that the old herbals agree that 'it is but lost time and labour to describe it."

Description

The true or Common Chamomile (Anthemis nobilis) is a low-growing plant, creeping or trailing, its tufts of leaves and flowers a foot high. The root is perennial, jointed and fibrous, the stems, hairy and freely branching, are covered with leaves which are divided into thread-like segments, the fineness of which gives the whole plant a feathery appearance. The blooms appear in the later days of summer, from the end of July to September, and are borne solitary on long, erect stalks, drooping when in bud. With their outer fringe of white ray-florets and yellow centres, they are remarkably like the daisy. There are some eighteen white rays arranged round a conical centre, botanically known as the receptacle, on which the yellow, tubular florets are placed- the centre of the daisy is, however, considerably flatter than that of the Chamomile.

All the Chamomiles have a tiny, chaffy scale between each two florets, which is very minute and has to be carefully looked for but which all the same is a vital characteristic of the genus Anthemis. The distinction between A. nobilis and other species of Anthemis is the shape of these scales, which in A. nobilis are short and blunt.

The fruit is small and dry, and as it forms, the hill of the receptacle gets more and more conical.

The whole plant is downy and greyishgreen in color. It prefers dry commons and sandy soil, and is found wild in Cornwall, Surrey, and many other parts of England.

Small flies are the chief insect-visitors to the flowers.

History

The fresh plant is strongly and agreeably aromatic, with a distinct scent of apples - a characteristic noted by the Greeks, on account of which they named it 'ground-apple' - kamai (on the ground) and melon (an apple) - the origin of the name Chamomile. The Spaniards call it 'Manzanilla," which signifies 'a little apple," and give the same name to one of their lightest sherries, flavoured with this plant.

When walked on, its strong, fragrant scent will often reveal its presence before it is seen. For this reason it was employed as one of the aromatic strewing herbs in the Middle Ages, and used often to be purposely planted in green walks in gardens. Indeed walking over the plant seems specially beneficial to it.

'Like a camomile bed -
The more it is trodden
The more it will spread,"

The aromatic fragrance gives no hint of its bitterness of taste.

The Chamomile used in olden days to be looked upon as the 'Plant's Physician," and it has been stated that nothing contributes so much to the health of a garden as a number of Chamomile herbs dispersed about it, and that if another plant is drooping and sickly, in nine cases out of ten, it will recover if you place a herb of Chamomile near it.

Parts Used Medicinally

The whole plant is odoriferous and of value, but the quality is chiefly centred in the flower-heads or capitula, the part employed medicinally, the herb itself being used in the manufacture of herb beers.

Both single and double flowers are used in medicine. It is considered that the curative properties of the single, wild Chamomile are the more powerful, as the chief medical virtue of the plant lies in the central disk of yellow florets, and in the cultivated double form the white florets of the ray are multiplied, while the yellow centre diminishes. The powerful alkali contained to so much greater extent in the single flowers is, however, liable to destroy the coating of the stomach and bowels, and it is doubtless for this reason that the British Pharmacopeia directs that the 'official' dried Chamomile flowers shall be those of the double, cultivated variety.

The double-flowered form was already well known in the sixteenth century. It was introduced into Germany from Spain about the close of the Middle Ages.

Chamomile was largely cultivated before the war in Belgium, France and Saxony and also in England, chiefly in the famous herbgrowing district of Mitcham. English flowerheads are considered the most valuable for distillation of the oil, and during the war the price of English and foreign Chamomile reached an exorbitant figure.

The 'Scotch Chamomile' of commerce is the Single or Wild Chamomile, the yellow tubular florets in the centre of the head being surrounded by a variable number of white, ligulate or strap-shaped ray florets. The 'English Chamomile' is the double form, with all or nearly all the florets white and ligulate. In both forms the disk or receptacle is solid and conical, densely covered with chaffy scales, and both varieties, but especially the single, have a strong aromatic odor and a very bitter taste.

Cultivation and Preparation for Market

Chamomile requires a sunny situation. The single variety, being the wild type, flourishes in a rather dry, sandy soil, the conditions of its natural habits on wild, open common-land, but the double-flowered Chamomile needs a richer soil and gives the heaviest crop of blooms in moist, stiffish black loam.

Propagation may be effected by seed, sown thinly in May in the open and transplanting when the seedlings are large enough to permanent quarters, but this is not to be recommended, as it gives a large proportion of single-flowered plants, which, as stated above, do not now rank for pharmaceutical purposes as high as the double-flowered variety, though formerly they were considered more valuable.

The usual manner of increasing stock to ensure the double-flowers is from 'sets," or runners of the old plants. Each plant normally produces from twelve to fourteen sets, but may sometimes give as many as from twenty-five to fifty. The old plants are divided up into their sets in March and a new plantation formed in well-manured soil, in rows 2 1/2 feet apart, with a distance of 18 inches between the plants. Tread the small plants in firmly, it will not hurt them, but make them root better. Keep them clean during the summer by hand-weeding, as hoeing is apt to destroy such little plants. They will require no further attention till the flowers are expanded and the somewhat tedious process of picking commences.

In autumn, the sets may be more readily rooted by placing a ring of good light soil about 2 or 3 inches from the centre of the old plant and pressing it down slightly.

Chemical Constituents

The active principles are a volatile oil, of a pale bluecolour (becoming yellow by keeping), a little Anthemic acid (the bitter principle), tannic acid and a glucoside.

The volatile oil is yielded by distillation, but is lost in the preparation of the extract. Boiling also dissipates the oil.

Medicinal Action and Uses

Tonic, achic, anodyne and antispasmodic. The official preparations are a decoction, an infusion, the extract and the oil.

The infusion, made from 1 OZ. of the flowers to 1 pint of boiling water and taken in doses of a tablespoonful to a wineglass, known popularly as Chamomile Tea, is an old-fashioned but extremely efficacious remedy for hysterical and nervous affections in women and is used also as an emmenagogue. It has a wonderfully soothing, sedative and absolutely harmless effect. It is considered a preventive and the sole certain remedy for nightmare. It will cut short an attack of delirium tremens in the early stage. It has sometimes been employed in intermittent fevers.

Chamomile Tea should in all cases be prepared in a covered vessel, in order to prevent the escape of steam, as the medicinal value of the flowers is to a considerable extent impaired by any evaporation, and the infusion should be allowed to stand on the flowers for 10 minutes at least before straining off.

Combined with ginger and alkalies, the cold infusion (made with 1/2 oz. of flowers to 1 pint of water) proves an excellent stomachic in cases of ordinary indigestion, such as flatulent colic, heartburn, loss of appetite, sluggish state of the intestinal canal, and also in gout and periodic headache, and is an appetizing tonic, especially for aged persons, taken an hour or more before a principal meal. A strong, warm infusion is a useful emetic. A concentrated infusion, made eight times as strong as the ordinary infusion, is made from the powdered flowers with oil of chamomile and alcohol and given as a stomachic in doses of 1/2 to 2 drachms, three times daily.

Chamomile flowers are recommended as a tonic in dropsical complaints for their diuretic and tonic properties, and are also combined with diaphoretics and other stimulants with advantage.

An official tincture is employed to correct summer diarrhea in children. Chamomile is used with purgatives to prevent griping, carminative pills being made from the essential essence of the flowers. The extract, in doses of 10 to 15 grains, combined with myrrh and preparations of iron, also affords a powerful and convenient tonic in the form of a pill. The fluid extract of flowers is taken in doses of from 1/2 to 1 drachm; the oil, B.P. dose, 1/2 to 3 drops.

Apart from their employment internally, Chamomile flowers are also extensively used by themselves, or combined with an equal quantity of crushed poppy-heads, as a poultice and fomentation for external swelling, inflammatory pain or congested neuralgia, and will relieve where other remedies have failed, proving invaluable for reducing swellings of the face caused through abscesses. Bags may be loosely stuffed withflowers and steeped well in boiling water before being applied as a fomentation. The antiseptic powers of Chamomile are stated to be 120 times stronger than sea-water. A decoction of Chamomile flowers and poppyheads is used hot as fomentation to abscesses - 10 parts of Chamomile flowers to 5 of poppy capsules, to 100 of distilled water.

The whole herb is used chiefly for making herb beers, but also for a lotion, for external application in toothache, earache, neuralgia, etc. One ounce of the dried herb is infused in 1 pint of boiling water and allowed to cool. The herb has also been employed in hot fomentations in cases of local and intestinal inflammation.

Culpepper gives a long list of complaints for which Chamomile is 'profitable," from agues and sprains to jaundice and dropsy, stating that 'the flowers boiled in Iye are good to wash the head," and tells us that bathing with a decoction of Chamomile removes weariness and eases pain to whatever part of the body it is employed. Parkinson, in his Earthly Paradise (1656), writes:

'Camomil is put to divers and sundry users, both for pleasure and profit, both for the sick and the sound, in bathing to comfort and strengthen the sound and to ease pains in the diseased."

Turner says:

'It hath floures wonderfully shynynge yellow and resemblynge the appell of an eye . . . the herbe may be called in English, golden floure. It will restore a man to hys color shortly yf a man after the longe use of the bathe drynke of it after he is come forthe oute of the bathe. This herbe is scarce in Germany but in England it is so plenteous that it groweth not only in gardynes but also VIII mile above London, it groweth in the wylde felde, in Rychmonde grene, in Brantfurde grene.... Thys herbe was consecrated by the wyse men of Egypt unto the Sonne and was rekened to be the only remedy of all agues."

The dried flowers of A. nobilis are used for blond dyeing, and a variety of Chamomile known as Lemon Chamomile yields a very fine essential oil.

GERMAN CHAMOMILE

Botanical: Matricaria chamomilla (LINN.)
Family: N.O. Compositae
Synonym: Wild Chamomile.
Part Used: Flowers.

The German Chamomile, sometimes called the Wild Chamomile, has flower-heads about 3/4 inch broad, with about fifteen white, strap shaped, reflexed ray florets and numeroustubular yellow, perfect florets. It is frequent in cornfields and so remarkably like the Corn Chamomile (Anthemis arvensis) that it is often difficult to distinguish it from that plant, but it is not ranked among the true Chamomiles by botanists because it does not possess the little chaffy scales or bracts between its florets; also the conical receptacle, or disk, on which the florets are arranged is hollow, not solid, like that of the Corn Chamomile. It may also be distinguished from A. cotula and Matricaria inodora, the Mayweeds, by the lapping-over scales of its involucre surrounding the base of the flower-head not being chaffy at the margin, as in those species. It has a strong smell, somewhat like that of the official Common Chamomile (A. nobilis), but less aromatic, whereas the Corn Chamomile which it so closely resembles is scentless.

Constituents

The flowers of the German Chamomile, though aromatic, have a very bitter taste. They contain a volatile oil, a bitter extractive and little tannic acid.

Medicinal Action and Uses

Carminative, sedative and tonic. The infusion of 1/2 oz. of the dried flowers to 1 pint of boiling water may be given freely in teaspoonful doses to children, for whose ailments it is an excellent remedy. It acts as a nerve sedative and also as a tonic upon the gastro-intestinal canal. It proves useful during dentition in cases of earache, neuralgic pain, stomach disorders and infantile convulsions. The flowers may also be used externally as a fomentation.

Preparations

Fluid extract: dose, 1/4 to 1 drachm.

STINKING CHAMOMILE

Botanical: Anthemis cotula (LINN.)
Family: N.O. Compositae
Synonyms: Mayweed. Maruta Cotula. Dog Chamomile. Maruta Foetida. Dog-Fennel.
Part Used: Whole herb.

Stinking Chamomile or Stinking Mayweed (Anthemis cotula), an annual, common in waste places, resembles the true Chamomile, having large solitary flowers on erect stems, with conical, solid receptacles, but the white florets have no membraneous scales at their base. It is distinguished from the other Chamomiles and closely allied genera by its foetid odor, which Gerard calls 'a naughty smell." This disagreeable smell, and the resemblance to fennel of its much-cut leaves gains it its other name of 'Dog's Fennel." The whole plant, not only the flowers, has this intense odor and is penetrated by an acrid juice that often will blister the hand which gathers it. Writers on toxicology have classed this plant amongst the vegetable poisons.

Medicinal Action and Uses

Tonic, antispasmodic, emmenagogue and emetic.

The whole herb is used (for drying, see FEVERFEW). Like true Chamomile, a strong decoction will produce vomiting and sweating. In America it is used in country districts as a sudorific in colds and chronic rheumatism. The infusion made from 1 OZ. of the dried herb in a pint of boiling water and taken warm in wine glassful doses has been used with success in sick headache and in convalescence from fevers. It was formerly used in scrofula and hysteria and externally in fomentations. A weaker infusion taken to a moderate extent acts as an emetie.

CHASTE TREE

Botanical: Agnus castus
Family: N.O. Verbenaceae
Part Used: The ripe berries.
Habitat: Shores of the Mediterranean.

Description

A deciduous shrub of free spreading habit, young shoots covered with a fine grey down; leaves opposite, composed of five to seven radiating leaflets borne on a main stalk 1 to 2 1/2 inches long, leaflets linear, lance-shaped, toothed, dark green above, grey beneath with a very close felt; stalks of leaflets 1/4 inch or less long- flowers fragrant, produced in September or October, in whorls on slender racemes 3 to 6 inches long, sometimes branched; the berries somewhat like peppercorns, dark purple, halfcovered by their sage-green calyces, yellowish within, hard, having an aromatic odor; taste warm, peculiar. The seeds were once held in repute for securing chastity, and the Athenian matrons in the sacred rites of Ceres used to string their couches with the leaves.

Medicinal Action and Uses

The fresh ripe berries are pounded to a pulp and used in the form of a tincture for the relief of paralysis, pains in the limbs, weakness, etc.

Other Species

Vitex trifolia, the three-leaved Chaste Tree, has similar properties.

CHAULMOOGRA

Botanical: Taraktogenos kurzii (KING)
Family: N.O. Bixaceae
Synonyms: Chaulmugra. Chaulmogra.
Part Used: The oil from the seeds.

Description

Seeds are ovoid, irregular and angular, 1 to 1 1/4 inches long, 1 inch wide, skin smooth, grey, brittle; kernel oily and dark brown. A fatty oil is obtained by expression, known officially as Gynocardia oil in Britain, as Oleum Chaulmoograe in the U.S.A.

Constituents

The oil contains chaulmoogric acid and palmitic acid, and the fatty oil has been found to yield glycerol, a very small quantity of phytosterol and a mixture of fatty acids.

Medicinal Action and Uses

Employed internally and externally in the treatment of skin diseases, scrofula, rheumatism, eczema, also in leprosy, as a counterirritant for bruises, sprains, etc., and sometimes applied to open wounds and sores. Also used in veterinary practice. Dose of oil, 5 or 10 to 60 minims. Gynocardia Ointment, I.C.A.

Other Species

The seeds of Gynocardia odorata have been erroneously given as the source of the oil.

Some of the commercial oil on the market probably comes from the allied species Hydnocarpus.

CHEKEN

Botanical: Eugenia cheken (MOL.)

Family: N.O. Myrtaceae

Synonyms: Arryan. Myrtus Chekan.

Part Used: Leaves.

Habitat: Chile.

Description

The flowers grow in the axils of the leathery leaves, white with a fourparted calyx, four petals and numerous stamens; the berry is crowned by the calyx, one or two-celled, containing one or two seeds. The leaves nearly sessile, oval, 1 inch long, smooth, slightly wrinkled, aromatic, astringent, and bitter.

Constituents

Volatile oil, tannin and four principles, viz. Chekenon, Chekenin, Chekenetin, and Cheken bitter, an amorphous, soluble bitter substance. The virtues of the leaves appear to be in the volatile oil they contain and in their tannin.

Medicinal Action and Uses

Most useful in the chronic bronchitis of elderly people and in chronic catarrh of the respiratory organs. Dose: Fluid extract, 1 to 2. fluid drachms.

CHENOPODIUMS

Family: N.O. Chenopodiaceae
Synonyms: Goosefoots. Wormseeds. Spinach. Glassworts. Sea Beets.

The Chenopodiaceae, or Goosefoot order, is a large family of homely and more or less succulent herbs-common weeds in most temperate climates, usually growing on the seashore and on salt marshes and on waste or cultivated ground.

The tribe derives its distinctive name from the Greek words, chen (a goose) and pous (a foot), in allusion to the supposed resemblance borne by the leaves of most of its members to the webbed feet of the goose. The leaves are entire, lobed or toothed, often more or less triangular in shape.

The minute flowers - which are wind fertilized - are without petals, bisexual and borne in dense axillary or terminal clusters or spikes. The small fruit is membraneous and one-seeded, often enclosed by the persistent calyx, which frequently is inflated.

Most of these plants contain large quantities of iron in the form of digestible organic compounds and many of the species provide soda in abundance.

Ten species of Chenopodium occur in Britain, one of which, C. Bonus-Henricus, has been much cultivated as a pot-herb, under the name of English Mercury and All Good. The Garden Orache and the Arrach, the Sea Beet and the Glassworts are other native plants belonging to this large family, which has about 600 members.

The seeds of C. Quinoa (Linn.), of the Andean region of South America, there constitute the staple and principal food of millions of the native inhabitants.

Quinoa is a perennial, indigenous to the high tableland of the Cordilleras, where, at the conquest by the Spaniards, it was the only farinaceous grain used as food. The plant is from 4 to 6 feet high and has many angular branches, dull glaucous leaves, of a triangular outline on long, narrow stalks, and flowers forming large, compact, branched heads and succeeded by minute, strong, flat seeds, of a black, white or red color.

The Quinoa has been introduced into Europe, but though large crops have been grown in France, the grain has an unpleasant acrid taste and will hardly be used as human food when anything better can be got, though the leaves make a pleasant vegetable, like spinach.

But in Peru, Chile and Bolivia, Quinoa is largely cultivated for its nutritious seeds, which are produced in great abundance and are made into soup and bread, and when fermented with millet, make a kind of beer. They are called 'Little Rice."

The seeds are prepared by boiling in water, like rice or oatmeal, a kind of gruel being the result, which is seasoned with Chile pepper and other condiments; or the grains are slightly roasted, like coffee, boiled in water and strained, the brown-coloured broth thus prepared being seasoned as in the first process. This second preparation is called Carapulque, and is said to be a favorite dish with the ladies of Lima, but, as already stated, in whatever way prepared, Quinoa is unpalatable to strangers, though it is probably a nutritious article of food, due to the amount of albumen it contains.

Two varieties are cultivated, one producing very pale seeds, called the White or Sweet variety, which is that used as food, and a dark-red fruited one, called the Red Quinoa. Both kinds contain an amaroid (or bitter substance), in specially large amounts in the bitter variety, which is reputed anthelmintic and emetic. By repeated washings, the substance is removed and the seeds can then be used as a food, like the 'sweet' variety.

A sweetened decoction of the fruit is used medicinally, as an application to sores and bruises, and cataplasms are also made from it.

The grain is said to be excellent for poultry and the plant itself to form good green food for cattle.

CHERRY LAUREL

POISON
Botanical: Prunus laurocerasus (LINN,)
Family: N.O. Rosaceae
Part Used: The leaves.
Habitat: Asia Minor; cultivated in Europe.

Description

A small evergreen tree rising 15 to 20 feet, with long, spreading branches which, like the trunk, are covered with a smooth blackish bark. Leaves oval, oblong, petiolate, from 5 to 7 inches in length, acute, finely toothed, firm, coriaceous, smooth, beautifully green and shiny, with oblique nerves and yellowish glands at the base. Flowers small, white, strongly odorous, disposed in simple axillary racemes. Fruit an oval drupe, similar in shape and structure to a black-cherry, the odor of hydrocyanic acid may be detected in almost all parts of the tree and especially in the leaves when bruised.

Constituents

Prulaurasin (laurocerasin) is the chief constituent of the leaves. This has been obtained in long, slender, acicular, bitter crystals, closely resembling amygdalin, but not identical with it. The leaves yield an average of 0.1 per cent of hydrocyanic acid, young leaves yielding more than the

Medicinal Action and Uses

Sedative, narcotic. The leaves possess qualities similar to those of hydrocyanic acid, and the water distilled from them is used for the same purpose as that medicine. Of value in coughs, whooping-cough, asthma, and in dyspepsia and indigestion.

Dosage

Cherry Laurel Water, B.P., 1/2 to 2 fluid drachms.

CHERRY STALKS

Botanical: Prunus avium and Other Species (LINN.)

Family: N.O. Rosaceae
Part Used: Fruit stalks.
Habitat: Britain, Clermond Ferrand in France, and other parts of the Continent.

Description

The fruit stalks of all species are used, their distinctive characteristics are stalks 1 3/4 inch long, very thin and enlarged at one end.

Medicinal Action and Uses

Astringent, tonic. Used in bronchial complaints anaemia, and for looseness of bowels, in the form of an infusion or decoction. 1/2 oz. of the stalks to a pint of water.

CHERRY, WILD

Botanical: Prunus serotina (EHRL.)
Family: N.O. Rosaceae
Synonyms: Virginian Prune. Black Cherry.
Parts Used: Bark of root, trunk and branches.
Habitat: North America generally, especially in Northern and Central States.

Description

This tree grows from 50 to 80 feet high, and 2 to 4 feet in diameter. The bark is black and rough and separates naturally from the trunk. Wood polishes well, as it is fine-grained and compact, hence it is much used by cabinet-makers. Leaves deciduous, 3 to 5 inches long, about 2 inches wide, on petioles which have two pairs of reddish glands, they are obovate, acuminate, with incurved short teeth, thickish and smooth and glossy on upper surface; flowers bloom in May, and are white, in erect long terminal racemes, with occasional solitary flowers in the axils of the leaves. Fruit about the size of a pea, purply-black, globular drupe, edible with bitterish taste, is ripe in August and September. The tree is most abundant and grows to its full size in the south-western States. The root-bark is of most value, but that of the trunk and branches is also utilized. This bark must be freshly collected each season as its properties deteriorate greatly if kept longer than a year. It has a short friable fracture and in commerce it is found in varying lengths and widths 1 to 8 inches, slightly curved, outer bark removed, a reddish-fawn color. These fragments easily powder. It has the odor of almonds, which almost disappears on drying, but is renewed by maceration. Its taste is aromatic, prussic, and bitter. It imparts its virtues to water or alcohol, boiling impairs its medicinal properties.

Constituents

Starch, resin, tannin, gallic acid, fatty matter, lignin, red coloring matter, salts of calcium, potassium, and iron, also a volatile oil associated with hydrocyanic acid by distillation of water from the bark

Medicinal Action and Uses

Astringent tonic, pectoral, sedative. It has been used in the treatment of bronchitis of various types. Is valuable in catarrh, consumption nervous cough, whooping-cough, and dyspepsia.

Dosages

Syrup, B.P. and U.S.P., 1 to 4 drachms. Tincture, B.P., 1/2 to 1 drachm. Infusion, U.S.P., 2 oz. Fluid extract, 1/2 to 1 drachm. Prunin, 1 to 3 grains.

Adulterant

A spurious cherry bark has been noted which may be distinguished by the fact that no hydrocyanic acid is found when macerated with water.

CHERRY, WINTER

Botanical: Physalis alkekengi (LINN.)
Family: N.O. Solonacea
Synonyms: Alkekengi officinale. Coqueret. Judenkirsche. Schlutte. Cape Gooseberry. Strawberry Tomato.
Parts Used: The fruits and the leaves.
Habitat: Europe. China and Cochin-China. An escape in the United States.

Description

The name of Physalis is derived from the Greek phusa (a bladder), for the five-cleft calyx greatly increases in size after the corolla falls off, thus enclosing the fruit in a large, leafy bladder. The plant bears smooth, dark-green leaves and yellowish-white flowers. The fruit is a round, red berry, about the size of a cherry, containing numerous flat seeds, kidney-shaped. It will grow freely in any garden, but sufficient is found growing wild for medicinal purposes.

The leaves and capsules are the most bitter parts of the plant. The epicarp and calyx include a yellow coloring matter which has been used for butter.

The berries are very juicy, with a rather acrid and bitter flavor. In Germany, Spain and Switzerland they are eaten freely, as are other edible fruits. By drying they shrink, and fade to a brownish-red.

Constituents

Physalin, a yellowish, bitter principle, has been isolated by extracting an infusion of the plant with chloroform. Lithal is sold as an extract of the berries to which lithium salt has been added. The fruit contains citric acid.

Medicinal Action and Uses

The berries are aperient and diuretic, are employed in gravel, suppression of urine, etc., and are highly recommended in fevers and in gout. Ray stated that a gouty patient had prevented returns of the disorder by taking eight berries at each change of the moon. Dioscorides claimed that they would cure epilepsy. The country people often use them both for their beasts and for themselves, and especially for the after-effects of scarlet fever.

The leaves and stems are used for the malaise that follows malaria, and for weak or anaemic persons they are slightly tonic. A strong dose causes heaviness and constipation, but sometimes they have cured colic followed by diarrhea.

While not so prompt in its action as sulphate of quinine, the powder is a valuablefebrifuge.

The leaves, boiled in water, are good for soothing poultices and fomentations.

Dosage

From 6 to 12 berries, or 1/2 an oz. of the expressed juice.

Other Species

P. viscosa (Ground Cherry or Yellow Henbane) can be used in a similar manner.

P. somnifera is a narcotic. The leaves are used in India, steeped in warm castoroil, as an application to carbuncles and other inflammatory swellings. The seeds are used to coagulate milk. Kunth states that the leaves have been found with Egyptian mummies.

The plant sold in pots as Winter Cherry is Solanum pseudo-capsicum.

CHESTNUT, HORSE

Botanical: Æsculus hippocastanum
Family: N.O. Sapindaceae
Synonym: Hippocastanum vulgare (Gaertn.).
Parts Used: Bark and fruit.

The Horse Chestnut, Aesculus hippocastanum, which has also been known as Hippocastanum vulgare (Gaertn.), is an entirely different tree from the Sweet Chestnut, to which it is not even distantly related, and is of much more recent importation to English soil. It is a native of northern and central parts of Asia, from which it was introduced into England about the middle of the sixteenth century.

The name Aesculus (from esca, food) was applied originally to a species of oak, which according to Pliny, was highly prized for its acorns, but how it came to be transferred to the Horse Chestnut is very uncertain; perhaps, as Loudon suggests, it was given ironically, because its nuts bear a great resemblance, externally, to those of the Sweet Chestnut, but are unfit for food. Hippocastanum (the specific name of the common sort) is a translation of the common name, which was given - Evelyn tells us - 'from its curing horses brokenwinded and other cattle of coughs." Some writers think that the prefix 'horse' is a corruption of the Welsh gwres, meaning hot, fierce, or pungent, e.g. 'Horse-chestnut' = the bitter chestnut, in opposition to the mild, sweet one.

The tree is chiefly grown for ornamental purposes,

in towns and private gardens and in parks, and forms fine avenues, which in the spring, when the trees are in full bloom, present a beautiful sight.

Description

The trunk of the tree is very erect and columnar, and grows very rapidly to a great height, with widely spreading branches. The bark is smooth and greyish-green in color: it has been used with some success in dyeing yellow. The wood, being soft and spongy, is of very little use for timber.

It is often used for packing-cases.

The sturdy, many-ribbed boughs and thick buds of the Horse Chestnut make it a conspicuous tree even in winter. The buds are protected with a sticky substance: defended by fourteen scales and gummed together, thus no frost or damp can harm the leaf and flower tucked safely away within each terminal bud, which develops with startling rapidity with the approach of the first warm days after the winter. The bud will sometimes develop the season's shoot in the course of three or four weeks. The unfolding of the bud is very rapid when the sun melts the resin that binds it so firmly together.

The large leaves are divided into five or seven leaflets, spreading like fingers from the palm of the hand and have their margins finely toothed. All over the small branches may be found the curious marks in the shape of minute horse-shoes, from which, perhaps, the tree gets its name. They are really the leaf scars. Wherever a bygone leaf has been, can be traced on the bark a perfect facsimile of a horse-shoe, even to the seven nail markings, which are perfectly distinct. And among the twigs may be found some with an odd resemblance to a horse's foot and fetlock.

The flowers are mostly white, with a reddish tinge, or marking, and grow in dense, erect spikes. There is also a dull red variety, and a less common yellow variety, which is a native of the southern United States, but is seldom seen here.

The fruit is a brown nut, with a very shining, polished skin, showing a dull, rough, pale-brown scar where it has been attached to the inside of the seed-vessel, a large green husk, protected with short spines, which splits into three valves when it falls to the ground and frees the nut.

Cultivation

The Horse Chestnut is generally raised from the nuts, which are collected in the autumn and sown in the early spring. The nuts should be preserved in sand during the winter, as they may become mouldy and rot. If steeped in water, they will germinate more quickly. They will grow 3 foot the first summer and require little care, being never injured by the cold of this climate. They thrive in most soils and situations, but do best in a good, sandy loam.

Part Used Medicinally

The bark and the fruit, from both of which a fluid extract is made. The bark is stripped in the spring and dried in the sun, or by slight artificial heat, and when dry, occurs in commerce in flattened pieces, 4 to 5 inches long and about 1 to 1 1/2 inch broad-about 1 to 1 1/4 inch thick, greyish-brown externally, showing corky elongated warts, and on the inner surface pinkish-brown, finely striated longitudinally. The bark is odourless, but has a bitter astringent taste.

Medicinal Action and Uses

The bark has tonic, narcotic and febrifuge properties and is used in intermittent fevers, given in an infusion of 1 OZ. to the pint, in tablespoonful doses, three or four times daily. As an external application to ulcers, this infusion has also been used with success.

The fruits have been employed in the treatment of rheumatism and neuralgia, and also in rectal complaints and for hemorrhoids.

Preparations

Fluid extract, fruit, 5 to 20 drops. Fluid extract, bark, 1/2 to 2 drachms.

Horse Chestnuts as Fodder

In Eastern countries considerable use is made of

Horse Chestnuts for feeding horses and cattle, and cattle are said to eat them with relish, though pigs will not touch them. The method of utilizing them is to first soak them in lime-water, which deprives them of the well-known bitter flavor inherent in the nuts, and then to grind them to a meal and mix them with the ordinary provender.

CONSTITUENTS

Analysis has shown that the nuts contain 3.04 per cent. water; 2.66 per cent. ash; 10.99 crude protein; oil, 5.34 per cent.; and 73 97 per cent. carbohydrates. Experiments conducted at Wye College proved that the most satisfactory way to prepare the Horse Chestnuts as food for animals was to soak partly crushed nuts in cold water overnight, then boil them for half an hour or so and strain off the water. The nuts were then dried, partially husked and reduced to a meal, which, though slightly bitter, had a pleasant taste and appearance. The meal was fed to a calf, a sheep and two pigs. The calf received up to 5 lb. of the meal per day and made good increase in live weight, and the sheep suffered no ill effects, but the pig refused to eat the food containing the meal. It is concluded that Horse Chestnuts are not poisonous to any of the farm animals experimented with, within the limits of what they can be induced to eat, and that they form a highly nutritious food. Chestnut meal is a fairly concentrated food, and contains about 14 per cent of starch, it being calculated that 1 Ib. of Horse Chestnut meal would be equivalent to 1 Ib. 1 OZ. of feeding barley, 1 lb. 4 OZ. of oats, 1 lb. 8 oz. of bran, and 3 lb. 5 OZ. of good meadow hay.

Experiments made during the Great War proved that for every ton of Horse Chestnuts which are harvested, half a ton of grain can be saved for human consumption, and thus the Horse Chestnuts, though totally unfit for human food, can be utilized indirectly to increase the national food supply.

The genus Pavia is so closely allied as to be now generally grouped with the Aesculus. The Red Buckeye (Ae. pavia) is a handsome small tree with dense and large foliage, together with bright red flowers in large loose clusters in early summer. Sometimes it rises from 15 to 20 feet high, but some of its varieties are only low-spreading or trailing shrubs. The Yellow Buckeye (Ae. flava) is common and sometimes 40 feet high. It has somewhat the habit of the Red Horse Chestnut (Ae. rubicunda), but has smoother leaves. The DWARF HORSE CHESTNUT (Ae. parviflora) is a handsome shrub, 6 to 10 feet high, flowering in later summer. Its foliage is much like that of other Aesculi, and its small, white, fragrant flowers are in long, erect plume-flowers.

CHESTNUT, SWEET

Botanical: Castanea vesca (GÆRTN.)
Family: N.O. Cupuliferae
Synonyms: Fagus Castanea. Sardian Nut. Jupiter's Nut. Husked Nut. Spanish Chestnut.
Parts Used: Leaves and fruit.

The Sweet Chestnut (Castanea vesca or Fagus castanea) has been with some reason described as the most magnificent tree which reaches perfection in Europe.

It grows so freely in this country that it has been by some authorities considered a true native, its claim resting chiefly upon the use of what was for centuries supposed to be Chestnut timber in very ancient buildings, such as the roof of Westminster Hall and the Parliament House of Edinburgh. It is now, however, recognized that the wood of Chestnut loses all virtue of durability when over fifty years old, and though the tree is of very quick growth, the beams in question could not have been grown in fifty years, so it has been proved that they are of Durmast Oak, which closely resembles Chestnut both in grain and color.

It is now generally accepted that the Chestnut is really a native of sunnier skies than ours, but was probably introduced into England by the Romans. Before then it was introduced into Europe from Sardis, in Asia Minor, whence the fruit was called the 'Sardian Nut." From Italy and Greece it seems to have spread itself over the greater part of temperate Europe, ripening its fruit and sowing itself wherever the vine flourishes.

In France, Italy and Spain it attains a great size. Theophrastus called it the 'Euboean Nut' from Eubcea, now Negropont, where it was very abundant.

The famous Tortworth Chestnut, in Gloucestershire, was a landmark in the boundary records compiled in the reign of John, and was already known as the Great Chestnut of Tortworth in the days of Stephen. This enormous tree at 5 feet from the ground measured over 50 feet in circumference in 1720, and was still flourishing some years ago. Many of the trees forming the vast Chestnut forests on the slopes of Mount Etna are said to be even larger. In the Mediterranean region the Chestnut flourishes luxuriantly.

Description

The tree grows very erect when planted among others, is firmly set and massive, the trunk columnar, tapering little, upstanding to the summit. When standing alone, it spreads its branches firmly on every side. Its bark is dark grey in color, thick and deeply furrowed: the furrows run longitudinally, but in age tend to twist, often then presenting almost the appearance of thick strands in a great cable.

The handsome, narrow leaves are large and glossy, somewhat leathery in texture, 7 to 9 inches in length, about 2 1/2 inches broad, tapering to a point at each end, the margins with distant, sharp-pointed, spreading teeth, arranged alternately on the twig. They remain on the trees late in autumn, turning to a golden color, and are then very beautiful, especially as they are not so liable to be insecteaten as are the leaves of the oak. They make useful litter.

The flowers appear after the leaves, in late spring or early summer, and are arranged in long catkins of two kinds. Some of the catkins bear only male flowers, each with eight stamens, and these mature first, the ripe pollen having a rather sickly odor. Other catkins have both kinds of flowers, the majority of them being pollen-bearing, but having also, near the twig from which they spring, the female or fruit-producing flowers in clusters, two or three flowers together in a four-lobed prickly involucre, which later grows completely together and becomes the thick, leathery hull which covers the ripening seeds. The fruit hangs in clusters of these forbidding-looking burs - the brown nuts, which are roundish in shape, drawn up to a point and flattened on one side, being thus enclosed in a kind of casket protected by spines .

Uses

In this country, as a rule not more than one of these nuts matures, and as they rarely come to great perfection, nearly all of those used are imported, mostly from Spain whence they are also called Spanish Chestnuts. The larger and better sorts, called Marones, are the produce of Italy, France, Switzerland and southern Germany, in which countries, especially in southern France and Italy, it forms an important article of diet, constituting in Italy a considerable proportion of the food of the peasantry.

They make an excellent stuffing for turkey, also roast pheasant, which is one of the few forms in which they are eaten here, apart from simply being roasted. Evelyn spoke of them as 'delicacies for princes and a lusty and masculine food for rusticks, and able to make women well-complexioned," and then not unnaturally lamented that in England they are chiefly given to swine.

The meal of the Chestnut has also been used for whitening linen cloth and for making starch. The best kind, the Marones, contain 15 per cent sugar, and by expression yield a thick syrup, from which in turn a very usable sugar can be derived. This variety in France forms the favorite sweetmeat: Marons glacés.

Chestnut makes excellent timber. Though in old age the wood is brittle and liable to crack, when in a growing stage, having very little sap wood, it contains more timber of a durable quality than an oak of the same dimensions, and young chestnuts have proved more durable than oak for woodwork that has to be partly in the ground, such as stakes and fences. It is used for many other purposes, such as pit-props and wine-barrels and formerly Chestnut timber was used indiscriminately with oak for the construction of houses, mill-work and household furniture. In hop-growing districts it is in great demand for poles, and a coppice of prime chestnut is worth over L. 50 (pounds sterling) per acre. It makes excellent underwood and is quick growing. We read of an abbot in the reign of Henry II having a grant made to him of 'tithes of Chestnuts in the Forest of Dean," and in modern days extensive plantings of Chestnuts have been made in the same great forest.

The usual method of propagation is by well-selected nuts, but if the tree is grown with the object of fruit-bearing, grafting is the best method. This is done in foreign countries and the method has been adopted in Devonshire. The grafted trees - called marronniers by the French - are, however, unfit for timber. The most suitable soil for Chestnut trees is a sandy loam, with a dry bottom, but they will grow in any soil, provided the subsoil be dry.

The Chestnut takes its name, Castanea, from a town of the name of Castanis in Thessaly, near where the tree grew in great abundance. It has the same name in different forms in all the European languages.

Part Used Medicinally

The leaves, picked in June and July when they are in best condition and dried. They have also been used in the fresh state.

Chestnut leaves have no odor, but an astringent taste.

Medicinal Action and Uses

In some places Chestnut leaves are used as a popular remedy in fever and ague, for their tonic and astringent properties.

Their reputation rests, however, upon their efficacy in paroxysmal and convulsive coughs, such as whooping-cough, and in other irritable and excitable conditions of the respiratory organs. The infusion of 1 OZ. of the dried leaves in a pint of boiling water is administered in tablespoonful to wine glassful doses, three or four times daily.

Culpepper says:

'if you dry the chestnut, both the barks being taken away, beat them into powder and make the powder up into an electuary with honey, it is a first-rate remedy for cough and spitting of blood.

Recipes

Chestnut Soup

Scald, peel and scrape 50 large chestnuts; put these into a stewpan with 2 OZ. of butter, an onion, 4 lumps of sugar, and a little pepper and salt, and simmer the whole over a slow fire for three-quarters of an hour; then bruise the chestnuts in a mortar; remove the pulp into a stewpan, add a quart of good brown gravy, and having rubbed the purée through a Tammy, pour it into a stewpan; make it hot and serve with fried crusts.

Chestnut Pudding

Put 12 OZ. of chestnut farina into a stewpan, and add 6 oz. of pounded sugar, a spoonful of vanilla sugar, a pinch of salt, 4 oz. of butter, and a pint of milk; stir this over the fire till it thickens, and then quicken the motion of the spoon until the paste leaves the sides of the stewpan; it must then be removed from the fire, and the yolks of 6 eggs incorporated therewith- then mix in gently the 6 whites whipped firm, and use this preparation to fill a plain mould spread inside with butter; place it on a baking-sheet, and bake it in an oven of moderate heat for about an hour; when done, turn it out on its dish, pour some diluted apricot jam round it, and serve.

CHICKWEED

Botanical: Stellaria media (CYRILL.)
Family: N.O. Caryophyllaceae
Synonyms: Starweed. Star Chickweed. Alsine media (Linn.). Passerina
(French) Stellaire.
(German) Augentrosgräs.
Part Used: Herb.

Habitat

It has been said that there is no part of the world where the Chickweed is not to be found. It is a native of all temperate and north Arctic regions, and has naturalized itself wherever the white man has settled, becoming one of the commonest weeds.

From the Groundsel, we naturally from association of ideas turn to the Chickweed, though it is in no way botanically allied to the Groundsel.

Several plants have been named Chickweed, one of them a plant belonging to the Purslane family and four species of Cerastium - the Mouse Ear Chickweeds - but the name especially belongs to the plant in question, Stellaria media, the ubiquitous garden weed, of which our caged birds are as fond as they are of Groundsel, a taste shared by young chickens, to whose diet it makes a wholesome addition.

Chickweed is a most variable plant. Gerard enumerates no less than thirteen species, but the various forms are nowadays merely considered deviations from the one type. Hooker gives three varieties which have been named by other botanists as separate species.

Description

The stem is procumbent and weak, much branched, often reaching a considerable length, trailing on the ground, juicy, pale green and slightly swollen at the joints. Chickweed is readily distinguished from the plants of the same genus by the line of hairs that runs up the stem on one side only, which when it reaches a pair of leaves is continued on the opposite side. The leaves are succulent, egg-shaped, about 1/2 inch long and 1/4 inch broad, with a short point, pale green and quite smooth, with flat stalks below, but stalkless above. They are placed on the stem in pairs. The small white star-like flowers are situated singly in the axils of the upper leaves. Their petals are narrow and deeply cleft, not longer than the sepals. They open about nine o'clock in the morning and are said to remain open just twelve hours in bright weather, but rain prevents them expanding, and after a heavy shower they become pendent instead of having their faces turned up towards the sun, though in the course of a few days rise again. The flowers are already in bloom in March and continue till late in the autumn. The seeds are contained in a little capsule fitted with teeth which close up in wet weather, but when ripe are open and the seeds are shaken out by each movement of the plant in the breeze this being one of the examples of the agency of the wind in the dispersal of seeds, which is to be seen in similar form in the capsules of poppy, henbane, campion and many other common plants.

The Chickweed is also an instance of what is termed the 'Sleep of Plants," for every night the leaves approach each other, so that their upper surfaces fold over the tender buds of the new shoots, and the uppermost pair but one of the leaves at the end of the stalk are furnished with longer leafstalks than the others, so that they can close upon the terminating pair and protect the tip of the shoot.

The young leaves when boiled can hardly be distinguished from spring spinach, and are equally wholesome. They may also be used uncooked with young Dandelion leaves to form a salad.

The custom of giving Chickweed to birds is a very old one, for Gerard tells us:

'Little birds in cadges (especially Linnets) are refreshed with the lesser Chickweed when they loath their meat whereupon it was called of some "Passerina." "

Both wild and caged birds eat the seeds as well as the young tops and leaves. Pigs like Chickweed, and also rabbits; cows and horses will eat it; sheep are indifferent to it, but goats refuse to touch it.

Part Used Medicinally

The whole herb, collected between May and July, when it is in the best condition, and dried in the same manner as Groundsel. It is used both fresh and dried.

Medicinal Action and Uses

Demulcent, refrigerant. It is held in great repute among herbalists, used mostly in the form of an ointment.

The fresh leaves have been employed as a poultice for inflammation and indolent ulcers with most beneficial results. A poultice of Chickweed enclosed in muslin is a sure remedy for a carbuncle or an external abscess. The water in which the Chickweed is boiled should also be used to bathe the affected part.

Gerard tells us that:

'the leaves of Chickweed boyled in water very soft, adding thereto some hog's grease, the powder of Fenugreeke and Linseed, and a few roots of Marsh Mallows, and stamped to the forme of Cataplasme or pultesse, taketh away the swelling of the legs or any other part . . . in a word it comforteth, digesteth, defendeth and suppurateth very notably."

He says that 'the leaves boyled in vinegar and salt are good against mangines of the hands and legs, if they be bathed therewith."

Combined with Elecampane, Chickweed has also been recommended as a specific for hydrophobia, and the juice, taken internally, for scurvy.

The plant chopped and boiled in lard makes a fine green cooling ointment, good for piles and sores, and cutaneous diseases. It has also been employed as an application for ophthalmia.

A decoction made with the fresh plant is good for constipation, and an infusion of the dried herb is efficacious in coughs and hoarseness. The dose of the fluid extract is 10 to 60 drops.

Culpepper calls it 'a fine, soft, pleasing herb, under the dominion of the Moon," and goes on to tell us that:

'It is found to be as effectual as Purslain to all the purposes whereunto it serveth, except for meat only. The herb bruised, or the juice applied, with cloths or sponges dipped therein to the region of the liver, and as they dry to have fresh applied, doth wonderfully temper the heat of the liver and is effectual for all impostumes and swellings whatsoever; for all redness in the face, wheals, pushes, itch or scabs, the juice being either simply used, or boiled in hog's grease; the juice or distilled water is of good use for all heat and redness in the eyes ... as also into the ears.... It helpeth the sinews when they are shrunk by cramps or otherwise, and extends and makes them pliable again, by using the following methods, viz.: Boil a handful of Chickweed and a handful of dried red-rose leaves, but not distilled, in a quart of muscadine, until a fourth part be consumed; then put to them a pint of oil of trotters, or sheep's feet, let them boil a good while, still stirring them well, which being strained, anoint the grieved part therewith warm against the fire, rubbing it well with your hand, and bind also some of the herb, if you choose, to the place, and with God's blessing it will help in three times dressing."

Chickweed water is an old wives' remedy for obesity.

CHICORY

Botanical: Cichorium intybus (LINN.)
Family: N.O. Compositae
Synonyms: Succory. Wild Succory. Hendibeh. Barbe de Capucin.
Part Used: Root.

Habitat

Wild Chicory or Succory is not uncommon in many parts of England and Ireland, though by no means a common plant in Scotland. It is more common on gravel or chalk, especially on the downs of the south-east coast, and in places where the soil is of a light and sandy nature, when it is freely to be found on waste land, open borders of fields and by the roadside, and is easily recognized by its tough, twig-like stems, along which are ranged large, bright blue flowers about the size and shape of the Dandelion. Sir Jas. E. Smith, founder of the Linnean Society, says of the tough stems: 'From the earliest period of my recollection, when I can just remember tugging ineffectually with all my infant strength at the tough stalks of the wild Succory, on the chalky hills about Norwich...."

Description

It is a perennial, with a tap root like the Dandelion. The stems are 2 to 3 feet high, the lateral branches numerous and spreading, given off at a very considerable angle from the central stem, so that the general effect of the plant, though spreading, is not rich and full, as the branches stretch out some distance in each direction and are but sparsely clothed with leaves of any considerable size. The general aspect of the plant is somewhat stiff and angular.

The lower leaves of the plant are large and spreading - thickly covered with hairs, something like the form of the Dandelion leaf, except that the numerous lateral segments or lobes are in general direction about at a right angle with the central stem, instead of pointing downwards, as in similar portions of the leaf of the Dandelion. The terminal lobe is larger and all the segments are coarsely toothed. The upper leaves are very much smaller and less divided, their bases clasping the stems.

The flowerheads are numerous, placed in the axils of the stem-leaves, generally in clusters of two or three. When fully expanded, the blooms are rather large and of a delicate tint of blue: the color is said to specially appeal to the humble bee. They are in blossom from July to September. However sunny the day, by the early afternoon every bloom is closed, its petal-rays drawing together. Linnaeus used the Chicory as one of the flowers in his floral Clock at Upsala, because of its regularity in opening at 5 a.m. and closing at 10 a.m. in that latitude. Here it closes about noon and opens between 6 and 7 in the morning.

History

It has been suggested that the name Succory came from the Latin succurrere (to run under), because of the depth to which the root penetrates. It may, however be a corruption of Chicory, or Ctchorium, a word of Egyptian origin, which in various forms is the name of the plant in practically every European language. The Arabian physicians called it 'Chicourey." Intybus, the specific name of the Chicory, is a modification of another Eastern name for the plant - Hendibeh. The Endive, an allied but foreign species (a native of southern Asia and northern provinces of China) derives both its common and specific names from the same word. The Endive and the Succory are the only two species in the genus Cichorium. There is little doubt that the Cichorium mentioned by Theophrastus as in use amongst the ancients was the wild Chicory, since the names by which the wild plant is known in all the languages of modern Europe are merely corruptions of the original Greek word, while there are different names in the different countries for the Garden Endive.

Succory was known to the Romans and eaten by them as a vegetable or in salads, its use in this way being mentioned by Horace, Virgil, Ovid, and Pliny.

On the Continent, Chicory is much cultivated, not only as a salad and vegetable, but also for fodder and more especially for the sake of its root, which though woody in the wild state, under cultivation becomes large and fleshy, with a thick rind, and is employed extensively when roasted and ground, for blending with coffee.

In this country Chicory has been little grown. There was an attempt in 1788 to introduce its cultivation here as fodder, it being grown largely for that purpose in France, especially for sheep, but it would seem not to have met with success and has not been grown as a farm crop, though it furnishes abundance of good fodder at a time when green food is scarce, growing very quickly, two cuttings being possible in the first year and three in subsequent years, the produce being said to be superior on the whole to Lucerne. Although this plant, being succulent, seldom dries well for hay in this country, it seems valuable as fresh food for horses, cows and sheep: rabbits are fond of it. There has been an attempt since the war to re-introduce the cultivation of Chicory, and it has been successfully grown at the experimental farm of the University College of North Wales at Bangor, and at Kirton, Lincolnshire, for the first time for forty years, was reported in March, 1917, to be yielding 20 tons per acre.

When grown for a forage crop, it should be sown during the last week in May, or first week in June, in drills about 15 inches apart, the plants being afterwards singled to from 6 inches to 8 inches in the row. About 5 lb. of seed will be needed for the acre. If sown too early the plant is likely to bolt. So grown, the crop of leaves can be cut in autumn to be fed to stock of all kinds, such as poultry, rabbits, cows, etc., and in following years, if the crop is kept clean, the foliage may be mown off three or four times. So grown it should of course never be allowed to seed.

On the Continent, especially in Belgium, the young and tender roots are boiled and eaten with butter like parsnips, and form a very palatable vegetable.

Uses

The leaves are used in salads, for which they are much superior to Dandelion. They may be cut and used from young plants, but are generally blanched, as the unblanched leaves are bitter. This forced foliage is termed by the French Barbe de Capucin and forms a favorite winter salad, much eaten in France and Belgium. A particularly fine strain is known as Witloof, in Belgium, where smallholders make a great feature of this crop and excel in its cultivation. The young blanched heads also form a good vegetable for cooking, similar to Sea Kale.

Enormous quantities of the plant are cultivated on the Continent, to supply the grocer with the ground Chicory which forms an ingredient or adulteration to coffee. In Belgium, Chicory is sometimes even used as a drink without admixture of coffee. For this purpose, the thick cultivated root is sliced kiln-dried, roasted and then ground. It differs from coffee in the absence of volatile oil, rich aromatic flavor, caffeine and caffeotannic acid, and in the presence of a large amount of ash, including silica. When roasted, it yields 45 to 65 per cent of soluble extractive matter. Roasted Coffee yields only 21 to 25 per cent of soluble extract, this difference affording a means of approximately determining the amount of Chicory in a mixture.

When infused, Chicory gives to coffee a bitterish taste and a dark color. French writers say it is contrastimulante, and serves to correct the excitation caused by the principles of coffee, and that it suits bilious subjects who suffer from habitual constipation, but is ill-adapted for persons whose vital energy soon flags, and that for lymphatic or bloodless persons its use should be avoided.

Cultivation

Chicory is a hardy perennial and will grow in almost any soil. For use as a salad, the plant may be easily cultivated in the kitchen garden. Sow the seed in May or June, in drills about 1 inch deep, about 12 inches apart, and thin out the young plants to 6 or 8 inches apart in the rows; when well up, water in very dry weather.

For blanching, dig up in October as many as may be needed, and after cutting off the leaves, it is well to let the roots be exposed to the air for a fortnight or three weeks; they should then be planted in deep boxes or pots of sand or light soil, leaving 8 inches between the soil and the top of the box. A cover of some sort is put on the box to exclude the light and the box put into a warm place, either in a warm green-house, under the stage, or, being so hardy, they may be successful in a moderately warm cellar and shed from which frost is excluded. Deprived of light, the young oncoming leaves become blanched and greatly elongated, and in this state are cut and sent to the market. If light is totally debarred, as it should be, the produce will be of a beautiful creamy white color, soft and nearly destitute of the bitter flavor present when the plants are grown in the open air.

The fresh root is bitter, with a milky juice which is somewhat aperient and slightly sedative, suiting subjects troubled with bilious torpor, whilst, on good authority, the plant has been pronounced useful against pulmonary consumption.

A decoction of 1 OZ. of the root to a pint of boiling water, taken freely, has been found effective in jaundice, liver enlargements, gout and rheumatic complaints, and a decoction of the plant, fresh gathered, has been recommended for gravel.

Syrup of Succory is an excellent laxative for children, as it acts without irritation.

An infusion of the herb is useful for skin eruptions connected with gout.

The old herbalists considered that the leaves when bruised made a good poultice for swellings, inflammations and inflamed eyes, and that 'when boiled in broth for those that have hot, weak and feeble stomachs doe strengthen the same." Tusser (1573) considered it - together with Endive - a useful remedy for ague, and Parkinson pronounced Succory to be a 'fine, cleansing, jovial plant."

Chicory when taken too habitually, or freely, causes venous passive congestion in the digestive organs within the abdomen and a fullness of blood in the head. If used in excess as a medicine it is said to bring about loss of visual power in the retina.

From the flowers a water was distilled to allay inflammation of the eyes. With violets, they were used to make the confection, 'Violet plates," in the days of Charles II.

The seeds contain abundantly a demulcent oil, whilst the petals furnish a glucoside which is colorless unless treated with alkalies, when it becomes of a golden yellow. The leaves have been used to dye blue.

SWINE'S CHICORY (Arnoseris pusilla, Gaertn.), also known as Lamb's Succory, is a cornfield weed belonging to a closely related genus. All its leaves are radical, and it has small heads of yellow flowers on leafless, branched flower-stalks. It has no therapeutic uses.

To obtain roots of a large size, the ground must be rich, light and well manured.

Part Used Medicinally

The root. When dried - in the same manner as Dandelion it is brownish, with tough, loose, reticulated white layers surrounding a radiate, woody column. It often occurs in commerce crowned with remains of the stem. It is in odorous and of a mucilaginous and bitter taste.

Constituents

A special bitter principle, not named, inulin and sugar.

Medicinal Action and Uses

Chicory has properties similar to those of Dandelion, its action being tonic, laxative and diuretic.

CHINA

Botanical: Smilax China (LINN.)
Family: N.O. Liliaceae
Habitat: China, Japan and East Indies.

Description

A climbing shrub with tuberous roots, stems prickly, leaves stalked and veined, with a tendril on each side of the leaf stalks. The flowers have globular heads, sessile in the axils of the leaves, Tubers cylindrical, irregular, 4 to 6 inches long, 2 inches thick, slightly flattened, having short knotty branches, with a rust-coloured shiny bark, sometimes smooth, may be wrinkled, internally pale fawn color, mealy, small resin cells, no odor, taste indifferent, afterwards slightly bitter and acrid, not unlike ordinary sarsaparilla.

Medicinal Action and Uses

Alterative, diaphoretic, tonic. China Smilax is used for the same purposes and has much the same properties as the official Sarsaparilla. In large doses it causes nausea and vomiting, especially valuable in weakened and depraved conditions due to a poisoned state of the blood, it is a useful alterative in old syphilitic cases and in chronic rheumatism; it is also used for certain skin diseases. It was introduced into China in A.D. 1535, when it was considered an infallible remedy for gout; in that country the roots are eaten as a food. With alum the root gives a yellow dye and with sulphate of iron a brown color.

The name Smilax was used by the Greeks to denote a poisonous tree, but some authorities consider it is derived from 'Smile," meaning cutting or scratching, having reference to the rough prickly nature of the plant.

Preparations

The compound syrup is mostly used to form a vehicle for the administration of mercury and iodide of potassium. Dose, 1/2 to 1 drachm.

The smoke from sarsaparilla has been highly recommended for asthma.

Other Species

The rootstocks of Smilax Pseudo-China are made into a sort of beer in South Carolina. They are also used to fatten pigs. In Persia the young shoots of some of these species are eaten as asparagus.

CHIRETTA

Botanical: Swertia chirata (BUCH.-HAM.)
Family: N.O. Gentianaceae
Synonyms: Chirata. Indian Gentian. Indian Balmony.
Part Used: Herb.
Habitat: Northern India, Nepal.

Description

This plant first came into notice in Britain in 1829, and in 1839 was admitted to the Edinburgh Pharmacopoeia. It is an annual, about 3 feet high; branching stem; leaves smooth entire, opposite, very acute, lanceolate; flowers numerous; peduncles yellow; one-celled capsule. The whole herb is used and collected when flower is setting for seed and dried.

Constituents

Two bitter principles, Ophelic acid and Chiratin, the latter in larger proportion.

Medicinal Action and Uses

The true Chiretta has a yellowish pith, is extremely bitter and has no smell, an overdose causes sickness and a sense of oppression in the stomach. It acts well on the liver, promoting secretion of bile, cures constipation and is useful for dyspepsia. It restores tone after illness.

Dosages and Preparations

Dried plant, 5 to 30 grains. Infusion of Chiretta, B.P., 1/2 to 1 fluid drachm. Fluid extract, 1/2 to 1 draehm. Solid extract, 4 to 8 grains.

Other Species

In Indian bazaars where Chiretta is much more used than in England, the name Chirata is given to manykinds of Gentian-like plants. The one that is most in use among them is Ophelia augustifolia, the hill Chirata. It can easily be recognized by the stem being hollow, without pith and lower part of stem square. Another adulterant is Andrographis paniculata, also a native of India, one of the Acanthaceae; this in the dried state looks more like a bundle of broomtops, but is used a great deal in India as it has two valuable bitter tonic principles, Andrographolide and Halmeghin.

CHIVES

Botanical: Allium schoenoprasum (LINN.)
Family: N.O. Liliaceae
Synonyms: Cives.
(French) Ail civitte
(Old French) Petit poureau
Part Used: Herb.

Habitat

The Chive is the smallest, though one of the finest-flavoured of the Onion tribe, belonging to the botanical group of plants that goes under the name of Allium, which includes also the Garlic, Leek and Shallot. Though said to be a native of Britain, it is only very rarely found growing in an uncultivated state, and then only in the northern and western counties of England and Wales and in Oxfordshire. It grows in rocky pastures throughout temperate and northern Europe. De Candolle says: 'This species occupies an extensive area in the northern hemisphere. It is found all over Europe from Corsica and Greece to the south of Sweden, in Siberia as far as Kamschatka and also in North America. The variety found in the Alps is the nearest to the cultivated form." Most probably it was known to the Ancients, as it grows wild in Greece and Italy. Dodoens figures it and gives the French name for it in his days: 'Petit poureau," relating to its rush-like appearance. In present day French it is commonly called 'Ail civitte." The Latin name of this species means 'Rush-Leek."

Description

The plant is a hardy perennial. The bulbs grow very close together in dense tufts or clusters, and are of an elongated form, with white, rather firm sheaths, the outer sheath sometimes grey.

The slender leaves appear early in spring and are long, cylindrical and hollow, tapering to a point and about the thickness of a crowsquill. They grow from 6 to 10 inches high.

The flowering stem is usually nipped off with cultivated plants (which are grown solely for the sake of the leaves, or 'grass'), but when allowed to rise, it seldom reaches more than a few inches to at most a foot in height. It is hollow and either has no leaf or one leaf sheathing it below the middle. It supports a close globular head, or umbel, of purple flowers; the numerous flowers are densely packed together on separate, very slender little flower-stalks, shorter than the flowers themselves, which lengthen slightly as the fruit ripens, causing the heads to assume a conical instead of a round shape. The petals of the flowers are nearly half an inch long; when dry, their pale-purple color, which has in Parts a darker flush, changes to rose-color. The anthers (the pollen-bearing part of the flower) are of a bluish-purple color. The seed-vessel, or capsule, is a little larger than a hemp seed and is completely concealed within the petals, which are about twice its length. The small seeds which it contains are black when ripe and similar to Onion seeds.

The flowers are in blossom in June and July, and in the most cold and moist situations will mature their seeds, though rarely allowed to do so under cultivation.

Cultivation

The Chive will grow in any ordinary garden soil. It can be raised by seed, but is usually propagated by dividing the clumps in spring or autumn. In dividing the clumps, leave about six little bulbs together in a tiny clump, which will spread to a fine clump in the course of a year, and may then be divided. Set the clumps from 9 inches to a foot apart each way. For a quick return, propagation by division of the bulb clumps is always to be preferred.

The green from the clumps can be cut three or four times in the season. When required for use, each clump may be cut in turn, fairly close to the ground. The leaves will soon grow again and be found more tender each time of cutting. By carefully cropping, the 'grass' can be obtained quite late in the season, until the early frosts come, when it withers up and disappears through the winter, pushing up again in the first warm days of February. For early crops, a little 'grass' can be forced on the clumps by placing cloches or a 'light' over them.

Beyond weeding between the clumps, no further care or attention is needed after division. Beds should be re-planted at least once in three or four years.

If it is desired to produce seed, grow two plantations, one for producing 'grass' for use, and the other to be left to flower and set seed, as you cannot get the two crops - 'grass' and seed, off the one set of plants.

Uses

The Chive contains a pungent volatile oil, rich in sulphur, which resent in all the Onion tribe and causes their distinctive smell and taste.

It is a great improvement to salads - cut fresh and chopped fine-and may be put not only into green salads, but also into cucumber salad, or sprinkled on sliced tomatoes.

Chives are also excellent in savoury omelettes, and may be chopped and boiled with potatoes that are to be mashed, or chopped fresh and sprinkled, just before serving, on mashed potatoes, both as a garnish and flavoring. They may also be put into soup, either dried, or freshly cut and finely chopped, and are a welcome improvement to homemade sausages, croquettes, etc., as well as an excellent addition to beefsteak puddings and pies.

Chives are also useful for cutting up and mixing with the food of newly-hatched turkeys.

Parkinson mentions Chives as being cultivated in his garden, among other herbs.

CICELY, SWEET

Botanical: Myrrhis odorata (SCOP.)
Family: N.O. Umbelliferae

Synonyms: British Myrrh. Anise. Great (Sweet) Chervil. Sweet Chervil. Smooth Cicely. Sweet Bracken. Sweet-fern. Sweet-Cus. Sweet-Humlock. Sweets. The Roman Plant. Shepherd's Needle. Smoother Cicely. Cow Chervil.
Parts Used: The whole plant and seeds.

Habitat

Mountain pastures from the Pyrenees to the Caucasus. In Britain, in the hilly districts of Wales, northern England and Scotland.

Description

The name Myrrhis odorata is derived from the Greek word for perfume, because of its myrrh-like smell.

It is a native of Great Britain, a perennial with a thick root and very aromatic foliage, on account of which it was used in former days as a salad herb, or boiled, when the root, leaves, and seed were all used. The leaves are very large, somewhat downy beneath, and have a flavor rather like Anise, with a scent like Lovage. The first shoots consist of an almost triangular, lacey leaf, with a simple wing curving up from each side of its root. The stem grows from 2 to 3 feet high, bearing many leaves, and white flowers in early summer appear in compound umbels.In appearance it is rather like Hemlock, but is of a fresher green color. The fruit is remarkably large, an inch long, dark brown, and fully flavoured. The leaves taste as if sugar had been sprinkled over them. It is probable that it is not truly a wild plant, as it is usually found near houses, where it may very probably be cultivated in the garden. Sweet Cicely is very attractive to bees; in the north of England it is said that the seeds are used to polish and scent oak floors and furniture. In Germany they are still very generally used in cookery. The old herbalists describe the plant as 'so harmless you cannot use it amiss." The roots were supposed to be not only excellent in a salad, but when boiled and eaten with oil and vinegar, to be 'very good for old people that are dull and without courage; it rejoiceth and comforteth the heart and increaseth their lust and strength."

Medicinal Action and Uses

Aromatic, stomachic, carminative and expectorant. Useful in coughs and flatulence, and as a gentle stimulant for debilitated stomachs. The fresh root may be eaten freely or used in infusion with brandy or water. A valuable tonic for girls from 15 to 18 years of age. The roots are antiseptic, and a decoction is used for the bites of vipers and mad dogs The distilled water is said to be diuretic, and helpful in pleurisy, and the essence to be aphrodisiac. The decoction of roots in wine is also said to be effective for consumption, in morning and evening doses of 4 to 8 OZ., while the balsam and ointment cure green wounds, stinking ulcers, and ease the pain of gout.

The medicinal properties resemble those of the American variety.

Chervil, or Scandix Cerefolium (fam. Umbelliferae), a native of southern Europe and the Levant, is used only in cookery, and used in the French bouquet of herbs known as 'fines herbes."

American Sweet Cicely (fam. Apicceae) or Ozmorrhiza longistylis. This plant grows in various parts of the United States, on lowlying, moist lands, flowering in May and June. The root has a sweet smell and taste, resembling aniseed and yields its properties to water or diluted alcohol.

CINERARIA MARITIMA

Botanical: Senecio maritima (LINN.)

Family: N.O. Compositae

Synonym: Dusty Miller.

Part Used: Juice of the leaves.

Habitat: Shores of the Mediterranean. Also found on the maritime rocks of Holyhead.

Description

The word 'Cineraria' means ashy grey, a mixture of black and white coloring resulting in the beautiful color of the plant which grows sparsely in the author's garden at Chalfont St. Peter. This plant is perennial, propagated by cuttings, layers, or seeds. It belongs to the groundsel or ragwort family, of which there are nearly 900 different species known to botanists. The species takes its name from Senex (an old man) in allusion to the white hairy pappus which crowns the achenes. The leaves are about 6 inches long, 2 inches wide, pinnately divided; flowers yellow.

Medicinal Action and Uses

The fresh juice is said to remove cataract. A few drops of the fresh juice are dropped into the eye.

CINNAMON

Botanical: Cinnamomum zeylanicum (NEES.)
Family: N.O. Lauraceae
Synonym: Laurus Cinnamomum.
Part Used: Bark.

Habitat

Ceylon, but grows plentifully in Malabar, Cochin-China, Sumatra and Eastern Islands. Has also been cultivated in the Brazils, Mauritius, India, Jamaica, etc.

Description

Grows best in almost pure sand, requiring only 1 per cent of vegetable substance; it prefers a sheltered place, constant rain, heat and equal temperature. The Dutch owned the monopoly of the trade of the wild produce, and it was not cultivated until 1776, owing to Dutch opposition and the belief that cultivation would destroy its properties.

Cinnamon is now largely cultivated. The tree grows from 20 to 30 feet high, has thick scabrous bark, strong branches, young shoots speckled greeny orange, the leaves petiolate, entire, leathery when mature, upper side shiny green, underside lighter; flowers small white in panicles; fruit, an oval berry like an acorn in its receptacle, bluish when ripe with white spots on it, bigger than a blackberry; the root-bark smells like cinnamon and tastes like camphor, which it yields on distillation. Leaves, when bruised, smell spicy and have a hot taste; the berry tastes not unlike Juniper and has a terebine smell; when ripe, bruised and boiled it gives off an oily matter which when cool solidifies and is called cinnamon suet.

The commercial Cinnamon bark is the dried inner bark of the shoots.

Cinnamon has a fragrant perfume, taste aromatic and sweet; when distilled it only gives a very small quantity of oil, with a delicious flavor.

Constituents

0 to 10 per cent of volatile oil, tannin, mucilage and sugar.

Medicinal Action and Uses

Carminative, astringent, stimulant, antiseptic; more powerful as a local than as a general stimulant; is prescribed in powder and infusion but usually combined with other medicines. It stops vomiting, relieves flatulence, and given with chalk and astringents is useful for diarrhea and hemorrhage of the womb.

Preparations and Dosages

Cinnamon Water, B.P., 1 to 2 fluid ounces. Tincture of Cinnamon, B.P., 1/2 to 1 drachm. Oil, B.P., 1/2 to 3 drops. Comp. Powd. Arom., B.P., 10 to 40 grains. Spirit, B.P., 5 to 20 drops.

Other Species

Cinnamon Cassia is often substituted for it it possesses much the same qualities and constituents but is inferior. See CASSIA.

C. Culiawan. Native of Amboyna- the bark has the flavor of cloves.

C. iners. Native of Malabar, seeds useful for fevers and dysentery; bark employed as a condiment.

C. nitidum. Dried leaves are said to furnish the aromatic called 'folid Malabathri."

CINNAMON, WHITE

Botanical: Canella alba (MURRAY)
Family: N.O. Canellaceae
Synonyms: Canella. White Wood. Wild Cinnamon. Canellae Cortex.
Part Used: The bark, deprived of its corky layer and

dried.
Habitat: The West Indies and Florida.

Description

A straight tree, from 10 to 50 feet in height, branched only at the top. The bark is whitish and the leaves alternate, oblong, thick, and of a dark, shining, laurel green. The flowers are small, and seldom open. They are of a violet color, and grow in clusters at the tops of the branches. The fruit is an oblong berry containing four kidney-shaped seeds, and turns from green to blue and then to a glossy black. The wild pigeons of Jamaica eat the fruit, and their flesh is flavoured by them. The whole tree is aromatic, and if the flowers are dried, then softened again in warm water, they have a fragrance resembling musk. Canella was first introduced into Britain in 1600. The Spaniards, on seeing it in America, thought it was a species of cinnamon, and brought it to Europe as 'white cinnamon."

The corky layer of the bark can be gently beaten off, and the inner bark is dried, and exported chiefly from the Bahamas.

In commerce the bark is found in quills or twisted pieces, of a pale orange-brown, with characteristic markings scars, or spots. The fracture is short, granular, and whitish. The odor is agreeable, resembling cloves and cinnamon, and the taste is pungent, bitter, and acrid.

The negroes and Caribs use it as a condiment or spice, and it is sometimes added by smokers to their tobacco to remove the unpleasant odor and make their rooms fragrant.

Constituents

A volatile oil, gum, starch, canellin, bitter extractive, resin, albumen, mannite, etc. The oil has a pungent, aromatic taste, and contains eugenol, cineol, and terpenes. There is no tannin.

Medicinal Action and Uses

An aromatic bitter, useful in enfeebled conditions of the stomach, and often given with other medicines. It was formerly given in scurvy. The powder is used with aloes as a stimulating purgative. It is often sold as a substitute for winter's bark, but it contains no tannic acid, or oxide of iron, both of which are present in the other.

Dosage

10 to 40 grains of the powder.

Other Species

C. axillaris of Brazil. Thought by some authorities to be the source of Malambo bark and Matias bark.

CLARY, COMMON

Botanical: Salvia sclarea (LINN.)
Family: N.O. Labiatae
Synonyms: Clarry. Orvale. Toute-bonne. Clear Eye. See Bright. Eyebright.
Parts Used: The herb and leaves, both fresh and dry.
Habitat: Middle Europe.

Common Clary, like the Garden Sage, is not a native of Great Britain, having first been introduced into English cultivation in the year 1562. It is a native of Syria Italy, southern France and Switzerland, but will thrive here upon almost any soil that is not too wet, though it will rot frequently upon moist ground in the winter.

Gerard, in 1597, describes and figures several varieties of Clary, under the names of Horminum and Gallitricum. He describes it as growing 'in divers barren places almost in every country, especially in the fields of Holborne neare unto Grayes Inne . . . and at the end of Chelsea." It must have become acclimatized very quickly if it was found 'in divers barren places' before the close of the sixteenth century, less than forty years after its introduction into the country.

Salmon, in 1710, in The English Herbal, gives a number of varieties of the Garden Clary, which he calls Horminum Hortense, in distinction to Horminum Sylvestre, the Wild Clary, subdividing it into the Common Clary (H. commune), the True Garden Clary of Dioscorides (H. sativum verum Dioscorides), the Yellow Clary (Calus Jovis), and the

Small or German Clary (H. humile Germanicum or Gallitricum alterum Gerardi). It is interesting to note that this last variety, being termed Gerardi, indicates that Gerard classified this species when it was first brought over from the Continent, evidently taking great pains to trace its history, giving in his Herball its Greek name and its various Latin ones. That Clary was known in ancient times is shown by the second variety, the True Garden Clarv being termed Dioscoridis.

Description

The Common Garden Clary is a biennial plant, its square, brownish stems growing 2 to 3 feet high, hairy and with few branches. The leaves are arranged in pairs, almost stalkless, and are almost as large as the hand, oblong and heart-shaped, wrinkled, irregularly toothed at the margins and covered with velvety hairs. The flowers are in a long, loose, terminal spike, on which they are set in whorls. The lipped corollas, similar to the Garden Sage, but smaller, are of a pale blue or white. The flowers are interspersed with large coloured, membraneous bracts, longer than the spiny calyx. Both corollas and bracts are generally variegated with pale purple and yellowish-white. The seeds are blackish brown, 'contained in long toothed husks," as an old writer describes the calyx. The whole plant possesses a very strong, aromatic scent, somewhat resembling that of Tolu, while the taste is also aromatic, warm and slightly bitter.

History

According to Ettmueller, this herb was first brought into use by the wine merchants of Germany, who employed it as an adulterant, infusing it with Elder flowers, and then adding the liquid to the Rhenish wine, which converted it into a Muscatel. It is still called in Germany Muskateller Salbei (Muscatel Sage).

Waller (1822) states it was also employed in this country as a substitute for Hops, for sophisticating beer, communicating considerable bitterness and intoxicating property, which produced an effect of insane exhilaration of spirits, succeeded by severe headache. Lobel says:

'Some brewers of Ale and Beere doe put it into their drinke to make it more heady, fit to please drunkards, who thereby, according to their several dispositions, become either dead drunke, or foolish drunke, or madde drunke."

In some parts of the country, a wine has been made from the herb in flower, boiled with sugar, which has a flavor not unlike Frontiniac.

Though employed in ancient times and in the Middle Ages for its curative properties, it seems to have fallen into disuse as a medicinal plant, though revived to a certain extent towards the end of the nineteenth century.

The English name Clary originates in the Latin specific name sclarea, a word derived from clarus (clear). This name Clary was gradually modified into 'Clear Eye," one of the popular names and generally explained from the fact that the seeds have been employed for clearing the sight, being so mucilaginous that a decoction from them placed in the eye would 'clear' it from any small foreign body, the presence of which might have caused irritation.

Although the Garden Clary has much fallen into disuse as a medicine, there is a big trade done in it now, mainly in France, for the extraction of its oil as a perfume fixer, and there is undoubtedly a big future ahead for it for this purpose, not only on the Continent, but also in this country.

Uses

The leaves are used to adulterate digitalis. The dried root and the seeds were formerly used in domestic medicine.

Cultivation

Clary is propagated by seed, which should be sown in the spring. When fit to move, the seedlings should be transplanted to an open piece of ground, a foot apart each way, if required in large quantities. After the plants have taken root, they will require no further care but to be kept free of weeds. The winter and spring following, the leaves will be in perfection. As the plant is a biennial only, dying off the second summer, after it has ripened its seeds, there should be young plants annually raised for use.

Constituents

Salvia Sclarea yields an oil with a highly aromatic odor, resembling that of ambergris. It is known commercially as Clary Oil, or Muscatel Sage, and is largely used as a fixer of perfumes. Pinene, cineol, and linalol have been isolated from this oil.

French Oil of Clary has a specific gravity of 0.895 to 0.930, and is soluble in two volumes of 80 per cent. alcohol. German oil of Clary has a specific gravity of 0.910 to 0.960, and is soluble in two volumes of 90 per cent alcohol.

Medicinal Action and Uses

Antispasmodic, balsamic, carminative, tonic, aromatic, aperitive, astringent and pectoral.

It has mostly been employed in disordered states of the digestion, as a stomachic, and has also proved useful in kidney diseases.

The seeds when soaked in water for a few minutes form a thick mucilage, which is efficacious in removing particles of dust from the eye. Gerard says:

'It purgeth them exceedingly from the waterish humerous rednesse, inflammation, and drives other maladies or all that happens unto the eies and takes away the paine and smarting thereof, especially being put into the eies one seed at a time and no more."

Culpepper tells us:

'For tumors, swellings, &c., make a mucilage of the seeds and apply to the spot. This will also draw splinters and thorns out of the flesh.... For hot inflammation and boils before they rupture, use a salve made of the leaves boiled with hot vinegar, honey being added later till the required consistency is obtained."

He recommends a powder of the dry roots taken as snuff to relieve headache, and 'the fresh leaves, fried in butter, first dipped in a batter of flour, eggs, and a little milk, serve as a dish to the table that is not unpleasant to any and exceedingly profitable."

The juice of the herb drunk in ale and beer, as well as the ordinary infusion, has been recommended as very helpful in all women's diseases and ailments.

In Jamaica, where the plant is found, it was much in use among the negroes, who considered it cooling and cleansing for ulcers, and also used it for inflammations of the eyes. A decoction of the leaves boiled in coconut oil was used by them to cure the stings of scorpions. Clary and a Jamaican species of Vervain form two of the ingredients of an aromatic warm bath sometimes prescribed there with benefit.

For violent cases of hysteria or wind colic, a spirituous tincture has been found of use, made by macerating in warm water for fourteen days, 2 OZ. of dried Clary leaves and flowers, 1 OZ. of Chamomile flowers, 1/2 oz. bruised Avens root, 2 drachms of bruised Caraway and Coriander seeds, and 3 drachms of bruised Burdock seeds, adding 2 pints of proof spirit, then filtering and diluting with double quantity of water - a wine glassful being the dose.

CLARY, WILD ENGLISH

Botanical: Salvia Verbenaca
Synonyms: Vervain Sage. Oculus Christi.
Parts Used: Leaves and seeds.

Salvia Verbenaca, the Wild English Clary, or Vervain Sage, is a native of all parts of Europe and not uncommon in England in dry pastures and on roadsides, banks and waste ground, especially near the sea, or on chalky soil. It is a smaller plant than the Garden Clary, but its medicinal virtues are rather more powerful.

Description

The perennial root is woody, thick and long, the stem 1 to 2 feet high, erect and with the leaves in distant pairs, the lower shortly stalked, and the upper ones stalkless. The radical leaves lie in a rosette and have foot-stalks 1 1/2 to 4 inches long, their blades about the same length, oblong in shape, blunt at their ends and heart-shaped at the base, wavy at the margins, which are generally indented by five or six shallow, blunt lobes on each side, and their surfaces much wrinkled. The whole plant is aromatic, especially when rubbed, and is rendered conspicuous by its long spike of purplish-blue flowers, first dense, afterwards becoming rather lax. The whorls of the spike are sixflowered, and at the base of each flower are two heart-shaped, fringed, pointed bracts. The calyx is much larger than the corolla. The plant is in bloom from June to August. The seeds are smooth, and like the Garden Clary produce a great quantity of soft, tasteless mucilage, when moistened. Because, if put under the eyelids for a few moments, the tears dissolve this mucilage, which envelopes any dust and brings it out safely, old writers called this plant 'Oculus Christi," or 'Christ's Eye."

Medicinal Action and Uses

'A decoction of the leaves," says Culpepper, 'being drank, warms the stomach, also it helps digestion and scatters congealed blood in any part of the body."

This Clary was thought to be more efficacious to the eye than the Garden variety.

'The distilled water strengthening the eyesight, especially of old people," says Culpepper, 'cleaneth the eyes of redness waterishness and heat: it is a gallant remedy for dimness of sight, to take one of the seeds of it and put it into the eyes, and there let it remain till it drops out of itself, the pain will be nothing to speak on: it will cleanse the eyes of all filthy and putrid matter; and repeating it will take off a film which covereth the sight."

CLEMATIS

POISON
Botanical: Clematis recta
Family: N.O. Ranunculaceae
Synonyms: Upright Virgin's Bower. Flammula Jovis.
Parts Used: The roots, stems.
Habitat: Europe.

Description

A perennial plant, stem about 3 feet high, leafy, striated, herbaceous, greenish or reddish; leaves large opposite, leaflets five to nine pubescent underneath, petioled; flowers, white in upright stiff terminal umbels, peduncles several times ternate; seeds dark brown, smooth, orbicular, much compressed, tails long yellowish, plumose; time for collecting when beginning to flower.

The leaves and flowers have an acrid burning taste, the acridity being greatly diminished by drying.

Medicinal Action and Uses

The leaves and flowers when bruised irritate the eyes and throat giving rise to a flow of tears and coughing; applied to the skin they produce inflammation and vesication, hence the name Flammula Jovis. They are diuretic and diaphoretic, and are useful locally and internally in syphilitic, cancerous and other foul ulcers. Best suited to fair people, much used by homoeopathists for eye affections, gonorrhoeal symptoms and inflammatory conditions.

Dosages

1 to 2 grains of the extract a day. 30 to 40 grains of the leaves in infusion a day.

Antidotes

Camphor moderates the too violent effects of the drug. Bryonia is said to appease the toothache caused by clematis.

Other Species

Clematis flammula (Sweet-scented Virgin's Bower) is cultivated in gardens, together with C. Vitalba (Travellers' Joy) and C. Virginia (Common Virgin's Bower). C. Viorna (Leather Flower) and C. crispa has been sometimes used in place of C. recta. C. flammula is said to contain an alkaloid, Clematine, a violent poison. From the bruised roots and stems of C. vitalba, boiled for a few minutes in water and then digested for a while in sweet oil, a preparation is made used as a cure for itch, this variety is also said to contain Clematine.

CLIVERS

Botanical: Galium aparine (LINN.)
Family: N.O. Rubiacece

Synonyms: Cleavers. Goosegrass. Barweed. Hedgeheriff. Hayriffe. Eriffe. Grip Grass. Hayruff. Catchweed. Scratweed. Mutton Chops. Robin-run-in-the-Grass. Loveman. Goosebill. Everlasting Friendship.
Part Used: Herb.

Habitat

It is abundant as a hedgerow weed, not only throughout Europe, but also in North America, springing up luxuriantly about fields and waste places.

The natural order Rubiaceae, to which the Madder (Rubia tinctoria) and our common wild plants, the Clivers, the Bedstraws and Sweet Woodruff belong, comprises upwards of 3,000 species. Many of these are of the highest utility to man, both as food and medicine, among the former the coffee-tree, Coffea Arabica, is perhaps of the first importance. The valuable drug quinine is furnished by several species of Cinchona, a South American genus, and drugs of similar properties are derived from other plants of the same tribe, while Ipecacuanha is the powdered root of another member of this order, growing in the forests of Brazil. Many species growing in tropical climates are moreover noted for the beauty and fragrance of their flowers.

Our British representatives are of a very different character, being all herbaceous plants, with slender, angular stems, bearing leaves arranged in whorls, or rosettes and small flowers. From the star-like arrangement of their leaves, all these British species have been assigned to the tribe Stellatae of the main order Rubiaceae. All the members of this tribe, numbering about 300, grow in the cold and temperate regions of the Northern Hemisphere.

Of the fifteen British representatives of the tribe Stellatae, eleven bear the name of Galium (the genus of the Bedstraws), and perhaps the commonest of these is the annual herb Galium aparine, familiarly known as Clivers or Goosegrass, though it rejoices in many other popular names in different parts of the country.

The angles of its quadrangular stalks and leaves are covered with little hooked bristles, which attach themselves to passing objects, and by which it fastens itself in a ladder-like manner to adjacent shrubs, so as to push its way upwards through the dense vegetation of the hedgerows into daylight, its rough, weak stems then struggling over and through all the other wayside plants, often forming matted masses.

The narrow, lance-shaped leaves - about 1/2 inch long and 1/4 inch broad - are arranged in rosettes or whorls, six or eight together, and are rough all over both margins and surface, the prickles pointing backwards. The flowers two or three together, spring from the axils of the leaves and are small and star-like, either white or greenish-white. They are followed by little globular seed-vessels, about 8 inch in diameter, covered with hooked bristles and readily adhering, like the leaves, to whatever they touch. By clinging to the coat of any animal that touches them, the dispersal of the seeds is ensured.

Most of the plant's popular names are connected with the clinging nature of the herb. Some of its local names are of very old origin, being derived from the Anglo-Saxon 'hedge rife," meaning a taxgatherer or robber, from its habit of plucking the sheep as they pass near a hedge. The old Greeks gave it the name Philanthropon, from its habit of clinging. The specific name of the plant, aparine, also refers to this habit, being derived from the Greek aparo (to seize). Clite, Click, Clitheren, Clithers are no doubt various forms of Cleavers, and Loveman is merely an Anglicized version of Philanthropon. Its frequent name, Goosegrass, is a reference to the fact that geese are extremely fond of the herb. It is often collected for the purpose of giving it to poultry. Horses, cows and sheep will also eat it with relish.

The seeds of Clivers form one of the best substitutes for coffee; they require simply to be dried and slightly roasted over a fire, and so prepared, have much the flavor of coffee. They have been so used in Sweden. The whole plant gives a decoction equal to tea.

We learn from Dioscorides that the Greek shepherds of his day employed the stems of this herb to make a rough sieve, and it is rather remarkable that Linnaeus reported the same use being made of it in Sweden, in country districts, as a filter to strain milk; the stalks are still used thus in Sweden.

The plant is inodorous, but has a bitterish and somewhat astringent taste.

The roots will dye red, and if eaten by birds will tinge their bones.

Part Used Medicinally

The whole plant root excepted, gathered in May and June, when just coming into flower.

Chemical Constituents

Chlorophyll, starch and three distinct acids, viz. a variety of tannic acid, which has been named galitannic acid, citric acid and a peculiar acid named rubichloric acid.

Medicinal Action and Uses

Diuretic, tonic, alterative, aperient.

In old Herbals it is extolled for its powers, and it is still employed in country districts, both in England and elsewhere, as a purifier of the blood, the tops being used as an ingredient in rural 'spring drinks."

Fluid extract: dose, 1/2 to 1 drachm.

Modern herbalists and homeopaths still recognize the value of this herb, and as an alterative consider it may be given to advantage in scurvy, scrofula, pso riasis and skin diseases and eruptions generally. The expressed juice is recommended, in doses of 3 oz. twice a day, but as it is a rather powerful diuretic, care should be taken that it is not given where a tendency to diabetes is manifested. Its use, however, is recommended in dropsical complaints, as it operates with considerable power upon the urinary secretion and the urinary organs. It is given in obstructions of these organs, acting as a solventof stone in the bladder.

The dried plant is often infused in hot water and drunk as a tea, 1 OZ. of the dried herb being infused to 1 pint of water. This infusion, either hot or cold, is taken frequently in wine-glassful doses.

The same infusion has a most soothing effect in cases of insomnia, and induces quiet, restful sleep.

A wash made from Clivers is said to be useful for sunburn and freckles, a decoction or infusion of the fresh herb being used for this purpose, applied to the face by means of a soft cloth or sponge.

The herb has a special curative reputation with reference to cancerous growths and allied tumors, an ointment being made from the leaves and stems wherewith to dress the ulcerated parts, the expressed juice at the same time being used internally.

Clivers was also used as an ointment for scalds and burns in the fourteenth century, under the name of Heyryt, Cosgres, Clive and Tongebledes (Tonguebleed), the latter doubtless from its roughness due to the incurved hooks all over the plant.

It was later used for colds, swellings, etc., the whole plant being rather astringent, and on account of this property being of service in some bleedings, as well as in diarrhea. Clivers tea is still a rural remedy for colds in the head.

The crushed herb is applied in France as a poultice to sores and blisters.

Gerard writes of Clivers as a marvellous remedy for the bites of snakes, spiders and all venomous creatures, and quoting Pliny, says: 'A pottage made of Cleavers, a little mutton and oatmeal is good to cause lankness and keepe from fatnesse."

Culpepper recommends Clivers for earache.

CLOVER, RED

Botanical: Trifolium pratense (LINN.)
Family: N.O. Leguminosae
Synonyms: Trefoil. Purple Clover.
Part Used: Blossoms.

Habitat

Abundant in Britain, throughout Europe, Central

and Northern Asia from the Mediterranean to the Arctic Circle and high up into the mountains.

Description

A perennial, but of short duration, generally abundant on meadow land of a light sandy nature, where it produces abundant blossom, forming an excellent mowing crop. Not of great value as a bee plant - the bees not working it for so long as they will the white variety.

Several stems 1 to 2 feet high, arising from the one root, slightly hairy; leaves ternate, leaflets ovate, entire, nearly smooth, ending in long point often lighter coloured in centre, flowers red to purple, fragrant, in dense terminal ovoid or globular heads.

Medicinal Action and Uses

The fluid extract of Trifolium is used as an alterative and antispasmodic. An infusion made by 1 OZ. to 1 pint of boiling water may with advantage be used in cases of bronchial and whooping-cough. Fomentations and poultices of the herb have been used as localapplications to cancerous growths.

Dosages

1 drachm of fluid extract, 1 to 2 drachms of infusion.

CLOVES

Botanical: Eugenia caryophyllata (THUMB.)
Family: N.O. Myrtaceae
Synonym: Eugenia Aromatica.
Part Used: Undeveloped flowers.
Habitat: Molucca Islands, Southern Philippines.

Description

A small evergreen tree, pyramidal, trunk soon divides into large branches covered with a smooth greyish bark; leaves large, entire, oblong, lanceolate (always bright green color), which stand in pairs on short foot-stalks, when bruised very fragrant. Flowers grow in bunches at end of branches.

At the start of the rainy season long greenish buds appear; from the extremity of these the corolla comes which is of a lovely rosy peach color; as the corolla fades the calyx turns yellow, then red. The calyces, with the embryo seed, are at this stage beaten from the tree and when dried are the cloves of commerce. The flowers have a strong refreshing odor. If the seeds are allowed to mature, most of the pungency is lost. Each berry has only one seed. The trees fruit usually about eight or nine years after planting. The whole tree is highly aromatic. The spice was introduced into Europe from the fourth to the sixth century.

The finest cloves come from Molucca and Pemba, where the trees grow better than anywhere else, but they are also imported from the East and West Indies, Mauritius and Brazil.

In commerce the varieties are known by the names of the localities in which they are grown. Formerly Cloves were often adulterated, but as production increased the price lowered and fraud has decreased. Cloves contain a large amount of essential oil which is much used in medicine. When of good quality they are fat, oily, and dark brown in color, and give out their oil when squeezed with the finger-nail. When pale color and dry, they are of inferior quality and yield little oil. Clove stalks are some times imported, and are said to be strongerand more pungent even than the Cloves.

Clove trees absorb an enormous amount of moisture, and if placed near water their weight is visibly increased after a few hours; dishonest dealers often make use of this knowledge in their dealings, and the powdered stems are often sold as pure powdered Cloves.

Constituents

Volatile oil, gallotannic acid; two crystalline principles - Caryophyllin, which is odourless and appears to be a phylosterol, Eugenin; gum, resin, fibre.

Medicinal Action and Uses

The most stimulating and carminative of all aromatics; given in powder or infusion for nausea emesis, flatulence, languid indigestion and dyspepsia, and used chiefly to assist the action of other medicines.

The medicinal properties reside in the volatile oil. The oil must be kept in dark bottles in a cool place. If distilled with water, salt must be added to raise the temperature of ebullition and the same Cloves must be distilled over and over again to get their full essence.

The oil is frequently adulterated with fixed oil and oil of Pimento and Copaiba. As a local irritant it stimulates peristalsis. It is a strong germicide, a powerful antiseptic, a feeble local anaesthetic applied to decayed teeth, and has been used with success as a stimulating expectorant in phthisis and bronchial troubles. Fresh infusion of Cloves contains astringent matter as well as the volatile oil. The infusion and Clove water are good vehicles for alkalies and aromatics.

Dosages

Fluid extract, 5 to 30 drops. Oil extract, 1 to 5 drops. Infusion, B.P., 1/2 to 1 OZ.

COCA, BOLIVIAN

POISON
Botanical: Erythroxylon Coca (LAMK.)
Family: N.O. Linaceae
Synonyms: Cuca. Cocaine.
Part Used: Leaves.
Habitat: Bolivia and Peru; cultivated in Ceylon and Java.

Description

Small shrubby tree 12 to 18 feet high in the wild state and kept down to about 6 feet when cultivated. Grown from seeds and requires moisture and an equable temperature. Starts yielding in eighteen months and often productive over fifty years. The leaves are gathered three times a year, the first crop in spring, second in June, and third in October; must always be collected in dry weather. There are two varieties in commerce, the Huanuco Coca, or Erythroxylon Coca, which comes from Bolivia and has leaves of a brownish-green color, oval, entire and glabrous, with a rather bitter taste, and Peruvian Coca, the leaves of which are much smaller and a pale-green color. Coca leaves deteriorate very quickly in a damp atmosphere, and for this reason the alkaloid is extracted from the leaves in South America before exportation. The Coca shrubs of India and Ceylon were originally cultivated from plants sent out there from Kew Gardens and grown from seeds.

Constituents

Coca leaves contain the alkaloids Cocaine, Annamyl Cocaine, andTruxilline or Cocamine. As a rule the Truxillo or Peruvian leaves contain more alkaloid than the Bolivian, though the latter are preferred for medicinal purposes. Java Coca contains tropacocaine and four yellow crystalline glucosides in addition to the other constituents.

Medicinal Action and Uses

The actions of Coca depend principally on the alkaloid Cocaine, but the whole drug is said to be more stimulating and to have a mild astringency. In Peru and Bolivia the leaves are extensively chewed to relieve hunger and fatigue, though the habit eventually ruins the health. Coca leaves are used as a cerebral and muscle stimulant, especially during convalescence, to relieve nausea, vomiting and pains of the stomach without upsetting the digestion. A tonic in neurasthenia and debilitated conditions. The danger of the formation of the habit, however, far outweighs any value the drug may possess, and use of Coca in any form is attended with grave risks. Cocaine is a general protoplasmic poison, having a special affinity for nervous tissue; it is a powerful local anaesthetic, paralysing the sensory nerve fibres. To obtain local cutaneous anaesthesia the drug is injected hypodermically. Applied to the eye it dilates the pupil and produces complete local anaesthesia. It is a general excitant of the central nervous system and the brain, especially the motor areas producing a sense of exhilaration and an incitement to effort; large doses cause hallucinations, restlessness, tremors and convulsions. Those acquiring the Cocaine habit suffer from emaciation, loss of memory, sleeplessness and delusions.

Preparations and Dosages

Elixir Coca, B.P.C., 1 to 4 fluid drachms. Extract of Coca, B.P.C., 2 to 10 grains. Liquid extract of Coca, B.P., 1/2 to 1 fluid drachm. Fluid extract of

Coca, U.S.P., 30 minims. Tincture of Coca, B.P.C., 1/2 to 1 fluid drachm. Coca Wine, B.P.C., 2 to 4 fluid drachms. Wine of Coca,, U.S.P., 4 fluid drachms. Cocaine, P.B., 1/20 to 1/2 grain.

Adulterants

Coca leaves have sometimes been adulterated with those of Jaborandi.

Poisoning Antidotes

Cocaine rarely enters the system through the alimentary canal, therefore the use of a stomach pump, emetics or chemical antidotes is not usual; strong coffee should be given as a stimulant by mouth or rectum and measures taken to prevent cardiac failure.

COCCULUS, INDICUS

POISON
Botanical: Anamirta paniculata (COLEBR.)
Family: N.O. Menispermaceae
Synonyms: Levant Nut. Fish Berry.
Part Used: Dried fruit.
Habitat: India, Ceylon, Malabar.

Description

A poisonous climbing plant with ash-coloured corky bark, leaves stalked, heart-shaped, smooth, underside pale with tufts of hair at the junctions of the nerves and at the base of the leaves, the flowers are pendulous panicles, male and female blooms on different plants; fruit round and kidney shaped, outer coat thin, dry, browny, black and wrinkled, inside a hard white shell divided into two containing a whitish seed, crescent shaped and very oily.

Constituents

The chief constituent is the bitter, crystalline, poisonous substance, picrotoxin; the seed also contains about 50 per cent. of fat.

Medicinal Action and Uses

The powdered berries are sometimes used as an ointment for destroying lice; the entire fruits are used to stupefy fish, being thrown on the water for that purpose. Picrotoxin is a powerful convulsive poison used principally to check night sweats in phthisis by its action in accelerating respiration, but it is not always successful. It was at one time used to adulterate beers, increasing their reputation as intoxicants; it is an antidote in Morphine poisoning.

Preparations

Fluid extract, 1/4 to 1 drop. Picrotoxin, B.P.

COCILLANA BARK

Botanical: Guarea rusbyi (BRIT.)
Family: N.O. Meliaceae
Synonyms: Sycocarpus Rusbyi. Guarea trichiliodes.
Part Used: Bark.
Habitat: Cuba.

Description

A large Bolivian tree; flowers in axillary clusters; bark ashy grey on the older trees on account of lichen growths; the inner bark is generally thicker than the outer; fracture, coarse fibrous splinters; odor musk like; taste distinctive, astringent and nauseous; leaves pinnate and of peculiar growth, as the lower leaflets fall young ones grow at the end of the same leaf-stalk, which elongates, the lower outer portion becomes woody with an outer bark and a thin pith inside and grows into a branch.

Medicinal Action and Uses

The bark causes vomiting, and often prostration and nausea. In action very like ipecacuanha, but a more stimulating expectorant. Used with success in the treatment of bronchitis and pulmonary complaints.

Preparations

Fluid extract: dose, 5 to 20 drops.

COCKLEBUR

Botanical: Xanthium spinosum (LINN.)
Family: N.O. Annuals in group of Ambroisecae of the Compositae
Synonym: Spiny Clot Burr.
Part Used: The whole plant.

Habitat

South Europe and naturalized in America near sea-coast, Central Asia northwards to the Baltic and many other parts of the globe.

Description

Xanthic flowers belong to a type which are yellow in color and can become white or red but never blue. These plants are spread as weeds or cultivated over a great part of the world. Stem annual, from 1 to 3 feet high, much branched and many spined; these are straw-coloured and divided about 1/4 inch from their base into three slender branches, diverging and sharp. Leaves lanceolate, acute, tapering to short leaf-stalks with two lobes at base; underside is covered with a thick white down. Flowers small, monoecious, those at apex sterile, while the fertile ones are at the base of the branchlets. Fruit, a rough burr with a short beak at the apex and covered densely with hooked prickles.

Medicinal Action and Uses

A valuable and sure specific in the treatment of hydrophobia. An active styptic, local and general. Fluid extract, 1 to 2 drachms. 10 grains of the powdered plant, four times daily.

Other Species

Xanthium Strumarium, a coarse erect annual, 1 to 2 feet high, leaves on long stalks, large broadly heart-shaped, coarsely toothed or angular on both sides. Flower heads, greenish yellow, terminal clusters on short racemes, upper ones male, lower female, forming when in fruit ovoid burrs covered with hooked prickles. The short stout conical beaks erect or curved inwards. It is not a British plant, though is sometimes found there and in Ireland.

COFFEE

Botanical: Coffea arabica (LINN.)
Family: N.O. Rubiaceae
Synonym: Caffea.
Parts Used: Seeds, leaves, caffeine.

Habitat

South-west point of Abyssinia. and cultivated throughout the tropics.

Description and History

The name Coffee is derived from Caffa, a province of Abyssinia. In its wild state the tree grows to a height of 30 feet, but in cultivation it is kept shorter to expedite picking; it has evergreen leaves, smooth and shiny on the upper side, dark green under and paler, 6 inches long, 2 1/2 inches wide; flowers in dense clusters at base of leaves, white and very decorative, but only lasting in bloom two days; berries red and fleshy like small cherries, each berry two-seeded, convex on one side, flat on the other with a long furrowed line running lengthways and covered with a thin parchment which has to be winnowed or milled before roasting, after the outer pulp has been removed by a machine. The roasting develops the volatile oil and peculiar acid to which the aromas and flavors are due. The Coffee shrub was introduced into Arabia early in the fifteenth century from Abyssinia, and for two centuries Arabia supplied the world's Coffee; at the end of the seventeenth century the Dutch introduced the plant into Batavia, and from there a plant was presented to Louis XIV in 1714. All the Coffee now imported from Brazil has been imported from that single plant. The European use of Coffee dates from the sixteenth century when it was introduced into Constantinople, and a century later in 1652 the first Coffee shop was opened in London. In 1858 the quantity imported into the United Kingdom was over sixty million pounds. In Turkey the consumption is enormous, and so necessary is it considered that the refusal to supply a reasonable amount to a Turk's wife is considered a legal cause for divorce.

Constituents of Roasted Coffee

Oil, wax, caffeine, aromatic oil, tannic acid, caffetannic acid, gum, sugar, protein.

Medicinal Action and Uses

An active brain stimulant, which produces sleeplessness, hence its great value in narcotic poisoning; in acute cases is injected into the rectum. Very valuable in cases of snake-bite, helping to ward off the terrible coma. It also exerts a soothing action on the vascular system, preventing a too rapid wasting of the tissues of the body; these effects are not only due to the volatile oil but to the caffeine it contains. The Malays infuse the leaves, which contain even more caffeine than the berries. Caffeine is valuable for heart disease, ascites and pleuritic effusion and combines well with digitalis; also valuable in cases of inebrity; is a powerful diuretic, but loses its effect with use.

Dose

Preparation Caffeine, 1 to 5 grains.

COHOSH, BLACK

Botanical: Cimicifuga racemosa (NUTT.)
Family: N.O. Ranunculaceae
Synonyms: Black Snake Root. Rattle Root. Squaw Root. Bugbane.
Part Used: Root.

Habitat

A native of North America, where it grows freely in shady woods in Canada and the United States. It is called Black Snake Root to distinguish it from the Common Snake Root (Aristolochia serpentaria).

Description

The seeds are sent annually to Europe, and should be sown as soon as the season will permit. It flowers in June or early in July, but does not perfect seed in England, though it thrives well in moist shady borders and is perfectly hardy. It is a tall, herbaceous plant, with feathery racemes of white blossoms, 1 to 3 feet long, which being slender, droop gracefully. The fruits are dry.

The plant produces a stout, blackish rhizome (creeping underground stem), cylindrical, hard and knotty, bearing the remains of numerous stout ascending branches. It is collected in the autumn after the fruit is formed and the leaves have died down, then cut into pieces and dried. It has only a faint, disagreeable odor, but a bitter and acrid taste.

The straight, stout, dark brown roots which are given off from the under surface of the rhizome are bluntly quadrangular and furrowed. In the dried drug, they are brittle, broken off usually quite close to the rhizome. In transverse section, they show several wedge-shaped bundles of porous, whitish wood. A similar section of the rhizome shows a large dark-coloured, horny pith, surrounded by a ring of numerous pale wedges of wood, alternately with dark rays, outside which is a thin, dark, horny bark.

Constituents

The chief constituent of Cimicifuga root is the amorphous resinous substance known as Cimicifugin, or Macrotin, of which it contains about 18 per cent but the bitter taste is due to a crystalline principle named Racemosin. The drug also contains two resins, together with fat, wax starch, gum, sugar and an astringent substance.

Medicinal Action and Uses

Astringent, emmenagogue, diuretic, alterative, expectorant. The root of this plant is much used in America in many disorders, and is supposed to be an antidote against poison and the bite of the rattlesnake. The fresh root, dug in October, is used to make a tincture.

In small doses, it is useful in children's diarrhea.

In the paroxyms of consumption, it gives relief by allaying the cough, reducing the rapidity of the pulse and inducing perspiration. In whooping-cough, it proves very effective.

The infusion and decoction have been given with success in rheumatism.

In infantile disorders, it is given in the form of syrup. It is said to be a specific in St. Vitus' Dance of children. Overdoses produce nausea and vomiting.

Preparations

Fluid extract, U.S.P., 15 to 30 drops. Fluid extract, B.P., 5 to 30 drops. Tincture, U.S.P., 1 drachm. Tincture, B.P., 15 to 60 drops. Cimicifugin, 1 to 6 grains. Powdered extract, U.S.P., 4 grains.

COHOSH, BLUE

Botanical: Caulophyllum thalictroides (MICH.)
Family: N.O. Berberidaceae
Synonyms: Pappoose Root. Squawroot. Blueberry Root.
Part Used: Root.
Habitat: United States and Canada.

Description

A handsome perennial plant, growing in low rich, moist, soil in swamps and near running streams, smooth and glaucous, and bears in May and June a panicle of small yellowish green flowers and one or two seeds about the size of a large pea, which ripen in August. These are sometimes roasted and boiled in water, and given as a decoction resembling coffee.

The berries are dry and mawkish; the root is a hard thick, irregular, knotty, contorted caudex, one to several inches long, with long slender radicles up to 8 inches long, externally yellowy brown, internally whitish to yellow, with a central pith running longitudinally; taste, sweetish-bitter, then acrid and pungent, with a slightly (pungent) fragrant odor; yields its properties to alcohol, water or glycerine.

Constituents

Gum, starch, salts, extractive, phosphoric acid, soluble resin, greenish-yellow coloring matter, and a body analogous to Saponin.

Medicinal Action and Uses

Emmenagogue, antispasmodic, diuretic, diaphoretic and anthelmintic. Said to be successfully used in rheumatism, dropsy, epilepsy, hysteria and uterine inflammation, specially for chronic cases. It is sometimes combined with Mitchella repens and Eupatoria aromatica. In use it is preferable to Ergot, expediting delivery, where delay results from debility, fatigue or want of uterine nervous energy.

Doses

Decoction or Infusion. 1 OZ. of root to 1 pint of boiling water, macerated for 1/2 hour. Dose, 2 to 4 fluid ounces three or four times a day.

Tincture

3 oz. of finely powdered root to 1 pint of alcohol, allowed to soak for two weeks, then well shaken and filtered. Dose, 1/2 fluid drachm to 2 fluid drachms. Fluid extract, 10 to 30 drops. Solid extract, 5 to 10 grains. Caulophyllum, 2 to 5 grains.

COLTSFOOT

Botanical: Tussilago Farfara (LINN.)
Family: N.O. Compositae
Synonyms: Coughwort. Hallfoot. Horsehoof. Ass's Foot. Foalswort. Fieldhove. Bullsfoot. Donnhove. (French) Pas d'âne
Parts Used: Leaves, flowers, root.

Habitat

Coltsfoot grows abundantly throughout England, especially along the sides of railway banks and in waste places, on poor stiff soils, growing as well in wet ground as in dry situations. It has long-stalked, hoof-shaped leaves, about 4 inches across, with angular teeth on the margins. Both surfaces are covered, when young, with loose, white, felted woolly hairs, but those on the upper surface fall off as the leaf expands. This felty covering easily rubs off and before the introduction of matches, wrapped in a rag dipped in a solution of saltpetre and dried in the sun, used to be considered an excellent tinder.

Description

The specific name of the plant is derived from Farfarus, an ancient name of the White Poplar, the leaves of which present some resemblance in form and color to those of this plant. There is a closer resemblance, however, to the leaves of the Butterbur, which must not be collected in error; they may be distinguished by their more rounded outline, larger size and less sinuate margin.

After the leaves have died down, the shoot rests and produces in the following February a flowering stem, consisting of a single peduncle with numerous reddish bracts and whitish hairs and a terminal, composite yellow flower, whilst other shoots develop leaves, which appear only much later, after the flower stems in their turn have died down. These two parts of the plant, both of which are used medicinally, are, therefore, collected separately and usually sold separately.

The root is spreading, small and white, and has also been used medicinally.

An old name for Coltsfoot was Filius ante patrem (the son before the father), because the star-like, golden flowers appear and wither before the broad, sea-green leaves are produced.

The seeds are crowned with a tuft of silky hairs, the pappus, which are often used by goldfinches to line their nests, and it has been stated were in former days frequently employed by the Highlanders for stuffing mattresses and pillows.

The underground stems preserve their vitality for a long period when buried deeply, so that in places where the plant has not been observed before, it will often spring up in profusion after the ground has been disturbed. In gardens and pastures it is a troublesome weed, very difficult to extirpate.

Parts Used

The leaves, collected in June and early part of July, and, to a slighter extent, the flower-stalks collected in February.

Constituents

All parts of the plant abound in mucilage, and contain a little tannin and a trace of a bitter amorphous glucoside. The flowers contain also a phytosterol and a dihydride alcohol, Faradial.

Medicinal Action and Uses

Demulcent, expectorant and tonic. One of the most popular of cough remedies. It is generally given together with other herbs possessing pectoral qualities, such as Horehound, Marshmallow, Ground Ivy, etc.

The botanical name, Tussilago, signifies 'cough dispeller," and Coltsfoot has justly been termed 'nature's best herb for the lungs and her most eminent thoracic." The smoking of the leaves for a cough has the recommendation of Dioscorides, Galen, Pliny, Boyle, and other great authorities, both ancient and modern, Linnaeus stating that the Swedes of his time smoked it for that purpose. Pliny recommended the use of both roots and leaves. The leaves are the basis of the British Herb Tobacco, in which Coltsfoot predominates, the other ingredients being Buckbean, Eyebright, Betony, Rosemary, Thyme, Lavender, and Chamomile flowers. This relieves asthma and also the difficult breathing of old bronchitis. Those suffering from asthma, catarrh and other lung troubles derive much benefit from smoking this Herbal Tobacco, the use of which does not entail any of the injurious effects of ordinary tobacco.

A decoction is made of 1 OZ. of leaves, in 1 quart of water boiled down to a pint, sweetened with honey or liquorice, and taken in teacupful doses frequently. This is good for both colds and asthma.

Coltsfoot tea is also made for the same purpose, and Coltsfoot Rock has long been a domestic remedy for coughs.

A decoction made so strong as to be sweet and glutinous has proved of great service in scrofulous cases, and, with Wormwood, has been found efficacious in calculus complaints.

The flower-stalks contain constituents similar to those of the leaves, and are directed by the British Pharmacopeia to be employed in the preparation of Syrup of Coltsfoot, which is much recommended for use in chronic bronchitis.

In Paris, the Coltsfoot flowers used to be painted as a sign on the doorpost of an apothecarie's shop.

Culpepper says:

'The fresh leaves, or juice, or syrup thereof, is good for a bad dry cough, or wheezing and shortness of breath. The dry leaves are best for those who have their rheums and distillations upon their lungs causing a cough: for which also the dried leaves taken as tobacco, or the root is very good. The distilled water hereof simply or with elder-flowers or nightshade is a singularly good remedy against all agues, to drink 2 OZ. at a time and apply cloths wet therein to the head and stomach, which also does much good being applied to any hot swellings or inflammations. It helpeth St. Anthony's fire (erysypelas) and burnings, and is singular good to take away wheals."

One of the local names for Coltsfoot, viz. Donnhove, seems to have been derived from Donn, an old word for horse, hence Donkey (a little horse). Donnhove became corrupted to Tun-hoof as did Hay-hove (a name for Ground Ivy) to ale-hoof.

The plant is so dissimilar in appearance at different periods that both Gerard and Parkinson give two illustrations: one entitled 'Tussilago florens, Coltsfoot in floure," and the other, 'Tussilaginous folia, the leaves of Coltsfoot," or 'Tussilago herba sine flore."

'Coltsfoot hath many white and long creeping roots, from which rise up naked stalkes about a spanne long, bearing at the top yellow floures; when the stalke and seede is perished there appeare springing out of the earth many broad leaves, green above, and next the ground of a white, hoarie, or grayish color. Seldom, or never, shall you find leaves and floures at once, but the floures are past before the leaves come out of the ground, as may appear by the first picture, which setteth forth the naked stalkes and floures, and by the second, which porttraiteth the leaves only."

Pliny and many of the older botanists thought that the Coltsfoot was without leaves, an error that is scarcely excusable, for, notwithstanding the fact that the flowers appear in a general way before the leaves, small leaves often begin to make their appearance before the flowering season is over.

Pliny recommends the dried leaves and roots of Coltsfoot to be burnt, and the smoke drawn into the mouth through a reed and swallowed, as a remedy for an obstinate cough, the patient sipping a little wine between each inhalation. To derive the full benefit from it, it had to be burnt on cypress charcoal.

COLUMBINE

Botanical: Aquilegia vulgaris (LINN.)
Family: N.O. Ranunculaceae
Synonym: Culverwort (Saxon).
Parts Used: Leaves, root, seeds.

The Columbine, though a wild flower in this country, found occasionally in woods and copses, and in open clearings (generally on a calcareous soil), is more familiar as a garden plant.

Description

From its branching and fibrous root, which is blackish and rather stout, springs a large tuft of leaves, dark and bluish green on the upper surfaces and greyish beneath. These lowest leaves are on long foot-stalks and are large, having a terminal group of three leaflets, and below them on each side another group of three leaflets. The stem-leaves get gradually smaller, the higher they grow up the stem, the uppermost being without stalks and merely threelobed. The flower stems are 1 to 2 feet high, erect and slender, often reddish in color, branching into a loose head of flowers, which are 1 1/2 to 2 inches in diameter and drooping.

The only variety in which the flowers are not drooping is Aquilegia parviflora, which Ledebour describes with the flowers perfectly erect.

When growing wild, the flowers are usually blue or dull purple, occasionally white. The Columbine may be distinguished from all other British flowers, by having each of its five petals terminated in an incurved, hornlike spur. The petals are tubular and dilated at the other extremity.

The flowers are perfumed like hay.

The plant is in blossom throughout May and June. Its fruit is composed of five carpels, cylindrical in form, with pointed ends like a cluster of little peapods, each carpel (or seed vessel) containing many smooth, dark-coloured seeds, which are freely shed when ripe, so that the parent plant is generally the centre of a little colony of seedlings.

The generic name of Aquilegia is derived from the Latin aquila (an eagle), the spurs of the flowers being considered to resemble an eagle's talons. The popular name, Columbine, is from the Latin columba (a dove or pigeon), from the idea that the flowers resemble a flight of these birds. A still older name, Culverwort, has the same reference wort being the Saxon word for a plant and culfre meaning a pigeon.

The Columbine is a favorite old-fashioned garden-flower, being mentioned by Tusser (1580) among a list of flowers suitable 'for windows and pots', Parkinson, in 1629, speaks of the many varieties grown in gardens.

It was one of the badges of the House of Lancaster and also of the family of Derby. The flower is referred to in Hamlet and in one of Ben Jonson's poems:

'Bring cornflag, tulip and Adonis flower,
Fair Oxeye, goldylocks and columbine."

Medicinal Action and Uses

Astringent. It has been employed on the continent, but according to Linnaeus, with very unsatisfactory results, children having sometimes been poisoned by it when given in too large doses. It is no longer used.

Culpepper tells us:

'The leaves of Columbine are successfully used in lotions for sore mouths and throats.... The Spaniards used to eat a piece of the root thereof in a morning fasting many days together, to help them when troubled with stone. The seed taken in wine with a little saffron removes obstructions of the liver and is good for the yellow jaundice."

COLUMBO, AMERICAN

Botanical: Frasera Carolinensis (WALT.)
Family: N.O. Gentianaceae
Synonyms: American Calumba. American Colombo. Radix Colombo Americanae. Frasera Walteri. Frasera Canadensis. Faux Colombo.
Part Used: The dried root.

Habitat

Middle and Southern United States and west of the Alleghanies.

Description

Frasera Carolinensis is chiefly known as an occasional substitute for Calurnba Root, or Jateorrhiza Colurnba, a native of Mozambique. The English name is derived from the African Kalumb.

It is a plant of from 4 to 9 feet in height, with a smooth, erect stem, bearing lanceolate leaves in whorls, and yellowish-white flowers in terminal panicles. The roots are triennial, horizontal, long, and yellow. They should be collected in the autumn of the second or the spring of the third year and cut into transverse slices before being dried. When sliced longitudinally they have been put on the market as American Gentian, and when fresh, their properties closely resemble Gentiana Lutea, the European Yellow Gentian. The sliced root as found in the market has a reddish-brown epidermis, yellow cortex and spongy centre. The taste is slightly bitter and saccharine. It may be distinguished from true Colombo Root by the absence of concentric circles, and the smaller, thicker slices.

Constituents

The root contains a peculiar acid, bitter extractive, gum, pectin, glucose, wax, resin, fatty matter, and yellowcolouring matter.

It may be distinguished from Calumba by the absence of starch (though it contains tannin), and by its change of color when treated with sulphate of iron, remaining unchanged by tincture of iodine or galls. It has not the pectine of gentians.

Medicinal Uses

Tonic, cathartic, emetic stimulant. When dried it is a simple bitter that may be used in a similar way to gentian. In its fresh state it is cathartic and emetic.

Dosages

Of powder, 1 to 3 grains. Of infusion of 1 fluid ounce to 1 pint of boiling water - 2 fluid ounces a day.

Other Species

Coscinium fenestratum is the Columbowood or false Columbo of Ceylon.

COMBRETUM

Botanical: Combretum sundaicum (MIF.)
Family: N.O. Combretaceae Myrobalans
Synonym: Jungle Weed.
Parts Used: Roasted leaves, stalks.

Habitat

Malay Peninsula and Sumatra, and the tropical regions of both Hemispheres

Description

Leaves odourless, taste astringent.

Medicinal Action and Uses

The leaves and stalks roasted have long been used in China in the form of a decoction, as a cure for the opium habit, the daily dose of opium is added to a decoction of the leaves and the patient is given 1 fluid ounce of the mixture every four hours.

Constituents

Combretum contains a large proportion of tannic acid and traces of a glucoside.

COMFREY

Botanical: Symphytum officinale (LINN.)
Family: N.O. Boraginaceae
Synonyms: Common Comfrey. Knitbone. Knitback. Consound. Blackwort. Bruisewort. Slippery Root. Boneset. Yalluc (Saxon). Gum Plant. Consolida. Ass Ear.
Parts Used: Root, leaves.

Habitat

A native of Europe and temperate Asia; is common throughout England on the banks of rivers and ditches, and in watery places generally.

This well-known showy plant is a member of the Borage and Forget-me-not tribe, Boraginaceae.

The plant is erect in habit and rough and hairy all over. There is a branched rootstock, the roots are fibrous and fleshy spindle-shaped, an inch or less in diameter and up to a foot long, smooth, blackish externally, and internally white, fleshy and juicy.

Description

The leafy stem, 2 to 3 feet high, is stout, angular and hollow, broadly winged at the top and covered with bristly hairs. The lower, radical leaves are very large, up to 10 inches long, ovate in shape and covered with rough hairs which promote itching when touched. The stem-leaves are decurrent, i.e. a portion of them runs down the stem, the body of the leaf being continued beyond its base and point of attachment with the stem. They decrease in size the higher they grow up the stem, which is much branched above and terminated by one-sided clusters of drooping flowers, either creamy yellow, or purple, growing on short stalks. These racemes of flowers are given off in pairs, and are what is known as scorpoid in form, the curve they always assume suggesting, as the word implies, the curve of a scorpion's tail, the flowers being all placed on one side of the stem, gradually tapering from the fully-expanded blossom to the final and almost imperceptible bud at the extremity of the curve, as in the Forget-meNot. The corollas are bell-shaped, the calyx deeply five-cleft, narrow to lance-shaped, spreading, more downy in the purpleflowered type. The fruit consists of four shining nutlets, perforated at the base, and adhering to the receptacle by their base. Comfrey is in bloom throughout the greater part of the summer, the first flowers opening at the end of April or early May.

The creamy yellow-flowered form is stated by Hooker to be Symphytum officinale proper, and the purple flowered he considered a variety and named it S. officinale, var patens. The botanist Sibthorpe makes a definite species of it under the name patens.

There is another species, S. tuberosum, found in wet places from North Wales, Stafford and Lincoln northwards into Scotland, and most common in the south of Scotland, though absent from Ireland.

In this form, the stem is scarcely branched and but

slightly winged, the bases of the leaves being hardly at all continued down the stem. Though also covered with hairs, the latter are not so bristly. The root-stock is short and horizontal with slender root fibres. This is a much smaller plant, the stem rarely more than a foot high, rather slender and leafy. The lower radical leaves are much as in S. officinale in form, but with longer footstalks. The flowers, creamy-yellow in color though about the same size as those of S. officinale, are in much smaller masses.

The Common Comfrey is abundantly met with in England, but is rare in Scotland; the tuberous Comfrey is commonly found in Scotland, but is seldom met with in England, the northern counties of England and North Wales being its extreme southern limit, so that except in the narrow zone of country common to both, there will be no possibility of mistaking the one species for the other.

The variety of S. officinale, with a purplish flower, is more common in many parts of the Continent than in England. The purple and yellowish flowers are not found mixed where the plants grow wild: the difference in color is permanent in plants raised from seed.

[In the water-meadows which form such a well-known feature in South Wilts, especially in the valleys round about Salisbury, Common Comfrey is abundant, and the flowers vary in color from creamy-white to a pretty rose-pink; while the purple sort is the commonest. - Note by a Wiltshire writer.]

A variety with flowers of a rich blue color S. Asperimum, Prickly Comfrey, was introduced into this country from the Caucasus in 1811 as a fodder plant. This species is the largest of the genus, rising to 5 feet and more, with prickly stems and bold foliage, the leaves very large and oval, the hairs on them having bulbous bases. It was extensively recommended as a green food for most animals, it being claimed for it that it contained a considerable amount of flesh-forming substances, and was, moreover, both preventative and curative of foot and mouth disease in cattle. It has the advantage of producing large crops, two at least in a season, if cut before the flowers quite expand, and in favourable circumstances even more, so that 40 to 50 tons of green food per acre might be reckoned on. At the time of its introduction, a number of farmers and smallholders planted it. It was found, however that though horses, cattle and pigs would eat it, they never took kindly to it as a forage. Horses in time of scarcity will eat it in small quantities in the green state, though do not care for it dried. It is a useful food in the green state for pigs of all ages, but it takes a little time for them to get used to it. Its feeding value, however, has been proved to be not so very much more than that of grass and though it grows luxuriantly in all moist situations, where the soil is pretty good, it is not adapted for either dry or poor land.

Formerly country people cultivated Comfrey in their gardens for its virtue in wound healing, and the many local names of the plant testify to its long reputation as a vulnerary herb - in the Middle Ages it was a famous remedy for broken bones. The very name, Comfrey, is a corruption of con firma, in allusion to the uniting of bones it was thought to effect, and the botanical name, Symphytum, is derived from the Greek symphyo (to unite).

Cultivation

Comfrey thrives in almost any soil or situation, but does best under the shade of trees.

Propagation may be effected either by seed or by division of roots in the autumn: the roots are very brittle, and the least bit of root will start growing afresh. They should be planted about 2 1/2 feet apart each way, and will need no further care except to keep them clear from weeds.

As a green crop they will yield largely if well-rotted manure be dug between the rows when dressing for winter.

As an ornamental plant, Comfrey is often introduced into gardens, from which it is very difficult to eradicate it when it has once established itself, a new plant arising from any severed portion of the root.

Parts Used Medicinally

The root and leaves, generally collected from wild plants.

Comfrey leaves are sometimes found as an adulteration to Foxglove leaves, which they somewhat resemble, but may be distinguished by the smaller veins not extending into the wings of the leaf-stalk, and by having on their surface isolated stiff hairs. They are also more lanceolate than Foxglove leaves.

Constituents

The chief and most important constituent of Comfrey root is mucilage, which it contains in great abundance, more even than Marshmallow. It also contains from 0.6 to 0.8 per cent. of Allantoin and a little tannin. Starch is present in a very small amount.

Medicinal Action and Uses

Demulcent, mildly astringent and expectorant. As the plant abounds in mucilage, it is frequently given whenever a mucilaginous medicine is required and has been used like Marshmallow for intestinal troubles. It is very similar in its emollient action to Marshmallow, but in many cases is even preferred to it and is an ingredient in a large number of herbal preparations. It forms a gentle remedy in cases of diarrhea and dysentery. A decoction is made by boiling 1/2 to 1 OZ. of crushed root in 1 quart of water or milk, which is taken in wine glassful doses, frequently.

For its demulcent action it has long been employed domestically in lung troubles and also for quinsy and whooping-cough. The root is more effectual than the leaves and is the part usually used in cases of coughs. It is highly esteemed for all pulmonary complaints, consumption and bleeding of the lungs. A strong decoction, or tea, is recommended in cases of internal hemorrhage, whether from the lungs, stomach, bowels or from bleeding piles -to be taken every two hours till the hemorrhage ceases, in severe cases, a teaspoonful of Witch Hazel extract being added to the Comfrey root tea.

A modern medicinal tincture, employed by homeopaths, is made from the root with spirits of wine, 10 drops in a tablespoonful of water being administered several times a day.

Comfrey leaves are of much value as an external remedy, both in the form of fomentations, for sprains, swellings and bruises, and as a poultice, to severe cuts, to promote suppuration of boils and abscesses, and gangrenous and ill-conditioned ulcers . The whole plant, beaten to a cataplasm and applied hot as a poultice, has always been deemed excellent for soothing pain in any tender, inflamed or suppurating part. It was formerly applied to raw, indolent ulcers as a glutinous astringent. It is useful in any kind of inflammatory swelling.

Internally, the leaves are taken in the form of an infusion, 1 OZ. of the leaves to 1 pint of boiling water.

Fluid extract: dose, 1/2 to 2 drachms.

The reputation of Comfrey as a vulnerary has been considered due partly to the fact of its reducing the swollen parts in the immediate neighborhood of fractures, causing union to take place with greater facility. Gerard affirmed: 'A salve concocted from the fresh herb will certainly tend to promote the healing of bruised and broken parts." Surgeons have declared that the powdered root, if dissolved in water to a mucilage, is far from contemptible for bleedings and fractures, whilst it hastens the callus of bones under repair. Its virtues as a vulnerary are now attributed to the Allantoin it contains. According to Macalister (British Medical Journal, Jan. 6, 1912), Allantoin in aqueous solution in strengths of 0.3 per cent has a powerful action in strengthening epithelial formations, and is a valuable remedy not only in external ulceration, but also in ulcers of the stomach and duodenum. Comfrey Root is used as a source of this cell proliferant Allantoin, employed in the dealing of chronic wounds, burns, ulcers, etc., though Allantoin is also made artificially.

The following is from the Chemist and Druggist of August 13, 1921:

'Allantoin is a fresh instance of the good judgment

of our rustics, especially of old times, with regard to the virtues of plants. The great Comfrey or consound, though it was official with us down to the middle of the eighteenth century, never had a very prominent place in professional practice; but our herbalists were loud in its praise and the country culler of simples held it almost infallible as a remedy for both external and internal wounds bruises, and ulcers, for phlegm, for spitting of blood, ruptures, hemorrhoids, etc. For ulcers of the stomach and liver especially, the root (the part used) was regarded as of sovereign virtue. It is precisely for such complaints as these that Allantoin, obtained from the rhizome of the plant, is now prescribed. One old Syrupus de Symphyto was a rather complicated preparation. Gerard has a better formula, also a compound, which he highly recommends for ulcers of the lungs. The old Edinburgh formula is the simplest and probably the best: Fresh Comfrey leaves and fresh plantain leaves, of each lb.ss.; bruise them and well squeeze out the juice, add to the dregs spring water lb.ij.; boil to half, and mix the strained liquor with the expressed juice; add an equal quantity of white sugar and boil to a syrup."

Culpepper says:

'The great Comfrey ("great" to distinguish it from the "Middle Comfrey" - another name for the Bugle) restrains spitting of blood. The root boiled in water or wine and the decoction drank, heals inward hurts, bruises, wounds and ulcers of the lungs, and causes the phlegm that oppresses him to be casily spit forth.... A syrup made there of is very effectual in inward hurts, and the distilled water for the same purpose also, and for outward wounds or sores in the fleshy or sinewy parts of the body, and to abate the fits of agues and to allay the sharpness of humours. A decoction of the leaves is good for those purposes, but not so effectual as the roots. The roots being outwardly applied cure fresh wounds or cuts immediately, being bruised and laid thereto; and is specially good for ruptures and broken bones, so powerful to consolidate and knit together that if they be boiled with dissevered pieces of flesh in a pot, it will join them together again."

He goes on to describe its curative effect on hemorrhoids and continues:

'The roots of Comfrey taken fresh, beaten small and spread upon leather and laid upon any place troubled with the gout presently gives ease: and applied in the same manner it eases pained joints and tends to heal running ulcers, gangrenes, mortifications, for which it hath by often experience been found helpful."

The young leaves form a good green vegetable, and are not infrequently eaten by country people. When fully grown they become, however, coarse and unpleasant in taste. They have been used to flavor cakes and other food.

In some parts of Ireland Comfrey is eaten as a cure for defective circulation and poverty of blood, being regarded as a perfectly safe and harmless remedy.

Comfrey roots, together with Chichory and Dandelion roots, are used to make a well-known vegetation 'Coffee," that tastes practically the same as ordinary coffee, with none of its injurious effects.

A strong decoction has been used on the Continent for tanning leather, and in Angora a sort of glue is got from the common Comfrey, which is used for spinning the famous fleeces of that country.

In that inimitable little book by Russell George Alexander, called A Plain Plantain, in which he quotes from an old MS. inscribed 'Madam Susanna Avery, Her Book, May ye 12th Anno Domini 1688," we find the following reference to Comfrey: 'From the French conserve, Latin conserva - healing: conserves - to boil together; to heal. A Wound Herb." 'The roots," says a sixteenthcentury writer, 'heal all inwarde woundes and burstings," and Baker (Jewell of Health, 1567) says: 'The water of the Greater Comferie druncke helpeth such as are bursten, and that have broken the bone of the legge." In cookery, the leaves gathered young may be used as a substitute for Spinach; the young shoots have been eaten after blanching by forcing them to grow through heaps of earth.

CONDURANGO

Botanical: Gonolobus Condurango (NICHOLS)
Family: N.O. Asclepiadaceae
Synonyms: Condurango Blanco. Marsdenia Condurango.
Part Used: Bark.
Habitat: Ecuador, South America.

Description

The product of an asclepiadaceous vine about 30 feet long and 2 feet in diameter. The bark is beaten with a mallet to separate it from the stem when it has been sun-dried. In commerce it occurs in quilled pieces 2 to 4 inches long and 1/2 inch in diameter. External surface, pale greyish brown to dark brown, nearly smooth, more or less scaly and roughened, with numerous warts or lenticels, the scales soft with sometimes a brownish-black fungus on them, inner side whity brown and longitudinally striate; fracture short, fibrous, granular; odor slightly aromatic, specially in the fresh drug; taste bitter and aromatic; yields not more than 12 per cent of ash.

Constituents

A large quantity of tannin, a glucoside and an alkaloid resembling strychnine in its action.

Medicinal Action and Uses

Diuretic stomachic, alterative. Has been regarded as a potential remedy for cancer and is useful in the early stages, but has no effect in the progress of the disease. There are many varieties of the plant, and the species experimented with in cancer is the Condurango blanco, which may be considered a genuine C. Cortex. It is largely used in South America as an alterative in chronic syphilis and is of great benefit.

It increases the circulation.

Dose

Fluid extract, 1/2 to 1 drachm.

Caution

Overdoses produce convulsions, ending in paralysis, vertigo and disturbed sight.

CONTRAYERVA

Botanical: Dorstenia Contrayerva (LINN.)
Family: N.O. Urticaceae
Synonyms: Dorstenia Houstoni (LINN.).
Part Used: Root.
Habitat: Native of Mexico, West Indies and Peru.

Description

Name derived from a Spanish-American word signifying counterpoison or antidote. It is probable that the root sold as Contrayerva is derived from several species of Dorstenia, others being Dorstenia Houstoni and D. Drabena, the former growing near Campeachy, the latter near Vera Cruz. The official root is the product of D. Brasiliensis and comes from Brazil. The commercial root is oblong, 1 or 2 inches long, thickness varies, hard rough solid, outside reddish brown, paler inside, odor aromatic, taste warm, bitter, pungent, rootlets notas strong as main tubes. The root properties are extracted by alcohol and boiling water, and makes a very mucilaginous decoction.

Constituents

Cajupine and contrayerbine.

Medicinal Action and Uses

Stimulant, tonic, and diaphoretic; given in cases of low fevers, typhoid, dysentery, diarrhea, and other illnesses needing a stimulant.

Dose

1/2 drachm of powdered root, or 1 oz. to 1 pint infused in boiling water.

CONVOLVULUS, FIELD

Botanical: Convolvulus arvensis (LINN.)
Family: N.O. Convolvulaceae
Synonyms: Cornbind. Ropebind. Withywind. Bearwind. Jack-run'-in'-the-Country. Devil's Garters. Hedge Bells.
Parts Used: Root, root resin.

Although the blossoms of the Field Convolvulus (C. arvensis) are some of the prettiest and daintiest of our native wild-flowers, the plant which bears them ranks among the most troublesome of weeds to the farmer not only creeping up his hedges, but strangling his corn and spreading over everything within its reach. In North America it has intruded as a most unwelcome immigrant, persistently covering the ground with its trailing stems.

Its roots run very deeply into the ground and extend over a large area. It is, therefore, extremely difficult to extirpate, for the long roots are brittle and readily snap, and any portion left in the ground will soon grow as vigorously as ever and send up shoots to the surface, so that in a very brief time it is again spreading over the ground and climbing over everything in its way.

Its delicate creeping stems grow with great rapidity, either when found on banks trailing along the ground amidst the grass or climbing wherever they find a support. Their ends swing slowly and continuously in circles and twine round anything with which they may happen to come in contact. It has been found that a Bindweed stem in favourable circumstances will make a complete revolution in about 1 3/4 hours, which explains the rapidity of its growth.

The generic name of the plant is derived from the Latin convolvo (to intertwine), and is descriptive of its general growth, for it does not, like many climbers, support itself by tendrils, but the whole plant twists itself tightly round the object that supports it - ordinarily a stalk of corn, or some other plant or object of similar size: it is never found twining round anything of bulky dimensions, such as gate-posts, etc. Its English name, Bindweed, is similarly given it for its habit of twining round and matting together all other plants near it. The Latin specific name, arvensis, is derived from arvum (a cornfield), because this species of Convolvulus, though commonly enough met with in waste places, is one of the characteristic flowers of the cornfield.

Professor Henslow remarks that this Field Convolvulus invariably twines round some stalk or object of small diameter.

Description

It is a perennial and has a long period of blooming, generally beginning to flower about the first week of June, and being found in blossom throughout the summer and autumn months. The leaves are arrow-shaped in form, but often very variable, the extremity of the leaf being in some cases far more acute than in others, and the lobes at the base more elongated. They are placed singly along the stem at very regular intervals.

From the axils of the leaves - the points at which their stalks join the main stemspring the flower-stalks, one to each leaf all up the stem. These flower-stalks often fork into two smaller ones, each bearing a bud. One of these lesser stalks is almost invariably smaller than the other, bearing a bud in an earlier stage of development, so that although the buds occur in pairs on the flower-stem, the flowers never expand at the same time, but always appear singly. At the junction of the flower-stalk and the main stem are a pair of very small scale-like bracts.

The flowers have trumpet-shaped corollas which vary a great deal in color - in some plants they are almost white, whilst in others the normal pink becomes almost crimson. On the underside are five dark pink rays. In the bud the petals are folded into five pleats, the outermost part of the fold being these deep pink rays. At the bottom of the flower are what appear to be the mouths of five tubes, or pipes, running downwards, the tubes being formed by the flattened filaments of the stamens being joined to the corolla tube and yet projecting ridge-like into the flower. Flowers with tubes like these are known as 'revolver flowers," because of the resemblance to the barrels of a revolver: the Gentians are another example. These tubes lead to the nectar which is contained in five small sacs, one at the base of each tube. To get to the honey an insect has to thrust its proboscis down each tube in turn, but whilst doing so, he knocks against the pollen in the anther placed just above it, and by carrying that pollen to the next flower it effects its cross-fertilization. In spite of this arrangement, it is a strange and unexplained fact that the flowers seldom set seeds, though the open corollas are visited by many insects, attracted by the nectar and by the faint perfume of vanilla that characterizes it. The failure to set seed is, however, quite compensated for by the vitality of its widely spreading, much branched roots, on which it chiefly depends for its propagation.

The Convolvulus is very sensitive to weather conditions, always closing in rain, to open again with the return of sunshine. It also closes at night. Its blossoms give a deep yellow or orange tint to water, which is heightened by alum and alkalies.

It is found wild throughout Europe, in Siberia, China, Persia and India, in North America where it has been introduced, and in Chile.

COOLWORT

Botanical: Tiarella Cordifolia (LINN.)
Family: N.O. Saxifragaceae
Synonyms: Foam Flower. Mitrewort
Part Used: Whole herb.
Habitat: North America from Canada to Virginia.

Description

Perennial, forms a neat little edging with tiny white spiraea-like flowers, buds tinged pink, grows in the author's garden, and, given air and sunlight, in a light rich soil thrives well. It has simple leaves spotted and veined deep red; basal leaves turn a rich red orange. Needs dividing every second year. Seeds are few, sub-globose. Taste slightly stringent, odourless.

Medicinal Action and Uses

Tonic, diuretic. Of value in gravel and other diseases of the bladder, and as a tonic in indigestion and dyspepsia, corrects acidity and aids the liver.

Dose

For an infusion or decoction, 1 OZ. to the pint of water; take freely 4 oz. of the infusion two or three times daily till conditions improve.

COPAIBA

Botanical: Copaifera Langsdorffii (DESF.)
Family: N.O. Leguminosae
Synonyms: Copaiva. Balsam Copaiba. Copaiba officinalis.
Part Used: Oleoresin.
Habitat: Brazil and north of South Africa.

Description

An oleoresin obtained from a South American species of Copaiba, by an incision in the trunk. It was first noticed in England in 1625, in a work published by Purchas. There are many species in South America, all yielding Copaiba- a single tree is said to yield about 40 litres. The first yield is clear, colorless and very thin, but in contact with the air its consistency soon becomes thicker and yellower. It is most largely collected from Para and Maranhao in Brazil, and is brought to this country in small casks and barrels; large quantities also come from Maracaibo in Venezuela, and it is also exported from Angostura, Cayenne, Rio Janeiro and some of the West Indian Islands. The variety that comes from Venezuela is more viscid and darker in color.

Constituents

Volatile oil, resin. Amorphous resin acids and resenes.

Copaiba is a clear transparent liquid of the consistency of olive oil, pale yellow with a peculiar but not unpleasant odor, taste bitterish, hot and nauseous; the substance it most closely resembles is turpentine. As it contains no benzoic acid, it cannot properly be called a resin.

Medicinal Action and Uses

Stimulant, diuretic, carminative, laxative; in large doses purgative, causing nausea, vomiting, strangury, bloody urine and fever. A good remedy for chronic catarrh and bronchitis, as it assists expectoration and is antiseptic; is given with advantage in leucorrhoea, chronic cystitis, diarrhea and hemorrhoids. It is chiefly used in gonorrhea (though not advocated for chronic cases), often combined with cubebs and sandal. It has also been recommended externally for chilblains. Both the volatile oil and resin are greatly altered when expelled in the urine, and when precipitated by nitric acid might be mistaken for albumen; it is considered a valuable hydragogue diuretic in obstinate dropsy.

It creates an irritant action on the whole mucous membrane, imparts a peculiar odor to the urine and breath, causes an eruption resembling measles attended with irritation and tingling; it is the resin, not the oleoresin, that is used as a diuretic.

Preparations and Dosages

Oil, B.P., 5 to 20 drops. For obstinate dropsy, 15 to 20 grains three times daily. Usually taken in pill or capsule form (10 to 15 minims), or in the form of an emulsion.

CORIANDER

Botanical: Coriandrum sativum (LINN.)
Family: N.O. Umbelliferae
Parts Used: Fruit and fresh leaves.

Habitat

Coriander, an umbelliferous plant indigenous to southern Europe, is found occasionally in Britain in fields and waste places, and by the sides of rivers. It is frequently found in a semi-wild state in the east of England, having escaped from cultivation.

Description

It is an annual, with erect stems, 1 to 3 feet high, slender and branched. The lowest leaves are stalked and pinnate, the leaflets roundish or oval, slightly lobed. The segments of the uppermost leaves are linear and more divided. The flowers are in shortly-stalked umbels, five to ten rays, pale mauve, almost white, delicately pretty. The seed clusters are very symmetrical and the seeds fall as soon as ripe. The plant is bright green, shining, glabrous and intensely foetid.

Gerard described it as follows:

'The common kind of Coriander is a very striking herb, it has a round stalk full of branches, two feet long. The leaves are almost like the leaves of the parsley, but later on become more jagged, almost like the leaves of Fumitorie, but a great deal smaller and tenderer. The flowers are white and grow in round tassels like Dill."

The inhabitants of Peru are so fond of the taste and smell of this herb that it enters into almost all their dishes, and the taste is often objectionable to any but a native. Both in Peru and in Egypt, the leaves are put into soup.

The seeds are quite round like tiny balls. They lose their disagreeable scent on drying and become fragrant- the longer they are kept, the more fragrant they become.

Coriander was originally introduced from the East, being one of the herbs brought to Britain by the Romans. As an aromatic stimulant and spice, it has been cultivated and used from very ancient times. It was employed by Hippocrates and other Greek physicians.

The name Coriandrum, used by Pliny, is derived from koros, (a bug), in reference to the foetid smell of the leaves.

Pliny tells us that 'the best (Coriander) came from Egypt," and from thence no doubt the Israelites gained their knowledge of its properties.

The Africans are said to have called this herb by a similar name (goid), which Gesenius derives from a verb (gadad), signifying 'to cut," in allusion to the furrowed appearance of the fruit.

It is still much used in the East as a condiment, and forms an ingredient in curry powder.

In the northern countries of Europe, the seeds are sometimes mixed with bread, but the chief consumption of Coriander seed in this country is in flavoring certain alcoholic liquors, for which purpose it is largely grown in Essex. Distillers of gin make use of it, and veterinary surgeons employ it as a drug for cattle and horses. The fruit is the only part of the plant that seems to have any medical or dietetical reputation.

Confectioners form from the seeds little, round pink and white comfits for children.

It is included in the British Pharmacopeia, but it is

chiefly used to disguise unpleasant medicine.

A power of conferring immortality is thought by the Chinese to be a property of the seeds.

Turner says (1551): “”Coriandre layd to wyth breade or barly mele is good for Saynt Antonyes fyre” (the erysipelas: so called because it was supposed to have been cured by the intercession of St. Anthony). Coriander cakes are seldom made now.”

Cultivation

Coriander likes a warm, dry, light soil, though it also does well in the somewhat heavy soil of Essex.

Sow in mild, dry weather in April, in shallow drills, about 1/2 inch deep and 8 or 9 inches apart, and cover it evenly with the soil. The seeds are slow in germinating. The seeds may also be sown in March, in heat, for planting out in May.

As the seeds ripen, about August, the disagreeable odor gives place to a pleasant aroma, and the plant is then cut down with sickles and when dry the fruit is threshed out.

The best land yields on an average 15 cwt. per acre. It is grown to a small extent in the Eastern counties, but more especially in Essex. It is also cultivated in various parts of Continental Europe, and in northern Africa, Malta and India.

Parts Used

The fruit, and sometimes for salads and soups - the fresh leaves.

The fruit (so-called seeds) are of globular form, beaked, finely ribbed, yellowish-brown 1/5 inch in diameter, with five longitudinal ridges, separable into two halves (the mericarps), each of which is concave internally and shows two broad, longitudinal oil cells (vittae). The seeds have an aromatic taste and, when crushed, a characteristic odor.

Constituents

Coriander fruit contains about 1 per cent of volatile oil, which is the active ingredient. It is pale yellow or colorless, and has the odor of Coriander and a mild aromatic taste. The fruit yields about 5 per cent of ash and contains also malic acid, tannin and some fatty matter.

Coriander fruit of the British Pharmacopoeia is directed to be obtained from plants cultivated in Britain, the fruit before being submitted to distillation being brushed or bruised.

The English-grown are said to have the finest flavor, though the Russian and German are the richest in oil. The Mogadore are the largest and brightest, but contain less oil, and the Bombay fruit, which are also large, are distinguished by their oval shape and yield the least oil of any.

Medicinal Action and Uses

Stimulant, aromatic and carminative. The powdered fruit, fluid extract and oil are chiefly used medicinally as flavoring to disguise the taste of active purgatives and correct their griping tendencies. It is an ingredient of the following compound preparations of the Pharmacopeia: confection, syrup and tincture of senna, and tincture and syrup of Rhubarb, and enters also into compounds with angelica gentian, jalap, quassia and lavender. As a corrigent to senna, it is considered superior to other aromatics.

If used too freely the seeds become narcotic.

Coriander water was formerly much esteemed as a carminative for windy colic.

Preparations

Powdered fruit: dose, 10 to 60 grains. Fluid extract, 5 to 30 drops. B.P.: dose, 1/2 to 3 drops.

Recipes

‘Lucknow’ Curry Powder

1 OZ. ginger, 1 OZ. Coriander seed, 1 OZ. cardamum seed, 1/4 oz. best Cayenne powder, 3 oz. turmeric.

Have the best ingredients powdered at the druggist’s into a fine powder and sent home in different papers. Mix them well before the fire, then put the mixture into a widemouthed bottle, cork well, and keep it in a dry place. - (From an old Family Cookerybook in the author's possession.)

CORKWOOD TREE

Botanical: Duboisia myoporoides
Family: N.O. Solanaceae
Synonym: Duboisia.
Part Used: Leaves.
Habitat: New South Wales and Queensland, Australia; New Caledonia.

Description

A tall glabrous shrub or small tree, flowers, axillary clusters, white with two-lipped calyx; corolla, funnel-shaped; limb, five parted; five stamens within the corolla (two long and two short); one rudimentary ovary, two many-ovalled compartments and fruit berry-like; leaves, inodorous and bitter taste. Another species, Duboisia Hoopwoodii, contains an acrid liquid alkaloid, Piturine, which is said to be identical with nicotine; it is largely used by the natives of Central Australia rather in the same way that the Indians use Coca leaves. It is obtained from the leaves and twigs, which are collected while the flowers are in bloom in August; the natives smoke and chew it for its stimulating effect, which enables them to work at high pressure without food.

Constituents

Alkaloidal sulphates, mainly hyoscyamine and hyoscine.

Medicinal Action and Uses

Sedative, hypnotic and mydriatic (of variable strength), which augments the activity of the respiratory system. Its alkaloid, Sulphate of Duboisia, is sometimes used as a substitute for atropine. The homeopaths use the tincture and the alkaloid for paralysis and eye affections; a red spot interfering with vision is an indication for its use. It is antidoted by coffee and lemon-juice.

CORN COCKLE

Botanical: Agrostemna Githago
Lychnis Githago
Family: N.O. Caryophyllaceae
Synonyms: Corn Pink. Corn Campion. Ray. Nigella. Zizany. Darnel. Tare. Gith. Lychnis. Githage. Agrostemma. Pseudo-melanthium. Lolium.
Part Used: Seeds.

Description

A well-known Corn weed, with large entire purple petals.

'An annual herb of the Pink family; one of the Campions. The tall, slender stem, 2 to 4 feet high, has a dense coat of white hairs. The narrow, lance-shaped leaves, 4 to 5 inches in length, are produced in pairs and their stalkless bases meet around the stem. The large solitary flowers have very long stalks which issue from the axils of the leaves. They are 1 1/2 and 2 inches broad, with purple petals which have pale streaks ("honey guides"), showing the way to the mouth of the tube. There are no scales round the mouth. But the striking feature of the flower which distinguishes it from the Campions is the woolly calyx with its five strong ridges and five long green teeth that far exceed the length of the petals; in the open flower they take their place between the petals, and seem to serve as preliminary alighting perches for the butterflies and moths by which the flowers are pollinated. Nectar is secreted at the bottom of the tube, whose depth makes the flower unsuitable for bees. The flower is at first male, the anthers shedding their pollen before the stigmas are mature; they are so disposed at the mouth of the tube that the nectar-seekers push their faces among them and pick up pollen. On visiting a flower that is a day or two older and has become female, the stigmas occupying the mouth are in the way to receive it by a similar process. Sometimes, smaller flowers are produced in addition, which are entirely female, for the stamens are not developed. The flowers bloom from June to August, and are succeeded by a large, oval capsule, opening by five teeth, and containing about 2 dozen large black seeds. The seeds contain an irritant poison, and sometimes cause trouble through being eaten by domestic animals, and by getting into milling corn and thence into the family loaf." - (Trees and Flowers of the Countryside.)

Corn Cockle is not used in alopathic medicine today, but according to Hill, if used long enough, it was considered a cure for dropsy and jaundice.

In homeopathy a trituration of the seeds has been found useful in paralysis and gastritis.

CORNFLOWER

Botanical: Centaurea Cyanus (LINN.)
Family: N.O. Compositae
Synonyms: Bluebottle. Bluebow. Hurtsickle. Blue Cap.
(French) Bluet.
Part Used: Flowers.

Centaurea Cyanus, the Cornflower, with its star-like blossoms of brilliant blue, is one of our most striking wild-flowers, though it is always looked on as an unwelcome weed by the farmer, for not only does it by its presence withdraw nourishment from the ground that is needed for the corn, 'but its tough stems in former days of hand-reaping were wont to blunt the reaper's sickle, earning it the name of 'Hurt Sickle':

"Thou blunt'st the very reaper's sickle and so
In life and death becom'st the farmer's foe."

The Latin name, Cyanus, was given the Cornflower after a youthful devotee of the goddess Flora (Cyanus), whose favorite flower it was, and the name of the genus is derived from the Centaur, Chiron, who taught mankind the healing virtue of herbs.

It has long been cultivated as a garden plant, in several colors as well as white. C. montana, a perennial form, is frequent in gardens.

Description

In the wild condition it is fairly common in cultivated fields and by roadsides. The stems are 1 to 3 feet high, tough and wiry, slender, furrowed and branched, somewhat angular and covered with a loose cottony down. The leaves, very narrow and long, are arranged alternately on the stem, and like the stem are covered more or less with white cobwebby down that gives the whole plant a somewhat dull and grey appearance. The lower leaves are much broader and often have a roughly-toothed outline. The flowers grow solitary, and of necessity upon long stalks to raise them among the corn. The bracts enclosing the hard head of the flower are numerous, with tightly overlapping scales, each bordered by a fringe of brown teeth. The inner disk florets are small and numerous, of a pale purplish rose color. The bright blue ray florets, thatform the conspicuous part of the flower, are large, widely spread, and much cut into.

Part Used Medicinally

The flowers are the part used in modern herbal medicine and are considered to have tonic, stimulant and emmenagogue properties, with action similar to that of Blessed Thistle.

A water distilled from Cornflower petals was formerly in repute as a remedy for weak eyes. The famous French eyewash, 'Eau de Casselunettes," used to be made from them. Culpepper tells us that the powder or dried leaves of the Bluebottle is given with good success to those that are bruised by a fall or have broken a vein inwardly. He also informs us that, with Plantain, Horsetail, or Comfrey,

"it is a remedy against the poison of the scorpion and resisteth all venoms and poisons. The seeds or leaves (or the distilled water of the herb) taken in wine is very good against the plague and all infectious diseases, and is very good in pestilential fevers: the juice put into fresh or green wounds doth quickly solder up the lips of them together, and is very effectual to heal all ulcers and sores in the mouth."

The expressed juice of the petals makes a good blue ink; if expressed and mixed with alum-water, it may be used in water-color drawing. It dyes linen a beautiful blue, but the color is not permanent.

The dried petals are used by perfumers for giving color to pot-pourri.

CORN, INDIAN

Botanical: Zea Mays (LINN.)

Family: N.O. Graminaceae
Synonym: Maize.
Part Used: Seeds.

Habitat

South America; also cultivated in other parts of America, in the West Indian Islands, Australia, Africa, India, etc., and now in France.

Description

A monoecious plant. Male flowers in terminal racemes; spikelets, two-flowered glumes nearly equal, herbaceous, terminating in two sharp points; females, axillary in the sheaths of the leaves. The spikes or ears proceed from the stalls at various distances from the ground, and are closely enveloped in several thin leaves, forming a sheath called the husk; the ears consist of a cylindrical substance, a pith called the cob; on this the seeds are ranged in eight rows, each row having thirty or more seeds. From the eyes or germs of the seeds proceed individual filaments of a silky appearance and bright green color; these hang from the point of the husk and are called 'the silk." The use of these filaments or stigmata is to receive the farina which drops from the flowers, and without which the flowers would produce no seed. As soon as this has been effected, the tops and 'the silk' dry up. The maize grains are of varying color - usually yellow, but often ranging to black.

Constituents

Starch, sugar, fat, salts, water, yellow oil, maizenic acid, azotized matter, gluten, dextrine, glucose, cellulose, silica, phosphates of lime and magnesia, soluble salts of potassa and soda.

Medicinal Action and Uses

Diuretic and mild stimulant. A good emollient poultice for ulcers, swellings, rheumatic pains. An infusion of the parched corn allays nausea and vomiting in many diseases. Cornmeal makes a palatable and nutritious gruel and is an excellent diet for convalescents.

Preparations

A liquid extract is official in U.S.A. and B.P.C.

Other Species

There is only one distinct species, but there are several varieties resulting from difference of soil, culture and climate. Five of these have been described by Stendel - and all are natives of South America. Some of the finest cobs have been raised in Australia, and the plant is also extensively grown in many parts of Africa and India for consumption. Maize is easily digested by the human body, and when cooked as porridge is called by the Americans 'Mush." Hominy, samp and cerealine are all starchy preparations of split maize. Corn bread contains much more nourishment thanwheaten bread, and is suitable for those suffering from kidney or liver diseases. Maizend or cornflour is prepared from the grains and represents only the fat-forming and heat producing constituents of the grain without mineral salts. It contains only 18 grains of proteids to the pound. Mexicans of today are very skilful in making fermented liquors from maize. One preparation called 'Chicka' resembles beer and cider, and a spirituous liquor called 'Pulque de Mahis," made from the juice of the stalk of the maize, forms an important article of commerce.

CORN SALAD

Botanical: Valerianella olitoria (MOENCH)
Family: N.O. Caryophylleae
Synonyms: Lamb's Lettuce. Valerian locusta (Linn.). White Pot Herb. Lactuca agnina.
(French) Loblollie. Mâche. Doucette. Salade de Chanoine. Salade de Prêtre.
Part Used: Herb.

Closely allied to the Valerians are the members of the genus Valerianella (the name signifying 'little Valerian'), the chief representative of which, V. olitoria (Moench), the Lamb's Lettuce or Corn Salad, was named by Linnaeus, Valeriana Locusta. At one time the plant was classed with the lettuces and called Lactuca agnina, either, as old writers tell us, from appearing about the lambing season, or because it is a favorite food of lambs. The young leaves in spring and autumn are eaten as a salad and are excellent.

This little plant is a common weed in waste ground

and cultivated land especially corn fields, having been long cultivated in gardens and at present found in an apparently wild state. Gerard says: 'We know the Lamb's Lettuce as Loblollie; and it serves in winter as a salad herb among others none of the worst." He tells us that the Dutch called it 'White Pot Herb' (probably in distinction from the 'Black Pot Herb' (Alexander's Smyrnium olusatrum), and that foreigners using it while in England led to its cultivation in our gardens. It is now not much grown here, and is much more known on the Continent, and has long been a favorite salad plant in France under the name of Mâche, Doucette and Salade de Chanoine, and also as Salade de Prêtre, from its being generally eaten in Lent.

Description

It is now common and generally distributed throughout Great Britain, a small, annual, bright-green plant, with succulent stems, 6 to 12 inches high, generally forking from the very base, or at least within the lowest quarter of their height. The first leaves, springing from the root, are 1 to 3 inches long, bluntly lance-shaped scarcely-stalked, generally decaying early. The stem leaves are quite stalkless, often stem-clasping. The flowers are minute and are greenish-white in appearance, arranged in close, rounded, terminal heads, surrounded by narrow bracts, the tiny corolla is pale lilac, but so small that the heads of flowers do not give the appearance of any color.

Cultivation

When cultivated in gardens, Lamb's Lettuce may be sown in rows all through the autumn, winter and early spring, so as to produce a constant succession of crops. A small portion of garden earth sown with the seeds in August, will supply an excellent portion of the salad throughout the winter. The younger the leaves, the better they taste in salad.

Medicinal Action and Uses

This herb was in request by country folk in former days as a spring medicine, and a homeopathic medicinal tincture is made from the fresh root.

Several other species are found in this country, either indigenous or introduced accidentally with the seeds of the plants described, but they are not common. Some botanists assign these species to the genus Fedia, the name of which is of uncertain derivation.

CORN SILK

Botanical: Zea Mays (LINN.)
Family: N.O. Graminaceae
Part Used: Flower pistils.
Habitat: Sub-tropical countries of the world. and cultivated in warm climates.

Description

The stigmas (fine soft, yellowish threads) from the female flowers of maize from 4 to 8 inches long and of a light green, purplish red, yellow or light brown color, stigmas bifid; the segments very slender, frequently unequal, nearly odourless, faintly sweetish taste.

Constituents

Maizenic acid is present in the dried corn silk; also fixed oil, resin, chlorophyl, sugar-gum extractive albuminoids phlobaphine salt, cellulose and water.

Medicinal Action and Uses

A mild stimulant, diuretic and demulcent, useful in acute and chronic cystitis and in the bladder irritation of uric acid and phosphatic gravel; has also been employed in gonorrhea. In action like Holy Thistle.

Preparations and Dosages

Infusion 1 in 10), 2 fluid ounces. Fluid extract of maize stigmas, B.P.C., 1 to 2 fluid drachms. Syrup of maize stigmas, B.P.C., 2 to 4 fluid drachms. Mazenic is given in doses of 1/8 grain.

COSTMARY

Botanical: Tanacetum balsamita (LINN.)
Family: N.O. Compositae
Synonyms: Alecost. Balsam Herb. Costmarie. Mace. Balsamita.
(French) Herbe Sainte-Marie.
Part Used: Leaves.

Closely allied to the Tansy is another old English herb - Costmary (Tanacetum balsamita, Linn.). The whole of this plant emits a soft balsamic odor - pleasanter and more aromatic than that of Tansy - to which fact it owes its name of balsamita, and we find it referred to by Culpepper and others as the 'Balsam Herb." In some old herbals it appears as Balsamita mas, Maudlin, Achillea ageratum, being Balsamita foemina.

It is a native of the Orient, but has now become naturalized in many parts of southern Europe and was formerly to be found in almost every garden in this country, having been introduced into England in the sixteenth century - Lyte, writing in 1578, said it was then 'very common in all gardens." Gerard, twenty years later, says 'it groweth everywhere in gardens," and Parkinson mentions it among other sweet herbs in his garden, but it has now so completely gone out of favour as to have become a rarity, though it may still occasionally be found in old gardens, especially in Lincolnshire, where it is known as 'Mace."

In distinction to the feathery leaves of its near relative, the Tansy, the somewhat long and broad leaves of Costmary are entire, their margins only finely toothed. The stems rise 2 to 3 feet from the creeping roots and bear in August, at their summit, heads of insignificant yellowish flowers in loose clusters, which do not set seed in this country.

Cultivation

The plant will thrive in almost every soil or situation, but will do best on dry land.

Propagation is effected by division of the roots in early spring, or in autumn, planting 2 feet apart, in a dry, warm situation. As the roots creep freely, the plants will probably spread over the intervening spaces in a couple of years and need dividing and transplanting every second or third year.

Grown in the shade, Costmary goes strongly to leaf, but will not flower.

Medicinal Action and Uses

On account of the aroma and taste of its leaves, Costmary was much used to give a spicy flavoring to ale - whence its other name, Aletcost. Markham (The Countrie Farmer, 1616) says that 'both Costmarie' and Avens 'give this savour."

The fresh leaves were also used in salads and in pottage, and dried are often put into potpourri, as they retain their aroma. Our great-grandmothers used to tie up bundles of Costmary with Lavender 'to Iye upon the toppes of beds, presses, etc., for sweet scent and savour."

The name Costmary is derived from the Latin costus (an Oriental plant), the root of which is used as a spice and as a preserve, and 'Mary," in reference to Our Lady. In the Middle Ages, the plant was widely associated with her name and was known in France as Herbe Sainte-Marie.

It was at one time employed medicinally in this country, having somewhat astringent and antiseptic properties, and had a place in our Pharmacopeia until 1788, chiefly as an aperient, its use in dysentery being especially indicated.

Green's Universal Herbal (1532) stated, 'A strong infusion of the leaves to be good in disorders of the stomach and head," and much celebrated for its efficacy as an emmenagogue.

Salmon (171O), among other uses, recommends the juice of the herb as a diuretic and 'good in cases of Quotidien Ague," and continues:

'The powder of the leaves is a good stomatick and may be taken from 1/2 to 1 dram morning and night. I commend it to such as are apt to have the gout to fly upwards into the stomach. It is astringent, resists poison and the bitings of venomous beasts and kills worms in human bodies. The oil by insolation or boiling in Olive oil warms and comforts preternatural coldness, discusses swellings and gives ease in gout, sciatica and other like pains. The Cataplasm draws out the fire in Burnings, being applied before they are blistered. The spirituous tincture helps a weak and disaffected liver, strengthens the nerves, head and brain."

Culpepper speaks of its being 'astringent to the stomach' and:

'strengthening to the liver and all other inward parts; and taken in whey works more effectually. Taken fasting in the morning it is very profitable for pains in the head that are continual, and to stay, dry up, and consume all thin rheums or distillations from the head into the stomach, and helps much to digest raw humours that are gathered therein. . . . It is an especial friend and help to evil, weak and cold livers. The seed is familiarly given to children for the worms, and so is the infusion of the flowers in white wine given them to the quantity of two ounces at a time."

And before Culpepper's days, Gerard had said:

'The Conserve made with leaves of Costmaria and sugar doth warm and dry thebraine and openeth the stoppings of the same; stoppeth all catarrhes, rheumes and distillations, taken in the quantitie of a beane."

We find this plant mentioned in a very composite old recipe 'for a Consumption," called 'Aqua Composita," in which it is spelt 'Coursemary." Also in an 'Oyntment," for 'bruises, dry itches, streins of veins and sinews, scorchings of gunpowder, the shingles, blisters, scabs and vermine."

An ointment made by boiling the herb in olive oil with Adder's Tongue and thickening the strained liquid with wax and resin and turpentine was considered to be very valuable for application to sores and ulccrs.

Achillea ageratum (Linn.), the Maudlin or Sweet Milfoil, a native of Italy and Spain, introduced into England in 1570, an aromatic plant with a sweet smell and a bitter taste, and yellow, tansy-like flowers, was used by the earlier herbalists for the same purposes as Costmary. Culpepper speaks of it growing in gardens and having the same virtues as Costmary, but by the time of Linnzeus its use was obsolete. Both Costmary and Maudlin were much used to make 'sweete washing water."

COTO

Botanical: Botanical source unknown
Family: Possibly N.O. Lauracea
Part Used: The bark.
Habitat: Bolivia.

Description

A bark bearing this name came into the London drug market about 1893. The bark of a rubiaceous plant (Palicourea densiflors), known as Coto, is employed in Brazil for rheumatism, but it is not known if this is the true Bolivian plant; the outer surface is irregular, of a cinnamon brown color. It is sold in pieces of 4 to 6 inches long, 3 inches wide and about 1 inch thick, and is sometimes covered with an adherent corry surface, free from lichens. The inner cross-sections of the bark are covered with yellowish spots, the odor is aromatic and much stronger if bruised, taste hot and biting; in powdered form the smell is very pungent. This description conforms with the barks sold in the American markets, but other barks are used under the same name, the chief being Paracote bark; this has an agreeable spicy taste, but is not so strong-smelling or tasting, and has deep white furrows on the surface.

Constituents

Coto bark contains a volatile alkaloid, a pungent aromatic volatile oil, a light brown soft resin, and a hard brown resin, starch, gum, sugar, tannin, Cal. Oxalate and three acids, acetic, butyric and formic.

Medicinal Action and Uses

Antiseptic, astringent. Coto bark is irritating to the skin applied externally. If taken internally it gives constant violent pain and vomiting. Its chief use is in diarrhea, but it has a tendency to produce inflammation, so must be used with great caution, it is said to lessen peristaltic action. Paracota bark resembles it in action, but is much less powerful. In Japan, paracota bark has been successfully employed for cholera by hypodermic injection of 3 grains of paracotoin. The value of cotoin in diarrhea is established, and it is also used for catarrhal diarrhea and for diarrhea in tubercular ulceration of typhoid fever. Has also a specific action on the alimentary canal, dilating the abdominal vessels and hastening absorption.

Preparations and Dosages

Cotoin, 1 to 3 grains. Fluid extract, 5 to 15 drops. Powdered coto, 2 to 15 grains.

COTTON ROOT

Botanical: Gossypium herbaceum (LINN.)
Family: N.O. Malvaceae
Part Used: Bark of root and of other cultivated species.

Habitat

Asia Minor, and cultivated in U.S.A. and Egypt, India, Mediterranean.

Description

Gossypium herbaceum is the indigenous species in India, and yields the bulk of the cotton of that country. It is also grown in the south of Europe, and other countries bordering on the Mediterranean Persia, etc. The seeds are woolly and yield a very short stapled cotton, while G. Barbadense gives the Sea Island, or long-stapled cotton, this latter being indigenous to America. The two varieties are recognized in the U.S.A. G. Barbadense, the best species was introduced from the Bahamas in 1785 and only grows in the low islands and sea-coast of Georgia and South Carolina. The upland Georgian, Bowed or short-stapled cotton, which forms the bulk of American cotton, is the produce of the upland or inner districts of the Southern States. Its staple is only about 1 1/4 inch long, and it adheres firmly to the seed, which is covered with short down. Egyptian cotton and Bourbon are likewise referrable to this species.

G. herbaceum is a biennial or triennial plant with branching stems 2 to 6 feet high, palmate hairy leaves, lobes lanceolate and acute flowers with yellow petals, and a purple spot in centre, leaves of involucre serrate, capsule when ripe splits open and shows a loose white tuft surrounding the seeds and adhering firmly to outer coating; it requires warm weather to ripen its seeds, which they do not do north of Virginia.

The crushed seeds give a fixed, semi-drying oil used in making soap, etc. The flowering time ends in September, and a month or so earlier the tops are cut off in order to ripen and send the sap back to the capsules. The pods are about the size of a walnut, and are collected by hand as they ripen;the cotton is also separated by hand and packed in bales. In the Levant the seeds are often used as food. An acre may be expected to produce 240 to 300 lb. of cotton.

The herbaceous part of the plant contains much mucilage and has been utilized as a demulcent. Cotton seeds have been used in the Southern States for intermittent fever with great success. The root and stem-bark deteriorates with age, so only newly harvested material should be used. The root-bark of commerce consists of thin flexible bands of quilled pieces covered with a browny yellow periderm, odor not strong, taste slightly acid.

Constituents

A peculiar acid resin, odourless and insoluble in water, absorbing oxygen when exposed, then changes to a red color. The bark also contains sugar, gum, tannin, fixed oil, chlorophyll.

Medicinal Action and Uses

Mainly used as an abortifacient in place of ergot, being not so powerful but safer; it was used largely in this way by the slaves in the south. It not only increases the contractions of the uterus in labour, but also is useful in the treatment of metrorrhagia, specially when dependent on fibroids; useful also as an ecbolic; of value in sexual lassitude. A preparation of cotton seed increases milk of nursing mothers.

Preparations

Boil 4 OZ. of the inner bar of the root in 1 quart of water down to 1 pint: dose, 1 full wineglass (4 oz.) every thirty minutes. Fluid extract, U.S.D., 1 to 2 drachms. Gossipium, 1 to 5 grains. Solid extract, 15 to 20 grains. Liquid extract of cotton root bark, B.P.C., 1/2 to 1 fluid drachm. Tinc. Gossipii, B.P.C., 1/2 to 1 fluid drachm. Decoction of cotton root bark, B.P.C., 1/2 to 2 fluid ounces (as an emmenagogue or to check hemorrhages).

COWHAGE

Botanical: Mucuna pruriens (LINN.)
Family: N.O. Leguminosae
Synonyms: Dolichos pruriens. Stizolobium pruriens. Mucuna prurita. Setae Siliquae Hirsutae. Cowage. Cowitch. Couhage. Kiwach.
(French) Cadjuet. Pois velus. Pois à gratter. Liane à gratter. Pois pouilleux. Ceil de bourrique.
(German) Kratzbohnen. Kuhkratze.
Parts Used: The hairs of the pod, seeds.
Habitat: Tropical regions, especially East and West Indies.

Description

The name of the genus, Mucuna, is that of a Brazilian species mentioned by Marggraf in 1648, and pruriens refers to the itching caused on the skin by the hairs. The popular name, variously spelt, is from the Hindustani.

Travellers in the tropics know the plants well on account of their annoying seed-pods, covered with stinging hairs which are easily shaken off, and cause great irritation. They are found in Asia, America, Africa, and the Fiji Islands.

M. pruriens is a leguminous climbing plant, with long, slender branches, alternate, lanceolate leaves on hairy petioles, 6 to 12 inches long, with large, white flowers, growing in clusters of two or three, with a bluish-purple, butterfly-shaped corolla.

The pods or legumes, hairy, thick, and leathery, averaging 4 inches long, are shaped like violin sound-holes, and contain four to six seeds. They are of a rich dark brown color, thickly covered with stiff hairs, about 1/1O inch long, which are the official part. In commerce they are found in a loose mass mixed with pieces of the pericarp.

When young and tender, the legumes are cooked and eaten in India.

Constituents

The hairs are usually filled with air, but sometimes contain granular matter, with tannic acid and resin. No tincture or decoction is effective.

Medicinal Action and Uses

A mechanical anthelmintic. The hairs, mixed with syrup, molasses, or honey, pierce the bodies of intestinal worms, which writhe themselves free from the walls, so that a brisk cathartic will bring them away. It is usually a safe remedy, but enteritis has sometimes followed its use. It has little effect upon tape-worm, but is good for Ascaris lumbricoides and in slightly less degree for the smaller Oxyuris vermicularis.

In the form of an ointment, Mucuna has been used as a local stimulant in paralysis and other affections, acting like Croton oil. A decoction of the root or legumes is said to have been used in dropsy as a diuretic and for catarrh, and in some parts of India an infusion is used in cholera.

It is a good medium for the application of such substances as muriate of morphia. In the proportion of 7 to 8 grains of cowhage to an ounce of lard, it should be rubbed in for from 10 to 20 minutes. It brings out flat, white pimples, which soon disappear. Oil relieves the heat and irritation caused on the skin.

The seeds are said to be aphrodisiac.

Dosage

For an adult, a tablespoonful, and for a child a teaspoonful, for three consecutive mornings, after which a brisk cathartic should be given.

Other Species

M. urens, or Dolichos urens (M. prurita),the seeds of which, called Horse-eye beans, round and brownish, are used as a substitute for Calabar beans. Some authorities regard this East Indian variety as a distinct species, being larger than M. pruriens.

COWSLIP

Botanical: Primula veris (LINN.)
Family: N.O. Primulaceae
Synonyms: Herb Peter. Paigle. Peggle. Key Flower. Key of Heaven. Fairy Cups. Petty Mulleins. Crewel. Buckles. Palsywort. Plumrocks. Mayflower. Pass-

word. Artetyke. Drelip. Our Lady's Keys. Arthritica.
(Anglo-Saxon) Cuy lippe.
(Greek) Paralysio.

Many of the Primrose tribe possess active medicinal properties. Besides the Cowslip and the Primrose, this family includes the little Scarlet Pimpernel (Anagallis), as truly a herald of warm summer weather as the Primrose is of spring, the Yellow Loosestrife and the Moneywort (Lysimachia vulgaris and Nummularia), the handsome Water Violet (Hottonia) and the nodding Cyclamen or Sowbread, all of which have medicinal value to a greater or lesser degree. Less important British members of the group are the Chaffweed (Centunculus minimus), one of the smallest among British plants, the Chickweed Wintergreen (Trientalis), the Sea Milk-wort (Glaux maritima), which has succulent salty leaves and has been used as a pickle, and the Common Brookweed or Water Pimpernel (Samolus).

The botanical name of the order, Primulaceae, is based on that of the genus Primula, to which belong not only those favorite spring flowers of the country-side, the Primrose, Cowslip, and their less common relative the Oxlip, but also the delicately-tinted greenhouse species that are such welcome pot plants for our rooms in mid-winter.

Linnaeus considered the Primrose, Cowslip and Oxlip to be but varieties of one species, but in this opinion later botanists have not followed him, though in all essential points they are identical.

Description

Quite early in the spring, the Cowslip begins to produce its leaves. At first, each is just two tight coils, rolled backwards and lying side by side; these slowly unroll and a leaf similar to that of a Primrose, but shorter and rounder, appears. All the leaves lie nearly flat on the ground in a rosette, from the centre of which rises a long stalk, crowned by the flowers, which spring all from one point, in separate little stalks, and thus form an 'umbel."The number of the flowers in an umbel varies very much in different specimens.

We quote the following from Familiar Wild Flowers:

'It is a curious fact that the inflorescence of the Primrose is as truly umbellate as that of the Cowslip, though in the former case it can only be detected by carefully tracing the flower stems to their base, when all will be found to spring from one common point. In some varieties of the Primrose the umbel is raised on a stalk, as in the Cowslip. This form is sometimes called Oxlip; it is by some writers raised to the dignity of an independent position as a true and distinct species. . . . Primrose roots may at times be met with bearing both forms, one or more stalked umbels together with a number of the ordinary type of flower."

The sepals of the flowers are united to form pale green crinkled bags, from which the corolla projects, showing a golden disk about inch across with scalloped edges, the petals being united into a narrow tube within the calyx. On the yellow disk are five red spots, one on each petal.

'In their gold coats spots you see,
These be rubies fairy favours
In those freckles lie their savours."

The Midsummer Night's Dream refers to the old belief that the flower held a magic value for the complexion.

The origin of Cowslip is obscure: it has been suggested that it is a corruption of'Cow's Leek," leek being derived from the Anglo-Saxon word leac, meaning a plant (comp. Houseleek).

In old Herbals we find the plant called Herb Peter and Key Flower, the pendent flowers suggesting a bunch of keys, the emblem of St. Peter, the idea having descended from old pagan times, for in Norse mythology the flower was dedicated to Frcya, the Key Virgin, and was thought to admit to her treasure palace. In northern Europe the idea of dedication to the goddess was transferred with the change of religion, and it became dedicated to the Virgin Mary, so we find it called 'Our Lady's Keys' and 'Key of Heaven," and 'Keyflower' remains still the most usual name.

The flowers have a very distinctive and fresh fragrance and somewhat narcotic juices, which have given rise to their use in making the fermented liquor called Cowslip Wine, which had formerly a great and deserved reputation and is still largely drunk in country parts, being much produced in the Midlands. It is made from the 'peeps," i.e. the yellow petal rings, in the following way: A gallon of 'peeps' with 4 lb. of lump sugar and the rind of 3 lemons is added to a gallon of cold spring water. A cup of fresh yeast is then included and the liquor stirred every day for a week. It is then put into a barrel with the juice of the lemons and left to 'work." When 'quiet," it is corked down for eight or nine months and finally bottled. The wine should be perfectly clear and of a pale yellow color and has almost the value of a liqueur. In certain children's ailments, Cowslip Wine, given in small doses as a medicine, is particularly beneficial.

Young Cowslip leaves were at one time eaten in country salads and mixed with other herbs to stuff meat, whilst the flowers were made into a delicate conserve. Cowslip salad from the petals, with white sugar, is said to make an excellent and refreshing dish.

Children delight in making Cowslip Balls, or 'tosties," from the flowers. The umbels are picked off close to the top of the main flowerstalk and about fifty to sixty are hung across a string which may be stretched for convenience between the backs of two chairs. The flowers are then pressed carefully together and the string tied tightly so as to collect them into a ball. Care must be taken to choose only such heads or umbels in which all the flowers are open, as otherwise the surface of the ball will be uneven.

Part Used Medicinally

The yellow corolla is alone needed, no stalk or green part whatever is required, only the yellow part, plucked out of the green calyx.

Constituents

The roots and the flowers have somewhat of the odor of Anise, due to their containing some volatile oil identical with Mannite. Their acrid principle is Saponin.

Medicinal Action and Uses

Sedative, antispasmodic.

In olden days, Cowslip flowers were ingreat request for homely remedies, their special value Iying in strengthening the nerves and the brain, and relieving restlessness and insomnia. The Cowslip was held good 'to ease paines in the head and is accounted next with Betony, the best for that purpose."

Cowslip Wine made from the flowers, as above described, is an excellent sedative. Also, 1 lb. of the freshly gathered blossom infused in 1 1/2 pint of boiling water and simmered down with loaf sugar to a fine yellow syrup, taken with a little water is admirable for giddiness from nervous debility or from previous nervous excitement, and this syrup was formerly given against palsy.

In earlier times, the Cowslip was considered beneficial in all paralytic ailments, being, as we have seen, often called Palsy Wort or Herba paralysis. The root was also called in old Herbals Radix arthritica, from its use as a cure for muscular rheumatisrm.

In A Plain Plantain (Russell G. Alexander) we read:

'Cowslip water was considered to be good for the memory, and Cowslips of Jerusalem for mitigating "hectical fevers." Mrs. Raffald (English Housekeeper, 1778) gives a recipe for the wine. "For the future," says the poet Pope, in one of his letters, "I'll drown all high thoughts in the Lethe of Cowslip Wine" (which is pleasantly soporific). Our Lady's Cowslip is Gagea lutea."

The old writers give a long list of ills that may be remedied by application of the roots or leaves of the plant; the juice of the flowers 'takes off spots and wrinkles from the face and other vices of the skin," the water of the flowers being 'very proper medicine for weakly people."

Turner says:

'Some weomen we find, sprinkle ye floures of cowslip wt whyte wine and after still it and wash their faces wt that water to drive wrinkles away and to make them fayre in the eyes of the worlde rather than in the eyes of God, Whom they are not afrayd to offend."

Formerly an ointment was made from the flowers as a cosmetic. Culpepper says:

'Our city dames know well enough the ointment or distilled water of it adds to beauty or at least restores it when lost. The flowers are held to be more effectual than the leaves and the roots of little use. An ointment being made with them taketh away spots and wrinkles of the skin, sunburnings and freckles and promotes beauty; they remedy all infirmities of the head coming of heat and wind, as vertigo, false apparitions, phrensies, falling sickess, palsies, convulsions, cramps, pains in the nerves, and the roots ease pains in the back and bladder. The leaves are good in wounds and the flowers take away trembling. Because they strengthen the brains and nerves and remedy palsies, the Greeks gave them the name Paralysio. The flowers preserved or conserved and a quantity the size of a nutmeg taken every morning is a sufficient dose for inward diseases, but for wounds, spots, wrinkles and sunburnings an ointment is made of the leaves and hog's lard."

A later writer, Hill (1755), tells us that when boiled in ale, the powdered roots were taken with success by country folk for giddiness, wakefulness and similar nervous troubles for which the syrup made from the flowers was also taken.

The usual dose of the dried and powdered flowers is 15 to 20 grains.

From Hartman's Family Physitian, 1696:

'Another way to make Cowslip Wine

'Having boil'd your Water and Sugar together, pour it boiling hot upon your Cowslips beaten, stir them well together, and let them stand in a Vessel close cover'd till it be almost cold; then put into it the Yest beaten with the Juice of Lemons; let it stand for two days, then press it out with as much speed as you can, and put it up into a Cask, and leave a little hole open, for the working; when it hath quite done working stop it up close for a Month or Six Weeks, then Bottle it. Cowslip Wine is very Cordial, and a glass of it being drank at night Bedward, causes sleep and rest. . . ."

The Bird's-eye Primrose (Primula farinosa) is a plant of mountain slopes and pastures, and may be met with on the mountain ranges of Europe and Asia. It is not uncommon in the northern counties of England, though much less common in Scotland.

Gerard, in his Herball, says:

"These plants grow very plentifully in moist and squally grounds in the North parts of England, as in Harwood, neere to Blackburne in Lancashire, and ten miles from Preston in Aundernesse; also at Crosby, Ravensnaith, and Craig-close in Westmorland. They likewise grow in the meadows belonging to a village in Lancashire neere Maudsley called Harwood, and at Hasketh, not far from thence, and in many other places of Lancashire, but not on this side Trent' (Gerard writes as a Londoner) 'that I could ever have certain knowledge of. Lobel reporteth, That Doctor Penny, a famous Physition of our London Colledge, did find them in these Southerne Parts."

Specimens of the Bird's-eye Primrose growing in the North of Scotland, in Caithness and the Orkney Islands, and in other localities bordering on the sea, vary from the typical form of the plant in being of stouter habit and much smaller, in having leaves of broader proportions and flowers of a deeper purple; and some botanists are inclined to distinguish this variety by creating it an independent species, and calling it the ScotchBird's-eye (P. Scotica), while others are content to consider it but a variety from the type, and label it P. farinosa, var. Scotica.

All the hardy varieties of Primula, whether Primrose, Cowslip, Polyanthus or Auricula, may be easily propagated by dividing the roots of old plants in autumn. New varieties are raised from seed, which should be sown as soon as ripe, in leaf-mould, and pricked out into beds when large enough.

Among the many splendid flowers that are grown in our greenhouses none shows more improvement under the fostering hand of the British florist than the Chinese Primula which originally had small, inconspicuous flowers, but now bears trusses of magnificent blooms ranging from the purest white to the richest scarlet and crimson. The Star Primulas, which have attained an even greater popularity in late years, are considered perhaps even more elegant, being looser in growth and carrying their plentiful blossoms in more graceful, if not more beautiful trusses. Both varieties are among the most beautiful of our winter-flowering plants, the toothed and lobed, somewhat heart-shaped leaves being extremely handsome with their crimson tints.

Seeds of these greenhouse Primulas should be sown in the spring in gentle heat, the soil used being very fine and pleasantly moist. The seedlings must be pricked off and potted out as necessary, with a view to ensuring sturdy, healthy growth.

P. obconica is a slightly varying type of these greenhouse Primulas, the leaves approaching more the shape of those of the common Primrose, the plants are exceedingly floriferous and graceful, the full trusses of delicate lilac flowers are borne on tall slender stems and care must be used in the handling of it, as the leaves sometimes cause an eruption like eczema. Homeopaths make a tincture from this species.

The broad, thick leaves of the Auricula (P. auricula), a frequent garden plant in this country, though not native to Great Britain, are used in the Alps as a remedy for coughs.

In its native state the Auricula is said to be either yellow or white. It is the skill of the gardener which has brought it to its present purple and brown. It was formerly known as Mountain Cowslip, or Bear's Ears.

COW-WHEAT

Botanical: Melampyrum pratense (LINN.)
Family: N.O. Scrophulariaceae
Synonyms: Horse Floure. Triticum vaccinium.
Part used: Herb.

Description

The Cow-wheat (Melampyrum pratense, Linn.) is an annual, with slender, branched stems, about a foot high, bearing stalkless, narrow, tapering, smooth leaves in distant pairs, each pair at right angles to those that are next to it, and long-tubed, pale yellow flowers which are placed in the axils of the upper leaves in pairs, all turning one way. The corolla is four times as long as the calyx, and the lower lip longer than the upper standing sharply out instead of hanging downwards as in most labiate flowers. The color is somewhat between the delicate pale yellow of the primrose and the rich bright yellow of the buttercup. The plant is in flower from June to September.

Cow-wheat is said to afford fodder for cattle, though not cultivated in this country for that purpose. Linnaeus states that when cows are fed in fields where the Meadow Cow-wheat is abundant, the butter yielded by their milk is peculiarly rich and of a brilliant yellow color, but in England the plant grows more frequently in the undergrowth of woods and thickets than in meadows, abounding in nearly all copses and woods throughout Great Britain.

The name of Cow-wheat is said to be derived from an extraordinary notion prevalent in some country districts among the peasantry of the Middle Ages, that the small seeds were capable of being converted into wheat, a supposition probably originating in the sudden appearance of the plants among corn, on land that had been recently cleared of wood.

Another reason for the meaning of Melampyrum is given in Lindley's Treasury of Botany, i.e. it refers to an ancient belief that the seeds, when mixed with grains of wheat and ground into flour tended to make the bread black.

The seeds, which bear some little resemblance to wheat, are generally eaten by swine, though they will not touch the herb. Cows and sheep are extremely fond of the plant, and Dr. Prior explains the name of the plant on the score that though its seed resembles wheat, it is only fit for cows. In old Herbals, we find it named 'Horse Floure' and also Triticum vaccinium. The generic name is derived from the Greek melas (black) and pyros (wheat), because the seeds made bread black when mixed with them.

Dodonaeus tells us that 'the seeds of this herb taken in meate or drinke troubleth the braynes, causing headache and drunkennesse."

CRANESBILL ROOT, AMERICAN

Botanical: Geranium maculatum (LINN.)
Family: N.O. Geraniaceae
Synonyms: Alum Root. Spotted Cranesbill. Wild Cranesbill. Storksbill. Alum Bloom. Wild Geranium. Chocolate Flower. Crowfoot. Dove's-foot. Old Maid's Nightcap. Shameface.
Parts Used: Dried rhizome, leaves.

Habitat

Flourishes in low grounds and woods from Newfoundland to Manitoba, south to Georgia, Missouri and in Europe.

Description

A perennial, grows from 1 to 2 feet high. The entire plant is erect and unbranched, more or less covered with hairs; the leaves deeply parted, each division again cleft and toothed, flowering April to June, color pale to rosy purple, petals veined and woolly at base, fruit a beaked capsule, divided into five cells, each cell containing one seed, the root stocks 2 to 4 inches long thick with numerous branches for the next growth, outside brown, white and fleshy inside when fresh, when dried it turns to a darkish purple inside; no odor, taste strongly astringent, contains much tannin which is most active just before the plant flowers. This is the time the root should be collected for drying.

Constituents

Tannic and gallic acid, also starch, sugar, gum, pectin and coloring matter.

Medicinal Action and Uses

Styptic, astringent, tonic. Used for piles and internalbleeding. Excellent as an injection for flooding and leucorrhoea, and taken internally for diarrhea, children's cholera, chronic dysentery; a good gargle.

The leaves are also used and give the greatest percentage of tannin and should be collected before the plant seeds.

Dosages

15 to 30 grains. Infusion, 1 OZ. herb to 1 pint water. Fluid extract, 1/2 to 1 drachm. Geranin, 1 to 3 grains.

Other Species

The English herb Geranium dissectum has similar properties.

CRAWLEY ROOT

Botanical: Corallorhiza odontorhiza (NUTT.)
Family: N.O. Orchidaceae
Synonyms: Dragon's Claw. Coral Root. Chicken Toe.
Part Used: The root.
Habitat: Indigenous to the United States, from Maine to Carolina westward.

Description

This parasitic plant has been used by herbalists for centuries. It grows in rich woods at the roots of trees.

It is singular and leafless, with muchbranched and toothed coral-like root-stocks, the root being a collection of fleshy, articulated tubers, the scape about 14 inches high, fleshy, smooth, striate, with a few long purplish-brown long sheaths, the flowers, 10 to 20, greenish brown in color, on a long spike, blooming from July to October, with a large, reflexed, ribbed, oblong capsule.

The root is the official part; it is small and dark, with a strong nitrous smell and a slightly bitter mucilaginous astringent taste, the fracture is short and presents under the microscope a frosted granular appearance.

Medicinal Action and Uses

Crawley Root is one of the most certain, quick and

powerful diaphoretics, but its scarcity and high price prevents it being more generally used. It promotes perspiration without producing any excitement in the system, so is of value in pleurisy, typhus fever and other inflammatory diseases. In addition to being a powerful diaphoretic, its action has a sedative effect. It has been found efficacious inacute erysipelas, cramps, nightsweats, flatulence and hectic fevers generally, and combines tonic, sedative, diaphoretic and febrifuge properties without weakening the patient, its valuable properties being most marked in low stages of fever.

Dosage

20 to 30 grains of powdered root given in very hot water every two or three hours. The powder should be kept in wellstoppered bottles as it is subject to deterioration from insects.

Combined with the resin of Blue Cohosh, it is an excellent remedy for amenorrhoea, dismenorrhoea, afterbirth pains, suppression of lochia and for febrile conditions of the parturient period, and combined with extract of Leptandra or Podophyllum resin, it acts well on the bowels and liver, and if mixed with Dioscorea is excellent for bilious and flatulent colic.

Fluid extract, 15 to 30 drops.

Other Species

It is considered that the varieties Corallorhiza multiflora, C. Wisteriana, C. verna and C. innata possess similar properties.

CROSSWORT

Botanical: Galium cruciata (SCOPOLI)
Family: N.O. Rubiaceae
Parts Used: Herb, leaves.

Description

The Crosswort (Galium cruciata, Scopoli), like G. verum, has yellow flowers, but they are not so showy, being only in short clusters of about eight together, in the axils of the upper whorls of leaves and of a dull, pale yellow. The stems are slender and scarcely branched, 1 to 2 feet long, and bear soft and downy leaves oblong in shape, arranged four in a whorl, hence the name Crosswort.

Medicinal Action and Uses

This species though now practically unused, was considered a very good wound herb for both inward and outward wounds. A decoction of the leaves in wine was also used for obstructions in the stomach or bowels and to stimulate appetite. It was also recommended as a remedy for rupture, rheumatism and dropsy.

We have only one representative in Great Britain of the genus Rubia (name from Latin ruber, red), from which this large natural order takes its name, namely the Wild Madder (R. peregrina, Linn.), common in bushy places in the south-west of England.

It is a long, straggling, perennial plant, many feet in length, with remarkably rough stems and leaves, the latter glossy above and growing in whorls of four to six, their margins recurved and bearing prickles, which are also present on the angles of the stem and the midribs of the leaves, the plant being otherwise smooth.

The flowers, in bloom from June to August, are yellowish-green and grow in loose panicles. They are followed by black berries, about as large as currants, which remain attached to the plant till late in winter.

The properties of this native Wild Madder are not made use of, although it yields a good dye, said to be but little inferior to that of the cultivated species, R. tinctorum, the Dyer's Madder, formerly a plant of much greater importance than it is now, owing to the researches of chemical science having discovered an easier source of the important dye it yields.

CROTON

Botanical: Croton tiglium (WILLD,)
Family: N.O. Euphorbiaceae
Synonyms: Tiglium Seeds. Klotzsch.
Part Used: The oil from ripe seeds.

Description

A small tree or shrub with a few spreading branches bearing alternate petiolate leaves which are ovate, acuminate, serrate, smooth, dark green on upper surface paler beneath and furnished with two glands at base. Flowers in erect terminal racemes, scarcely as long as the leaf, the lower female, upper male, straw-coloured petals. Fruit a smooth capsule of the size of a filbert, three cells, each containing a single seed; these seeds resemble castor beans in size and structure, oblong, rounded at the extremities with two faces; the kernel or endosperm is yellowish brown and abounds in oil. The oil is obtained by expression from the seeds previously deprived of the shell.

Constituents

Croton oil consists chiefly of the glycerides of stearic, palmitic, myristic, lauric and oleic acids; there are also present in the form of glycerin ethers the more volatile acids as formic, acetic, isobutyric and isovalerianic acids. The active principle is believed to be Crotonic acid, which is freely soluble in alcohol.

Medicinal Action and Uses

A powerful drastic purgative, in large doses apt to excite vomiting and severe griping pains capable of producing fatal effects. It acts with great rapidity, frequently evacuating the bowels in less than an hour. The dose is very small; a drop placed on the tongue of a comatose patient will generally operate It is chiefly employed in cases of obstinate constipation, often being successful where other drugs have failed. Applied externally, it produces inflammation of the skin attended with pustular eruption, and has been used as a counter-irritant in rheumatism gout, neuralgia, bronchitis, etc. It should be diluted with three parts of olive oil, soap liniment or other vehicle and applied as a liniment. Must always be used with the greatest care and should never be given to children or pregnant women.

Preparations and Dosage

Dose of the oil, 1/2 to 1 minim on a lump of sugar Collodium Crotons B.P.C., a powerful counter-irritant and vesicant. Liniment of Croton oil, B.P., seldom used owing to the painful inflammation which may be produced.

CROWFOOT, CELERY-LEAVED

Botanical: Ranunculus sceleratus (LINN.)
Family: N.O. Ranunculaceae
Synonym: Marsh Crowfoot.
Part Used: Whole plant.

Habitat

The Celery-leaved Crowfoot is widely spread throughout Britain, growing in watery places and muddy ditches, flowering during July and August.

Description

The root is annual. The plant itself is of a pale, shining, yellowishgreen color, juicy and very glabrous except the flower-stalks and upper part of the stem, which are occasionally hairy. The flowers are numerous, small and of a palish yellow.

This species is easily distinguished by its broad, shining, lower leaves, which are on long stalks, the blades palmate, and cut into three divisions, which are notched and toothed. The stem is thick, hollow, furrowed and bears small sessile leaves, divided into three narrow parts, hardly toothed at all. The small, pale yellow flowers, about 1/4 inch across, are succeeded by smooth, oblong seed-heads.

Medicinal Action and Uses

One of the most virulent of native plants: bruised and applied to the skin, it raises a blister and creates a sore by no means easy to heal. When chewed, it inflames the tongue and produces violent effects. Even the distilled water is intensely acrimonious, and as it cools, deposits crystals which are insoluble, and have the curious property of being inflammable. Yet if the plant be boiled and the water thrown away, it is said to be not unwholesome, the peasants of Wallachia eating it thus as a vegetable. When made into a tincture, given in small diluted doses, it proves curative of stitch in the side and neuralgic pains between the ribs.

CROWFOOT, UPRIGHT MEADOW

Botanical: Ranunculus acris (LINN.)
Family: N.O. Ranunculaceae

Synonyms: Gold Cup. Grenouillette.
Part Used: Whole herb.

Habitat

This Buttercup is a native of meadows and pastures in all the northern parts of Europe, and is very common in England, flowering in June and July.

The Upright Meadow Crowfoot, a familiar plant in our hay-fields, is recognized at once from all other Buttercups or Crowfoots by its tall flower-stalks not being furrowed, and its fruit-base, or receptacle, not being hairy. The stems are hollow, round, more or less covered with soft, silky hairs and very freely branching towards their summits, where they are terminated by numerous goldenyellow flowers.

Description

The leaves vary a good deal in form, according to their position on the plant: the lower leaves are on long petioles (foot-stalks) and are comprised of numerous wide-spreading and deeply divided segments; the upper leaves are small, composed of few segments, simple in form and few in number. The root is perennial, though the plant itself dies down each autumn, and has many long, white fibres.

The petals of the flower are bright, shining yellow; the calyx is composed of five greenish-yellow spreading sepals. The centre of the flower, as in other Buttercups, is a clustering mass of stamens round the smooth, green immature seed-vessels, which develop into a round head of numerous small bodies called achenes.

Most of the Crowfoots are known to be acrid and some even to be poisonous, but this plant receives its Latin specific name of acris from its supposed intensity of acridity, for all parts of it are intensely acrid. It has been stated that even pulling it up and carrying it some little distance, has produced considerable inflammation in the palm of the hand, and that cattle will not readily eat it in the green state, and if driven by hunger to feed on it, their mouths become sore and blistered. According to Linnaeus, sheep and goats eat it, but cattle, horses and pigs refuse it. When made into hay, it loses its acrid quality, but then seems to be too hard and and stalky to yield much nourishment. The notion that the butter owes its yellow color to the prevalence of buttercups in the meadows, is quite groundless - it is the richness of the pasture that communicates this color to the butter and not these flowers which the cattle seldom or never touch willingly.

Miss Pratt (Familiar Wild Flowers) states:

'Instances are common in which the wanderer in the meadow has lain down to sleep with a handful of these flowers beside him, and has awakened to find the skin of his cheek pained and irritated to a high degree, by the acrid blossoms having lain near it."

Poetically, the associations of this plant are numerous. Gay tells us in The Shepherd's Oracle that it was worn by lovers at betrothal time, and its golden color was dedicated to Hymcn in classical history. In France, it is termed the grenouillette, a name similar in meaning to its Latin generic name Ranunculus, a reference to the moist meadows in which it usually grows. In the astrological Herbals it was deemed a plant of Mars, on account of its acrid, fiery nature.

Old authors say:

'this fiery and hot-spirited herb is not fit to be given inwardly, but that an ointment of the leaves and flowers will raise a blister and may be applied to the nape of the neck to draw rheum from the eyes," and that mixed with a little mustard it raises a blister as perfectly as the Spanish Fly.

Medicinal Action and Uses

The juice of the leaves takes away warts, and bruised together with the roots will act as a caustic. In violent headaches where pain is confined to one part, a plaster made of them often affords instant relief, and they have been used in gout with great success.

The fresh leaves formed part of a famous cure for cancer, practised by a Mr. Plunkett in 1794.

Thornton, in his Herbal of 100 years ago, says if

a decoction of the plant be poured on ground containing worms, 'they will be forced to rise from their concealment."

CUBEBS

Botanical: Piper cubeba (LINN.)
Family: N.O. Piperaceae
Synonym: Tailed Pepper.
Part Used: The dried, full-grown, unripe fruit.
Habitat: Java, Penang, and other parts of East Indies.

Description

A climbing perennial plant, with dioecious flowers in spikes. The fruit is a globose, pedicelled drupe. It is extensively grown in the coffee plantations, well shaded and supported by the coffee trees. Odor aromatic and characteristic- taste strongly aromatic and pungent and somewhat bitter. Commercial Cubebs are often adulterated with other fruits containing a volatile oil, but with very different properties. There is no evidence that the plant was known to the ancients, though it was probably brought into Europe by the Arabians, who doubtless employed the fruit as pepper.

Constituents

10 to 18 per cent of volatile oil, also resins, amorphous cubebic acid and colorless crystalline cubebin. By extraction with ether yields about 22 per cent of oleoresin.

Medicinal Action and Uses

Stimulant, carminative, much used as a remedy for gonorrhea, after the first active inflammatory symptoms have subsided; also used in leucorrhoea, cystitis, urethritis, abscesses of the prostate gland, piles and chronic bronchitis.

Preparations and Dosages

Infusion: 1 OZ. of Cubebs to 1 pint of water is sometimes used as an injection in discharge from the vagina. In the treatment of gonorrhea it is usually given in capsule form combined with copaiba, etc. Powdered fruit: dose, 1/2 to 1 drachm. Oil, 5 to 30 drops. Fluid extract, 1/4 to 1 drachm.

Cubebs should be freshly prepared as the oil evaporates; the powder is often adulterated with pimento. The crushed fruit should turn crimson with the addition of sulphuric acid and give a mace-like smell; this experiment will detect any adulteration.

CUCKOO-PINT

Botanical: Arum maculatum
Family: N.O. Araceae
Synonyms: Lords and Ladies. Arum. Starchwort. Adder's Root. Bobbins. Friar's Cowl. Kings and Queens. Parson and Clerk. Ramp. Quaker. Wake Robin.
Part Used: Root.

The Arum family, Aroidae, which numbers nearly 1,000 members, mostly tropical, and many of them marsh or water plants, is represented in this country by a sole species, Arum maculatum (Linn.), familiarly known as Lords and Ladies, or Cuckoo-pint.

Description

The flowering organs are contained in a sheath-like leaf called a spathe, within which rises a long, fleshy stem, or column called the spadix, bearing closely arranged groups of stalkless, primitive flowers. At the base are a number of flowers each consisting of a pistil only. Above these is a belt of sterile flowers, each consisting of only a purplish anther. Above the anther is a ring of glands, terminating in short threads The spadix is then prolonged into a purple; club-like extremity.

The bright leaves, conspicuous by their glossiness and purple blotches, and their halberd-like shape, are some of the first to emerge from the ground on the approach of spring, and may then be noticed under almost every hedge in shady situations; the pale green spathe is a still more striking object when it appears in April and May.

In autumn, the lowest ring of flowers form a cluster of bright scarlet, attractive berries, which remain long after the leaves have withered away, and on their short, thick stem alone mark the situation of the plant. In pite of their very acrid taste, they have sometimes been eaten by children, with most injurious results, being extremely poisonous. One drop of their juice will cause a burning sensation in the mouth and throat for hours. In the case of little children who have died from eating the berries, cramp and convulsions preceded death if no medical aid had been obtained.

The Arum has large tuberous roots, somewhat resembling those of the Potato, oblong in shape, about the size of a pigeon's egg, brownish externally, white within and when fresh, fleshy yielding a milky juice, almost insipid to the taste at first, but soon producing a burning and pricking sensation. The acridity is lost during the process of drying and by application of heat, when the substance of the tuber is left as starch. When baked, the tubers are edible, and from the amount of starch, nutritious. This starch of the root, after repeated washing, makes a kind of arrowroot, formerly much prepared in the Isle of Portland, and sold as an article of food under the name of Portland Sago, or Portland Arrowroot, but now obsolete. For this purpose, it was either roasted or boiled, and then dried and pounded in a mortar, the skin being previously peeled.

Arum starch was used for stiffening ruffs in Elizabethan times, when we find the name Starchwort among the many names given to the plant. Gerard says:

'The most pure and white starch is made of the rootes of the Cuckoo-pint, but most hurtful for the hands of the laundresse that have the handling of it, for it chappeth, blistereth, and maketh the hands rough and rugged and withall smarting."

This starch, however, in spite of Gerard's remarks, forms the Cyprus Powder of the Parisians, who used it as a cosmetic for the skin, and Dr. Withering says of this cosmetic formed from the tuber starch, that 'it is undoubtedly a good and innocent cosmetic'; and Hogg (Vegetable Kingdom, 1858) reported its use in Italy to remove freckles from the face and hands.

In parts of France, a custom existed of turning to account the mucilaginous juice of the plant as a substitute for soap, the stalks of the plant when in flower being cut and soaked for three weeks in water, which was daily poured off carefully and the residue collected at the bottom of the pan, then dried and used for laundry work.

Withering quotes Wedelius for the supposition that it was this plant, under the name of Chara, on which the soldiers of Caesar's army subsisted when encamped at Dyrrhachium.

A curious belief is recorded by Gerard as coming from Aristotle, that when bears were half-starved with hibernating and had lain in their dens forty days without any nourishment, but such as they get by 'sucking their paws," they were completely restored by eating this plant.

The roots, according to Gilbert White, are scratched up and eaten by thrushes in severe snowy seasons, and the berries are devoured by several kinds of birds, particularly by pheasants. Pigs which have eaten the fresh tubers suffered, but none died, though it acts as an irritant and purgative. As the leaves when bruised give out a disagreeable odor, they are not spontaneously eaten by animals, who quickly refuse them.

Constituents

The fresh tuber contains a volatile, acrid principle and starch, albumen, gum, sugar, extractive, lignin and salts of potassium and calcium. Saponin has been separated, also a brownish, oily liquid alkaloid, resembling coniine in its properties, but less active.

Arum leaves give off prussic acid when injured, being a product of certain glucosides contained, called cyanophoric glucosides.

Collection and Uses

The tubers for medicinal use should be dug up in autumn, or in early spring, before the leaves are fully developed. If laid in sand in a cellar, they can be preserved in sound condition for nearly a year.

When not needed for use in the fresh state, they

can be dried slowly in very gentle heat and sliced. The dried slices are reduced to powder and kept in the cool, in stoppered bottles.

The fresh root when beaten up with gum, is recommended as a good pill mass, retaining all the medicinal properties.

The Arum had formerly a great reputation as a drug, in common with all other plants containing acrid or poisonous principles.

The dried root was recommended as a diuretic and stimulant, but is no longer employed. The British Domestic Herbal describes a case of alarming dropsy with great constitutional exhaustion treated most successfully with a medicine composed of Arum and Angelica, which cured in about three weeks.

The juice of the fresh tuber is purgative, but too violently so to be safely administered, and its use for this purpose has now been abandoned. Other uses of the tuber are, however, advocated in herbal medicine. Preparations were once official in the Dublin Pharmacopeia, and are also recommended by Homeopathy. A homeopathic tincture is prepared from the plant, and its root, which proves curative in diluted doses for a chronic sore throat with swollen mucous membranes and hoarseness, and likewise for a feverish sore throat.

An ointment made by stewing the fresh sliced tuber with lard is stated to be an efficient cure for ringworm, though the fresh sliced tuber applied to the skin produces a blister. The juice of the fresh plant when incorporated with lard has also been applied locally in the treatment of ringworm.

Other Species

The AMERICAN ARUM (Arum triphyllum, Limn), Dragon Root, has similar characters and properties to the above.

Synonym: Wild Turnip. Jack-in-the-Pulpit.

It is very common in eastern North America, in moist places, where it is known as Indian Turnip, Wild Turnip, Jack-in-thePulpit, Devil's Ear, Pepper Turnip, Wake Robin, etc.

It grows 1 to 3 feet high; a green spathe, broadly striped with brown purple, arches over and encloses the spadix. The corm is smaller than the English species, 1/2 to 2 inches broad and about half as high. It is very acrid when fresh, but loses this property when cooked, or partially when dried.

For the drug market it is collected in the early spring, transversely sliced and dried, and is employed in both herbal and homeopathic treatment.

It has acrid, stimulant, diaphoretic and expectorant properties, and is said to be useful when taken immediately after eating, to assist digestion and promote assimilation. It is considered a stimulant to the lungs in consumption, asthma and chronic forms of lung complaints, and to be of great value in hoarseness, coughs, asthma, rheumatism and lung diseases.

Owing to its acrimony, it is usually given in powder in honey or syrup, or mixed with fine sugar.

In the absolutely fresh state, both English and American Arums are violent irritants to the mucous membrane, producing when chewed, intense burning to the mouth and throat, and if taken internally, causing violent gastro-enteritis, which may end in death.

Dose

Powdered root 10 to 30 grains.

The ITALIAN ARUM drug of Southern Europe is derived from the Mediterranean A. Italicum (Mill.), which is found also in the Isle of Wight. It has the same poisonous properties.

That of Asia Minor, with similar properties, is A. dioscorides, Sib.

In A. Italicum and some of the other species, the spadix which supports the flowers disengages a quantity of heat, sufficient to be felt by the hand that touches it. Lamarck mentions an extraordinary degree of heat evolved by A. maculatum about the time when the sheath is about to open.

The DRAGON ARUM of the ancients was probably Amorphophallus campanulatus (Pol.) of the East Indies, whose corm-like rhizome gives rise yearly to one enormous leaf and an equally gigantic inflorescence. Its dirty red and yellow color and foetid smell attract numbers of carrion flies, by which it is fertilized; they are often so deceived as to lay their eggs on the spadix.

The Arrow poison, Maschi, of Guiana, is supposed to come from a species of Arum.

On account of their starch, the rhizomes and tubers of many other species of this family are used as foods, or the starches are extracted. Even those which are poisonous may be thus employed, since cooking usually destroys their toxicity.

The most important, edible product is the corm of Calocasia antiquorum (Schott) (syn. Caladium, or A. esculentum, Linn.), Taro, which is one of the most largely used of tropical foods. Other species are similarly used. It abounds in starch and is much used as an article of food by the natives of Hawaii and other Pacific Islands. In the natural state, both the foliage and roots of Taro have all the pungent acrid qualities that mark the genus to which the plant belongs, but these are so dissipated by cooking that they become mild and palatable with no peculiar flavor more than belongs to good bread. The islanders bake the root in ovens in the same way as Bread Fruit, then beat it into a mass like dough, called Poe.

In India, a liniment is made of the root of Calocasia macrorhiza and Gingilie oil, and used by the native practitioners for frictions to cure intermittent fevers.

In South America, A. Indicum, the Mankuchoo and Manguri of Brazil, is much cultivated about the huts of the natives for its esculent stem and pendulous tubers.

Arum Arrowroot is derived from A. Dracunculus (Linn.), being something like Tapioca.

The root of A. montanum is used in India to poison tigers. The roots of A. lyratum furnish an article of diet to the natives of the Circar mountains. They require, however, to be carefully boiled several times, and dressed in a particular manner, to divest them of a somewhat disagreeable taste.

A. Dracunculus is sometimes cultivated in gardens for the sake of its large pedate leaves, its spotted stem and handsome purple spadix. It is well, however, to advise those intending to add this plant to their gardens that though its lurid and striking spadix forms a handsome feature in a border yet its odor is decidedly strong and unpleasant resembling that of putrid meat, a fact which is evidently perceived by insects who swarm to it, especially in hot weather.

CUCUMBER

Botanical: Cucumis sativa (LINN.)
Family: N.O. Cucurbitaceae
Synonym: Cowcumber.
Part Used: The whole fruit peeled and unpeeled, raw and cooked.
Habitat: Native of East Indies. First cultivated in Britain about 1573.

Description

In the East this trailing annual plant has been extensively cultivated from some 3,000 years and spread westward. It was known to the Greeks (the Greek name being sikuos) and to the Romans. According to Pliny, the Emperor Tiberius had it on his table daily, summer and winter. Pliny describes the Italian fruit as very small, probably like our gherkin; the same form is figured in Herbals of the sixteenth century, but states, 'if hung in a tube while in blossom, the Cucumber will grow to a most surprising length." In Bible history, the Israelites in the wilderness complained to Moses that they missed the luxuries they had in Egypt, 'Cucumbers and Melons," and Hasselquist in his travels (middle of eighteenth century) states: 'they still form a great part of the food of the lower-class people in Egypt serving them for meat, drink and physic." Isaiah, speaking of the desolation of Judah says: 'The daughter of Zion is left as a cottage in a vineyard, as a lodge in a garden of cucumbers." The Cucumber of the Scriptures is, however, by some authorities considered to be a wild form of Cucumis melo, the melon.

The Cucumber has been long known in England, where it was common in the time of Edward III (1327), then fell into disuse and was forgotten till the reign of Henry VIII, but not generally cultivated here till the middle of the seventeenth century. It is too well known to need description.

Constituents

The dietary value of Cucumber is negligible, there being upwards of 96 per cent water in its composition.

Medicinal Action and Uses

Cucumber seeds possess similar properties to those of the allied Pumpkin (Cucurbita Pepo, Linn.) which are distinctly diuretic, but mainly employed as a very efficient taeniacide, 1 to 2 oz. of the seed, thoroughly ground and made into an electuary with sugar, or into an emetic with water, being taken fasting, followed in from 1 to 2 hours by an active purge. The resin has been given in doses of 15 grains.

Cucumber seeds are much smaller than Pumpkin seeds, relatively narrower and thicker and with almost no marginal groove. The emulsion made by bruising Cucumber seeds and rubbing them up with water was formerly thought to possess considerable virtue and was much used in catarrhal affections and diseases of the bowels and urinary passages.

Recipes

As a cosmetic, Cucumber is excellent for rubbing over the skin to keep it soft and white. It is cooling, healing and soothing to an irritated skin, whether caused by sun, or the effects of a cutaneous eruption, and Cucumber juice is in great demand in various forms as a cooling and beautifying agent for the skin. Cucumber soap is used by many women, and a Cucumber wash applied to the skin after exposure to keen winds is extremely beneficial. This lotion is made as follows:

Cucumber Lotion

Peel 1 or 2 large Cucumbers, cut them into slices, and place them in a double boiler, which should be closely covered. Cook them slowly until they are soft. Then put the pieces into a fine linen bag and squeeze them until all the juice has been extracted. Add to the extracted juice one-fourth of rectified spirits of wine (or whisky) and one-third of Elder-flower water. Shake the mixture well and pour into small bottles ready for use.

Another Cucumber Lotion for Sunburn

Chop up a Cucumber and squeeze out the juice with a lemon-squeezer. Mix this with a quantity of glycerine and rose-water mixed together in equal parts.

Cucumber juice is used in the preparation of Glycerine and Cucumber creams. After expression and clarification, it is treated with alcohol, benzoin or salicylic acids being added as preservatives.

Emollient ointments prepared from the Cucumber were formerly considerably employed in irritated states of the skin, but they have been largely superseded by non-fatty cosmetics. The most frequently used preparation of Cucumber at the present time is the cosmetic preparation known as Cucumber Jelly, which is used as a soothing application in roughness of the skin, etc. It consists of a jelly of tragacanth, quince seeds or some similar mucilaginous drug, flavoured with Cucumber juice, which imparts to the preparation a characteristic odor.

The lotion sold in the shops as Glycerinc and Cucumber sometimes contain Cucumber juice, but more frequently this is conspicuous by its absence.

The French make an ointment of Cucumber, using it like cold cream, called 'Pomade aux Concombres," made with Cucumber juice, lard, veal suet, Balsam of Tolu in alcohol, and rose-water.

Other Cucumber Ointment Recipes

1. Take 7 lb. green Cucumbers, 24 oz. pure lard and 15 oz. veal suet. Grate the washed Cucurnbers to

a pulp, express and strain the juice. Cut the suet into small pieces, heat over a water bath till melted then add the lard and when melted, strain through muslin into an earthen vessel capable of holding a gallon and stir until thickening commences, when one-third of the juice is to be added and the whole beaten with a spatula till the odor has been almost wholly extracted. Decant the portion which separates, then add, consecutively, the remaining two-thirds of the juice and decant similarly. Then close the jar closely and place in a water bath till the fatty matter entirely separates from the juice. The green coagulum floating on the surface is now removed and the jar put in a cool place that the ointment may solidify. Then separate the crude ointment from the liquid on which it floats, melt again, strain and put up in closely-sealed glass jars. A layer of rose-water on its surface will aid preservation.

2. Incorporate 1 part of distilled Spirit of Cucumbers with 7 parts of benzoinated lard. The spirit is made by distilling a mixture of 1 part of grated Cucumbers with 3 parts of diluted alcohol, returning the first 2 parts or distillates which come over. This spirit is permanent and ointment or cream made from it keeps well.

Cucumber Milk is made of the following ingredients: 1 OZ. soap, 1 OZ. olive oil, 1 OZ. wax, 1 OZ. spermaceti 1 lb. almonds, 4 1/2 pints freshly expressed Cucumber juice, 1 pint extract of Cucumber, 2 lb. alcohol.

Use in Perfumery

The peculiarly refreshing odor of Cucumber has found application in perfumery. Various products belonging under this head requiring the odor of Cucumber - it being used in blending certain bouquet perfumes - this plant is to be included among the aromatic plant in a wider sense.

Extract of Cucumber may be prepared as follows:

To 8 lb. Cucumbers, take 5 quarts of alcohol. The Cucumbers are peeled, cut into thin slices and macerated in the warm alcohol. If the odor is not strong enough in the alcohol after some days, it is poured over some more fresh slices, the macerated residue is expressed and at the end of the operation all the liquors are united and filtered.

Concentrated Cucumber perfume is made by the repeated extraction of the freshly sliced fruit with strong alcohol and subsequent concentration by distillation in vacuo. It is naturally very expensive.

Other Species

The SIKKIM CUCUMBER (C. sativa, var. sikkimensis) is a large-fruited form, reaching 15 inches long by 6 inches thick, grown in the Himalayas. The fruit, produced abundantly, is reddish brown, marked with yellow and is eaten both raw and cooked.

The WEST INDIAN GHERKIN is C. anguria a plant with slender vines and very abundant, small, egg-shaped green fruit, covered with warts and prickles. It is the principal ingredient in West Indian pickles and is also used there in soups and frequently eaten green, but is far inferior to the common Cucumber.

C. flexuosum is the SNAKE CUCUMBER: it grows to a great length and may be used either raw or pickled.

The Squirting Cucumber, Ecballium Elaterium, furnishes the drug Elaterium.

The fruits of C. trigonis (Roxb.), 'Karit," C. Hardwickii, Royle (the Hill Colocynth of India), and C. prophetarum (Linn.) of Arabia (the last-named containing the bitter substance prophetin, which occurs also in Elaterium) are largely employed as purgatives.

A less bitter variety of Karit is said to be eaten after the removal of its bitter principle by maceration in water.

C. myriocarpus (Naud.), a small gourd of South Africa, is used by the Kaffirs as an emetic in the form of the fruit-pulp, 20 grains being found to produce nausea and purgation after several hours. Larger quantities produce vomiting with some blood and considerable salivation. Its active principle has been called Myriocarpin.

The INDIAN CUCUMBER, or Cucumber Root, is the rhizome of Medeola virginiana (Linn.) a member of the order Liliaceae, reputed to be hydragogue and diuretic and therefore used in dropsies. In its fresh state it is somewhat Cucumber-like in taste.

The Bitter Cucumber is another name for Colocynth (Citrullus colocynthis, Schrader).

The Cucumber Tree, so called from the resemblance of the young fruits to small cucumbers, is Magnolia virginiana, var. acuminata (Linn.), the Mountain Magnolia. It has shortly acuminate leaves and yellowish-green flowers, 3 to 4 inches across, with a peculiar bluish tinge. The wood of the tree is yellow and is used for bowls. The bark was formerly official, with that of other species of Magnolia, in the United States Pharmacopeia, employed for its tonic, stimulant and diaphoretic properties and, like other bitters, employed in the treatment of malarial fever and considered a valuable remedy for rheumatism. Dose of the recently-dried bark is 1/2 to 1 drachm, frequently repeated; of the tincture, 1 fluid drachm.

CUCUMBER, SQUIRTING

Botanical: Ecballium elaterium
Family: N.O. Cucurbitaceae
Synonyms: Momordica Elaterium. Wild Cucumber.
Habitat: Europe, cultivated in Britain.

Description

A perennial plant but in Britain an annual, with a large fleshy root from which rise several round, thick stems, branching and trailing like the Common Cucumber but without tendrils; leaves heartshaped, rough; flower-stalks auxillary; male flowers in clusters with bell-shaped, yellow green veined corollas, females solitary; fruit a small elliptical greenish gourd covered with soft triangular prickles. The fruits forcibly eject their seeds together with a mucilaginous juice, a phenomenon due to endormosis. The plant flowers in July. The fruit is collected just before it ripens and is left until it matures and ejects the seeds and juice; this must not be artificially hastened or the product will be injured; the juice is then dried in flakes and sent to the market as Elaterium. The flakes often bear the impress of the muslin on which they were dried.

Constituents

Elaterin; a green resin, starch, lignin, and saline matter.

Medicinal Action and Uses

A powerful hydragogue cathartic, and in large doses excites nausea and vomiting. If administered too frequently it operates with great violence on both the stomach and bowels producing inflammation and possibly fatal results. It also increases the flow of urine, and is of some use in the treatment of dropsy, especially when oedema is due to disease of the kidney. There is a case on record of a French doctor who suffered severely from carrying some of the seeds in his hat from the Jardin des Plante to his Paris lodging.

Preparations and Dosages

It must be used with the greatest caution; because of its variability Elaterium should not be employed, preference always being given to the official Elaterin. 'Elaterium, 1/10 to 1/2 grain. Elacterin, 1/40 to 1/10 grain. Compound powder of Elacterin = Elaterin in fine powder, 1 part milk, sugar in fine powder 39 parts; dose, 1 to 4 grains.

Poisons and Antidotes

As for Bitter Apple.

CUDBEAR

Botanical: Rocella tinctoria
Family: N.O. Lichenes
Habitat: Maritime rocks of Madeira. The Azores, Canary and Cape de Verde Islands.

Cudbear is a purplish-red powder prepared from a species of the Rocella tinctoria, Lecanora Acharius and other lichens. It is an alcoholic or agueous preparation of a deep red color, which is lightened by the addition of acids and changed to a purplish red by alkalies. It yields about 35 per cent of ash, mostly sodium chloride.

Action and Uses

Employed for coloring purposes as a dye. Cudbear is very difficult to extract, so the liquid preparations are rarely uniform in color, and for this reason powdered Cudbear is generally used. The powder is made from an ammoniacal infusion of the lichen evaporated to dryness and then reduced to powder. In pharmacy it is sometimes used as a test for alkalies and acids.

R. tinctoria is the lichen from which Litmus is obtained. The lichen is boiled with water, containing chalk in suspension, and then concentrated in vacuum; it is then dried, freed from impurities and put in large vats together with the liquor and ammonia. It is kept at 25 to 30 degrees F. for two or three months and then dried and powdered.

CUDWEED

Botanical: Graphalium uliginosum
Family: N.O. Compositae
Synonyms: Cotton Weed. March Everlasting.
Part Used: Herb.
Habitat: Marshy places in most parts of Europe.

Description

Stalk branched, diffused; flowers crowded, termina tiny; leaves elliptical, tapering into a long foot-stalk, slightly downy and greenish above, whitish and more downy underneath. The ends of the branches crowded with nurnerous heads of nearly sessile flowers which appear in August.

Medicinal Action and Uses

Quinsy, gargle astringent, infusion 1 OZ. to 1 pint boiling water taken internally in wine glassful; also used as a gargle.

Fluid extract: Dose, 1/2 to 1 drachm.

CUMIN

Botanical: Cuminum cyminum (LINN.)
Family: N.O. Umbelliferae
Synonym: Cumino aigro (Malta).
Part Used: Fruit.

Habitat

Cumin, besides being used medicinally, was in the Middle Ages one of the commonest spice of European growth. It is a small annual, herbaceous plant, indigenous to Upper Egypt, but from early times was cultivated in Arabia, India, China, and in the countries bordering on the Mediterranean.

Description

Its stem is slender and branched, rarely exceeding 1 foot in height and somewhat angular. The leaves are divided into long, narrow segments like Fennel, but much smaller and are of a deep green color, generally turned back at the ends. The upper leaves are nearly stalkless, but the lower ones have longer leafstalks. The flowers are small, rose-coloured or white, in stalked umbels with only four to six rays, each of which are only about 1/3 inch long, and bloom in June and July, being succeeded by fruit - the so-called seeds - which constitute the Cumin of pharmacy. They are oblong in shape, thicker in the middle, compressed laterally about 5 inch long, resembling Caraway seeds, but lighter in color and bristly instead of smooth, almost straight, instead of being curved. They have nine fine ridges, overlapping as many oil channels, or vittae. The odor and taste are somewhat like caraway, but less agreeable.

History

Cumin is mentioned in Isaiah xxvii. 25 and 27, and Matthew xxiii. 23, and in the works of Hippocrates and Dioscorides. From Pliny we learn that the ancients took the ground seed medicinally with bread, water or wine, and that it was accounted the best of condiments. The seeds of the Cumin when smoked, were found to occasion pallor of the face, whence the expression of Horace, exsangue cuminum, and Pliny tells us that the followers of the celebrated rhetorician Porcius Latro employed it to produce a complexion such as bespeaks application to study.

Cumin also symbolized cupidity among the Greeks: Marcus Aurelius was so nicknamed because of his avarice, and misers were jocularly said to have eaten Cumin.

In the thirteenth and fourteenth centuries, when it was much in use as a culinary spice, its average price in England per lb. was 2d., equivalent to 1s. 4d. at the present day.

Cumin has now gone out of use in European medicine, having been replaced by Caraway seed, which has a more agreeable flavor, but it is still used to some extent in India, in native medicine. Its principal employment is in veterinary medicine and as an ingredient in curry powder, for which purposes it is imported from Bombay and Calcutta, Morocco, Sicily and Malta. It is commonly sold in Malta, where they call it cumino aigro (hot Cumin), to distinguish it from Anise, which they term cumino dulce, or sweet Cumin.

Cultivation

Although we get nearly all our supplies from the Mediterranean, it would be perfectly feasible to grow Cumin in England, as it will ripen its fruit as far north as Norway. It is, however, rarely cultivated here, and seeds are generally somewhat difficult to obtain.

They should be sown in small pots, filled with light soil and plunged into a very moderate hot bed to bring up the plants. These should be hardened gradually in an open frame and transplanted into a warm border of good soil, preserving the balls of earth which adhere to the roots in the pots. Keep clean of weeds and the plants will flower very well and will probably perfect their seeds if the season should be warm and favourable.

The plants are threshed when the fruit is ripe and the 'seeds' dried in the same manner as Caraway.

Constituents

The strong aromatic smell and warm, bitterish taste of Cumin fruits are due to the presence of a volatile oil which is separated by distillation of the fruit with water, and exists in the proportion of 2 to 4 per cent. It is limpid and pale yellow in color, and is mainly a mixture of cymol or cymene and cuminic aldehyde, or cyminol, which is its chief constituent.

The tissue of the fruits contains a fatty oil with resin, mucilage and gum, malates and albuminous matter, and in the outerseed coat there is much tannin. The yield of ash is about 8 per cent.

Medicinal Action and Uses

Stimulant, antispasmodic, carminative. The older herbalists esteemed Cumin superior in comforting carminative qualities to Fennel or Caraway, but on account of its very disagreeable flavor, its medicinal use at the present day is almost confined to veterinary practice, in which it is employed as a carminative.

Formerly Cumin had considerable repute as a corrective for the flatulency of languid digestion and as a remedy for colic and dyspetic headache. Bruised and applied externally in the form of a plaster, it was recommended as a cure for stitches and pains in the side caused by the sluggish congestion of indolent parts, and it has been compounded with other drugs to form a stimulating liniment.

Bay-salt and Cumin-seeds mixed, is a universal remedy for the diseases of pigeons, especially scabby backs and breasts. The proportions of the remedy are: 1/4 lb. Baysalt, 1/4 lb. Common Salt, 1 lb. Fennel-seeds, 1 lb. Dill-seeds, 1 lb. Cumin-seeds, 1 OZ. Assafoetida; mix all with a little wheaten flour and some fine-worked clay; when all are well beaten together, put into two earthen pots and bake them in the oven. When cold, put them on the table in the dove-cote; the pigeons will eat it and thus be cured.

CUP PLANT

Botanical: Silphium perfoliatum
Family: N.O. Compositae
Synonyms: Indian Cup Plant. Ragged Cup.
Part Used: Root.
Habitat: Western States of America, Oregon, Texas.

Description

The chief features of the genus are the monaecious radiate heads, the ray florets strap-shaped and pistil bearing, the disc florets tubular and sterile, and the broad flat achenes, surrounded by a wing notched at the summit and usually terminating in two short awn-like teeth which represent the pappus. Its distinctive character is rhizome, cylindrical, crooked, rough, small roots, and transversed section shows large resin cells. Taste, persistent, acrid. The most interesting of the species is the Compass plant, so named from its tendency to point to the North. This plant is also known by the names of Pilot plant, Polar plant, Rosin and Turpentine weed, and like the Cup plant of another species, Silphium Loeve, with tuberous roots, which are a native food in the Columbia valley, is cultivated in English gardens. The Cup plant derives its name from the cup-like appearance of the winged stalks of its opposite leaves which are united.

Medicinal Action and Uses

Tonic, diaphoretic, alterative. Found useful in liver and spleen maladies, also in fevers, internal bruises, debility, ulcers, and a general alterative restorative. Gum is a stimulant and antispasmodic.

Dose

4 oz. of powdered root in decoction. Powder itself in 20-grain doses.

Other Species

S. Ginniferum or Rosin weed is said to bestimulating and antispasmodic, and yields resinous secretions like mastic; this resin is diuretic and imparts to the urine an aromatic odor. Its root is a good expectorant in pulmonary and catarrhal diseases and the Compass plant is said to be emetic.

CURRANT, BLACK

Botanical: Ribes nigrum (LINN.)
Family: N.O. Saxifragaceae
Synonyms: Quinsy Berries. Squinancy Berries.
Parts Used: Fruit, leaves, bark, roots.
Habitat: Europe.

Description

The Black Currant is occasionally found wild in damp woods as far north as the middle of Scotland, but is considered to be a true native only in Yorkshire and the Lake District - when found apparently wild in other parts of the country, its presence is due to the agency of birds. It is easily distinguished at all seasons by the strong perfume of its buds and leaves.

This shrub shows the only instance of a process by which double flowers may become single, by changing petals into stamina. It has a solitary, one-flowered peduncle at the base of the raceme, and its leaves are dotted underneath.

It was not so popular originally as the Red and White Currants, for Gerard describes the fruit as being 'of a stinking and somewhat loathing savour."

The berries are sometimes put into brandy like Black Cherries. The Russians make wine of them, with or without honey or spirits, while in Siberia a drink is made of the leaves which, when young, make common spirits resemble brandy. An infusion of them is like green tea, and can change the flavor of black tea. Goats eat the leaves, and bears especially like the berries, which are supposed to have medicinal properties not possessed by others of the genus.

Medicinal Uses

Diuretic, diaphoretic, febrifuge.

The juice can be boiled to an extract with sugar, when it is called Rob, and is used for inflammatory sore throats. Excellent lozenges are also prepared from it.

The infusion of the leaves is cleansing and diuretic, while an infusion of the young roots is useful in eruptive fevers and the dysenteric fevers of cattle.

The raw juice is diuretic and diaphoretic, and is an excellent beverage in febrile diseases.

A decoction of the bark has been found of value in calculus, dropsy, and haemorrhoidal tumors.

Recipes

Black Currant Jelly

It should not be made with too much sugar or its medicinal properties will be impaired. For a sore throat, take a tablespoonful of the jam or jelly; put it in a tumbler and fill the tumbler with boiling water. This 'Black Currant Tea' has a soothing, demulcent effect, taken several times in the day and drunk while hot.

A delicious wine can be made from the fruit. The following is a recipe from an old Cookery Book:

Black Currant Wine, very fine

To every 3 quarts of juice, put the same of water, unboiled; and to every 3 quarts of the liquor, add 3 lb . of very pure, moist sugar. Put it in a cask, preserving a little for filling up. Put the cask in a warm, dry room, and the liquor will ferment itself. Skim off the refuse, when the fermentation shall be over, and fill up with the reserved liquor. When it has ceased working, pour 3 quarts of brandy to 40 quarts of wine. Bung it close for nine months, then bottle it and drain the thick part through a jelly-bag, until it be clear, and bottle that. Keep it ten or twelve months.

Black Currant Cheese

is delicious and is made by putting equal parts of stalked currants and loaf sugar into a pan; place over low heat and stir until the sugar has dissolved, then bring slowly to the boil, stirring all the time. Remove all scum and simmer for an hour, stirring often. Rub the fruit through a hair sieve, return the puree to the pan, and stir until it boils, then put it into small pots and cover like jam.

CURRANT, RED

Botanical: Ribes rubrum (LINN.)
Family: N.O. Grossulariacae
Synonyms: Ribs. Risp. Reps.
Part Used: The fruits, especially the juice.
Habitat: Central and Northern Europe, and United States, Siberia and Canada.

Description

This plant is equally at home in hedges and ditches, trained against the wall of a house, or as a shrub cultivated in gardens. It has straggling stems, three to five lobed leaves, yellowish-green flowers, and fruit in pendulous racemes. The smooth berries are always red in the wild state, but cultivation has added the white and champagne or flesh-coloured varieties. The White and Red Dutch Currants are regarded as the best. The English name was given because the berries were like the Corinth or Zante Grape, the currant of the shops. There are between thirty and forty kinds of currant recognized in catalogues. The fruit is a favorite for tarts andjellies, and being a very hardy plant, is within the reach of all. The juice is a pleasant acid in punch, and was a favorite ingredient in the coffee-houses of Paris, where the sweetened juice is still preferred as a beverage, to syrup of almonds.

Constituents

The juice is said to contain citric acid, malic acid, sugar, vegetable jelly and jam.

Medicinal Action and Uses

Refrigerant, aperient, antiscorbutic. The juice forms a refreshing drink in fever, and the jelly, made from equal weights of fruit and sugar, when eaten with 'high' meats, acts as an anti-putrescent. The wine made from white 'red' currants has been used for calculous affections.

In some cases the fruit causes flatulence and indigestion. It has frequently given much help in forms of visceral obstruction. The jelly is antiseptic, and will ease the pain of a burn and prevent the formation of blisters, if applied immediately. Some regard the leaves as having emmenagogue properties.

Poison and Antidotes

In common with other acidulous fruits, they must be turned out of an open tin immediately into a glass or earthenware dish, or the action of the acid combining with the surrounding air will begin to engender a deadly metallic poison.

CYCLAMEN, IVY-LEAVED

Botanical: Cyclamen hederaefolium
Family: N.O. Primulaceae
Synonym: Sowbread.
Part Used: Tuherous root-stock used fresh when the plant is in flower.

The Cyclamens at first glance do not appear to have much similarity with Primulas, but certain structural points in common have caused them to be grouped in the same family.

There are eight members of the genus, distributed over Southern Europe, North Africa and Western Asia, one of which, Cyclamen hederaefolium, the Ivy-leaved Cyclamen or Sowbread, has been occasionally found in Kent and Sussex, but is generally considered to have been introduced accidentally, being really a native of Italy. Its large, tuberous rootstock, in common with that of C. Europaeum and of others found in the south of Europe, is intensely acrid, a quality that has caused its employment as a purgative.

Description

It occurs rarely in hedge banks and copses, flowering in September. The tuber, 1 to 3 inches in diameter, is turnip-shaped, brown in color and fibrous all over. The nodding rose-coloured or white flowers, which appear before the leaves, are placed singly on fleshy stalks, 4 to 8 inches high. The corolla tube is short, thickened at the throat, the lobes are bent back and are about an inch in length and red at the base. As the fruit ripens, the flower-stalk curls spirally and buries it in the earth. The name of the genus is derived from the Greek cyclos (a circle), either from the reflexed lobes of the corolla, or from the spiral form of the fruit-stalk. The leaves, appearing after the flowers, are somewhat heart-shaped, five to nine angled, in the manner of ivy leaves, dark green, with a white mottled border, often purple beneath, and spring straight from the root on longish stalks or petioles. They continue growing all the winter and spring till May, when they begin to decay, and in June are entirely dried up.

The apparently inappropriate name of this beautiful little plant, Sowbread, arises from its tuberous roots having afforded food for wild swine.

The favorite greenhouse Cyclamens flowering in the winter months, are varieties of a Persian species, C. Perscum, introduced into European horticulture in the middle of the eighteenth century.

Part Used Medicinally

The tuberous rootstock, used fresh, when the plant is in flower.

Constituents

Besides starch, gum and pectin, the tuber yields chemically cyclamin or arthanatin, having an action like saponin.

Medicinal Action and Uses

A homeopathic tincture is made from the fresh root, which applied externally as a liniment over the bowels causes purging.

Old writers tell us that Sowbread baked and made into little flat cakes has the reputation of being 'a good amorous medicine," causing the partaker to fall violently in love.

Although the roots are favorite food of swine, their juice is stated to be poisonous to fish.

Powdered root: dose, 20 to 40 grains.

The fresh tubers bruised and formed into a cataplasm make a stimulating application to indolent ulcers.

An ointment called 'ointment of arthainta' was made from the fresh tubers for expelling worms, and was rubbed on the umbilicus of children and on the abdomen of adults to cause emesis and upon the region over the bladder to increase urinary discharge.

D

DAFFODIL

Botanical: Narcissus Pseudo-narcissus
Family: N.O. Arnaryllidaceae
Synonyms: Narcissus. Porillon. Daffy-down-dilly. Fleur de coucou. Lent Lily.
Parts Used: Bulb, leaves, flowers.
Habitat: Europe, including Britain.

Description

The Common Daffodil, a representative of the Ajax group, grows wild in most European countries. Its green, linear leaves about a foot long, and golden, terminal flowers, are familiar in moist woods and country gardens.

The bulbs should be gathered during the winter, and the flowers when in full bloom, in dry weather, and dried quickly. The bulbs and not the flowers of other species are used.

Constituents

Professor Barger has given the following notes on the alkaloid of Narcissus Pseudo-narcissus. 'In 1910 Ewins obtained from the bulbs a crystalline alkaloid, to which he gave the name of narcissine, and on analysis found the formula to be C16H17ON." He notes that the alkaloid is characterized by great stability and cannot easily be decomposed. Ringer and Morshead found the alkaloid from resting bulbs acted like pilocarpine, while that from the flowering bulbs resembled atropine. Laidlaw tested Ewins' alkaloid on frogs and cats, but found no action similar to pilocarpine or atropine. 0.125 gram given by mouth to a cat caused vomiting, salivation and purgation. In 1920 Asahtna, Professor of Chemistry in the Tokyo College of Pharmacy, showed that narcissine is identical with Iycorine isolated from Lycoris radiata in 1899. The name narcissine has therefore been dropped. Lycorine is quite common in the N.O. Amaryllidaceae. It was found in Buphane disticha by Tutin in the Mellome Research Laboratory in 1911 (Journ. Chem. Soc. Transactions 99, page 1,240). It is generally present in quite small quantities, at most 0.1 to 0.18 per cent of the fresh material. Chemically, Iycorine or narcissine has some resemblance to hydrastine, and like it, contains a dioxymethylene group.

Medicinal Action and Uses

The following is a quotation from Culpepper:

'Yellow Daffodils are under the dominion of Mars, and the roots thereof are hot and dry in the third degree. The roots boiled and taken in posset drink cause vomiting and are used with good success at the appearance of approaching agues, especially the tertian ague, which is frequently caught in the springtime. A plaster made of the roots with parched barley meal dissolves hard swellings and imposthumes, being applied thereto; the juice mingled with honey, frankincense wine, and myrrh, and dropped into the ears is good against the corrupt and running matter of the ears, the roots made hollow and boiled in oil help raw ribed heels; the juice of the root is good for the morphew and the discolouring of the skin."

It is said by Galen to have astringent properties. It has been used as an application to wounds. For hard imposthumes, for burns, for strained sinews, stiff or painful joints, and other local ailments, and for 'drawing forth thorns or stubs from any part of the body' it was highly esteemed.

The Daffodil was the basis of an ancient ointment called Narcissimum.

The powdered flowers have been used as an emetic in place of the bulbs, and in the form of infusion or syrup, in pulmonary catarrh.

Dosages

Of powder, from 20 grains to 2 drachms as an emetic. Of extract, 2 to 3 grains.

Poison and Antidotes

It may be noted that Henry states that Iycorine or narcissine in warm-blooded animals acts as an emetic causing eventually collapse and death by paralysis of the central nervous system.

There have been several cases of poisoning by Daffodil bulbs which have been eaten in mistake for onions. In one case the points observed were: (1) the speedy action of the poison; (2) the fact that the high temperature did not destroy the toxicity of the poison; and (3) the relatively small quantity of Daffodil bulbs which caused the trouble.

Other Species

The bulbs of N. poeticus, N. odorus, and N. jonquilla possess similar acrid and emetic properties.

DAHLIAS

Botanical: Dahlia Variabilis
Family: N.O. Compositae
Synonym: Georgina.

The Dahlia is named after Dr. Dahl, a pupil of Linnaeus, but is also known, especially on the Continent, by the name 'Georgina." It is a native of Mexico, where it grows in sandy meadows at an elevation of 5,000 feet above the sea, and from whence the first plants introduced to England were brought by way of Madrid, in 1789, by the Marchioness of Bute. These having been lost, others were introduced, in 1804, by Lady Holland. These, too, perished, so fresh ones were obtained from France, when the Continent was thrown open by the Peace of 1814.

Constituents

The Inulin obtained in Dandelion and Chicory is also present in Dahlia tubers under the name of Dahlin. After undergoing a special treatment, Dahlia tubers and Chicory will yield the pure Laevulose that is sometimes called Atlanta Starch or Diabetic Sugar, which is frequently prescribed for diabetic and consumptive patients, and has been given to children in cases of wasting illness.

There was a very considerable business done in this product before the War by certain German firms. In a paper read at the Second International Congress of the Sugar Industry, held at Paris in 1908, it was stated that pure Laevulose is preferably made by the inversion of Inulin with dilute acids, and that the older process of preparation from invert sugar or molasses does not yield a pure product. The first step in the technical production of Laevulose is in the preparation of Inulin, and Dahlia tubers or Chicory root, which contain 6 to 12 per cent of Inulin are the most suitable material. Chicory root can readily be obtained in quantity, and Dahlia plants, if cultivated for the purpose, should yield in a few years a plentiful supply of cheap raw material.

For extraction of the Inulin, the roots or tubers are sliced, treated with milk of lime and steamed. The juice is then expressed and clarified by subsidence and filtration, the clear liquid being run into a revolving cooler until flakes are produced. These flakes are separated by a centrifugal machine, washed and decolorized, and the thus purified product finally treated with diluted acid, and so converted into Laevulose. This solution of Laevulose is neutralized and evaporated to a syrup in a vacuum pan.

Laevulose can be produced in this manner from Chicory roots and Dahlia tubers at an enormous reduction of price from the older methods of preparing it from molasses or sugar, the resultant product being moreover of absolute purity. Its sweet and pleasant taste are likely to make it used not only for diabetic patients, but also in making confectionery and for retarding crystallization of sugar products. It can also readily be utilized in the brewing and mineral water industries.

The research staff of one of the Scottish Universities during the War developed a process of extracting a valuable and much needed drug for the Army from Dahlia tubers, and was using as much material for the purpose as could be spared by growers.

DAISY, COMMON

Botanical: Bellis perennis (LINN.)
Family: N.O. Compositae
Synonyms: Bruisewort. (Scotch) Bairnwort. (Welsh) Llygad y Dydd (Eye of the Day).
Parts Used: Root, leaves.

The Common Daisy, which flowers from the earliest days of spring till late in the autumn, and covers the ground with its flat leaves so closely that nothing can grow beneath them, needs no detailed description.

It had once, in common with the Ox-Eye Daisy, a great reputation as a cure for fresh wounds, used as an ointment applied externally, and against inflammatory disorders of the liver, taken internally in the form of a distilled water of the plant.

The flowers and leaves are found to afford a certain amount of oil and ammoniacal salts.

Gerard mentions the Daisy, under the name of 'Bruisewort," as an unfailing remedy in 'all kinds of paines and aches," besides curing fevers, inflammation of the liver and 'alle the inwarde parts."

In 1771 Dr. Hill said that an infusion of the leaves was 'excellent against Hectic Fevers." The Daisy was an ingredient of an ointment much used in the fourteenth century for wounds, gout and fevers.

A strong decoction of the roots has been recommended as an excellent medicine in scorbutic complaints, it being stated, however, that the use of it must be continued for a considerable length of time before its effects will appear.

The taste of the leaves is somewhat acrid, notwithstanding which it has been used in some countries as a pot-herb. On account of the acrid juice contained in the leaves, no cattle will touch it, nor insects attack it.

The roots, too, have a penetrating pungency, containing some tannic acid, and there was once a popular superstition (to which Bacon refers) that if they be boiled in milk and the liquid given to puppies, the animals will grow no bigger.

According to some old writers, the generic name is derived from the Latin bellus (pretty or charming), though others say its name is from a dryad named Belidis. The common name is a corruption of the old English name 'day's-eye," and is used by Chaucer in that sense:

'Well by reason men it call maie

The Daisie, or else the Eye of the Daie."

In Scotland it is the 'Bairnwort," testifying to the joy of children in gathering it for daisy-chains.

There is a common proverb associated with the flower and its abundance in spring and early summer: 'When you can put your foot on seven daisies summer is come."

DAISY, OX-EYE

Botanical: Chrysanthemum leucanthemum (LINN.)
Family: N.O. Compositae
Synonyms: Great Ox-eye. Goldens. Marguerite. Moon Daisy. Horse Gowan. Maudlin Daisy. Field Daisy. Dun Daisy. Butter Daisy. Horse Daisy. Maudlinwort. White. Weed. Leucanthemum vulgare. (Scotch) Gowan.
Parts Used: Whole herb, flowers, root.

The Ox-Eye Daisy is a familiar sight in fields. In Somersetshire there is an old tradition connecting it with the Thunder God, and hence it is sometimes spoken of as the 'Dun Daisy."

It is to be found throughout Europe and Russian Asia. The ancients dedicated it to Artemis, the goddess of women, considering it useful in women's complaints. In Christian days, it was transferred to St. Mary Magdalen and called Maudelyn or Maudlin Daisy after her. Gerard terms it Maudlinwort.

The genus derives its name from the Greek words chrisos (golden) and anthos (flower), and contains only two indigenous species this and the Corn Marigold, in which the whole flower is yellow, not only the central disc of florets, as in the Daisy. The specific name of the Ox-Eye signifies 'white flower," being like the generic name, Greek in origin. The old northern name for the Daisy was Baldur's Brow, and this, with many other species of Chrysanthemum became dedicated to St. John.

Description

The plant generally grows from 1 to 2 feet high. The root is perennial and somewhat creeping; the stems, hard and wiry, furrowed and only very slightly branched. The leaves are small and coarsely toothed; those near the root are somewhat rounder in form than those on the stem, and are on long stalks, those on the stem are oblong and stalkless.

By the middle of May, the familiar yellowcentred white flower-heads commence to bloom, and are at their best till about the close of June, though isolated specimens may be met with throughout the summer, especially where undisturbed by the cutting of the hay, as on railway banks, where the plant flourishes well. Beneath each flower-head is a ring of green sheathing bracts, the involucre. These not only protect and support the bloom, but doubtless prevents insects trying to bite their way to the honey from below. They, as well as the rest of the plant, are permeated with an acrid juice that is obnoxious to insects.

The young leaves are said to be eaten in salads in Italy. According to Linnaeus, horses, sheep and goats eat the plant, but cows and pigs refuse it on account of its acridity.

Part Used Medicinally

The whole herb, collected in May and June, in the wild state, and dried. Also the flowers.

The taste of the dried herb is bitter and tingling, and the odor faintly resembles that of valerian.

Medicinal Action and Uses

Antispasmodic diuretic, tonic. Ox-Eye Daisy has been successfully employed in whooping-cough, asthma and nervous excitability.

As a tonic, it acts similarly to Chamomile flowers, and has been recommended for nightsweats. The flowers are balsamic and make a useful infusion for relieving chronic coughs and for bronchial catarrhs. Boiled with the leaves and stalks and sweetened with honey, they make an excellent drink for the same purpose. In America, the root is also employed successfully for checking the night-sweats of pulmonary consumption, the fluid extract being taken, 15 to 60 drops in water.

Externally, it is serviceable as a lotion for wounds, bruises, ulcers and some cutaneous diseases.

Gerard writes:

'Dioscorides saith that the floures of Oxeie made up in a seare cloth doe asswage and washe away cold hard swellings, and it is reported that if they be drunke by and by after bathing, they make them in a short time wellcoloured that have been troubled with the yellow jaundice."

Culpepper tells us that it is 'a wound herb of good respect, often used in those drinks and salves that are for wounds, either inward or outward' . . . and that it is 'very fitting to be kept both in oils, ointments, plasters and syrups." He also tells us that the leaves bruised and applied reduce swellings, and that

'a decoction thereof, with wall-wort and agrimony, and places fomented or bathed therewith warm, giveth great ease in palsy, sciatica or gout. An ointment made thereof heals all wounds that have inflammation about them."

Country people used formerly to take a decoction of the fresh herb in ale for the cure of jaundice.

DAMIANA

Botanical: Turnera aphrodisiaca (WILLD.)
Family: N.O. Turneraceae
Part Used: Leaves.
Habitat: Mexico, South Arnerica, Texas, West Indies.

Description

A small shrub; leaves smooth and pale green on upper side, underneath glabrous, with a few hairs on the ribs, ovolanceolate, shortly petiolate with two small glands at base; flowers yellow, rising singly from axils of the leaves, capsule one-celled splitting into three pieces; smell aromatic, taste characteristic, bitterish, aromatic and resinous.

Constituents

A greenish volatile oil, smelling like chamomile, amorhpous bitter principle Damianin, resins and tannin.

Medicinal Action and Uses

Mild purgative, diuretic, tonic, acting directly on the reproductive organs, stimulant, hypochondriastic, aphrodisiae.

Preparations

Fluid extract, 1/2 to 1 drachm. Solid extract, 5 to 10 grains. Often combined with Nux Vomica, Phosphorus, etc.

Other Species

Turnera opifera leaves are used as an infusion and given as an astringent and tonic by the natives of Brazil, also T. ulmifolia for its tonic and expectorant properties.

Aplopappus discoideus was formerly sold as Damiana, but can easily be detected, as the leaves are distinctly lanceolate, with only two or three teeth on either side.

DAMIANA, FALSE

Botanical: Aplopappus laricifolius
Family: N.O. Compositae
Synonyms: Aplopappus. Bigelovia Veneta.
Part Used: The leaves.
Habitat: Chili.

Description

The U.S.D. refers to Aplopappus discoideus as False Damiana. Gray refers to it as Bigelovia Veneta.

Constituents

A volatile oil, also a fatty oil which has the smell of the plant, brown acid, resin, tannin. The resin is peculiar in containing other resins.

Medicinal Action and Uses

It is used as a stimulant in flatulent dyspepsia and chronic inflammation with hemorrhage of the lower bowel. It is very useful in dysentery and in genito-urinary catarrh and as a stimulant expectorant; the tincture is useful for slowly healing ulcers.

Preparations and Dosages

A strong decoction is made by 1 part to 5 of water. 1 tablespoonful as a dose every two hours. Dose of the fluid extract, 5 to 20 minims.

DANDELION

Botanical: Taraxacum officinale (WEBER)
Family: N.O. Compositae
Synonyms: Priest's Crown. Swine's Snout.
Parts Used: Root, leaves.

The Dandelion (Taraxacum officinale, Weber, T. Densleonis, Desf; Leontodon taraxacum, Linn.), though not occurring in the Southern Hemisphere, is at home in all parts of the north temperate zone, in pastures, meadows and on waste ground, and is so plentiful that farmers everywhere find it a troublesome weed, for though its flowers are more conspicuous in the earlier months of the summer, it may be found in bloom, and consequently also prolifically dispersing its seeds, almost throughout the year.

Description

From its thick tap root, dark brown, almost black on the outside though white and milky within, the long jagged leaves rise directly, radiating from it to form a rosette Iying close upon the ground, each leaf being grooved and constructed so that all the rain falling on it is conducted straight to the centre of the rosette and thus to the root which is, therefore, always kept well watered. The maximum amount of water is in this manner directed towards the proper region for utilization by the root, which but for this arrangement would not obtain sufficient moisture, the leaves being spread too close to the ground for the water to penetrate.

The leaves are shiny and without hairs, the margin of each leaf cut into great jagged teeth, either upright or pointing somewhat backwards, and these teeth are themselves cut here and there into lesser teeth. It is this somewhat fanciful resemblance to the canine teeth of a lion that (it is generally assumed) gives the plant its most familiar name of Dandelion, which is a corruption of the French Dent de Lion, an equivalent of this name being found not only in its former specific Latin name Dens leonis and in the Greek name for the genus to which Linnaeus assigned it, Leontodon, but also in nearly all the languages of Europe.

There is some doubt, however, as to whether it was really the shape of the leaves that provided the original notion, as there is really no similarity between them, but the leaves may perhaps be said to resemble the angular jaw of a lion fully supplied with teeth. Some authorities have suggested that the yellow flowers might be compared to the golden teeth of the heraldic lion, while others say that the whiteness of the root is the feature which provides the resemblance. Flückiger and Hanbury in Pharmacographia, say that the name was conferred by Wilhelm, a surgeon, who was so much impressed by the virtues of the plant that he likened it to Dens leonis. In the Ortus Sanitatis, 1485, under 'Dens Leonis," there is a monograph of half a page (unaccompanied by any illustration) which concludes:

'The Herb was much employed by Master Wilhelmus, a surgeon, who on account of its virtues, likened it to "eynem lewen zan, genannt zu latin Dens leonis" (a lion's tooth, called in Latin Dens leonis)."

In the pictures of the old herbals, for instance, the one in Brunfels' Contrafayt Kreuterbuch, 1532, the leaves very much resemble a lion's tooth. The root is not illustrated at all in the old herbals, as only the herb was used at that time.

The name of the genus, Taraxacum, is derived from the Greek taraxos (disorder), and akos (remedy), on account of the curative action of the plant. A possible alternative derivation of Taraxacum is suggested in The Treasury of Botany:

'The generic name is possibly derived from the Greek taraxo ("I have excited" or "caused") and achos (pain), in allusion to the medicinal effects of the plant."

There are many varieties of Dandelion leaves; some are deeply cut into segments, in others the segments or lobes form a much less conspicuous feature, and are sometimes almost entire.

The shining, purplish flower-stalks rise straight from the root, are leafless, smooth and hollow and bear single heads of flowers. On picking the flowers, a bitter, milky juice exudes from the broken edges of the stem, which is present throughout the plant, and which when it comes into contact with the hand, turns to a brown stain that is rather difficult to remove.

Each bloom is made up of numerous strapshaped florets of a bright golden yellow. This strap-shaped corolla is notched at the edge into five teeth, each tooth representing a petal, and lower down is narrowed into a claw-like tube, which rests on the singlechambered ovary containing a single ovule. In this tiny tube is a copious supply of nectar, which more than half fills it, and the presence of which provides the incentive for the visits of many insects, among whom the bee takes first rank. The Dandelion takes an important place among honey-producing plants, as it furnishes considerable quantities of both pollen and nectar in the early spring, when the bees' harvest from fruit trees is nearly over. It is also important from the beekeeper's point of view, because not only does it flower most in spring, no matter how cool the weather may be, but a small succession of bloom is also kept up until late autumn, so that it is a source of honey after the main flowers have ceased to bloom, thus delaying the need for feeding the colonies of bees with artificial food.

Many little flies also are to be found visiting the Dandelion to drink the lavishly-supplied nectar. By carefully watching, it has been ascertained that no less than ninety-three different kinds of insects are in the habit of frequenting it. The stigma grows up through the tube formed by the anthers, pushing the pollen before it, and insects smearing themselves with this pollen carry it to the stigmas of other flowers already expanded, thus insuring cross-fertilization. At the base of each flower-head is a ring of narrow, green bracts the involucre. Some of these stand up to support the florets, others hang down to form a barricade against such small insects as might crawl up the stem and injure the bloom without taking a share in its fertilization, as the winged insects do.

The blooms are very sensitive to weather conditions: in fine weather, all the parts are outstretched, but directly rain threatens the whole head closes up at once. It closes against the dews of night, by five o'clock in the evening, being prepared for its night's sleep, opening again at seven in the morning though as this opening and closing is largely dependent upon the intensity of the light, the time differs somewhat in different latitudes and at different seasons.

When the whole head has matured, all the florets close up again within the green sheathing bracts that lie beneath, and the bloom returns very much to the appearance it had in the bud. Its shape being then somewhat reminiscent of the snout of a pig, it is termed in some districts 'Swine's Snout." The withered, yellow petals are, however soon pushed off in a bunch, as the seeds, crowned with their tufts of hair, mature, and one day, under the influence of sun and wind the 'Swine's Snout' becomes a large gossamer ball, from its silky whiteness a very noticeable feature. It is made up of myriads of plumed seeds or pappus, ready to be blown off when quite ripe by the slightest breeze, and forms the 'clock' of the children, who by blowing at it till all the seeds are released, love to tell themselves the time of day by the number of puffs necessary to disperse every seed. When all the seeds have flown, the receptacle or disc on which they were placed remains bare, white, speckled and surrounded by merely the drooping remnants of the sheathing bracts, and we can see why the plant received another of its popular names, 'Priest's Crown," common in the Middle Ages, when a priest's shorn head was a familiar object.

Small birds are very fond of the seeds of the Dandelion and pigs devour the whole plant greedily. Goats will eat it, but sheep and cattle do not care for it, though it is said to increase the milk of cows when eaten by them. Horses refuse to touch this plant, not appreciating its bitter juice. It is valuable food for rabbits and may be given them from April to September forming excellent food in spring and at breeding seasons in particular.

The young leaves of the Dandelion make an agreeable and wholesome addition to spring salads and are often eaten on the Continent, especially in France. The full-grown leaves should not be taken, being too bitter, but the young leaves, especially if blanched, make an excellent salad, either alone or in combination with other plants, lettuce, shallot tops or chives.

Young Dandelion leaves make delicious sandwiches, the tender leaves being laid between slices of bread and butter and sprinkled with salt. The addition of a little lemon-juice and pepper varies the flavor. The leaves should always be torn to pieces, rather than cut, in order to keep the flavor.

John Evelyn, in his Acetana, says: 'With thie homely salley, Hecate entertained Theseus." In Wales, they grate or chop up Dandelion roots, two years old, and mix them with the leaves in salad. The seed of a special broad-leaved variety of Dandelion is sold by seedsmen for cultivation for salad purposes. Dandelion can be blanched in the same way as endive, and is then very delicate in flavor. If covered with an ordinary flower-pot during the winter, the pot being further buried under some rough stable litter, the young leaves sprout when there is a dearth of saladings and prove a welcome change in early spring. Cultivated thus, Dandelion is only pleasantly bitter, and if eaten while the leaves are quite young, the centre rib of the leaf is not at all unpleasant to the taste. When older the rib is tough and not nice to eat. If the flower-buds of plants reserved in a corner of the garden for salad purposes are removed at once and the leaves carefully cut, the plants will last through the whole winter.

The young leaves may also be boiled as a vegetable, spinach fashion, thoroughly drained, sprinkled with pepper and salt, moistened with soup or butter and served very hot. If considered a little too bitter, use half spinach, but the Dandelion must be partly cooked first in this case, as it takes longer than spinach. As a variation, some grated nutmeg or garlic, a teaspoonful of chopped onion or grated lemon peel can be added to the greens when they are cooked. A simple vegetable soup may also be made with Dandelions.

The dried Dandelion leaves are also employed as an ingredient in many digestive or diet drinks and herb beers. Dandelion Beer is a rustic fermented drink common in many parts of the country and made also in Canada. Workmen in the furnaces and potteries of the industrial towns of the Midlands have frequent resource to many of the tonic Herb Beers, finding them cheaper and less intoxicating than ordinary beer, and Dandelion stout ranks as a favorite. An agreeable and wholesome fermented drink is made from Dandelions, Nettles and Yellow Dock.

In Berkshire and Worcestershire, the flowers are used in the preparation of a beverage known as Dandelion Wine. This is made by pouring a gallon of boiling water over a gallon of the flowers. After being well stirred, it is covered with a blanket and allowed to stand for three days, being stirred again at intervals, after which it is strained and the liquor boiled for 30 minutes, with the addition of 3 1/2 lb. of loaf sugar, a little ginger sliced, the rind of 1 orange and 1 lemon sliced. When cold, a little yeast is placed in it on a piece of toast, producing fermentation. It is then covered over and allowed to stand two days until it has ceased 'working," when it is placed in a cask, well bunged down for two months before bottling. This wine is suggestive of sherry slightly flat, and has the deserved reputation of being an excellent tonic, extremely good for the blood.

The roasted roots are largely used to form Dandelion Coffee, being first thoroughly cleaned, then dried by artificial heat, and slightly roasted till they are the tint of coffee, when they are ground ready for use. The roots are taken up in the autumn, being then most fitted for this purpose. The prepared powder is said to be almost indistinguishable from real coffee, and is claimed to be an improvement to inferior coffee, which is often an adulterated product. Of late years, Dandelion Coffee has come more into use in this country, being obtainable at most vegetarian restaurants and stores. Formerly it used occasionally to be given for medicinal purposes, generally mixed with true coffee to give it a better flavor. The ground root was sometimes mixed with chocolate for a similar purpose. Dandelion Coffee is a natural beverage without any of the injurious effects that ordinary tea and coffee have on the nerves and digestive organs. It exercises a stimulating influence over the whole system, helping the liver and kidneys to do their work and keeping the bowels in a healthy condition, so that it offers great advantages to dyspeptics and does not cause wakefulness.

Parts Used Medicinally

The root, fresh and dried, the young tops. All parts of the plant contain a somewhat bitter, milky juice (latex), but the juice of the root being still more powerful is the part of the plant most used for medicinal purposes.

History

The first mention of the Dandelion as a medicine is in the works of the Arabian physicians of the tenth and eleventh centuries, who speak of it as a sort of wild Endive, under the name of Taraxcacon. In this country, we find allusion to it in the Welsh medicines of the thirteenth century. Dandelion was much valued as a medicine in the times of Gerard and Parkinson, and is still extensively employed.

Dandelion roots have long been largely used on the Continent, and the plant is cultivated largely in India as a remedy for liver complaints.

The root is perennial and tapering, simple or more or less branched, attaining in a good soil a length of a foot or more and 1/2 inch to an inch in diameter. Old roots divide at the crown into several heads. The root is fleshy and brittle, externally of a dark brown, internally white and abounding in an inodorous milky juice of bitter, but not disagreeable taste.

Only large, fleshy and well-formed roots should be collected, from plants two years old, not slender, forked ones. Roots produced in good soil are easier to dig up without breaking, and are thicker and less forked than those growing on waste places and by the roadside. Collectors should, therefore only dig in good, free soil, in moisture and shade, from meadowland. Dig up in wet weather, but not during frost, which materially lessens the activity of the roots. Avoid breaking the roots, using a long trowel or a fork, lifting steadily and carefully. Shake off as much of the earth as possible and then cleanse the roots, the easiest way being to leave them in a basket in a running stream so that the water covers them, for about an hour, or shake them, bunched, in a tank of clean water. Cut off the crowns of leaves, but be careful in so doing not to leave any scales on the top. Do not cut or slice the roots or the valuable milky juice on which their medicinal value depends will be wasted by bleeding.

Cultivation

As only large, well-formed roots are worth collecting, some people prefer to grow Dandelions as a crop, as by this means large roots are insured and they are more easily dug, generally being ploughed up. About 4 lb. of seed to the acre should be allowed, sown in drills, 1 foot apart. The crops should be kept clean by hoeing, and all flower-heads should be picked off as soon as they appear, as otherwise the grower's own land and that of his neighbours will be smothered with the weed when the seeds ripen. The yield should be 4 or 5 tons of fresh roots to the acre in the second year. Dandelion roots shrink very much in drying, losing about 76 per cent of their weight, so that 100 parts of fresh roots yield only about 22 parts of dry material. Under favourable conditions, yields at the rate of 1,000 to 1,500 lb. of dry roots per acre have been obtained from second-year plants cultivated.

Dandelion root can only be economically collected when a meadow in which it is abundant is ploughed up. Under such circumstances the roots are necessarily of different ages and sizes, the seeds sowing themselves in successive years. The roots then collected after washing and drying, have to be sorted into different grades. The largest, from the size of a lead pencil upwards, are cut into straight pieces 2 to 3 inches long, the smaller side roots being removed, these are sold at a higher price as the finest roots. The smaller roots fetch a less price, and the trimmings are generally cut small, sold at a lower price and used for making Dandelion Coffee. Every part of the root is thus used. The root before being dried should have every trace of the leaf-bases removed as their presence lessens the value of the root.

In collecting cultivated Dandelion advantage is obtained if the seeds are all sown at one time, as greater uniformity in the size of the root is obtainable, and in deep soil free from stones, the seedlings will produce elongated, straight roots with few branches, especially if allowed to be somewhat crowded on the same principles that coppice trees produce straight trunks. Time is also saved in digging up the roots which can thus be sold at prices competing with those obtained as the result of cheaper labour on the Continent. The edges of fields when room is allowed for the plough-horses to turn, could easily be utilized if the soil is good and free from stones for both Dandelion and Burdock, as the roots are usually much branched in stony ground, and the roots are not generally collected until October when the harvest is over. The roots gathered in this month have stored up their food reserve of Inulin, and when dried present a firm appearance, whilst if collected in spring, when the food reserve in the root is used up for the leaves and flowers, the dried root then presents a shrivelled and porous appearance which renders it unsaleable. The medicinal properties of the root are, therefore, necessarily greater in proportion in the spring. Inulin being soluble in hot water, the solid extract if made by boiling the root, often contains a large quantity of it, which is deposited in the extract as it cools.

The roots are generally dried whole, but the largest ones may sometimes be cut transversely into pieces 3 to 6 inches long. Collected wild roots are, however, seldom large enough to necessitate cutting. Drying will probably take about a fortnight. When finished, the roots should be hard and brittle enough to snap, and the inside of the roots white, not grey

The roots should be kept in a dry place after drying, to avoid mould, preferably in tins to prevent the attacks of moths and beetles. Dried Dandelion is exceedingly liable to the attacks of maggots and should not be kept beyond one season.

Dried Dandelion root is 1/2 inch or less in thickness, dark brown, shrivelled, with wrinkles running lengthwise, often in a spiral direction; when quite dry, it breaks easily with a short, corky fracture, showing a very thick, white bark, surrounding a wooden column. The latter is yellowish, very porous, without pith or rays. A rather broad but indistinct cambium zone separates the wood from the bark, which latter exhibits numerous well-defined, concentric layers, due to the milk vessels. This structure is quite characteristic and serves to distinguish Dandelion roots from other roots like it. There are several flowers easily mistaken for the Dandelion when in blossom, but these have either hairy leaves or branched flower-stems, and the roots differ either in structure or shape.

Dried Dandelion root somewhat resembles Pellitory and Liquorice roots, but Pellitory differs in having oil glands and also a large radiate wood, and Liquorice has also a large radiate wood and a sweet taste.

The root of Hawkbit (Leontodon hispidus) is sometimes substituted for Dandelion root. It is a plant with hairy, not smooth leaves, and the fresh root is tough, breaking with difficulty and rarely exuding much milky juice. Some kinds of Dock have also been substituted, and also Chicory root. The latter is of a paler color, more bitter and has the laticiferous vessels in radiating lines. In the United States it is often substituted for Dandelion. Dock roots have a prevailing yellowish color and an astringent taste.

During recent years, a small form of a Dandelion root has been offered by Russian firms, who state that it is sold and used as Dandelion in that country. This root is always smaller than the root of T. officinale, has smaller flowers, and the crown of the root has often a tuft of brown woolly hairs between the leaf bases at the crown of the root, which are never seen in the Dandelion plant in this country, and form a characteristic distinction, for the root shows similar concentric, horny rings in the thick white bark as well as a yellow porous woody centre. These woolly hairs are mentioned in Greenish's Materia Medica, and also in the British Pharmaceutical Codex, as a feature of Dandelion root, but no mention is made of them in the Pharmacographia, nor in the British Pharmacopeia or United States Pharmacopeia, and it is probable, therefore, that Russian specimens have been used for describing the root, and that the root with brown woolly hairs belongs to some other species of Taraxacum.

Chemical Constituents

The chief constituents of Dandelion root are Taraxacin, acrystalline, bitter substance, of which the yield varies in roots collected at different seasons, and Taraxacerin, an acrid resin, with Inulin (a sort of sugar which replaces starch in many of the Dandelion family, Compositae), gluten, gum and potash. The root contains no starch, but early in the year contains much uncrystallizable sugar and laevulin, which differs from Inulin in being soluble in cold water. This diminishes in quantity during the summer and becomes Inulin in the autumn. The root may contain as much as 24 per cent. In the fresh root, the Inulin is present in the cell-sap, but in the dry root it occurs as an amorphodus, transparent solid, which is only slightly soluble in cold water, but soluble in hot water.

There is a difference of opinion as to the best time for collecting the roots. The British Pharmacopeia considers the autumn dug root more bitter than the spring root, and that as it contains about 25 per cent insoluble Inulin, it is to be preferred on this account to the spring root, and it is, therefore, directed that in England the root should be collected between September and February, it being considered to be in perfection for Extract making in the month of November.

Bentley, on the other hand, contended that it is more bitter in March and most of all in July, but that as in the latter month it would generally be inconvenient for digging it, it should be dug in the spring, when the yield of Taraxacin, the bitter soluble principle, is greatest.

On account of the variability of the constituents of the plant according to the time of year when gathered, the yield and composition of the extract are very variable. If gathered from roots collected in autumn, the resulting product yields a turbid solution with water; if from spring-collected roots, the aqueous solution will be clear and yield but very little sediment on standing, because of the conversion of the Inulin into Laevulose and sugar at this active period of the plant's life.

In former days, Dandelion Juice was the favorite preparation both in official and domestic medicine. Provincial druggists sent their collectors for the roots and expressed the juice while these were quite fresh. Many country druggists prided themselves on their Dandelion Juice. The most active preparations of Dandelion, the Juice (Succus Taraxaci) and the Extract (Extractum Taraxaci), are made from the bruised fresh root. The Extract prepared from the fresh root is sometimes almost devoid of bitterness. The dried root alone was official in the United States Pharmacopoeia.

The leaves are not often used, except for making Herb-Beer, but a medicinal tincture is sometimes made from the entire plant gathered in the early summer. It is made with proof spirit.

When collecting the seeds care should be taken when drying them in the sun, to cover them with coarse muslin, as otherwise the down will carry them away. They are best collected in the evening, towards sunset, or when the damp air has caused the heads to close up.

The tops should be cut on a dry day, when quite free of rain or dew, and all insect-eaten or stained leaves rejected.

Medicinal Action and Uses

Diuretic, tonic and slightly aperient. It is a general stimulant to the system, but especially to the urinary organs, and is chiefly used in kidney and liver disorders.

Dandelion is not only official but is used in many patent medicines. Not being poisonous, quite big doses of its preparations may be taken. Its beneficial action is best obtained when combined with other agents.

The tincture made from the tops may be taken in doses of 10 to 15 drops in a spoonful of water, three times daily.

It is said that its use for liver complaints was assigned to the plant largely on the doctrine of signatures, because of its bright yellow flowers of a bilious hue.

In the hepatic complaints of persons long resident in warm climates, Dandelion is said to afford very marked relief. A broth of Dandelion roots, sliced and stewed in boiling water with some leaves of Sorrel and the yolk of an egg, taken daily for some months, has been known to cure seemingly intractable cases of chronic liver congestion.

A strong decoction is found serviceable in stone and gravel: the decoction may be made by boiling 1 pint of the sliced root in 20 parts of water for 15 minutes, straining this when cold and sweetening with brown sugar or honey. A small teacupful may be taken once or twice a day.

Dandelion is used as a bitter tonic in atonic dyspepsia, and as a mild laxative in habitual constipation. When the stomach is irritated and where active treatment would be injurious, the decoction or extract of Dandelion administered three or four times a day, will often prove a valuable remedy. It has a good effect in increasing the appetite and promoting digestion.

Dandelion combined with other active remedies has been used in cases of dropsy and for induration of the liver, and also on the Continent for phthisis and some cutaneous diseases. A decoction of 2 OZ. of the herb or root in 1 quart of water, boiled down to a pint, is taken in doses of one wine glassful every three hours for scurvy, scrofula, eczema and all eruptions on the surface of the body.

Preparations and Dosages

Fluid extract, B.P., 1/2 to 2 drachms. Solid extract, B.P. 5 to 15 grains. Juice, B.P., 1 to 2 drachms. Leontodin, 2 to 4 grains.

Dandelion Tea

Infuse 1 OZ. of Dandelion in a pint of boiling water for 10 minutes; decant, sweeten with honey, and drink several glasses in the course of the day. The use of this tea is efficacious in bilious affections, and is also much approved of in the treatment of dropsy.

Or take 2 OZ. of freshly-sliced Dandelion root, and boil in 2 pints of water until it comes to 1 pint; then add 1 OZ. of compound tincture of Horseradish. Dose, from 2 to 4 OZ. Use in a sluggish state of the liver.

Or 1 OZ. Dandelion root, 1 OZ. Black Horehound herb, 1/2 OZ. Sweet Flag root, 1/4 OZ. Mountain Flax. Simmer the whole in 3 pints of water down to 1 1/2 pint, strain and take a wine glassful after meals for biliousness and dizziness.

For Gall Stones

1 OZ. Dandelion root, 1 OZ. Parsley root, 1 OZ. Balm herb, 1/2 OZ. Ginger root, 1/2 OZ. Liquorice root. Place in 2 quarts of water and gently simmer down to 1 quart, strain and take a wine glassful every two hours.

For a young child suffering from jaundice: 1 OZ. Dandelion root, 1/2 oz. Ginger root, 1/2 oz. Caraway seed, 1/2 oz. Cinnamon bark, 1/4 oz. Senna leaves. Gently boil in 3 pints of water down to 1 1/2 pint, strain, dissolve 1/2 lb. sugar in hot liquid, bring to a boil again, skim all impurities that come to the surface when clear, put on one side to cool, and give frequently in teaspoonful doses.

A Liver and Kidney Mixture

1 OZ. Broom tops, 1/2 oz. Juniper berries, 1/2 oz. Dandelion root, 1 1/2 pint water. Boil in gredients for 10 minutes, then strain and adda small quantity of cayenne. Dose, 1 tablespoonful, three times a day.

A Medicine for Piles

1 OZ. Long-leaved Plantain, 1 OZ. Dandelion root, 1/2 oz. Polypody root, 1 OZ. Shepherd's Purse. Add 3 pints of water, boil down to half the quantity, strain, and add 1 OZ. of tincture of Rhubarb. Dose, a wine glassful three times a day. Celandine ointment to be applied at same time.

In Derbyshire, the juice of the stalk is applied to remove warts.

DEER'S TONGUE

Botanical: Liatris odoratissima (WILLD.)
Family: N.O. Orchidaceae
Synonyms: Vanilla Leaf. Wild Vanilla. Trilissia odorata.
Part Used: Leaves.
Habitat: North America: cultivated in England.

Description

Herbaceous perennial plant, composite distinguished by a naked receptacle, oblong, imbricated, involucre, and a feathery pappus, fleshy basal leaves obolanceolate, terminating in a flattened stalk. Leaves of stem clasping at base. The leaves are used to flavor tobacco. Their perfume is largely due to Coumarin, which can be seen in crystals on the upper side of the smooth spatulate leaves. Most of the species are used medicinally.

Medicinal Action and Uses

Demulcent, febrifuge, diaphoretic.

Other Species

Liatris spicata has a warm bitterish taste and used as a local application for sore throat in the treatment of gonorrhea.

L. squarrosa, called 'the rattlesnake' because the roots are used to cure rattlesnake bite, a handsome plant with very long narrow leaves, and large heads of lovely purple flowers.

L. scariosa also used for snake-bite and recognized by the involucral scales which are margined with purple.

DILL

Botanical: Peucedanum graveolens (BENTH.)
Family: N.O. Compositae
Synonyms: Anethum graveolus. Fructus Anethi.
Part Used: Dried ripe fruit.

Dill is a hardy annual, a native of the Mediterranean region and Southern Russia. It grows wild among the corn in Spain and Portugal and upon the coast of Italy, but rarely occurs as a cornfield weed in Northern Europe.

The plant is referred to in St. Matthew XXiii., 23, though the original Greek name Anethon, was erroneously rendered Anise by English translators, from Wicklif (1380) downwards.

Dill is commonly regarded as the Anethon of Dioscorides. It was well known in Pliny's days and is often mentioned by writers in the Middle Ages. As a drug it has been in use from very early times. It occurs in the tenth-century vocabulary of Alfric, Archbishop of Canterbury.

The name is derived, according to Prior's Popular Names of English Plants, from the old Norse word, dilla (to lull), in allusion to the carminative properties of the drug.

Lyte (Dodoens, 1578) says Dill was sown in all gardens amongst worts and pot-herbs.

In the Middle Ages, Dill was also one of the herbs used by magicians in their spells, and charms against witchcraft.

In Drayton's Nymphidia are the lines:
'Therewith her Vervain and her Dill,
That hindereth Witches of their Will."

Culpepper tells us that:

'Mercury has the dominion of this plant, and therefore to be sure it strengthens the brain.... It stays the hiccough, being boiled in wine, and but smelled unto being tied in a cloth. The seed is of more use than the leaves, and more effectual to digest raw and vicious humours, and is used in medicines that serve to expel wind, and the pains proceeding therefrom...."

Description

The plant grows ordinarily from 2 to 2 1/2 feet high and is very like fennel, though smaller, having the same feathery leaves, which stand on sheathing foot-stalks, with linear and pointed leaflets. Unlike fennel, however, it has seldom more than one stalk and its long, spindle-shaped root is only annual. It is of very upright growth, its stems smooth, shiny and hollow, and in midsummer bearing flat terminal umbels with numerous yellow flowers, whose small petals are rolled inwards. The flat fruits, the so-called seeds, are produced in great quantities. They are very pungent and bitter in taste and very light, an ounce containing over 25,000 seeds. Their germinating capacity lasts for three years. The whole plant is aromatic.

The plant was placed by Linnaeus in a separate genus, Anethum, whence the name Fructus Anethi, by which Dill fruit goes in medicine. It is now included in the genus Peucedanum.

Cultivation

This annual is of very easy culture. When grown on a large scale for the sake of its fruits, it may be sown in drills 10 inches apart, in March or April, 10 lb. of the seed being drilled to the acre, and thinned out to leave 8 to 10 inches room each way Sometimes the seed is sown in autumn as soon as ripe, but it is not so advisable as spring sowing. Careful attention must be given to the destruction of weeds. The crop is considered somewhat exhaustive of soil fertility.

Harvesting

Mowing starts as the lower seeds begin, the others ripening on the straw. In dry periods, cutting is best done in early morning or late evening, care being taken to handle with the least possible shaking to prevent loss. The loose sheaves are built into stacks of about twenty sheaves, tied together. In hot weather, threshing may be done in the field, spreading the sheaves on a large canvas sheet and beating out. The average yield is about 7 cwt. of Dill fruits per acre.

The seeds are finally dried by spreading out on trays in the sun, or for a short time over the moderate heat of a stove, shaking occasionally.

Dill fruits are oval, compressed, winged about one-tenth inch wide, with three longitudinal ridges on the back and three dark lines or oil cells (vittae) between them and two on the flat surface. The taste of the fruits somewhat resembles caraway. The seeds are smaller, flatter and lighter than caraway and have a pleasant aromatic odor. They contain a volatile oil (obtained by distillation) on which the action of the fruit depends. The bruised seeds impart their virtues to alcohol and to boiling water.

Constituents

Oil of Dill is of a pale yellow color, darkening on keeping, with the odor of the fruit and a hot, acrid taste. Its specific gravity varies between 0.895 and 0.915. The fruit yields about 3.5 per cent of the oil, which is a mixture of a paraffin hydrocarbon and 40 to 60 per cent of d-carvone, with d-limonene. Phellandrine is present in the English and Spanish oils, but not to any appreciable extent in the German oil.

In spite of the difference in odor between Dill and Caraway oils, the composition of the two is almost identical, both consisting nearly entirely of limonene and carvone. Dill oil, however, contains less carvone than caraway oil.

English-distilled oils usually have the highest specific gravity, from 0.910 to 0.916, and are consequently held in the highest esteem.

Uses

As a sweet herb, Dill is not much used in this country. When employed, it is for flavoring soups, sauces, etc., for which purpose the young leaves only are required. The leaves added to fish, or mixed with pickled cucumbers give them a spicy taste.

Dill vinegar, however, forms a popular household condiment. It is made by soaking the seeds in vinegar for a few days before using.

The French use Dill seeds for flavoring cakes and pastry, as well as for flavoring sauces.

Perhaps the chief culinary use of Dill seeds is in pickling cucumbers: they are employed in this way chiefly in Germany where pickled cucumbers are largely eaten.

Medicinal Action and Uses

Like the other umbelliferous fruits and volatile oils, both Dill fruit and oil of Dill possess stimulant, aromatic, carminative and stomachic properties, making them of considerable medicinal value.

Oil of Dill is used in mixtures, or administered in doses of 5 drops on sugar, but its most common use is in the preparation of Dill Water, which is a common domestic remedy for the flatulence of infants, and is a useful vehicle for children's medicine generally.

Preparations

Dill water, 1 to 8 drachms. Oil, 1 to 5 drops.

Oil of Dill is also employed for perfuming soaps.

The British Pharmacopoeia directs that only the fruits from English-grown plants shall be employed pharmaceutically, and it is grown in East Anglia for that purpose. The Dill fruits of commerce are imported from central and southern Europe, the plant being largely cultivated in Germany and Roumania.

Considerable quantities of Dill fruit are imported from India and Japan - they are the fruits of a species of Peucedanum that has been considered by some botanists entitled to rank as a distinct species, P. Sowa (Kurz), but is included by others in the species, P. graveolens. Indian dill is widely grown in the Indies under the name of 'Soyah," its fruit and leaves being used for flavoring pickles. Its fruits are narrower and more convex than European dill, with paler, more distinct ridges and narrower wings.

The oils from both Japanese and Indian dill differ from European dill oil, in having a higher specific gravity (0.948 to 0.968), which is ascribed to the presence of dill apiol, and in containing much less carvone than the European oil. It should not be substituted for the official oil.

African dill oil is produced from plants grown from English imported seed. The fruits are slightly larger than the English fruits and a little paler in color, their odor closely resembling the English. The yield of oil is slightly larger than that of English fruits, and it is considered that if the fruits can be produced in Cape Colony, they should form a most useful source of supply.

Fennel and Dill Recipes

A Sallet of Fennel

'Take young Fennel, about a span long in the spring, tye it up in bunches as you do Sparragrass; when your Skillet boyle, put in enough to make a dish; when it is boyled and drained, dish it up as you do Sparragrass, pour on butter and vinegar and send it up." (From The Whole Body of Cookery Dissected, 1675, by William Tabisha.)

Fennel and Gooseberry Sauce

'Brown some butter in a saucepan with apinch of flour, then put in a few cives shred small, add a little Irish broth to moisten it, season with salt and pepper; make these boil, then put in two or three sprigs of Fennel and some Gooseberries. Let all simmer together till the Gooseberries are soft and then put in some Cullis." (From Receipt Book of Henry Howard, Cook to the Duke of Ormond, 1710.)

Dill and Collyflower Pickle

'Boil the Collyflowers till they fall inpieces; then with some of the stalk and worst of the flower boil it in a part of the liquer till pretty strong. Then being taken off strain it- and when settled, clean it from the bottom. Then with Dill, gross pepper, a pretty quantity of salt, when cold add as much vinegar as will make it sharp and pour all upon the Collyflower." (From Acetaria, a book about Sallets, 1680, by John Evelyn.)

To Pickle Cucumbers in Dill

'Gather the tops of the ripest dill and cover the bottom of the vessel, and lay a layer of Cucumbers and another of Dill till you have filled the vessel within a handful of the top. Then take as much water as you think will fill the vessel and mix it with salt and a quarter of a pound of allom to a gallon of water and poure it on them and press them down with a stone on them and keep them covered close. For that use I think the water will be best boyl'd and cold, which will keep longer sweet, or if you like not this pickle, doe it with water, salt and white wine vinegar, or (if you please) pour the water and salt on them scalding hot which will make them ready to use the sooner." (From Receipt Book of Joseph Cooper, Cook to Charles I, 1640.)

DITA BARK

Botanical: Alstonia scholaris (R. BR,)
Family: N.O. Apocynaceae
Synonyms: Devil's Bit. Pali-mara. Bitter Bark. Australian Fever Bush. Devil Tree.
Habitat: India. Moluccas. Philippines.

Description

The genus of Alstonia takes its name from Alston, a Professor of botany in Edinburgh. Grows 50 to 80 feet high, has a furrowed trunk, oblong stalked leaves 6 inches long, 2 to 4 inches wide, in whorls round stem, upper surface glossy, under one white, and marked with nerves running at right-angles to midrib; taste bitter, but no odor. A. constricta, belonging to the same order, is also recognized by the British Pharmacopeia; the bark is quite dissimilar however, and contains different alkaloids, slightly aromatic odor, taste very bitter, used for same purposes, mainly as a febrifuge in malarial fever, tonic and astringent, with much the same properties as Peruvian bark.

Constituents

The strongest alkaloids in A. scholaris bark are Ditamine, Echitanine, the latter in character resembling ammonia other constituents are echierin, echicaoutin echitin, and echitein - these are crystalline and Echiretin amorphous.

Constituents of A. constricta bark, alstonine and porphyrine, is colorless and amorphous; also contains porphyrosine and alstonidine.

Medicinal Action and Uses

Though Alstonia is used in India and Eastern Colonies for malarial conditions, its efficacy in this respect is not to be compared with cinchona bark, though it does not produce the bad effects cinchona does. It is also employed as a bitter tonic, vermifuge, and as a cure for chronic diarrhea and bowel complaints, both varieties are used.

Preparation

Dita bark: 1 part in 20 for B.P. infusion, 1/2 to 1 fluid ounce; 1 part in 8 Alcohol Tinc., B.P., 1/2 to 1 fluid drachm. Dose, 2 to 4 grains.

Other Species

The A. spectabilis, a habitat of Java, contains the same alkaloid as Dita bark, with the addition of a crystalline alkaloid, Alstonamine.

DOCKS

Family: N.O. Polygonaceae

The name Dock is applied to a widespread tribe of broad-leaved wayside weeds, having roots possessing astringent qualities united in some with a cathartic principle, rendering them valuable as substitutes for Rhubarb, a plant of the same family.

Although now, in common with the Sorrels, assigned to the genus Rumex, the Docks were formerly ranked as members of the genus Lapathum, this name being derived from the Greek word, lapazein (to cleanse), an allusion to the medicinal virtues of these plants as purgatives, the word still surviving in the name of one of the species, Rumex Hydrolapathum.

All the Docks resemble our Garden Rhubarb more or less, both in their general characteristics and in possessing much tannin.Most of them furnish rumicin, or crysophanic acid, which is useful in chronic scrofulous disorders.

The young leaves and shoots of several species of Dock may be eaten as pot-herbs, but are not very palatable, and have a slight laxative effect. 'Sour Docks' were considered formerly a good accompaniment to boiled beef, either hot or cold, but this was a popular name, not for the ordinary kinds of Docks, but for the closely allied Sorrel or Sorrel Dock (Rumex acetosa), whose herbage has a somewhat acid flavor. This, with its French variety, R. scutatus, has been much cultivated as a pot-herb.

PATIENCE DOCK

Botanical: Rumex alpinus
Synonyms:Herb Patience. Monk's Rhubarb. Passion's Dock.

This, although not considered a native plant, grows wild in some parts of the country, mostly by roadsides and near cottages, being originally a garden escape. It is a large plant, about 6 feet high, with very large, long, pointed leaves on thick hollow footstalks. The long stout root was also formerly used medicinally for its slight astringent qualities. It was considered good for jaundice.

It has a gentle laxative action. There are about ten or eleven kinds of native Docks.

ROUND LEAF DOCK

Botanical: Rumex obtusifolius
Synonyms: Common Wayside Dock. Butter Dock.

Description

It is a large and spreading plant, its stout stems 2 to 3 feet high, the leaves 6 to 12 inches long, with rather slender foot-stalks, the margins waved and the end or apex of the leaf rounded. The flowers are small, green and numerous, arranged in whorled spikes at the ends of the stem. In this, as in all the Docks, the flowers contain both stamens and pistils - the nearly-related Sorrels, on the contrary, having their stamens and pistils on different plants. This Dock is so coarse that cattle refuse to touch it. It is a troublesome weed, all the more because it prefers growing on good land, not thriving in poor soil. Its broad foliage serves also to lodge the destructive turnip fly. The leaves are often applied as a rustic remedy to burns and scalds and used for dressing blisters, serving also as a popular cure for Nettle stings.

The cure was accompanied by the words:

'Nettle in, Dock;
Dock in, Nettle out
Dock rub Nettle out,"

and is the origin of the saying: 'In Dock, out Nettle', to suggest inconstancy.

A tea made from the root was formerly given for the cure of boils. The plant is frequently called Butter Dock, because its cool leaves have often been used in the country for wrapping up butter for the market.

SHARP POINTED DOCK

Botanical: Rumex acetus

Description

A common plant like the Common Dock, but handsomer, and distinguished by its sharp-pointed leaves being narrower and longer. It grows about 3 feet high, having erect, round, striated stems and small greenish flowers, turning brown when ripe. The root has been used in drinks and decoctions for scurvy and as a general blood cleanser, and employed for outward application to cutaneous eruptions, in the form of an ointment, made by beating it up with lard.

Both the Round-leaved Dock and the Sharp-pointed Dock, together with the BLOODY-VEINED DOCK (Rumex sanguineus) (which is very conspicuous on account of its veins and foot-stalks abounding in a bloodcoloured juice), make respectively with their astringent roots a useful infusion against bleedings and fluxes, also with their leaves, a decoction curative of several chronic skin diseases.

THE YELLOW DOCK (Rumex crispus), the RED DOCK (R. aquaticus) and the GREAT WATER DOCK (R. Hydrolapathum) are, however, the species more generally used medicinally.

YELLOW DOCK

Botanical: Rumex crispus
Synonym: Curled Dock.

Description

The leaves are crisped at their edges. It grows freely in our roadside ditches and waste places. The roots are 8 to 12 inches long, about 1/2 inch thick, fleshy and usually not forked. Externally they are of a rusty brown and internally whitish, with fine, straight, medullary rays and a rather thick bark. It has little or no smell and a rather bitter taste. The stem is 1 to 3 feet high and branched, the leaves, 6 to 10 inches long.

Medicinal Action and Uses

The Yellow Dock is applicable to all the purposes for which the other species are used. The root has laxative, alterative and mildly tonic action, and can be freely used as a tonic and laxative in rheumatism, bilious complaints and as an astringent in piles, bleedings of the lungs, etc. It is largely prescribed for diseases of the blood, from a spring eruption, to scurvy, scrofula and chronic skin diseases. It is also useful in jaundice and as a tonic to the stomach and the system generally. It has an action on the bowels very similar to that of Rhubarb, being perhaps a little less active, but operating without pain or uneasiness.

Rumicin is the active principle of the Yellow Dock, and from the root, containing Chrysarobin, a dried extract is prepared officially, of which from 1 to 4 grains may be given for a dose in a pill. This is useful for relieving a congested liver, as well as for scrofulous skin diseases.

A syrup can be made by boiling 1/2 lb. crushed root in a pint of syrup, which is taken in teaspoonful doses. The infusion administered in wine glassful doses - is made by pouring 1 pint of boiling water on 1 OZ. of the powdered root. A useful homeopathic tincture is made from the plant before it flowers, which is of particular service to an irritable tickling cough of the upper air-tubes and the throat. It is likewise excellent for dispelling any obstinate itching of the skin. It acts like Sarsaparilla for curing scrofulous skin affections and glandular swellings.

To be applied externally for cutaneous affections, an ointment may be made by boiling the root in vinegar until the fibre is softened and then mixing the pulp with lard.

The seeds have been given with advantage in dysentery, for their astringent action.

The Yellow Dock has also been considered to have

a positive effect in restraining the inroads made by cancer in the human system, being used as an alterative and tonic to enfeebled condition caused by necrosis, cancer, etc. It has been used in diphtheria.

Preparations

Fluid extract, 30 to 60 drops. Solid extract, 5 to 15 grains. Rumin, 3 grains.

The roots are collected in March, being generally ploughed up.

RED DOCK

Botanical: Rumex aquaticus
Synonym: Water Dock

The Red Dock, or Water Dock (Rumex aquaticus), has properties very similar to those of the Yellow Dock. It is frequent in fields, meadows and ditches. Its rootstock is top-shaped, the outer surface blackish or dark brown, the bark porous and the pith composed of honeycomb-like cells, with a short zone of woody bundles separated by rays. It has an astringent and somewhat sweet taste, but no odor. The stem is 1 to 3 feet high, very stout; the leaves similar to those of the Yellow Dock, having also crisped edges, but being broader, 3 to 4 inches across.

Medicinal Action and Uses

This Dock has alterative, deobstruent and detergent action. Its powers as a tonic are, perhaps rather more marked than the previous species. For internal use, it is given in an infusion, in wine glassful doses. Externally it is used as an application for eruptive and scorbutic diseases, ulcers and sores, being employed for cleansing ulcers in affections of the mouth, etc. As a powder, it has cleansing and detergent effect upon the teeth.

The root of this and all other Docks is dried in the same manner as the Yellow Dock.

Preparation

Fluid extract, 30 to 60 drops.

GREAT WATER DOCK

Botanical: Rumex Hydrolapathum

The Great Water Dock (Rumex Hydrolapathum), the largest of all the Docks, 5 to 6 feet high, is frequent on river banks. It is a picturesque plant with several erect, furrowed stems arising from its thick, blackish root, each of which are branched in the upper part, and bear numerous green flowers in almost leafless whorls. The leaves are exceedingly large - 1 to 3 feet long, dull green, not shiny, lance-shaped and narrow, tapering at both ends, the lower ones heart-shaped at the base. It is much like Rumex acutus, but larger.

This Dock, also, has some reputation as an antiscorbutic, and was used by the ancients. The root is strongly astringent, and powdered makes a good dentifrice. It is this species that is said to be the Herba Britannica of Pliny. This name does not denote British origin - the plant not being confined to the British Isles - but is said to be derived from three Teutonic words: brit (to tighten), tan (a tooth), and ica (loose), thus expressing its power of bracing up loose teeth and spongy gums.

Miss Rohde (Old English Herbals) says:

'It is interesting to find that Turner identifies the Herba Britannica of Dioscorides and Pliny (famed for having cured the soldiers of Julius Caesar of scurvy in the Rhine country) with Polygonum bistorta, which he observed plentifully in Friesland, the scene of Pliny's observations. This herb is held by modern authorities to be Rumex aquaticus (Great Water Dock)."

As a stomach tonic the following decoction was formerly much in use: 2 oz. of the root sliced were put into 3 pints of water, with a little cinnamon or liquorice powder, and boiled down to a quart and a wine glassful taken two or three times a day. The astringent qualities of the root render it good in case of diarrhea, the seeds (as with the other Docks) having been used for the same purpose. The green leaves are reputed to be an excellent application for ulcers of the eyes.

Culpepper says of the Docks:

'All Docks are under Jupiter, of which the Red Dock, which is commonly called Bloodwort, cleanseth the blood and strengthens the liver, but the Yellow Dock root is best to be taken when either the blood or liver is affected by choler. All of them have a kind of cooling, drying quality: the Sorrel being most cool and the Bloodworts most drying. The seed of most kinds, whether garden or field, doth stay laxes and fluxes of all sorts, and is helpful for those that spit blood. The roots boiled in vinegar helpeth the itch, scabs and breaking out of the skin, if it be bathed therewith. The distilled water of the herb and roots have the same virtue and cleanseth the skin from freckles.... All Docks being boiled with meat make it boil the sooner; besides Bloodwort is exceeding strengthening to the liver and procures good blood, being as wholesome a pot-herb as any growing in a garden."

Another species of Rumex may also be termed of indirect medicinal use, for Turkey opium, as imported, comes in flattened masses enveloped in poppy leaves and covered with the reddish-brown, triangular winged fruit of a species of Rumex, to prevent the cakes adhering to one another.

DODDER

Botanical: Cuscuta Europaea
Family: N.O. Convolvulaceae
Synonyms: Beggarweed. Hellweed. Strangle Tare. Scaldweed. Devil's Guts.

Belonging to the same family as the Convolvulus is a small group of plants, the genus Cuscuta, that at first glance seem to have little in common with our common Bindweeds. All the members of this genus are parasites, with branched, climbing cord-like and thread-like stems, no leaves and globular heads of small wax-like flowers.

The seeds germinate in the ground in the normal manner and throw up thready stems, which climb up adjoining plants and send out from their inner surfaces a number of small vesicles, which attach themselves to the bark of the plant on which they are twining. As soon as the young Dodder stems have firmly fixed themselves, the root from which they have at first drawn part of their nourishment withers away, and the Dodder, entirely losing its connection with the ground, lives completely on the sap of its 'host," and participates of its nature.

One British species is very abundant on Furze, another on Flax, others on Thistles and Nettles, etc.

Cuscuta Epithymum, THE LESSER DODDER, is the species of Dodder that formerly was much used medicinally, and which is the commonest. It is parasitic on Thyme Heath, Milk Vetch, Potentilla and other small plants, but most abundant on Furze, which it often entirely conceals with its tangled masses of red, thread-like stems. The flowers are in dense, round heads, each flower small, light flesh-coloured and wax-like, the corolla bellshaped, four- to five-cleft. Soon after flowering, the stems turn dark brown and in winter disappear.

The Dodder which grows on Thyme, C. Epithemum, was often preferred to others.

The threads being boiled in water (preferably fresh gathered) with ginger and allspice produced a decoction used in urinary complaints, kidney, spleen and liver diseases for its laxative and hepatic action. It was considered useful in jaundice, as well as in sciatica and scorbutic complaints.

The juice of two Brazilian species of Dodder is given for hoarseness and spitting of blood and their powder applied to wounds, to hasten healing.

Other species of Dodder which more or less resemble the Lesser Dodder are C. Europaea, THE GREATER OR COMMON DODDER which is parasitical on Thistles and Nettles, and has stems as thick as twine, reddish or yellow, with pale orange-coloured flowers 1/2 to 3/4 inch in diameter; C. Epilinum, FLAX DODDER, parasitical on Flax, to crops of which it is sometimes very destructive, and with seeds of which it is supposed to have been introduced, C. Hassiaca, parasitical on Lucerne, and C. Trifolii, CLOVER DODDER, parasitical on Clover.

Both the Greater Dodder and the Lesser Dodder have been employed medicinally.

Culpepper tells us:

'All Dodders are under Saturn. We confess Thyme is of the hottest herb it usually grows upon, and therefore that which grows upon thyme is hotter than that which grows upon colder herbs; for it draws nourishment from what it grows upon, as well as from the earth where its root is, and thus you see old Saturn is wise enough to have two strings to his bow. This is accounted the most effectual for melancholy diseases, and to purge black or burnt color, which is the cause of many diseases of the head and brain, as also for the trembling of the heart, faintings, and swoonings. It is helpful in all diseases and griefs of the spleen and melancholy that arises from the windiness of the hypochondria. It purges also the reins or kidneys by urine; it openeth obstructions of the gall, whereby it profiteth them that have the jaundice; as also the leaves, the spleen; purging the veins of choleric and phlegmatic humours and cures children in agues, a little wormseed being added.

'The other Dodders participate of the nature of those plants whereon they grow: as that which hath been found growing upon Nettles in the west country, hath by experience been found very effectual to procure plenty of urine, where it hath been stopped or hindered."

Many of its popular and local names testify to the bad reputation it had among farmers, such as Beggarweed, Hellweed, Strangle Tare, and Scaldweed, the latter from the scalded appearance it gives to bean crops. The name 'Devil's Guts' shows how much its strangling threads were detested. An old writer comments:

'Hellweed grows upon tares more abundantly in some places, where it destroyeth the pulse, or at least maketh it much worse, and is called of the country people Hellweed, because they know not how to destroy it."

It was not only considered useful in jaundice but also in sciatica and scorbutic complaints. Gathered fresh and applied externally after being bruised, the plant has been found efficacious in dispersing scrofulous tumors. The whole plant, of whatever species, is very bitter, and an infusion acts as a brisk purge.

DOGWOOD, JAMAICA

Botanical: Piscidia erythrina (JACQ.)
Family: N.O. Leguminosae
Part Used: Bark.
Habitat: West Indies, Florida, Texas, Mexico, the northern part of South America.

Description

A tree with very valuable wood and with the foliage and habit of Lonchocarpus. The pods bear four projecting longitudinal wings. The pounded leaves- and young branches are used to poison fish the method followed is to fill an open crate with the branches, drop it into the water, and swill it about till the water is impregnated with the liquid from the leaves, etc.; this quickly stupefies the fish and enables the fishers to catch them quickly. In commerce the bark is found in quilled pieces 1 or 2 inches long and 1 inch thick. The outer surface yellow or greyish brown, inner surface lighter coloured or white, and if damp a peculiar blue color. Inside it is very fibrous and dark brown, taste very acrid and bitter, and produces burning sensation in mouth with a strong disagreeable smell like broken opium. In 1844 attention was called to its narcotic, analgesic and sudorific properties which are uncertain.

Constituents

Resin, fat, a crystallizable substance called piscidin and in the aqueous extract of the bark piscidic acid, and a bitter glucoside.

Medicinal Action and Uses

In some subjects it cures violent toothache, neuralgia and whooping-cough and promotes sleep, and acts as an antispasmodic in asthma. It also dilates the pupil and is useful in dysmenorrhoea and nervous debility. In other subjects it only causes gastric distress and nausea; over doses produce toxic effects.

PREPARATIONS AND DOSAGES

Fluid extract, 5 to 20 drops, which may be cautiously increased to 2 fluid drachms. Solid extract, 1 to 5 grains.

DRAGON'S BLOOD

Botanical: Daemomorops draco (BLUME)
Family: N.O. Palmaceae
Synonyms: Calamus Draco. Draconis Resina. Sanguis draconis. Dragon's Blood Palm. Blume.
Part Used: The resinous exudation of the fruits.
Habitat: Sumatra.

DESCRIPTION

Dragon's Blood, as known in commerce, has several origins, the substance so named being contributed by widely differing species. Probably the best known is that from Sumatra. Daemomorops Draco formerly known as Calamus Draco, was transferred with many others of the species to Daemomorops, the chief distinguishing mark being the placing of the flowers along the branches instead of their being gathered into catkins, as in those remaining under Calamus.

The long, slender stems of the genus are flexible, and the older trees develop climbing propensities. The leaves have prickly stalks which often grow into long tails and the bark is provided with many hundreds of flattened spines. The berries are about the size of a cherry, and pointed. When ripe they are covered with a reddish, resinous substance which is separated in several ways, the most satisfactory being by steaming, or by shaking or rubbing in coarse, canvas bags. An inferior kind is obtained by boiling the fruits to obtain a decoction after they have undergone the second process. The product may come to market in beads, joined as if forming a necklace, and covered with leaves (Tear Dragon's Blood), or in small, round sticks about 18 inches long, packed in leaves and strips of cane. Other varieties are found in irregular lumps, or in a reddish powder. They are known as lump, stick, reed, tear, or saucer Dragon's Blood.

USES

It is used as a coloring matter for varnishes, toothpastes, tinctures, plasters, for dyeing horn to imitate tortoiseshell, etc. It is very brittle, and breaks with an irregular, resinous fracture, is bright red and glossy inside, and darker red sometimes powdered with crimson, externally. Small, thin pieces are transparent.

CONSTITUENTS

Several analyses of Dragon's Blood have been made with the following results:

(1) 50 to 70 per cent resinous compound of benzoic and benzoyl-acetic acid, with dracoresinotannol, and also dracon alban and dracoresene.

(2) 56.8 per cent of red resin compounded of the first three mentioned above, 2.5 per cent of the white, amorphous dracoalban, 13.58 of the yellow, resinous dracoresene, 18.4 vegetable debris, and 8.3 per cent. ash.

(3) 90.7 per cent of red resin, draconin, 2.0 of fixed oil, 3.0 of benzoic acid, 1.6 of calcium oxalate, and 3.7 of calcium phosphate.

(4) 2.5 per cent of draco-alban, 13.58 of draco resen, 56.86 of draco resin, benzoic dracoresinotannol ester and benzoylaceticdracoresinotannol ester, with 18.4 of insoluble substances.

Dragon's Blood is not acted upon by water, but most of it is soluble in alcohol. It fuses by heat. The solution will stain marble a deep red, penetrating in proportion to the heat of the stonc.

MEDICINAL ACTION AND USES

Doses of 10 to 30 grains were formerly given as an astringent in diarrhea, etc., but officially it is never at present used internally, being regarded as inert.

The following treatment is said to have cured cases of severe syphilis. Mix 2 drachms of Dragon's Blood, 2 drachms of colocynth, 1/2 oz. of gamboge in a mortar, and add 3 gills of boiling water. Stir for an hour, while keeping hot. Allow to cool, and add while stirring a mixture of 2 OZ. each of sweet spirits of nitre and copaiba balsam.

Dosage

1/2 oz. for catharsis, followed by 1 drachm two or three times a day.

Other Species

The Malay varieties are from D. didynophyllos, D. micranthus and D. propinguus.

The Borneo variety is from D. draconcellus and others. 'Zanzibar Drop' or Socotrine Dragon's Blood is imported from Bombay and Zanzibar, and is the product of D. cinnabari. It has no scales, and like other nonSumatra varieties, is not soluble in benzene and carbon disulphide.

Dracaena Draco is a giant tree of the East Indies and Canary Islands, and shares with the baobab tree the distinction of being the oldest living representative of the vegetable kingdom, being much reverenced by the Guanches of the Canaries, who use its product for embalming in the fashion of the Egyptians.

The trunk cracks and emits a red resin used as 'tear' Dragon's Blood, now rarely seen in commerce.

Dracaena terminalis, or Chinese Colli, yields Chinese Dragon's Blood, used in China for its famous red varnish. In some countries a syrup, yielding sugar, is made from the roots (called Tii roots). An intoxicating drink can be made from it, and it has also been used in dysentery and diarrhea, and as a diaphoretic.

Pterocarpus Draco, of the East Indies and South America, yields a resin found, as Guadaloupe Dragon's Blood, in small irregular lumps.

Croton Draco or Mexican Dragon's Blood, is called Sangre del Drago, and is used in Mexico as a vulnerary and astringent. Others used are from:

Croton hibiscifolius of New Granada.

Croton sanguifolius of New Andalusia, and

Calamus rotang of the East Indies and Spanish America.

DROPWORT, HEMLOCK WATER

POISON
Botanical: Oenanthe crocata (LINN.)
Family: N.O. Umbelliferae
Synonyms: Horsebane. Dead Tongue. Five-Fingered Root. Water Lovage. Yellow Water Dropwort.
Part Used: Root.

The name Water Hemlock is, though incorrectly, often popularly applied to several species of Oenanthe, the genus of the Water Dropworts, which of all the British umbelliferous plants are the most poisonous.

The species most commonly termed Water Hemlock is Oenanthe crocata, the Hemlock Water Dropwort, a common plant in England, especially in the southern counties, in ditches and watering places, but not occurring in Scandinavia, Holland, Germany, Russia, Turkey or Greece.

Description

It is a large, stout plant, 3 to 5 feet high, the stems thick, erect, much branched above, furrowed, hollow, tough, dark green and smooth.

The roots are perennial and fleshy, of a pale yellow color. They have a sweetish and not unpleasant taste, but are virulently poisonous. Being often exposed by the action of running water near which they grow, they are thus easily accessible to children and cattle, and the plant should not be allowed to grow in places where cattle are kept, as instances are numerous in which cows have been poisoned by eating these roots. They have also occasionally been eaten in mistake, either for wild celery or water parsnip, with very serious results, great agony, sickness, convulsions, or even death resulting. While the root of the Parsnip is single and conical in form, that of Oenanthe crocata consists of clusters of fleshy tubers similar to those of the Dahlia, hence, perhaps, one of its popular names: Dead Tongue.

The author of Familiar Wild Flowers states that the name 'Dead Tongue' was given from the paralysing effect of this plant on the organs of speech.

No British wild plant has been responsible for more fatal accidents than the one in question: a party of workmen repairing a breach in a towing-path dug up the plants and ate the roots, mistaking them for parsnips; another party, working in a field, thought that a few of the leaves with their bread and cheese would prove a tasty relish: in each case death occurred within three hours. On another occasion eight boys ate the roots, and five died - and the other three had violent convulsions and lost their reason for many hours.

The plant has been used to poison rats and moles.

Both stem and root, when cut, exude a yellowish juice, hence the specific name of the plant and one of the common names (Yellow Water Dropwort) by which it is known. The juice will stain the hands yellow. The generic name, Oenanthe, is derived from the Greek ainos (wine) and anthos (a flower), from the wine-like scent of the flowers.

The leaves are somewhat celery-like in form, and the flowers are in bloom in June and July, and are borne in large umbels. There is considerable variety in the form of the leafsegments, the number of rays in the umbel, and of the involucre bracts. The lower leaves, with very short, sheathing footstalks, are large and spreading, reaching more than a foot in length, broadly triangular in outline and tripinnate. The leaflets are stalkless, 1 to 1 1/2 inch long, roundish, with a wedge-shaped base, deeply and irregularly lobed, dark green, paler and shining beneath. The upper leaves are much smaller, nearly stalkless, the segments narrower and acute.

This most poisonous of our indigenous plants is not official and has never been used to any extent in medicine, though in some cases it has been taken with effect in eruptive diseases of the skin, being given at first in small doses, gradually increased.

Great caution must be exercised in the use of the tincture. The dose of the tincture is 1 to 5 drops. The roots have likewise been used in poultices to whitlows and to foul ulcers, both in man and horned cattle.

DROPWORT, WATER

Botanical: Oenanthe phellandrium (LANK.)
Family: N.O. Umbelliferae
Synonyms: Water Fennel. Horsebane. Phellandrium aquaticum (Linn.).
Part Used: Fruit.

Oenanthe phellandrium (syn. Phellandrium aquaticum), the Fine-leaved Water Dropwort, known popularly as Water Fennel, is a common British plant in ditches and by the sides of ponds.

It is a biennial, flowering from July to September in its second year of growth.

Description

The stems are 2 to 3 feet high, very stout at the base, rising from fibrous roots. The leaves are divided into many fine segments, the lower ones submerged. The umbels are smaller than those of O. crocata and are on short stalks, springing either from the forks of the branches or from opposite the leaves.

The rootstock varies in appearance, according to the locality. If growing in deep or running water the rootstock and stem are long and slender; in other districts it is thicker and more erect. The variety that grows in deep running water is often considered a distinct species and is classed under O. fluviatilis.

O. phellandrium is less poisonous than O. crocata, but both produce ill-effects if eaten.

Constituents

The fruits yield from 1 to 2 1/2 per cent of an ethereal oil, known as Water Fennel Oil, a yellow liquid of strong, pleasant, characteristic odor and burning taste, its specific gravity 0.85 to 0.89, containing as its chief constituent about 80 per cent of the terpene Phellandrene.

Medicinal Action and Uses

The fruits have been used in chronic pectoral affections such as bronchitis, pulmonary consumption and asthma, also in dyspepsia, intermittent fever, obstinate ulcers, etc. The dose when given in powdered form is 5 or 6 grains to commence with, so repeated as to amount to a drachm in four hours. An alcoholic extract and essence of the fruits has also been recommended as a very valuable and active remedy in the relief of consumption and bronchitis.

In overdoses the fruits produce vertigo, intoxication and other narcotic effects.

Externally applied, the root has sometimes been used as a local remedy in piles. When eaten in mistake, like that of O. crocata, the results have sometimes proved fatal. The symptoms produced are those of irritation of the stomach, failure of circulation and great cerebral disturbance, indicated by giddiness, convulsions and coma.

The fresh leaves are injurious to cattle, producing a kind of paralysis when eaten. When dried, they lose their deleterious properties .

O. fistulosa, the Common Water Dropwort, is found in watery places. This has a mixture of slender and fleshy roots, and bears leaves with only a few narrow segments. It is also poisonous. A peculiar resinous principle, called cenanthin, has been found in this species.

Most of the other species of Oenanthe found both in Great Britain and in the United States are poisonous, although none appear to be as virulent as O. crocata. A few are, however, innocuous, and their roots, especially those of O. pimpinelloides, have been esteemed as food in certain districts. Burnett (Medical Botany) states 'they are replete with a bland farina and have something the flavor of a filbert."

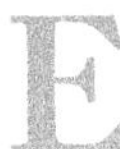

ECHINACEA

Botanical: Echinacea angustifolia (DE CANDOLLE)
Family: N.O. Compositae
Synonyms: Black Sampson. Coneflower. Niggerhead. Rudbeckia. Brauneria pallida (Nutt.).
Parts Used: Root, dried; also rhizome.
Habitat: America, west of Ohio, and cultivated in Britain.

Description

Named Echinacea by Linnaeus, and Rudbeckia, after Rudbeck, father and son, who were his predecessors at Upsala.

The flowers are a rich purple and the florets are seated round a high cone; seeds, four-sided achenes. Root tapering, cylindrical, entire, slightly spiral, longitudinally furrowed; fracture short, fibrous; bark thin; wood, thick, in alternate porous, yellowish and black transverse wedges, and the rhizome has a circular pith. It has a faint aromatic smell, with a sweetish taste, leaving a tingling sensation in the mouth not unlike Aconitum napellus, but without its lasting numbing effect.

Constituents

Oil and resin both in wood and bark and masses of inulin, inuloid, sucrose, vulose, betaine, two phytosterols and fatty acids, oleic, cerotic, linolic and palmatic.

Medicinal Action and Uses

Echinacea increases bodily resistance to infection and is used for boils, erysipelas, septicaemia, cancer, syphilis and other impurities of the blood, its action being antiseptic. It has also useful properties as a strong alterative and aphrodisiac. As an injection, the extract has been used for hemorrhoids and a tincture of the fresh root has been found beneficial in diphtheria and putrid fevers.

Other Species

Echinacea purpurea has similar properties to E. angustifolia; the fresh root of this is the part used.

ELDER

Botanical: Sambucus nigra (LINN.)
Family: N.O. Caprifoliaceae
Synonyms: Black Elder. Common Elder. Pipe Tree. Bore Tree. Bour Tree. (Fourteenth Century) Hylder, Hylantree. (Anglo-Saxon) Eldrum. (Low Saxon). Ellhorn. (German) Hollunder. (French) Sureau.
Parts Used: Bark, leaves, flowers, berries.

The Elder, with its flat-topped masses of creamy-white, fragrant blossoms, followed by large drooping bunches of purplish-black, juicy berries, is a familiar object in English countryside and gardens. It has been said, with some truth, that our English summer is not here until the Elder is fully in flower, and that it ends when the berries are ripe.

The word 'Elder' comes from the Anglo-Saxon word aeld. In Anglo-Saxon days we find the tree called Eldrun, which becomes Hyldor and Hyllantree in the fourteenth century. One of its names in modern German - Hollunder - is clearly derived from the same origin. In Low-Saxon, the name appears as Ellhorn. Æld meant 'fire," the hollow stems of the young branches having been used for blowing up a fire: the soft pith pushes out easily and the tubes thus formed were used as pipes - hence it was often called Pipe-Tree, or Bore-tree and Bour-tree, the latter name remaining in Scotland and being traceable to the Anglo-Saxon form, Burtre.

The generic name Sambucus occurs in the writings of Pliny and other ancient writers and is evidently adapted from the Greek word Sambuca, the Sackbut, an ancient musical instrument in much use among the Romans, in the construction of which, it is surmised, the wood of this tree, on account of its hardness, was used. The difficulty, however, of accepting this is that the Sambuca was a stringed instrument, while anything made from the Elder would doubtless be a wind instrument, something of the nature of a Pan-pipe or flute. Pliny records the belief held by country folk that the shrillest pipes and the most sonorous horns were made of Elder trees which were grown out of reach of the sound of cock-crow. At the present day, Italian peasants construct a simple pipe, which they call sampogna, from the branches of this plant.

The popular pop-gun of small boys in the country has often been made of Elder stems from which the pith has been removed, which moved Culpepper to declare: 'It is needless to write any description of this (Elder), since every boy that plays with a pop-gun will not mistake another tree for the Elder." Pliny's writings also testify that pop-guns and whistles are manufactures many centuries old!

History

A wealth of folk-lore, romance and superstition centre round this English tree. Shakespeare, in Cymbeline, referring to it as a symbol of grief, speaks slightingly of it as 'the stinking Elder," yet, although many people profess a strong dislike to the scent of its blossom, the shrub is generally beloved by all who see it. In countrysides where the Elder flourishes it is certainly one of the most attractive features of the hedgerow, while its old-world associations have created for it a place in the hearts of English people.

In Love's Labour Lost reference is made to the common medieval belief that 'Judas was hanged on an Elder." We meet with this tradition as far back in English literature as Langland's Vision of Piers Plowman (middle of the fourteenth century, before Chaucer):

'Judas he japed with Jewen silver
And sithen an eller hanged hymselve."

Why the Elder should have been selected as a gallows for the traitor Apostle is, considering the usual size of the tree, puzzling; but Sir John Mandeville in his travels, written about the same time, tells us that he was shown 'faste by' the Pool of Siloam, the identical 'Tree of Eldre that Judas henge himself upon, for despeyr that he hadde, when he solde and betrayed oure Lord." Gerard scouts the tradition and says that the Judas-tree (Cercis siliquastrum) is 'the tree whereon Judas did hange himselfe."

Another old tradition was that the Cross of Calvary was made of it, and an old couplet runs:

'Bour tree - Bour tree: crooked rong
Never straight and never strong;
Ever bush and never tree
Since our Lord was nailed on thee."

In consequence of these old traditions, the Elder became the emblem of sorrow and death, and out of the legends which linger round the tree there grew up a host of superstitious fancies which still remain in the minds of simple country folk. Even in these prosaic days, one sometimes comes across a hedge-cutter who cannot bring himself to molest the rampant growth of its spreading branches for fear of being pursued by ill-luck. An old custom among gypsies forbade them using the wood to kindle their camp fires and gleaners of firewood formerly would look carefully through the faggots lest a stick of Elder should have found its way into the bundle, perhaps because the Holy Cross was believed to have been fashioned out of a giant elder tree, though probably the superstitious awe of harming the Elder descended from old heathen myths of northern Europe. In most countries, especially in Denmark, the Elder was intimately connected with magic. In its branches was supposed to dwell a dryad, Hylde-Moer, the Elder-tree Mother, who lived in the tree and watched over it. Should the tree be cut down and furniture be made of the wood, Hylde-Moer was believed to follow her property and haunt the owners. Lady Northcote, in The Book of Herbs, relates:

'There is a tradition that once when a child was put in a cradle of Elder-wood, HyldeMoer came and pulled it by the legs and would give it no peace till it was lifted out Permission to cut Elder wood must always be asked first and not until Hylde-Moer has given consent by keeping silence, may the chopping begin."

Arnkiel relates:

'Our forefathers also held the Ellhorn holy wherefore whoever need to hew it down (or cut its branches) has first to make request "Lady Ellhorn, give me some of thy wood and I will give thee some of mine when it grows in the forest" - the which, with partly bended knees, bare head and folded arms was ordinarily done, as I myself have often seen and heard in my younger years."

Mr. Jones (quoted in The Treasury of Botany), in his Notes on Certain Superstitions in the Vale of Gloucester, cites the following, said to be no unusual case:

'Some men were employed in removing an old hedgerow, partially formed of Eldertrees. They had bound up all the other wood into faggots for burning, but had set apart the elder and enquired of their master how it was to be disposed of. Upon his saying that he should of course burn it with the rest, one of the men said with an air of undisguised alarm, that he had never heard of such a thing as burning Ellan Wood, and in fact, so strongly did he feel upon the subject, that he refused to participate in the act of tying it up. The word Ellan (still common with us) indicates the origin of the superstition."

In earlier days, the Elder Tree was supposed to ward off evil influence and give protection from witches, a popular belief held in widely-distant countries. Lady Northcote says:

'The Russians believe that Elder-trees drive away evil spirits, and the Bohemians go to it with a spell to take away fever. The Sicilians think that sticks of its wood will kill serpents and drive away robbers, and the Serbs introduce a stick of Elder into their wedding ceremonies to bring good luck. In England it was thought that the Elder was never struck by lightning, and a twig of it tied into three or four knots and carried in the pocket was a charm against rheumatism. A cross made of Elder and fastened to cowhouses and stables was supposed to keep all evil from the animals."

In Cole's Art of Simpling (1656) we may read how in the later part of the seventeenth century:

'in order to prevent witches from entering their houses, the common people used to gather Elder leaves on the last day of April and affix them to their doors and windows,"

and the tree was formerly much cultivated near English cottages for protection against witches .

The use of the Elder for funeral purposes was an old English custom referred to by Spenser,

'The Muses that were wont green Baies to weave,
Now bringen bittre Eldre braunches seare."
And Canon Ellacombe says that in the Tyrol:
'An Elder bush, trimmed into the form of a cross, is planted on a new-made grave, and if it blossoms, the soul of the person lying beneath it is happy."

Green Elder branches were also buried in a grave to protect the dead from witches and evil spirits, and in some parts it was a custom for the driver of the hearse to carry a whip made of Elder wood.

In some of the rural Midlands, it is believed that if a child is chastised with an Elder switch, it will cease to grow, owing, in this instance, to some supposed malign influence of the tree. On the other hand, Lord Bacon commended the rubbing of warts with a green Elder stick and then burying the stick to rot in the mud, and for erysipelas, it was recommended to wear about the neck an amulet made of Elder 'on which the sun had never shined."

In Denmark we come across the old belief that he who stood under an Elder tree on Midsummer Eve would see the King of Fairyland ride by, attended by all his retinue. Folkard, in Plant-Lore, Legends and Lyrics, relates:

'The pith of the branches when cut in round, flat shapes, is dipped in oil, lighted, and then put to float in a glass of water; its light on Christmas Eve is thought to reveal to the owner all the witches and sorcerers in the neighborhood';

and again,

'On Bertha Night (6th January), the devil goes about with special virulence. As a safeguard, persons are recommended to make a magic circle, in the centre of which they should stand, with Elderberries gathered on St. John's night. By doing this, the mystic Fern-seed may be obtained, which possesses the strength of thirty or forty men."

This is a Styrian tradition.

The whole tree has a narcotic smell, and it is not considered wise to sleep under its shade. Perhaps the visions of fairyland were the result of the drugged sleep! No plant will grow under the shadow of it, being affected by its exhalations.

Apart from all these traditions, the Elder has had from the earliest days a firm claim on the popular affection for its many sterling virtues.

Uses

Its uses are manifold and important. The wood of old trees is white and of a fine, close grain, easily cut, and polishes well, hence it was used for making skewers for butchers, shoemakers' pegs, and various turned articles, such as tops for angling rods and needles for weaving nets, also for making combs, mathematical instruments and several different musical instruments, and the pith of the younger stems, which is exceedingly light, is cut into balls and is used for electrical experiments and for making small toys. It is also considerably used for holding small objects for sectioning for microscopical purposes.

In a cutting of Worlidge's Mystery of Husbandry (dated 1675) the Elder is included in the 'trees necessary and proper for fencing and enclosing of Lands."

'A considerable Fence," he writes, 'may be made of Elder, set of reasonable hasty Truncheons, like the Willow and may be laid with great curiosity: this makes a speedy shelter for a garden from Winds, Beasts and suchlike injuries,"

though he adds and emphasizes with italics, 'rather than from rude Michers."

The word 'micher' is now obsolete, but it means a lurking thief, a skulking vagabond. By clipping two or three times a year, an Elder hedge may, however, be made close and compact in growth. There is an old tradition that an Elder stake will last in the ground longer than an iron bar of the same size, hence the old couplet:

'An eldern stake and a black thorn ether (hedge)
Will make a hedge to last for ever."

The leaves have an unpleasant odor when bruised, which is supposed to be offensive to most insects, and a decoction of the young leaves is sometimes employed by gardeners to sprinkle over delicate plants and the buds of the flowers to keep off the attacks of aphis and minute caterpillars. Moths are fond of the blossoms, but it was stated by Christopher Gullet (Phil. Trans., 1772, LXII) that if turnips, cabbages, fruit trees or corn be whipped with bunches of the green leaves, they gain immunity from blight. Though this does not sound a very practical procedure, there is evidently some foundation for this statement, as the following note which appeared in the Chemist and Druggist, January 6, 1923, would seem to prove:

'A liquid preparation for preventing, and also curing, blight in fruit trees, wherein the base is a liquid obtained by boiling the young shoots of the Elder tree or bush, mixed with suitable proportions of copper sulphate, iron sulphate, nicotine, soft soap, methylated spirit and slaked lime."

The leaves, bruised, if worn in the hat or rubbed on the face, prevent flies settling on the person. In order to safeguard the skin from the attacks of mosquitoes, midges and other troublesome flies, an infusion of the leaves may be dabbed on with advantage. Gather a few fresh leaves from the elder, tear them from their stalks and place them in a jug, pouring boiling water on them and covering them at once, leaving for a few hours. When the infusion is cold, it is fit for use and should be at once poured off into a bottle and kept tightly corked. It is desirable to make a fresh infusion often. The leaves are said to be valued by the farmer for driving mice away from granaries and moles from their usual haunts.

The bark of the older branches has been used in the Scotch Highlands as an ingredient in dyeing black, also the root. The leaves yield, with alum, a green dye and the berries dye blue and purple, the Juice yielding with alum, violet; with alum and salt, a lilac color.

The botanist finds in this plant an object of considerable interest, for if a twig is partially cut, then cautiously broken and the divided portions are carefully drawn asunder, the spiral air-vessels, resembling a screw, may be distinctly seen.

Linnaeus observed that sheep eat the leaves, also cows, but that horses and goats refuse it. If sheep that have the foot-rot can get at the bark and young shoots, they will cure themselves. Elderberries are eaten greedily by young birds and pigeons, but are said to have serious effects on chickens: the flowers are reported to be fatal to turkeys, and according to Linnaeus, also to peacocks.

Elder Flowers and Elder Berries have long been used in the English countryside for making many home-made drinks and preserves that are almost as great favorites now as in the time of our great-grandmothers. The berries make an excellent home-made wine and winter cordial, which improves with age, and taken hot with sugar, just before going to bed, is an old-fashioned and wellestablished cure for a cold.

In Kent, there are entire orchards of Elder trees cultivated solely for the sake of their fruit, which is brought regularly to market and sold for the purpose of making wine. The berries are not only used legitimately for making Elderberry Wine, but largely in the manufacture of so-called British wines - they give a red color to raisin wine - and in the adulteration of foreign wines. Judiciously flavoured with vinegar and sugar and small quantities of port wine, Elder is often the basis of spurious 'clarets' and 'Bordeaux." 'Men of nice palates," says Berkeley (Querist, 1735), 'have been imposed on by Elder Wine for French Claret." Cheap port is often faked to resemble tawny port by the addition of Elderberry juice, which forms one of the least injurious ingredients of factitious port wines. Doctoring port wine with Elderberry juice seems to have assumed such dimensions that in 1747 this practice was forbidden in Portugal, even the cultivation of the Elder tree was forbidden on this account. The practice proving so lucrative, however, is by no means obsolete, but as the berries possess valuable medicinal properties, this adulteration has no harmful results. The circumstances under which this was proved are somewhat curious. In 1899 an American sailor informed a physician of Prague that getting drunk on genuine, old, dark-red port was a sure remedy for rheumatic pains. This unedifying observation started a long series of investigations ending in the discovery that while genuine port wine has practically no anti-neuralgic properties, the cheap stuff faked to resemble tawny port by the addition of elderberry juice often banishes the pain of sciatica and other forms of neuralgia, though of no avail in genuine neuritis. Cases of cure have been instanced after many tests carried out by leading doctors in Prague and other centres abroad, the dose recommended being 30 grams of Elderberry juice mixed with 10 grams of port wine.

The Romans, as Pliny records, made use of it in medicine, as well as of the Dwarf Elder (Sambucus Ebulus). Both kinds were employed in Britain by the ancient English and Welsh leeches and in Italy in the medicine of the School of Salernum. Elder still keeps its place in the British Pharmacopoeia, the cooling effects of Elder flowers being well known. In many parts of the country, Elder leaves and buds are used in drinks, poultices and ointments.

John Evelyn, writing in praise of the Elder, says:

'If the medicinal properties of its leaves, bark and berries were fully known, I cannot tell what our countryman could ail for which he might not fetch a remedy from every hedge, either for sickness, or wounds."

'The buds boiled in water gruel have effected wonders in a fever, the spring buds are excellently wholesome in pattages; and small ale in which Elder flowers have been infused is esteemed by many so salubrious that this is to be had in most of the eatinghouses about our town."

He also, as we have seen, recommends Elder flowers infused in vinegar as an ingredient of a salad, 'though the leaves are somewhat rank of smell and so not commendable in sallet they are of the most sovereign virtue," and goes so far as to say, 'an extract composed of the berries greatly assists longevity. Indeed this is a catholicum against all infirmities whatever."

Some twenty years before Evelyn's eulogy there had appeared in 1644 a book entirely devoted to its praise: The Anatomie of the Elder, translated from the Latin of Dr. Martin Blockwich by C. de Iryngio (who seems to have been an army doctor), a treatise of some 230 pages, that in Latin and English went through several editions. It deals very learnedly with the medicinal virtues of the tree - its flowers, berries, leaves, 'middle bark," pith, roots and 'Jew's ears," a large fungus often to be found on the Elder (Hirneola auricula Judae), the name a corruption of 'Judas's ear," from the tradition, referred to above, that Judas hanged himself on the Elder. It is of a purplish tint, resembling in shape and softness the human ear, and though it occurs also on the Elm, it grows almost exclusively on Elder trunks in damp, shady places. It is curious that on account of this connexion with Judas, the fungus should have (as Sir Thomas Browne says) 'become a famous medicine in quinses, sore-throats, and strangulation ever since." Gerard says, 'the jelly of the Elder otherwise called Jew's ear, taketh away inflammations of the mouth and throat if they be washed therewith and doth in like manner help the uvula," and Salmon, writing in the early part of the eighteenth century, recommends an oil of Jew's ears for throat affections. The fungus is edible and allied species are eaten in China.

Evelyn refers to this work (or rather to the original by 'Blockwitzius," as he calls him!) for the comprehensive statement in praise of the Elder quoted above. It sets forth that as every part of the tree was medicinal, so virtually every ailment of the body was curable by it, from toothache to the plague. It was used externally and internally, and in amulets (these were especially good for epilepsy, and in popular belief also for rheumatism), and in every kind of form - in rob and syrup, tincture, mixture, oil, spirit, water, liniment, extract, salt, conserve, vinegar, oxymel, sugar, decoction, bath, cataplasm and powder. Some of these were prepared from one part of the plant only, others from several or from all. Their properties are summed up as 'desiccating, conglutinating, and digesting," but are extended to include everything necessary to a universal remedy. The book prescribes in more or less detail for some seventy or more distinct diseases or classes of diseases, and the writer is never at a loss for an authority - from Dioscorides to the Pharmacopoeias of his own day-while the examples of cures he adduces are drawn from all classes of people, from Emylia, Countess of Isinburg, to the tradesmen of Heyna and their dependants.

The interest in the Elder evinced about this period is also demonstrated by a tract on 'Elder and Juniper Berries, showing how useful they may be in our Coffee Houses," which was published with The Natural History of Coffee, in 1682.

Parts Used Medicinally

The bark, leaves, flowers and berries.

Bark

The Inner Bark should be collected in autumn, from young trees. It is best dried in a moderate sunheat, being taken indoors at night. When ready for use, it is a light grey, soft and corky externally, with broad fissures; white and smooth on the inner surface. The taste of the bark is sweetish at first, then slightly bitter and nauseous. It is without odor.

Chemical Constituents

The active principle of the bark is a soft resin, and an acidViburnic acid, which has been proved identical with Valeric acid. Other constituents are traces of a volatile oil, albumen, resin, fat, wax, chlorophyll, tannic acid, grape sugar, gum, extractive, starch, pectin and various alkaline and earthy salts. (According to an analysis by Kramer in 1881.)

Medicinal Action and Uses

The bark is a strong purgative which may be employed with advantage, an infusion of 1 OZ. in a pint of water being taken in wine glassful doses; in large doses it is an emetic. Its use as a purgative dates back to Hippocrates. It has been much employed as a diuretic, an aqueous solution having been found very useful in cardiac and renal dropsies. It has also been successfully employed in epilepsy.

An emollient ointment is made of the green inner bark, and a homeopathic tincture made from the fresh inner bark of the young branches, in diluted form, relieves asthmatic symptoms and spurious croup of children - dose, 4 or 5 drops in water.

Culpepper states:

'The first shoots of the common Elder, boiled like Asparagus, and the young leaves and stalks boiled in fat broth, doth mightily carry forth phlegm and choler. The middle or inward bark boiled in water and given in drink wortheth much more violently; and the berries, either green or dry, expel the same humour, and are often given with good success in dropsy; the bark of the root boiled in wine, or the juice thereof drunk, worketh the same effects, but more powerfully than either the leaves or fruit. The juice of the root taken, causes vomitings and purgeth the watery humours of the dropsy."

Though the use of the root is now obsolete, its juice was used from very ancient times to promote both vomiting and purging, and taken, as another old writer recommends, in doses of 1 to 2 tablespoonsful, fasting, once in the week, was held to be 'the most excellent purge of water humours in the world and very singular against dropsy." A tea was also made from the roots of Elder, which was considered an effective preventative for incipient dropsy, in fact the very best remedy for such cases .

Leaves

Elder leaves are used both fresh and dry.

Collect the leaves in June and July. Gather only in fine weather, in the morning, after the dew has been dried by the sun. Strip the leaves off singly, rejecting any that are stained or insect-eaten. Drying is then done in the usual manner.

Constituents

Elder Leaves contain an alkaloid Sambucine, a purgative resin and the glucoside Sambunigrin, which crystallizes in white, felted needles. Fresh Elder leaves yield about 0.16 per cent of hydrocyanic acid. They also contain cane sugar, invertin, a considerable quantity of potassium nitrate and a crystalline substance, Eldrin, which has also been found in other white flowering plants.

De Sanctis claims to have isolated the alkaloid Coniine from the branches and leaves of Sambucus nigra. Alpes (Proc. Amer. Pharm. Assoc., 1900) found undoubted evidence of an alkaloid in the roots of the American Elder (S. Canadensis), its odor being somewhat similar to that of coniine and also suggesting nicotine. This alkaloid was evidently volatile. It appeared to be much less abundant in the dried roots after some months keeping. The fresh root of S. Canadensis has been found extremely poisonous, producing death in children within a short time after being eaten with symptoms very similar to those of poisoning by Hemlock (Conium).

Uses

Elder leaves are used in the preparation of an ointment, Unguentum Sambuci Viride, Green Elder Ointment, which is a domestic remedy for bruises, sprains, chilblains, for use as an emollient, and for applying to wounds. It can be compounded as follows: Take 3 parts of fresh Elder leaves, 4 parts of lard and 2 of prepared suet, heat the Elder leaves with the melted lard and suet until the color is extracted, then strain through a linen cloth with pressure and allow to cool.

Sir Thomas Browne (1655) stated: 'The common people keep as a good secret in curing wounds the leaves of the Elder, which they have gathered the last day of April." The leaves, boiled soft with a little linseed oil, were used as a healing application to piles. An ointment concocted from the green Elderberries, with camphor and lard, was formerly ordered by the London College of Surgeons to relieve the same complaint. The leaves are an ingredient of many cooling ointments: Here is another recipe, not made from Elder leaves alone, and very much recommended by modern herbalists as being very cooling and softening and excellent for all kinds of tumors, swellings and wounds: Take the Elder leaves 1/2 lb., Plantain leaves 1/4 lb., Ground Ivy 2 oz., Wormwood 4 oz. (all green); cut them small, and boil in 4 lb. of lard, in the oven, or over a slow fire; stir them continually until the leaves become crisp, then strain, and press out the ointment for use.

Oil of Elder Leaves (Oleum Viride), Green Oil, or Oil of Swallows, is prepared by digesting 1 part of bruised fresh Elder leaves in 3 parts of linseed oil. In commerce, it is said to be generally coloured with verdigris.

Like the bark, the leaves are also purgative, but more nauseous than the bark. Their action is likewise expectorant, diuretic and diaphoretic. They are said to be very efficacious in dropsy. The juice of Elder leaves is stated by the old herbalists to be good for inflammation of the eyes, and 'snuffed up the nostrils," Culpepper declares, 'purgeth the brain." Another old notion was that if the green leaves were warmed between two hot tiles and applied to the forehead, they would promptly relieve nervous headache.

The use of the leaves, bruised and in decoction to drive away flies and kill aphides and other insect pests has already been referred to.

Flowers

Elder Flowers are chiefly used in pharmacy in the fresh state for the distillation of Elder Flower Water, but as the flowering season only lasts for about three weeks in June, the flowers are often salted, so as to be available for distillation at a later season, 10 per cent of common salt being added, the flowers being them termed 'pickled." They are also dried, for making infusions.

The flowers are collected when just in full bloom and thrown into heaps, and after a few hours, during which they become slightly heated the corollas become loosened and can then be removed by sifting. The Elder 'flowers' of pharmacy consist of the small white wheel-shaped, five-lobed, monopetalous corollas only, in the short tube of which the five stamens with very short filaments and yellow anthers are inserted. When fresh, the flowers have a slightly bitter taste and an odor scarcely pleasant. The pickled flowers, however, gradually acquire an agreeable fragrance and are therefore generally used for the preparation of Elder Flower Water. A similar change also takes place in the water distilled from the fresh flowers.

In domestic herbal medicines, the dried flowers are largely used in country districts and are sold by herbalists either in dried bunches of flowers, or sifted free from flower stalks. The flowers are not easily dried of good color. If left too late exposed to the sun before gathering, the flowers assume a brownish color when dried, and if the flower bunches are left too long in heaps, to cause the flowers to fall off, these heaps turn black. If the inflorescence is only partly open when gathered, the flower-heads have to be sifted more than once, as the flowers do not open all at the same time. The best and lightest coloured flowers are obtained at the first sifting, when the flowers that have matured and fallen naturally are free from stalks, and dried quickly in a heated atmosphere. They may be very quickly dried in a heated copper pan, being stirred about for a few minutes. They can also be dried almost as quickly in a cool oven, with the door open. Quickness in drying is essential.

The dried flowers, which are so shrivelled that their details are quite obscured, have a dingy, brownish-yellow color and a faint, but characteristic odor and mucilaginous taste. As a rule, imported flowers have a duller yellow color and inferior odor and are sold at a cheaper rate. When the microscope does not reveal tufts of short hairs in the sinuses of the calyx, the drug is not of this species. Most pharmacopoeias specify that dark brown or blackish flowers should be rejected. This appearance may be due to their having been collected some time after opening, to carelessness in drying, or to having been preserved too long.

The flowers of the Dwarf Elder, a comparatively uncommon plant in this country are distinguished from those of the Common Elder by having dark red anthers.

The flowers of the Yarrow (Achillea millefolium), and other composite plants, which have been used as adulterants of Elder flowers differ still more markedly in appearance and their presence in the drug is readily detected.

Constituents

The most important constituent of Elder Flowers is a trace of semisolid volatile oil, present to the extent only of 0.32, per cent possessing the odor of the flowers in a high degree. It is obtained by distilling the fresh flowers with water, saturating the distillate with salt and shaking it with ether. On evaporating the ethereal solution, the oil is obtained as a yellowish, buttery mass. Without ether, fresh Elder flowers yield 0.037 per cent of the volatile oil and the dried flowers 0.0027 per cent only.

Elder Flower Water (Aqua Sambuci) is an official preparation of the British Pharmacopoeia, which directs that it be made from 100 parts of Elder Flowers distilled with 500 parts of water (about 10 lb. to the gallon), and that if fresh Elder flowers are not obtainable, an equivalent quantity of the flowers preserved with common salt be used. The product has at first a distinctly unpleasant odor, but gradually acquires an agreeably aromatic odor, and it is preferable not to use it until this change has taken place.

Elder Flower Water is employed in mixing medicines and chiefly as a vehicle for eye and skin lotions. It is mildly astringent and a gentle stimulant. It is the Eau de Sureau of the Continent, Sureau being the French name of the Eider.

Here is a recipe that can be carried out at home: Fill a large jar with Elder blossoms, pressing them down, the stalks of course having been removed previously. Pour on them 2 quarts of boiling water and when slightly cooled, add 1 1/2 OZ. of rectified spirits. Cover with a folded cloth, and stand the jar in a warm place for some hours. Then allow it to get quite cold and strain through muslin. Put into bottles and cork securely.

Elderflower Water in our great-grandmothers' days was a household word for clearing the complexion of freckles and sunburn, and keeping it in a good condition. Every lady's toilet table possessed a bottle of the liquid, and she relied on this to keep her skin fair and white and free from blemishes, and it has not lost its reputation. Its use after sea-bathing has been recommended, and if any eruption should appear on the face as the effect of salt water, it is a good plan to use a mixture composed of Elder Flower Water with glycerine and borax, and apply it night and morning.

Elder Flowers, if placed in the water used for washing the hands and face, will both whiten and soften the skin-a convenient way being to place them in a small muslin bag. Such a bag steeped in the bathwater makes a most refreshing bath and a wellknown French doctor has stated that he considers it a fine aid in the bath in cases of irritability of the skin and nerves.

The flowers were used by our forefathers in bronchial and pulmonary affections, and in scarlet fever, measles and other eruptive diseases. An infusion of the dried flowers, Elder Flower Tea, is said to promote expectoration in pleurisy; it is gently laxative and aperient and is considered excellent for inducing free perspiration. It is a good oldfashioned remedy for colds and throat trouble, taken hot on going to bed. An almost infallible cure for an attack of influenza in its first stage is a strong infusion of dried Elder Blossoms and Peppermint. Put a handful of each in a jug, pour over them a pint and a half of boiling water, allow to steep, on the stove, for half an hour then strain and sweeten and drink in bed as hot as possible. Heavy perspiration and refreshing sleep will follow, and the patient will wake up well on the way to recovery and the cold or influenza will probably be banished within thirty-six hours. Yarrow may also be added.

Elder Flower Tea, cold, was also considered almost as good for inflammation of the eyes as the distilled Elder Flower Water.

Tea made from Elder Flowers has also been recommended as a splendid spring medicine, to be taken every morning before breakfast for some weeks, being considered an excellent blood purifier.

Externally, Elder Flowers are used in fomentations, to ease pain and abate inflammation. An old writer tells us:

'There be nothing more excellent to ease the pains of the hemorrhoids than a fomentation made of the flowers of the Elder and Verbusie, or Honeysuckle in water or milk for a short time. It easeth the greatest pain. "

A lotion, too, can be made by pouring boiling water on the dried blossoms, which is healing, cooling and soothing. Add 2 1/2 drachms of Elder Flowers to 1 quart of boiling water, infuse for an hour and then strain. The liquor can be applied as a lotion by means of a linen rag, for tumors boils, and affections of the skin, and is said to be effective put on the temples against headache and also for warding off the attacks of flies.

A salad of young Elder buds, macerated a little in hot water and dressed with oil, vinegar and salt, has been used as a remedy against skin eruptions.

Elder Vinegar made from the flowers is an old remedy for sore throat.

A good ointment is also prepared from the flowers by infusion in warm lard, useful for dressing wounds, burns and scalds, which is used, also, as a basis for pomades and cosmetic ointments, Elder Flower Ointment (Unguentum Sambuci) was largely used for wounded horses in the War - the Blue Cross made a special appeal for supplies - but it is also good for human use and is an old remedy for chapped hands and chilblains. Equal quantities of the fresh flowers and of lard are taken, the flowers are heated with the lard until they become crisp, then strained through a linen cloth with pressure and allowed to cool. For use as a Face Cream, the directions are a little more elaborate, but it is essentially the same: Melt lard in a pan then add a small cup of cold water and stir well. Simmer with the lid on for about an hour and finally let the mixture boil with the lid off until all the water has evaporated; this will have happened when, on stirring, no steam arises. Place on one side to cool a little and then pass the liquid fat through a piece of muslin so that it may be well strained and free from impurities. Take a quantity of Elder Flowers equal in weight to the lard and place these in the lard. Then boil up the mixture again, keeping it simmering for a good hour. At the end of that time, strain the whole through a coarse cloth and when cool, the ointment will be ready for use.

Elder Flowers, with their subtle sweet scent, entered into much delicate cookery, in olden days. Formerly the creamy blossoms were beaten up in the batter of flannel cakes and muffins, to which they gave a more delicate texture. They were also boiled in gruel as a fever-drink, and were added to the posset of the Christening feast.

Berries

All the other parts of the Elder plant, except the wood and pith, are more active than either the flowers or the fruit. Fresh Elder Berries are found to contain sudorific properties similar to those of the flowers, but weaker. Chemically, the berries furnish Viburnic acid, with an odorous oil, combined with malates of potash and lime. The fresh, ripe fruits contain Tyrosin.

The blue coloring matter extracted from them has been considerably used as an indication for alkalis, with which it gives a green color, being red with acids. (Alkalis redden some vegetable yellows and change some vegetable blues to green.) According to Cowie this coloring matter is best extracted in the form of a 20 per cent tincture from the refuse remaining after the expression of the first juice. The coloring matter is precipitated blue by lead acetate (National Standard Dispensatory, 1909.)

The Romans made use of Elderberry juice as a hair-dye, and Culpepper tells us that 'the hair of the head washed with the berries boiled in wine is made black."

English Elder Berries, as we have seen, are extensively used for the preparation of Elder Wine. French and other Continental Elder berries, when dried, are not liked for this purpose, as they have a more unpleasant odor and flavor, and English berries are preferred. Possibly this may be due to the conditions of growth, or variety, or to the presence of the berries of the Dwarf Elder. Aubrey (1626-97) tells us that:

'the apothecaries well know the use of the berries, and so do the vintners, who buy vast quantities of them in London, and some do make no inconsiderable profit by the sale of them."

They were held by our forefathers to be efficacious in rheumatism and erysipelas. They have aperient, diuretic and emetic properties, and the inspissated juice of the berries has been used as an alterative in rheumatism and syphilis in doses of from one to two drachms, also as a laxative in doses of half an ounce or more. It promotes all fluid secretions and natural evacuations.

For colic and diarrhea, a tea made of the dried berries is said to be a good remedy.

In The Anatomie of the Elder, it is stated that the berries of the Elder and Herb Paris are useful in epilepsy. Green Elderberry Ointment has already been mentioned as curative of piles.

After enumerating many uses of the Elder, Gerard says:

'The seeds contained within the berries, dried, are good for such as have the dropsie, and such as are too fat, and would faine be leaner, if they be taken in a morning to the quantity of a dram with wine for a certain space. The green leaves, pounded with Deeres suet or Bulls tallow are good to be laid to hot swellings and tumors, and doth assuage the paine of the gout."

Parkinson, physician to James I, also tells us of the same use of the seeds, which he recommends to be taken powdered, in vinegar.

Elderberry Wine has a curative power of established repute as a remedy, taken hot, at night, for promoting perspiration in the early stages of severe catarrh, accompanied by shivering, sore throat, etc. Like Elderflower Tea, it is one of the best preventives known against the advance of influenza and the ill effects of a chill. A little cinnamon may be added. It has also a reputation as an excellent remedy for asthma.

Almost from time immemorial, a 'Rob' (a vegetable juice thickened by heat) has been made from the juice of Elderberries simmered and thickened with sugar, forming an invaluable cordial for colds and coughs, but only of late years has science proved that Elderberries furnish Viburnic acid, which induces perspiration, and is especially useful in cases of bronchitis and similar troubles.

To make Elderberry Rob, 5 lb. of fresh ripe, crushed berries are simmered with 1 lb. of loaf sugar and the juice evaporated to the thickness of honey. It is cordial, aperient and diuretic. One or two tablespoonsful mixed with a tumblerful of hot water, taken at night, promotes perspiration and is demulcent to the chest. The Rob when made can be bottled and stored for the winter. Herbalists sell it ready for use.

'Syrup of Elderberries' is made as follows: Pick the berries when throughly ripe from the stalks and stew with a little water in a jar in the oven or pan. After straining, allow 1/2 oz. of whole ginger and 18 cloves to each gallon. Boil the ingredients an hour, strain again and bottle. The syrup is an excellent cure for a cold. To about a wine glassful of Elderberry syrup, add hot water, and if liked, sugar.

Both Syrup of Elderberries and the Rob were once official in this country (as they are still in Holland), the rob being the older of of the two, and the one that retained its place longer in our Pharmacopoeia. In 1788, its name was changed to Succus Sambuci spissatus, and in 1809 it disappeared altogether. Brookes in 1773 strongly recommended it as a 'saponaceous Resolvent' promoting 'the natural secretions by stool, urine and sweat," and, diluted with water, for common colds. John Wesley, in his Primitive Physick, directs it to be taken in broth, and in Germany it is used as an ingredient in soups.

There were six or seven robs in the old London Pharmacopeia, to most of which sugar was added. They were thicker than syrups, but did not differ materially from them; among them was a rob of Elderberries, and both Quincy and Bates had a syrup of

Elder.

An old prescription for sciatica (called the Duke of Monmouth's recipe) was compounded of ripe haws and fennel roots, distilled in white wine and taken with syrup of Elder.

The use of the juicy berries, not as medicine, but as a pleasant article of food, in jam, jelly, chutney and ketchup has already been described.

Medicinal Preparations

Fluid extract of bark, 1/2 to 1 drachm. Water, B.P.

Elder Wine Recipes

An old recipe for Elder Wine

'To every quart of berries put 2 quarts of water; boil half an hour, run the liquor and break the fruit through a hair sieve; then to every quart of juice, put 3/4 of a pound of Lisbon sugar, coarse, but not the very coarsest. Boil the whole a quarter of an hour with some Jamaica peppers, ginger, and a few cloves. Pour it into a tub, and when of a proper warmth, into the barrel, with toast and yeast to work, which there is more difficulty to make it do than most other liquors. When it ceases to hiss, put a quart of brandy to eight gallons and stop up. Bottle in the spring, or at Christmas. The liquor must be in a warm place to make it work."

The following recipe for making Elder Wine is given by Mrs. Hewlett in a work entitled Cottage Comforts:

'If two gallons of wine are to be made, get one gallon of Elderberries, and a quart of damsons, or sloes; boil them together in six quarts of water, for half an hour, breaking the fruit with a stick, flat at one end; run off the liquor, and squeeze the pulp through a sieve, or straining cloth; boil the liquor up again with six pounds of coarse sugar, two ounces of ginger, two ounces of bruised allspice, and one ounce of hops; (the spice had better be loosely tied in a bit of muslin); let this boil above half an hour; then pour it off, when quite cool, stir in a teacupful of yeast, and cover it up to work. After two days, skim off the yeast, and put the wine into the barrel, and when it ceases to hiss, which will be in about a fortnight, paste a stiff brown paper over the bung-hole. After this, it will be fit for use in about 8 weeks, but will keep 8 years, if required. The bag of spice may be dropped in at the bung-hole, having a string fastened outside, which shall keep it from reaching the bottom of the barrel."

Another Recipe

'Strip the berries, which must be quite ripe, into a dry pan and pour 2 gallons of boiling water over 3 gallons of berries. Cover and leave in a warm place for 24 hours; then strain, pressing the juice well out. Measure it and allow 3 pounds of sugar, half an ounce of ginger and 1/4 ounce of cloves to each gallon. Boil for 20 minutes slowly, then strain it into a cask and ferment when lukewarm. Let it remain until still, before bunging, and bottle in six months.

'If a weaker wine is preferred, use 4 gallons of water to 3 gallons of berries and leave for two days before straining.

'If a cask be not available, large stone jars will answer: then the wine need not be bottled."

Parkinson tells us that fresh Elder Flowers hung in a vessel of new wine and pressed every evening for seven nights together, 'giveth to the wine a very good relish and a smell like Muscadine." Ale was also infused with Elder flowers.

The berries make good pies, if blended with spices, and formerly used to be preserved with spice and kept for winter use in pies when fruit was scarce. Quite a delicious jam can also be made of them, mixed with apples, which has much the flavor of Blackberry jam. They mix to very great advantage with Crab Apple, or with the hard Catillac cooking Pear, or with Vegetable Marrow, and also with Blackberries or Rhubarb.

The Fruit Preserving Section of the Food Ministry issued during the War the following recipe for Elderberry and Apple Jam: 6 lb. Elderberries, 6 lb. sliced apples, 12 lb. sugar. Make a pulp of the apples by boiling in water till soft and passing through a coarse sieve to remove any seeds or cores. The Elderberries should also be stewed for half an hour to soften them. Combine the Apple pulp, berries and sugar and return to the fire to boil till thick.

Another Recipe

Equal quantities of Elderberries and Apples, 3/4 lb. sugar and one lemon to each pound of fruit. Strip the berries from the stalks, peel, core and cut up the apples and weigh both fruits. Put the Elderberries into a pan over low heat and bruise them with a wooden spoon. When the juice begins to flow, add the Apples and one-third of the sugar and bring slowly to the boil. When quite soft, rub all through a hair sieve. Return the pulp to the pan, add the rest of the sugar, the grated lemon rind and juice and boil for half an hour, or until the jam sets when tested. Remove all scum, put into pots and cover.

Elderberry Jam without Apples

To every pound of berries add 1/4 pint ofwater, the juice of 2 lemons and 1 lb. of sugar. Boil from 30 to 45 minutes, until it sets when tested. Put into jars and tie down when cold.

The Elderberry will, of course, also make a jelly. As it is a juicy fruit, it will not need the addition of any more liquid than, perhaps, a squeeze of lemon. Equal quantities of Elderberry juice and apple juice, and apple juice from peeling, will require 3/4 lb. of sugar to a pint. Elderberry Jelly is firm and flavorous, with a racy tang.

When the fruit is not quite ripe, it may be preserved in brine and used as a substitute for capers.

The juice from Elder Berries, too, was formerly distilled and mixed with vinegar for salad dressings and flavoring sauces. Vinegars used in former times frequently to be aromatized by steeping in them barberries, rosemary, rose leaves, gilliflowers, lavender, violets - in short, any scented flower or plant though tarragon is now practically the only herb used in this manner to any large extent.

Elderflower Vinegar

Take 2 lb. of dried flowers of Elder. If you use your own flowers, pluck carefully their stalks from them and dry them carefully and thoroughly. This done, place in a large vessel and pour over them 2 pints of good vinegar. Close the vessel hermetically, keep it in a very warm place and shake them from time to time. After 8 days, strain the vinegar through a paper filter. Keep in well-stoppered bottles.

This is an old-world simple, but rarely met with nowadays, but worth the slight trouble of making. It was well-known and appreciated in former days and often mentioned in old books; Steele, in The Tatler, says: 'They had dissented about the preference of Elder to Wine vinegar."

One seldom has the chance of now tasting the old country pickle made from the tender young shoots and flowers. John Evelyn, writing in 1664, recommends Elder flowers infused in vinegar as an ingredient of a salad. The pickled blossoms are said by those who have tried them to be a welcome relish with boiled mutton, as a substitute for capers. Clusters of the flowers are gathered in their unripened green state, put into a stone jar and covered with boiling vinegar. Spices are unnecessary. The jar is tied down directly the pickle is cold. This pickle is very good and has the advantage of costing next to nothing.

The pickle made from the tender young shoots - sometimes known as 'English Bamboo' - is more elaborate. During May, in the middle of the Elder bushes in the hedges, large young green shoots may be observed. Cut these, selecting the greenest, peel off every vestige of the outer skin and lay them in salt and water overnight. Each individual length must be carefully chosen, for while they must not be too immature, if the shoots are at all woody, they will not be worth eating, The following morning, prepare the pickle for the Mock Bamboo. To a quart of vinegar, add an ounce of white pepper, an ounce of ginger, half a saltspoonful of mace and boil all well together. Remove the Elder shoots from the salt and water, dry in a cloth and slice up into suitable pieces, laying them in a stone jar. Pour the boiling mixture over them and either place them in an oven for 2 hours, or in a pan of boiling water on the stove. When cold, the pickle should be green in color. If not, strain the liquor, boil it up again, pour over the shoots and repeat the process. The great art of obtaining and retaining the essence of the plant lies in excluding air from the tied-down jar as much as possible.

The young shoots can also be boiled in salted water with a pinch of soda to preserve the color, they prove beautifully tender, resembling spinach, and form quite a welcome addition to the dinner table.

Good use can be made of the berries for Ketchup and Chutney, and the following recipes will be found excellent.

Elderberry Chutney

2 lb. Elderberries, 1 large Onion, 1 pint vinegar, 1 teaspoonful salt, 1 teaspoonful ground ginger, 2 tablespoonsful sugar, 1 saltspoonful cayenne and mixed spices, 1 teaspoonful mustard seed.

Stalk, weigh and wash the berries; put them into a pan and bruise with a wooden spoon; chop the onion and add with the rest of the ingredients and vinegar. Bring to the boil and simmer till it becomes thick. Stir well, being careful not to let it burn as it thickens. Put into jars and cover.

Another Recipe

Rub 1 1/2 lb. of berries through a wire sieve, pound 1 onion, 6 cloves, 1/4 oz. ground ginger, 2 oz. Demerara sugar, 3 oz. stoned raisins, a dust of cayenne and mace, 1 teaspoonful salt and 1 pint vinegar. Put all in an enamelled saucepan and boil with the pulp of the berries for 10 minutes. Take the pan from the fire and let it stand till cold. Put the chutney into jars and cork securely.

Elderberry Ketchup

1 pint Elderberries, 1 OZ. shallots, 1 blade mace, 1/2 oz. peppercorns, 1 1/2 OZ. whole ginger, 1 pint vinegar.

Pick the berries (which must be ripe) from the stalks, weigh and wash them. Put them into an unglazed crock or jar, pour over the boiling vinegar and leave all night in a cool oven. Next day, strain the liquor from the berries through a cloth tied on to the legs of an inverted chair and put it into a pan, with the peeled and minced shallots, the ginger peeled and cut up small, the mace and peppercorns. Boil for 10 minutes, then put into bottles, dividing the spices among the bottles. Cork well.

All parts of the tree - bark, leaves, flowers and berries - have long enjoyed a high reputation in domestic medicine. From the days of Hippocrates, it has been famous for its medicinal properties.

ELDER, DWARF

Botanical: Sambucus Ebulus (LINN.)
Family: N.O. Caprifoliaceae
Synonyms: Danewort. Walewort. Blood Hilder.
(French) Hièble.
(German) Attichwurzel.
Part Used: Leaves.

Habitat

This species is found less frequently in hedges, but inclines to waste places, not infrequently among rubbish and the ruined foundations of old buildings. Gerard speaks of the 'dwarf Elder' growing 'in untoiled places plentifully in the lane at Kilburne Abbey by London." The celebrated natural historian of Selborne speaks of the Dwarf Elder as growing among the rubbish and ruined foundations of the Priory. Spots of equal interest with that of Selborne might be cited as favorite haunts of the Dwarf Elder. It grows profusely near Carisbrooke Castle, below the timeworn walls of Scarborough Castle, beside the old Roman Watling Street, where it is crossed by the footpath from Norton to Wilton, in Northamptonshire.

Its old names, Danewort and Walewort (walslaughter) are supposed to be traceable to an old belief that it sprang from the blood of slain Danes - it grows near Slaughterford in Wilts, that being the site of a great Danish battle. Another notion is that it was brought to England by the Danes and planted on the battlefields and graves of their slain countrymen. In Norfolk it still bears the name of Danewort and Blood Hilder (Blood Elder). In accounting for its English name, Sir J. E. Smith says: 'Our ancestors evinced a just hatred of their brutal enemies, the Danes, in supposing the nauseous, fetid and noxious plant before us to have sprung from their blood."

The Dwarf Elder differs from the Common Elder in being a herbaceous plant seldom exceeding 3 feet in height and dying back to the ground every year, spreading by underground shoots from the creeping root.

Description

In leaf, flower and subsequent berry it bears a close resemblance to the Common Elder tree; the stem, however, is not woody and the leaves are distinguished by having a stipule, or small leaf, at the base of the finely-toothed leaflets, which are more numerous than those of the Common Elder, usually seven in number, larger and narrower and sometimes lobed. The flowers are whiter than those of the Common Elder, the corollas splashed with crimson on the outside and have dark red anthers. They are in bloom in July and August, have a less aromatic smell and do not always bring their fruit, a reddishpurple berry, to perfect ripeness in this country. The berries are, however, often present among imported Continental dried elderberries, the species being much more common there than here. In France it is called Hièble, in Germany Attichwurzel.

Medicinal Action and Uses

Expectorant, diuretic, diaphoretic, purgative.

The Dwarf Elder has more drastic therapeutic action than the Common Elder, and it is only the leaves, or very occasionally the berries, that are used medicinally. The leaves are probably more used in herbal practice than those of Sambucus nigra, and are ingredients in medicines for inflammation of both kidney and liver. The drug is said to be very efficacious in dropsy. Dwarf Elder Tea, which has been considered one of the best remedies for dropsy, is prepared from the dried roots, cut up fine or ground to powder; the drug was much used by Kneipp.

The root, which is white and fleshy, has a nauseous, bitter taste and a decoction from it is a drastic purgative. Culpepper states that the decoction cures the bites of mad dogs and adders. The root-juice has been employed to dye hair black.

The leaves, bruised and laid on boils and scalds, have a healing effect, and boiled in wine and made into a poultice were employed in France to resolve swellings and relieve contusions.

A rob made from the berries is actively purgative.

An oil extracted from the seeds has been used as an application to painful joints.

Mice and moles are said not to come near the leaves, and in Silesia there is a belief that it prevents some of the diseases of swine, being strewn in sties.

In the United States, the name of Dwarf Elder is given to an entirely different plant, viz. Aralia hispida (N.O. Araliaceae). In Homeopathy, it is the American Dwarf Elder which is employed. There it is also called Bristly Sarsaparilla and Wild Elder. It is found growing in rocky places in North America.

The homeopaths use a tincture from the fresh, root and a fluid extract is also prepared from it. It has sudorific, diuretic and alterative properties and is regarded as very valuable in dropsy, gravel and in suppression of urine. It is particularly recommended as a diuretic in dropsy, being more acceptable to the stomach than other remedies of the same class.

The 'Prickly Elder' of America is a closely related species, A. spinosa, also known as False Prickly Ash (the real Prickly Ash being Xanthoxylum Americanum), which contains a glucoside named Aralin. A decoction of the plant is used for the same purposes as Sarsaparilla.

The 'Poison Elder' of America is again no Elder, but a Sumach, its other name being Swamp Sumach, botanically Rhus verni (Linn.). It is a handsome shrub or small tree, 10 to 15 feet high, growing in swamps from Canada to California, with very small greenish flowers and small greenish-white berries and is extremely poisonous. It was confounded by the older botanists with R. vernicifera (D.C.) of Japan, the Japanese lacquer tree, which has similar poisonous properties. Its synonym is R. venenata (D.C.) See SUMACH.

There is a tree called the 'Box Elder," mentioned by W. J. Bean in his Trees and Shrubs hardy in the British Isles; this is not a true Elder, however, but one of the American maples that yield sugar.

There are about half a dozen species of Elder hardy in Great Britain. The Common Elder (S. nigra), of which there are many varieties in cultivation, several of which are very ornamental, has leaves often very finely divided and jagged and variegated both with golden and silver blotches, a specially ornamental form being the 'golden cut-leaf Elder," and another with yellow berries; the American Elder (S. canadensis) (the flowers of which, together with those of S. nigra are official in the United States Pharmacopoeia) has berries smaller and deep purple rather than black, the leaves broader and the flowers more fragrant than our Common Elder, it never attains tree size, but is a shrub of from 6 to 10 feet in height; the Blue Elder (S. glauca), the intensely blue berries of which are used as a food, when cooked, in California; the Red-berried Elder (S. racemosa), a pretty species, native of Central and Southern Europe, cultivated in shrubberies, which flowers in March and towards the end of summer is highly ornamental, with large oval clusters of bright scarlet berries, is so attractive to birds that their beauty is rarely seen, except when cultivated close to a house; the Red-berried American Elder (S. rubens and S. melanocarpa).

Cultivation

The Elders like moisture and a loamy soil; given these, they are not difficult to accommodate. The pruning of the sorts grown for their foliage should be done before growth recommences.

They can be easily propagated by cuttings or by seeds, but the former being the most expeditious method is generally followed. The season for planting the cuttings is any time from September to March, and no more care is needed than to thrust the cuttings 6 to 8 inches into the ground. They will take root very quickly, and can be afterwards transplanted where they are to remain. If their berries are allowed to fall upon the ground, they will produce abundance of plants in the following summer.

Herbaceous kinds like S. Ebulus may be increased by dividing the rootstocks in early autumn or spring.

ELDER, DWARF, AMERICAN

Botanical: Aralia hispida
Family: N.O. Araliaceae
Habitat: New England to Virginia.

A perennial, stem 1 to 2 feet high, lower part woody and shrubby, beset with sharp bristles, upper part leafy and branching. Leaflets oblongovate, acute serrate, leaves bipinnate, many simple umbels, globose, axillary and terminal on long peduncles, has bunches of dark-coloured nauseous berries, flowers June to September. The whole plant smells unpleasantly. Fruit, black, round, one-celled, has three irregular-shaped seeds. The bark is used medicinally, but the root is the more active.

This plant must not be confused with the English Dwarf Elder (Sambucus Ebulus).

Medicinal Action and Uses

Sudorific in warm infusion - bark diuretic and alterative and has a special action on kidneys. Most valuable in urinary diseases, dropsy, gravel, suppression of urine, etc. A decoction of the fresh roots and juice are efficacious in dropsy, being a good hydragogue and also an emetic. Dose, decoction, 2 to 4 oz. three times daily.

ELECAMPANE

Botanical: Inula Helenium (LINN.)
Family: N.O. Compositae
Synonyms: Scabwort. Elf Dock. Wild Sunflower.
Horseheal. Velvet Dock.
(French) Aunée
(German) Alantwurzel
(Welsh) Marchalan
Part Used: Root.

Habitat

Elecampane is one of our largest herbaceous plants. It is found widely distributed throughout England, though can scarcely be termed common, occurring only locally, in damp pastures and shady ground. It is probably a true native plant in southern England, but where found farther north may have originally only been an escape from cultivation, as it was cultivated for centuries as a medicinal plant, being a common remedy for sicknesses in the Middle Ages. When present in Scotland, it is considered to have been introduced. Culpepper says:

'It groweth in moist grounds and shadowy places oftener than in the dry and open borders of field and lanes and other waste places, almost in every county in this country, but it was probably more common in his days, cultivation of it being still general."

It is found wild throughout continental Europe, from Gothland southwards, and extends eastwards in temperate Asia as far as Southern Siberia and North-West India. As a plant of cultivation, it has wandered to North America, where it has become thoroughly naturalized in the eastern United States, being found from Nova Scotia to Northern Carolina, and westward as far as Missouri, growing abundantly in pastures and along roadsides, preferring wet, rocky ground at or near the base of eastern and southern slopes.

Description

It is a striking and handsome plant. The erect stem grows from 4 to 5 feet high, is very stout and deeply furrowed, and near the top, branched. The whole plant is downy. It produces a radical rosette of enormous, ovate, pointed leaves, from 1 to 1 1/2 feet long and 4 inches broad in the middle velvety beneath, with toothed margins an borne on long foot-stalks; in general appearance the leaves are not unlike those of Mullein. Those on the stem become shorter andrelatively broader and are stem-clasping.

The plant is in bloom from June to August. The flowers are bright yellow, in very large, terminal heads, 3 to 4 inches in diameter, on long stalks, resembling a double sunflower. The broad bracts of the leafy involucre under the head are velvety. After the flowers have fallen, these involucral scales spread horizontally, and the removal of the fruit shows the beautifully regular arrangement of the little pits on the receptacle, which form a pattern like the engine-turning of a watch. The fruit is quadrangular and crowned by a ring of pale-reddish hairs - the pappus.

The plant springs from a perennial rootstock, which is large and succulent, spindleshaped and branching, brown and aromatic, with large, fleshy roots.

History

Elecampane was known to the ancient writers on agriculture and natural history, and even the Roman poets were acquainted with it, and mention Inula as affording a root used both as a medicine and a condiment. Horace, in the Eighth Satire, relates how Fundanius first taught the making of a delicate sauce by boiling in it the bitter Inula, and how the Romans, after dining too richly, pined for turnips and the appetizing Enulas acidas:

'Quum rapula plenus
Atque acidas mavult inulas."

Inula, the Latin classical name for the plant, is considered to be a corruption of the Greek word Helenion which in its Latinized form, Helenium, is also now applied to the same species. There are many fables about the origin of this name. Gerard tells us: 'It took the name Helenium of Helena, wife of Menelaus, who had her hands full of it when Paris stole her away into Phrygia." Another legend states that it sprang from her tears: another that Helen first used it against venomous bites; a fourth, that it took the name from the island Helena, where the best plants grew.

Vegetius Renatus about the beginning of the fifth century, calls it Inula campana, and St. Isidore, in the beginning of the seventh, names it Inula, adding 'quam Alam rustici vocant." By the mediaeval writers it was often written Enula. Elecampane is a corruption of the ante-Linnaean name Enula campana, so called from its growing wild in Campania.

The herb is of ancient medicinal repute, having

been described by Dioscorides and Pliny. An old Latin distich celebrates its virtues: Enula campana reddit praecordia sana (Elecampane will the spirits sustain). 'Julia Augustus," said Pliny, 'let no day pass without eating some of the roots of Enula, considered to help digestion and cause mirth." The monks equally esteemed it as a cordial. Pliny affirmed that the root 'being chewed fasting, doth fasten the teeth," and Galen that 'It is good for passions of the hucklebone called sciatica."

Dioscorides, in speaking of Castus root, related that it is often mixed with that of Elecampane, from Kommagene (N.W. Syria) (Castus, derived from Aplotaxis auriculata (D.C.), is remarkably similar to Elecampane, both in external appearance and structure. It is an important spice, incense and medicine in the East.)

Elecampane is frequently mentioned in the Anglo-Saxon writings on medicine current in England prior to the Norman Conquest; it is also the 'Marchalan' of the Welsh physicians of the thirteenth century, and was generally known during the Middle Ages.

It was formally cultivated in all private herb-gardens, as a culinary and medicinal plant, and it is still to be found in old cottage gardens. Not only was its root much employed as a medicine, but it was also candied and eaten as a sweetmeat. Dr. Fernie tells us, in Herbal Simples:

'Some fifty years ago, the candy was sold commonly in London as flat, round cakes being composed largely of sugar and coloured with cochineal. A piece was eaten each night and morning for asthmatical complaints, whilst it was customary when travelling by a river, to suck a bit of the root against poisonous exalations and bad air. The candy may still be had from our confectioners, but now containing no more of the plant Elecampane than there is of barley in Barley Sugar."

In Denmark, Elecampane is sometimes called Elf-Doc. Here one sometimes comes across the name Elf-Dock locally, also Elfwort.

Cultivation

Although Elecampane is no longer grown to any extent in England, it is still cultivated for medicinal use on the Continent, mainly in Holland, Switzerland and Germany, most largely near the German town of Colleda, not far from Leipzig.

It grows well in moist, shady positions, in ordinary garden soil, though it flourishes best in a good, loamy soil, the ground being damp, but fairly well-drained.

It is easily cultivated. Seeds may be sown, either when ripe, in cold frames, or in spring in the open. It is best propagated, however, by off-sets, taken in the autumn from the old root, with a bud or eye to each. These will take root very readily, and should be planted in rows about a foot asunder, and 9 or 10 inches distant in the rows. In the following spring, the ground should be kept clean from weeds, and if slightly dug in autumn, it will greatly promote the growth of the roots, which will be fit for use after two years' growth.

By cutting the root into pieces about 2 inches long, covering with rich, light, sandy soil and keeping in gentle heat during the winter, a good stock of plants can also be obtained.

Part Used Medicinally

The drug, Elecampane (Radix Inulae), consists of both rhizome or rootstock and roots. It is official in most pharmacopoeias.

For pharmaceutical use, the root is taken from plants two to three years old; when more advanced it becomes too woody. As a rule, it is dug in autumn.

Elecampane root has at first a somewhat glutinous taste, but by chewing, it becomes subsequently aromatic, and slightly bitter and pungent; it has an agreeably aromatic somewhat camphoraceous orris-like odor.

The distinguishing characteristics of Elecampane root to be noted by a student are:

Its horny, not starchy nature.

The presence of oil-glands.

The absence of well-marked radiate structure in the wood.

Most roots of similar appearance to Elecampane root, such as Belladonna, Dandelion and Marsh Mallow, are devoid of oil-glands. Belladonna, moreover, is distinguished from it by its starchy fracture, Dandelion by its thick, ringed bark, and Marsh Mallow by its radiate structure and fibrous, easily separated bark. Pellitory root, which has oil-glands, is distinguished by its yellow, radiate wood, distinctive odor and taste.

Constituents

The substance most abundantly contained in Elecampane root is Inulin, discovered by Valentine Rose, of Berlin in 1804, who named it Alantin (the German name of the plant is Alantwurzel; French, Aunée), but the title, Inulin proposed by Thompson, has been generally adopted. It has the same composition as starch, but stands to a certain extent in opposition to that substance, which it replaces in the rootsystem of Compositae. In living plants, Inulin is dissolved in the watery juice, and on drying, is deposited within the cells in amorphous masses, which in polarized light are inactive. It resembles starch in appearance, but differs from it in giving a yellow instead of a blue color with iodine, in being soluble in boiling water without forming a paste, and in being deposited unchanged from the hot aqueous solution when it cools. With nitric acid, Inula affords no explosive compound as starch does. By prolonged heat or the action of dilute acids, it is changed first to inulin then to levulin, and finally to levulose. It is only slightly changed to sugar by ferments.

Sachs showed in 1864 that by immersing the roots of Elecampane or Dahlia variabilis in alcohol and glycerine, Inulin may be precipitated in globular aggregations of needleshaped crystalline form.

Elecampane is the richest source of inulin.

The amount of Inulin varies according to the season, but is more abundant in the autumn. Dragendorff, who in 1870 made it the subject of a very exhaustive treatise, obtained from the root in October not less than 44 per cent, but in spring only 19 per cent, its place being taken by levulin, mucilage, sugar and several glucosides. Inulin is widely distributed in the perennial roots of Compositae, and has been met with in the natural orders Campanulacae, Goodeniaceae, Lobeliaceae, Stylidiaceae, and in the root of the White Ipecacuanha of Brazil, belonging to the order Violaceae.

Inulin is closely associated in Elecampane with Inulenin, obtainable in microscopical needles, slightly soluble in cold water and weak alcohol, and pseudo-inulin, which occurs in irregular granules, very soluble in hot water and weak, hot alcohol, but insoluble in cold alcohol.

It was observed by Le Febre as early as 1660 that when the root of Elecampane is subjected to distillation with water, a crystallizable substance collects in the head of the receiver, and similar crystals may be observed after carefully heating a thin slice of the root, and are often found as a natural efflorescence on the surface of roots that have been long kept. This was considered as a distinct body called Helenin, or Elecampane camphor, but the researches of Kallen in 1874 showed that it was resolvable into two crystallizable substances, which he named Helenin, a body without taste or color, and Alantcamphor, with a peppermint odor and taste. As a result of further research, it is considered that the crystalline mass yielded by Elecampane root on distillation with water in the proportion of 1 to 2 per cent, and associated with about 1 per cent volatile oil, consists of Alantolactone, iso-alantolactone and Alantolic acid, all of which are crystalline, nearly colorless, and have but slight odor and taste. The oily portion, Alantol, found in the distillate, a colorless liquid, has a peppermint-like odor.

Medicinal Action and Uses

Diuretic, tonic, diaphoretic, expectorant, alterative, antiseptic, astringent and gently stimulant. It was employed by the ancients in certain diseases of women, also in phthisis, in dropsy and in skin affections. Its name 'Scabwort' arose from the fact that a decoction of it is said to cure sheep affected with the scab, and the name 'Horse-heal' was given it from its reputed virtues in curing the cutaneous diseases of horses.

In herbal medicine it is chiefly used for coughs, consumption and other pulmonary complaints, being a favorite domestic remedy for bronchitis. It has been employed for many years with good results in chest affections, for which it is a valuable medicine as it is in all chronic diseases of the lungs asthma and bronchitis. It gives relief to the respiratory difficulties and assists expectoration. Its principal employment as a separate remedy is in acute catarrhal affections, and in dyspepsia attended with relaxation and debility, given in small, warm and frequently repeated doses. It is, however, seldom given alone, but most frequently preferred in combination with other medicines of a similar nature. It is best given in the form of decoction, the dose being a small teaspoonful, three times a day.

The root used not only to be candied and eaten as a sweetmeat, but lozenges were made of it. It has been employed in whooping-cough. It is sometimes employed in the form of a confection for piles, 1 OZ. of powdered root being mixed with 2 OZ. of honey.

In the United States, it has also been highly recommended, both for external use and internal administration in diseases of the skin, an old use of the root that has maintained its reputation for efficacy.

Externally applied, it is somewhat rubefacient, and has been employed as an embrocation in the treatment of sciatica, facial and other neuralgia.

Of late years, modern scientific research has proved that the claims of Elecampane to be a valuable remedy in pulmonary diseases has a solid basis. One authority, Korab, showed in 1885 that the active, bitter principle, Helenin, is such a powerful antiseptic and bactericide, that a few drops of a solution of 1 part in 10,000 immediately kills the ordinary bacterial organisms, being peculiarly destructive to the Tubercle bacillus. He gave it successfully in tubercular and catarrhal diarrhoeas, and praised it also as an antiseptic in surgery. In Spain it has been made use of as a surgical dressing. Obiol, in 1886, stated it to be an efficient local remedy in the treatment of diphtheria, the false membrane being painted with a solution of Helenin in Oil of Almond.

Medicinal Preparations

Powdered root 1/2 to 1 drachm. Fluid extract, 1/2 to 1 drachm. Inulin, 1 to 3 grains.

Gerard tells us: 'It is good for shortnesse of breathe and an old cough, and for such as cannot breathe unless they hold their neckes upright." And further:

'The root of Elecampane is with good success mixed with counterpoisons, it is a remedy against the biting of serpents, it resisteth poison. It is good for them that are bursten and troubled with cramps and convulsions."

And Culpepper says:

'The fresh roots of Elecampane preserved with sugar or made into a conserve, or a syrup, are very effectual to warm a cold windy stomach and stitches in the side, caused by spleen and to relieve cough, shortness of breath and wheezing in the lungs. The dried root made into powder and mixed with sugar, and taken, serveth the same purpose.... It cures putrid and pestilential fevers and even the plague. The roots and herbes beaten and put into new ale or beer and daily drunk, cleareth, strengtheneth and quickeneth the sight of the eyes. The decoction of the roots in wine or the juice taken therein, destroys worms in the stomach, and gargled in the mouth or the root chewed, fasteneth loose teeth and keeps them from putrefaction, and being drunk is good for spitting of blood, and it removes cramps or convulsions, gout, sciatica, pains in the joints, applied outwardly or inwardly, and is also good for those that are ruptured, or have any inward bruise. The root boiled well in vinegar, beaten afterwards and made into an ointment with hog's suet or oil of trotters is a most excellent remedy for scabs or itch in young or old the places also bathed and washed with the decoction doth the same; it heals putrid sores or cankers. In the roots of this herb lieth the chief effect for the remedies aforesaid. The distilled water of the leaves and roots together is very good to cleanse the skin of the face or other parts from any morphew, spots or blemishes and make it clear."

In Switzerland (Neufchâtel) Elecampane root is one of the substances used in the preparation of Absinthe, and it was also used for the same purpose in France. It furnishes the Vin d'Aulnée of the French.

A blue dye has been extracted from the root, bruised and macerated and mingled with ashes and whortleberries.

'The wine wherein the root of Elicampane hath steept," says Markham (Countrie Farme 1616), 'is singularly good against the colicke." A cordial was made from the plant by infusing Elecampane roots with sugar and currants in white port.

ELM, COMMON

Botanical: Ulmus campestris (LINN.)
Family: N.O. Urticaceae
Synonyms: Ulmi cortex. Broad-leaved Elm. Ulmus suberosa (var. Orme).
Part Used: The dried inner bark.
Habitat: Britain (not indigenous), Europe, Asia, North Africa.

Description

The Elms belong to the natural order Ulmaceae and to the genus Ulmus, which contains sixteen species, widely distributed throughout the north temperate zone, extending southwards as far as Mexico in the New World and the Sikkim Himalayas in the Old World.

The Common Elm (U. campestris, Linn.) is a doubtful native of England, found throughout the greater part of Europe, in North Africa, Asia Minor and eastwards to Japan.

It grows in woods and hedgerows, especially in the southern part of Britain and on almost all soils, thriving even in the smoky atmosphere of a city, but on a rich loam, in open, low-lying situations, attaining a height of 60 to 100 feet, even rising to 130 and 150 feet. In the first ten years of its growth the tree grows to 25 or 30 feet.

The branches are numerous and spreading, the bark rugged, the leaves alternate, ovate rough, doubly toothed and unequal at the base. The flowers are small and numerous appearing in March and April before the leaves, in purplish-brown tufts. If one of these tufts be examined, it will be found to be a short axis with a number of leaves, beginning two-ranked at the base, and going over to five-ranked above. There are no flowers in the axils of the lowest ten or twelve, in the axils of the upper leaves are flowers arranged in small cymes (in some species), but in U. campestris reduced to the one central flower. Each flower has a four-toothed, bell-shaped calyx surrounding four stamens and a onecelled ovary bearing two spreading hairy styles.

The seed-vessels are green, membraneous, one-seeded and deeply cleft, but the tree seldom perfects its seed in England, being propagated by root-suckers from old trees, or by layers from stools.

In age and size, the Elm closely approaches the Oak, but is more varied, a large number of named varieties being grown.

Uses

All parts of the tree, including sapwood, are used in carpentry. The wood is close-grained, free from knots, hard and tough, and not subject to splitting, but it does not take a high polish. It does not crack when once seasoned and is remarkably durable under water, being specially adapted for any purpose which requires exposure to wet. To prevent shrinking and warping in drying, it may be preserved in water or mud, but is best worked up soon after felling. In drying, the wood loses over 60 per cent of its weight.

Elm wood is used for keels and bilge planks, the blocks and dead eyes of rigging and ship's pumps, for coffins, wheels, furniture, turned articles and general carpenter's work. Elm boards are largely used for lining the interior of carts, wagons and wheelbarrows on account of the extreme toughness of the wood, and it has been much employed in the past for making sheds, most of the existing farm buildings being covered with elm. Previous to the common employment of cast-iron, Elm was very much in use for waterpipes.

The inner bark is very tough and is made into mats and ropes. The leaves and young shoots have been found a suitable food for live stock.

Elm Tree Disease

Investigations are at present being carried on as to the cause of a mysterious disease, known as the Dutch Elm disease, which is killing trees on many parts of the Continent. It first appeared in North Brabant in 1919, and spread until it is now all over Holland. By 1921, the disease was rampant in Belgium and in the same year it appeared in France, while in 1924 and 1925 it spread widely in Germany and it is also working havoc in Spain.

The first sign of the disease in trees up to thirty years old is a mass of dry twigs and leaves in the crown while the other parts are still green. Within a week, all the leaves of the tree may fall, or the leaves on one side of the tree may remain fresh, while on the other side they fall off. No cure has yet been discovered, and the tree eventually dies. Most investigators consider that the disease is caused by a fungus (Graphium ulmus), the infection being carried by spores blown from one tree to another.

To prevent the importation into Britain of this mysterious disease, the Ministry of Agriculture, early in 1927, prohibited live elms from the European mainland from being landed in England and Wales.

Constituents

Analyses of Elm wood show 47.8 per cent of lime, 21.9 of potash and 13.7 of soda.

A peculiar vegetable principle, called Ulmin or Ulmic Acid, was first discovered in the gummy substance which spontaneously exudes in summer from the bark of the Common Elm, becoming by the action of the air a dark-brown, almost black substance, without smell or taste, insoluble in cold sparingly soluble in boiling water, which it colors yellowish-brown, soluble in alcohol and readily dissolved by alkaline solutions.

The inner bark is very mucilaginous, and contains a little tannic acid which gives it a somewhat bitter and slightly astringent taste, it also contains a great deal of starch.

Medicinal Action and Uses

Tonic, demulcent, astringent and diuretic. Wasformerly employed for the preparation of an antiscorbutic decoction recommended in cutaneous diseases of a leprous character, such as ringworm. It was applied both externally and internally. Under the title of Ulmus the dried inner bark was official in the British Pharmacopoeia of 1864 and 1867 directions for the preparation of Decoc. Ulmi being as follows: Elm Bark 1 part, water 8 parts; boil for 10 minutes, strain, make up to 8 parts.

A homeopathic tincture is made of the inner bark, and used as an astringent.

Fluid extract, dose 2 to 4 oz. three or four times daily.

A medicinal tea was also formerly made from the flowers.

In Persia, Italy and the south of France, galls, sometimes the size of a fist, are frequently produced on the leaves. They contain a clear water called eau d'orme, which is sweet and viscid, and has been recommended to wash wounds, contusions and sore eyes. Culpepper tells us:

'the water that is found in the bladders on the leaves of the elm-tree is very effectual to cleanse the skin and make it fair."

Towards autumn, these galls dry, the insects in them die and there is found a residue in the form of a yellow or blackish balsam, called beaume d'ormeau, which has been recommended for diseases of the chest.

Other Species

A variety of the Common Elm, the CORK-BARKED ELM (U. campestris, var. suberosa), is distinguished chiefly by its thick, deeplyfissured bark, the corky excrescences along the branchlets causing them to appear much thicker than they really are. A North American species with this feature most pronounced is U. alata, which well deserves its name of the WINGED ELM.

The SCOTCH ELM, or WYCH ELM (U. montana, With. - formerly called U. glabra, Huds.), is indigenous to Britain and is the common Elm of the northern part of the island.

It is a beautiful tree, both in form and foliage, usually attaining a height of about 50 feet, though tall-growing specimens have been known to attain 120 feet.

It has drooping branches and a smoother thinner bark than U. campestris, its leaves equally rough on the upper surface, though rather downy beneath, are longer, wider and more tapering and more deeply notched. A further distinction is that whereas the seeds of the Common Elm are placed near the end of their oblong envelope, those of the Wych Elm are set in the centre of their envelope. Moreover, the Common Elm has a profuse undergrowth of young shoots round the base of the trunk and few are to be seen round that of the Wych Elm. This is probably the 'French Elm' of Evelyn. An upright form of it is called the 'Cornish Elm."

The wood, though more porous than that of the Common Elm, is tough and hardy when properly seasoned, and being very flexible when steamed, is well adapted for boat-building, though for the purposes of the wheelwright and millwright is inferior to that of the Common Elm. Branches of Wych Elm were formerly used for making bows and when forked were employed as divining rods. The bark of the young limbs is very tough and flexible, and is often stripped off in long ribands and used in Wales for securing thatch and other similar purposes.

On the leaves of U. chenensis, a number of galls are produced, which are used by the Chinese for tanning leather and dyeing.

ELM, SLIPPERY

Botanical: Ulmus fulva (MICH.)
Family: N.O. Urticaceae
Synonyms: Red Elm. Moose Elm. Indian Elm.
Part Used: The inner bark.
Habitat: The United States, Canada.

Description

The Slippery Elm is a small tree abundant in various parts of North America.

The branches are very rough, the leaves long, unequally toothed, rough with hairs on both sides, the leaf-buds covered with a dense yellow Wool. The flowers are stalkless.

The inner bark has important medicinal value and is an official drug of the United States Pharmacopoeia.

The bark, which is the only part used, is collected in spring from the bole and larger branches and dried. Large quantities are collected, especially in the lower part of the state of Michigan. As the wood has no commercial value, the tree is fully stripped and consequently dies.

The bark as it appears in commerce for use in medicine consists only of the inner bark or bast and is sold in flat pieces 2 to 3 feet long and several inches wide, but only about 1/8 to 1/16 of an inch in thickness. It is very tough and flexible, of a fine fibrous texture, finely striated longitudinally on both surfaces, the outer surface reddish-yellow, with patches of reddish brown, which are part of the outer bark adhering to the inner bast. It has an odor like Fenugreek and a very mucilaginous, insipid taste. The strips can be bent double without breaking: if broken, the rough fracture is mealy, strongly but finely fibrous. The clean transverse section shows numerous medullary rays and altemate bands of bast parenchyma, thus giving it a chequered appearance. A section moistened and left for a few minutes, and again examined, shows large swollen mucilage cells.

The powdered bark is sold in two forms: a coarse powder for use as poultices and a fine powder for making a mucilaginous drink. The disintegrated bark forms, when moistened, a flexible and spongy tissue, which is easily moulded into pessaries, teats, and suppositories.

It is recommended that ten-year-old bark should be used.

The powder should be greyish or fawncoloured. If dark or reddish, good results will not be obtained. The powdered bark is said to be often adulterated with damaged flour and other starchy substances.

Constituents

The principal constituent of the bark is the mucilage contained in large cells in the bast. This mucilage is very similar to that found in linseed. It is precipitated by solutions of acetate and subacetate of lead, although not by alcohol The mucilage does not dissolve, but only swells in water and is so abundant that 10 grains of the powdered bark will make a thick jelly with an ounce of water.

Microscopic examination of the tissue of the bark shows round starch grains and very characteristic twin crystals of Calcium oxalate.

Medicinal Action and Uses

Demulcent, emollient, expectorant, diuretic, nutritive. The bark of this American Elm, though not in this country as in the United States an official drug, is considered one of the most valuable remedies in herbal practice, the abundant mucilage it contains having wonderfully strengthening and healing qualities.

It not only has a most soothing and healing action on all the parts it comes in contact with, but in addition possesses as much nutrition as is contained in oatmeal, and when made into gruel forms a wholesome and sustaining food for infants and invalids. It forms the basis of many patent foods.

Slippery Elm Food is generally made by mixing a teaspoonful of the powder into a thin and perfectly smooth paste with cold water and then pouring on a pint of boiling water, steadily stirring meanwhile. It can, if desired, be flavoured with cinnamon, nutmeg or lemon rind.

This makes an excellent drink in cases of irritation of the mucous membrane of the stomach and intestines, and taken at night will induce sleep.

Another mode of preparation is to beat up an egg with a teaspoonful of the powdered bark, pouring boiling milk over it and sweetening it.

Taken unsweetened, three times a day, Elm Food gives excellent results in gastritis, gastric catarrh, mucous colitis and enteritis, being tolerated by the stomach when all other foods fail, and is of great value in bronchitis, bleeding from the lungs and consumption (being most healing to the lungs), soothing a cough and building up and preventing wasting.

A Slippery Elm compound excellent for coughs is made as follows: Cut obliquely one or more ounces of bark into pieces about the thickness of a match; add a pinch of Cayenne flavor with a slice of lemon and sweeten, infusing the whole in a pint of boiling water and letting it stand for 25 minutes. Take this frequently in small doses: for a consumptive patient, about a pint a day is recommended. It is considered one of the best remedies that can be given as it combines both demulcent and stimulating properties. Being mucilaginous, it rolls up the mucous material so troublesome to the patient and passes it down through the intestines.

In typhoid fever, the Slippery Elm drink, prepared as for coughs, is recommended, serving a threefold purpose, to cleanse, heal and strengthen, the patient being allowed to drink as much as desired until thirst has abated, and other remedies can be used. If the patient is not thirsty, a dose of 2 large tablespoonfuls every hour for an adult has been prescribed.

The bark is an ingredient in various lung medicines. A valuable remedy for Bronchitis and all diseases of the throat and lungs is compounded as follows: 1 teaspoonful Flax seed, 1 OZ. Slippery Elm bark, 1 OZ. Thoroughwort, 1 stick Liquorice, 1 quart water. Simmer slowly for 20 minutes. Strain and add 1 pint of the best vinegar and 1/2 pint of sugar. When cold, bottle. Dose: 1 tablespoonful two or three times a day.

In Pleurisy, the following is also recommended: Take 2 oz. each of Pleurisy root, Marsh Mallow root, Liquorice root and Slippery Elm bark. Boil in 3 pints of water down to 3 gills. Dose: 1/2 teaspoonful every half-hour, to be taken warm.

As a heart remedy, a pint of Slippery Elm drink has been prescribed alternately with Bugleweed compound.

Slippery Elm bark possesses also great influence upon diseases of the female organs.

It is particularly valuable both medicinally and as an injection in dysentery and other diseases of the bowels, cystitis and irritation of the urinary tract. The injection for inflammation of the bowels is made from an infusion of 1 OZ. of the powder to 1 pint of boiling water, strained and used lukewarm. Other remedies should be given at the same time.

An injection for diarrhea may also be made as follows: 1 drachm powdered Slippery Elm bark, 3 drachms powdered Bayberry, 1 drachm powdered Scullcap.

Pour on 1/2 pint of boiling water, infuse for half an hour, strain, add a teaspoonful of tincture of myrrh and use lukewarm.

As an enema for constipation, 2 drachms of Slippery Elm bark are mixed well with 1 OZ. of sugar, then 1/2 pint of warm milk and water and an ounce of Olive Oil are gently stirred in.

Injection for worms (Ascarides): 1/2 drachm Aloes powder, 1 drachm common salt, 1/2 drachm Slippery Elm powder (fine). When well mixed, add 1/2 pint warm water and sweeten with molasses, stirring well.

Slippery Elm mucilage is also prescribed to be mixed with Oil of Male Fern (2 oz. of the mucilage to 1 drachm of the oil) as a remedy for the expulsion of tapeworm

The Red Indians have long used this viscous inner bark to prepare a healing salve, and in herbal medicine a Slippery Elm bark powder is considered one of the best possible poultices for wounds, boils, ulcers, burns and all inflamed surfaces, soothing, healing and reducing pain and inflammation.

It is made as follows: Mix the powder with hot water to form the required consistency, spread smoothly upon soft cotton cloth and apply over the parts affected. It is unfailing in cases of suppurations, abscesses, wounds of all kinds, congestion, eruptions, swollen glands, etc. In simple inflammation, it may be applied directly over the part affected; to abscesses and old wounds, it should be placed between cloths. If applied to parts of the body where there is hair, the face of the poultice should be smeared with olive oil before applying.

In old gangrenous wounds, an excellent antiseptic poultice is prepared by mixing with warm water or an infusion of Wormwood, equal parts of Slippery Elm powder and very fine charcoal and applying immediately over the part.

A very valuable poultice in cases where it is desirable to hasten suppuration or arrest the tendency to gangrene is made by mixing the Slippery Elm powder with brewer's yeast and new milk.

Compound Bran poultice is made by mixing with hot vinegar equal quantities of wheaten Bran with Slippery Elm powder. This is an excellent poultice for severe rheumatic and gouty affections, particularly of the joints, synovitis etc.

Herbal poultices, generally made from the bruised, fresh leaves of special herbs, are frequently mixed with Slippery Elm and boiling water sufficient to give the mass consistency.

Marshmallow Ointment, one of the principal ointments used in herbal medicine, has a considerable proportion of Slippery Elm bark in its composition. It is made as follows: 3 oz. Marshmallow leaves, 2 OZ. Slippery Elm bark powder, 3 oz. Beeswax, 16 OZ. Lard. Boil the Marshmallow and Slippery Elm bark in 3 pints of water for 15 minutes. Express, strain and reduce the liquor to half a pint. Melt together the lard and wax by gentle heat, then add the extract while still warm, shake constantly till all are thoroughly incorporated and store in a cool place.

The bark of Slippery Elm is stated to preserve fatty substances from becoming rancid.

It has been asserted that a pinch of the Slippery Elm powder put into a hollow tooth stops the ache and greatly delays decay, if used as soon as there is any sign of decay.

Lozenges or troches containing 3 grains of Elm flavoured with methyl salicylate are used as a demulcent.

Preparations

Mucilage, U.S.P., made by digesting 6 grams of bruised Slippery Elm in 100 c.c. and heated in a closed vessel in a water-bath for 1 hour and then strained.

Other Species

Fremontia Californica, or Californian Slippery Elm, has bark with similar properties, and is used in the same way, but is not botanically related.

EMBELIA

Botanical: Embelia Ribes and robusta (BURM.)
Family: N.O. Myrsinaceae
Synonyms: Viranga. Birang-i-kabuli.
Part Used: Dried fruits.
Habitat: India, Indian Archipelago, Tropical Asia, Southern China, East Africa.

Description

A straggling shrub, almost a climber. The plant possesses petiolate leaves and has small, whity-pink flowers in racemes at ends of the branches. The berries (the drug) are minute, round, spherical fruits (not unlike peppercorns) and vary in color from red to black - those of E. Ribes have ovate, lanceolate smooth leaves and warty fruits, and are often sold to traders to adulterate pepper, which they so much resemble as to render it almost impossible to distinguish them by sight, or by any other means, as they possess a considerable degree of the spice flavor. The fruits of E. robusta, however, are longitudinally finely striated. Both fruit have often a short stalk and calyx fivepartite, removing this, a small hole is found in the fruit. The reddish seed, enclosed in a brittle pericarp, is covered by a thin membrane; when this is taken off, the seed is seen covered with light spots which disappear after immersion in water. The seed is horny, depressed at the base and has a ruminated endosperm. Taste, aromatic and astringent, with a slight pungency, owing to a resinous substance present in them.

Constituents

Embelic acid, found in golden-yellow lamellar crystals (this acid is soluble in chloroform, alcohol and benzene, but not in water) and a quinone, Embelia.

Medicinal Action and Uses

Anthelmintic, specially used to expel tapeworm, which are passed dead. In India and the Eastern Colonies the drug is given in the early morning, fasting, mixed with milk, and followed by a purgative. The dose is 1 to 4 drachms. The seeds are also made into an infusion, or ground to powder and taken in water or syrup, and being almost tasteless are not an unpleasant remedy.

Ammonium embelate is an effective taenicide for children: dose, 3 grains; adult dose, 6 or more grains.

The berries of E. robusta are considered cathartic.

Other Species

E. Basaal, an Indian variety, with larger elliptical leaves, more or less downy, is useful in various ways. The young leaves, in combination with ginger, are used as a gargle for sore throats, the dried bark of the root as a remedy for toothache, and the ground berries, mixed with butter or lard, made into an ointment and laid on the forehead for pleuritis.

EPHEDRA

Botanical: Ephedra vulgaris (RICH.)
Family: N.O. Gnetaceae
Synonyms: Ephedrine. Epitonin. Ma Huang.
Habitat: West Central China, Southern Siberia, Japan.

Description

It is found on sandy seashores and in temperate climates of both hemispheres. The plant has stamens and pistils on separate flowers--staminate flowers in catkins and a membraneous perianth, pistillate flowers terminal on axillary stalks, within a two-leaved involucre. Fruit has two carpels with a single seed in each and is a succulent cone, branches slender and erect, small leaves, scale-like, articulated and joined at the base into a sheath.

Constituents

Ephedrine is salt of an alkaloid and is in shining white crystals very soluble in water.

Medicinal Action and Uses

A sympathetic nerve stimulant resembling adrenaline, its effect on the unstriped muscular fibres is remarkable. It acts promptly in relieving swellings of the mucous membrane. It has valuable antispasmodic properties, acts on the air passages and is of benefit in asthma and hay fever; it is also employed for rheumatism; a 5 to 10 per cent solution has mydriatic properties, prophylactically used for low blood pressure in influenza, pneumonia, etc. Used in tablet form for oral or hypodermic administration and in ampuls for hypodermic, intramuscular and intravenous use. It can advantageously be used in solution with liquid paraffin, either alone or in conjunction with methol camphor and oil of thyme. Dose, 1/2 to 1 grain.

EUCALYPTUS

Botanical: Eucalyptus globulus (LABILLE.)
Family: N.O. Myrtaceae
Synonyms: Blue Gum Tree. Stringy Bark Tree.
Part Used: The oil of the leaves.

Habitat

Australia. Now North and South Africa, India, and Southern Europe.

The tree is indigenous with a few exceptions to Australia and Tasmania. The genus contains about 300 species and is one of the most characteristic genera of the Australian flora.

Description

The leaves are leathery in texture, hang obliquely or vertically, and are studded with glands containing a fragrant volatile oil. The flowers in bud are covered with a cup-like membrane (whence the name of the genus, derived from the Greek eucalyptos well-covered), which is thrown off as a lid when the flower expands. The fruit is surrounded by a woody, cupshaped receptacle and contains numerous minute seeds.

Eucalyptus trees are quick growers and many species reach a great height. Eucalyptus amygdalin (Labille) is the tallest known tree, specimens attaining as much as 480 feet, exceeding in height even the Californian Big Tree (Sequoia gigantea). Many species yield valuable timber, others oils, kino, etc.

There are a great number of species of Eucalyptus trees yielding essential oils, the foliage of some being more odorous than that of others, and the oils from the various species differing widely in character. It necessarily follows that the term Eucalyptus oil is meaningless from a scientific point of view unless the species from which it is derived is stated.

The Eucalyptus industry is becoming of economic importance to Australia, especially in New South Wales and Victoria. Many of the old species which give the oil of commerce have given way to other species which have been found to gave larger yields or better oils. About twenty-five species are at the present time being utilized for their oil.

The oils may be roughly divided into three classes of commercial importance: (1) the medicinal oils, which contain substantial amounts of eucalyptol (also known as cineol); (2) the industrial oils, containing terpenes, which are used for flotation purposes in mining operations; (3) the aromatic oils, such as E. citriodora, which are characterized by their aroma.

The British Pharmacopoeia describes Eucalyptus Oil as the oil distilled from the fresh leaves of E. globulus and other species.

E. globulus, the best-known variety (its name bestowed, it is said, by the French botanist De Labillardière, on account of the resemblance of its waxy fruit to a kind of button at that time worn in France), is the Blue Gum Tree of Victoria and Tasmania, where it attains a height of 375 feet, ranking as one of the largest trees in the world. It is also called the Fever Tree, being largely cultivated in unhealthy, low-lying or swampy districts for its antiseptic qualities.

The first leaves are broad, without stalks, of a shining whitish-green and are opposite and horizontal, but after four or five years these are succeeded by others of a more ensiform or sword-shaped form, 6 to 12 inches long, bluish-green in hue, which are alternate and vertical, i.e. with the edges turned towards the sky and earth, an arrangement more suited to the climate and productive of peculiar effects of light and shade. The flowers are single or in clusters, almost stalkless.

The Eucalyptus, especially E. globulus, has been successfully introduced into the south of Europe, Algeria, Egypt, Tahiti, South Africa and India, and has been extensively planted in California and also, with the object of lessening liability to droughts, along the line of the Central Pacific Railway.

It thrives in any situation, having a mean annual temperature not below 60 degrees F., but will not endure a temperature of less than 27 degrees F., and although many species of Eucalyptus will flourish out-of-doors in the south of England, they are generally grown, in this country, in pots as greenhouse plants.

It was Baron Ferdinand von Müller, the German botanist and explorer (from 1857 to 1873 Director of the Botanical Gardens in Melbourne), who made the qualities of this Eucalyptus known all over the world, and so led to its introduction into Europe, North and South Africa, California and the non-tropical districts of South America. He was the first to suggest that the perfume of the leaves resembling that of Cajaput oil, might be of use as a disinfectant in fever districts, a suggestion which has been justified by the results of the careful examination to which the Eucalyptus has been subjected since its employment in medicine. Some seeds, having been sent to France in 1857, were planted in Algiers and thrived exceedingly well. Trottoir, the botanical superintendent, found that the value of the fragrant antiseptic exhalations of the leaves in fever or marshy districts was far exceeded by the amazingly powerful drying action of the roots on the soil. Five years after planting the Eucalyptus, one of the most marshy and unhealthy districts of Algiers was converted into one of the healthiest and driest. As a result, the rapidly growing Eucalyptus trees are now largely cultivated in many temperate regions with the view of preventing malarial fevers. A noteworthy instance of this is the monastery of St. Paolo à la tre Fontana, situated in one of the most fever-stricken districts of the Roman Campagna. Since about 1870, when the tree was planted in its cloisters, it has become habitable throughout the year. To the remarkable drainage afforded by its roots is also ascribed the gradual disappearance of mosquitoes in the neighborhood of plantations of this tree, as at Lake Fezara in Algeria.

In Sicily, also, it is being extensively planted to combat malaria, on account of its property of absorbing large quantities of water from the soil. Recent investigations have shown that Sicilian Eucalyptus oil obtained from leaves during the flowering period can compete favourably with the Australian oil in regard to its industrial and therapeutic applications. Oil has also been distilled in Spain from the leaves of E. globulus, grown there.

In India, considerable plantations of E. globulus were made in 1863 in the Nilgiris at Ootacamund, but though a certain amount of oil is distilled there locally, under simple conditions, little attempt has hitherto been made to develop the industry on a commercial scale, Australia remaining the source of supply.

A great increase in Euealyptus cultivation has recently taken place in Brazil as a result of a decree published in 1919 awarding premiums and free grants of land to planters of Eucalyptus and other trees of recognized value for essence cultivation.

Constituents

The essential Oil of Eucalyptus used in medicine is obtained by aqueous distillation of the fresh leaves. It is a colorless or straw-coloured fluid when properly prepared, with a characteristic odor and taste, soluble in its own weight of alcohol. The most important constituent is Eucalyptol, present in E. globulus up to 70 per cent of its volume. It consists chiefly of a terpene and a cymene. Eucalyptus Oil contains also, after exposure to the air, a crystallizable resin, derived from Eucalyptol.

The British Pharmacopoeia requires Eucalyptus Oil to contain not less than 55 per cent, by volume, of Eucalyptol, to have a specific gravity 0.910 to 0.930 and optical rotation -10 degrees to 10 degrees. The official method for the determination of the Eucalptol depends on the conversion of this body into a crystalline phosphate, but numerous other methods have been suggested (see Parry, Essential Oils,

A small amount of medicinal oil is still distilled from E. globulus, but Its odor is less agreeable than those of many others. Today, E. polybractea (Silver Malee Scrub which is cultivated and the oil distilled near Bendigo in Victoria), containing 85 per cent of Eucalyptol, and E. Smithii (Gully Ash) are favorites for distillation. Among others frequently employed, E. Australiana yields a valuable medicinal oil and also E. Bakeri, a large shrub or pendulous willow-like tree, about 30 to 50 feet high, with very narrow leaves, found from northern New South Wales to central Queensland, known locally as the 'Malee Box." The oil from this species is of a bright reddish-yellow and contains 70 to 77 per cent of Eucalyptol and other aromatic substances identical with those found in E. polybractea.

The oil used for flotation purposes in the extraction of ores is known as that of E. amygdalina, and is probably derived from this tree as well as from E. dives. It is an oil containing little Eucalyptol and having a specific gravity from 0.866 to 0.885, and an optical rotation -59 to -75 degrees, its chief constituent is phellandrene, which forms a crystalline nitrate and is very irritating when inhaled. There is a considerable demand in New South Wales for the cheap phellandrene Eucalyptus oils for use in the mining industry in the separation of metallic sulphides from ores.

Of the perfume-bearing oils, that of E. citriodora, the CITRON-SCENTED GUM, whose leaves emit a delightful lemon scent, contains up to 98 per cent of citronellol and is much used in perfumery, fetching four times as much as the medicinal oils. E. Macarthurii ('Paddy River Box') contains up to 75 per cent of geranyl acetate, and as a source of geraniol this tree would probably repay cultivation: it is now receiving special attention in Australia, as it is a very rapid grower. E. odorata yields also an odorous oil used by soapmakers in Australia. E. Staigeriana, the Lemon-scented Iron Bark, has also a very pleasing scent, and the fragrance of the leaves of E. Sturtiana is similar to that of ripe apples.

There are a number of Eucalypts which contain a ketone known as piperitone, such as E. piperita. This body can be used in the synthesis of menthol, but it remains to be seen whether the process can be made a commercial success. E. dives (Peppermint Gum) and E. radiata (White Top Peppermint) yield oils with a strong peppermint flavor.

Details of an enormous number of the oils of Eucalyptus can be found in A Research on the Eucalypts, by Baker and Smith.

Medicinal Action and Uses

Stimulant, antiseptic, aromatic.

The medicinal Eucalyptus Oil is probably the most powerful antiseptic of its class, especially when it is old, as ozone is formed in it on exposure to the air. It has decided disinfectant action, destroying the lower forms of life. Internally, it has the typical actions of a volatile oil in a marked degree.

Eucalyptus Oil is used as a stimulant and antiseptic gargle. Locally applied, it impairs sensibility. It increases cardiac action.

Its antiseptic properties confer some antimalarial action, though it cannot take the place of Cinchona.

An emulsion made by shaking up equal parts of the oil and powdered gum-arabic with water has been used as a urethral injection, and has also been given internally in drachm doses in pulmonary tuberculosis and other microbic diseases of the lungs and bronchitis.

In croup and spasmodic throat troubles, the oil may be freely applied externally.

The oil is an ingredient of 'catheder oil," used for sterilizing and lubricating urethral catheters.

In large doses, it acts as an irritant to the kidneys, by which it is largely excreted, and as a marked nervous depressant ultimately arresting respiration by its action on the medullary centre.

For some years Eucalyptus-chloroform was employed as one of the remedies in the tropics for hookworm, but it has now been almost universally abandoned as an inefficient anthelmintic, Chenopodium Oil having become the recognized remedy.

In veterinary practice, Eucalyptus Oil is administered to horses in influenza, to dogs in distemper, to all animals in septicaemia. It is also used for parasitic skin affections.

Preparations

The dose of the oil is 1/2 to 3 minims. Eucalyptol may be given in similar doses and is preferable for purposes of inhalation, for asthma, diphtheria, sore throat, etc.

As a local application for ulcers and sores, 1 OZ. of the oil is added to 1 pint of lukewarm water. For local injections, 1/2 OZ. to the pint is taken.

The Fluid Extract is used internally, the dose 1/2 to 1 drachm, in scarlet fever, typhoid and intermittent fever.

Eucalyptol, U.S.P.: dose, 5 drops. Ointment, B.P.

Other Species

EUCALYPTUS GUM or KINO

E. nostrata and some other species ofEucalyptus yield Eucalyptus or Red Gum, a ruby-coloured exudation from the bark (to be distinguished from Botany Bay Kino).

Red Gum is a very powerful astringent and is given internally in doses of 2 to 5 grains in cases of diarrhea and pharyngeal inflammations. It is prepared in the form of tinctures, syrups, lozenges, etc.

Red Gum is official in Great Britain, being imported from Australia, though the Kino generally employed here as the official drug is derived from Pterocarpus Marsupium, a member of the order Leguminosae, East Indian, or Malabar Kino, and is administered in doses of 5 to 20 grains powdered, or 1/2 to 1 drachm of the tincture.

In veterinary practice, Red Gum is occasionally prescribed for diarrhea in dogs and is used for superficial wounds.

E. globulus, E. resinifera and other species yield what is known as Botany Bay Kino, an astringent, dark-reddish, amorphous resin, which is obtained in a semi-fluid state by making incisions in the trunk of the tree and is used for similar purposes

J. H. Maiden (Useful Native Plants of Australia, 1889) enumerates more than thirty species as Kino-yielding.

MANNA

From the leaves and young bark of E. mannifera, E. viminalis, E. Gunnii, var. rubida, E. pulverulenta, etc., a hard, opaque sweet substance is procured, containing melitose. The Lerp Manna of Australia is, however, of animal origin. See KINOS.

Ointments

Compound Resin Ointment, B.P.C. Resin 20; Oil of Eucalyptus by weight, 15; Hard paraffin, 10; Soft paraffin, 55.

Eucalyptus Ointment (Benn's Botanic Doctor's Adviser). Elder Oil, 12 OZ.; White Wax, 2 OZ.; Spermaceti, 1 1/2 oz.; Eucalyptus Oil, 2 drachms; Wintergreen Oil, 20 drops.

A good ointment for the skin, containing antiseptic and healing properties. It produces very satisfactory results in scurf, chapped hands, chafes, dandruff, tender feet, enlargements of the glands, spots on the chest, arms, back and legs, pains in the joints and muscles.

Apply a piece of clean cotton or lint to wounds after all dirt is washed away. For aches and pains rub the part affected well and then cover with lint. Repeat two or three times, taking a blood-purifying mixture at the same time.

EYEBRIGHT

Botanical: Euphrasia officinalis (LINN.)
Family: N.O. Scrophulariaceae
Synonyms: Euphrasia.
(French) Casse-lunette.
(German) Augentröst.
Part Used: Herb.

The Eyebright is the only British species of a genus containing twenty species distributed over Europe, Northern and Western Asia and North America.

Description

It is an elegant little plant, 2 to 8 inches high, an annual, common on heaths and other dry pastures, especially on a chalky soil, and flowering from July to September, with deeply-cut leaves and numerous, small, white or purplish flowers variegated with yellow.

It varies much in size and in the color of the corolla, which changes to quite white and yellow. On the mountains and near the sea, or in poor soil, it is often a tiny plant, only an inch or so high, with the stem scarcely branched, but in rich soil it assumes the habit of a minute shrub and forms a spreading tuft, 8 or 9 inches high. The leaves, also, are sometimes almost round, and at other times pointed and narrow, their margins, however, always deeply cut into teeth. The variability of the Eyebright has led to much discussion as to how many species of it are known: continental botanists define numerous species, but our botanists follow Bentham and Hooker, who considered that there is only one very variable species, with three principal varieties: officinalis proper, in which the corolla lip equals or exceeds the tube and the bracts of the flower-spike are broad at the base; gracilis, more slender, the corolla lip shorter than the tube, and the flower-spike bracts narrowed at the base, and maritima, found on the shores of the Shetland Islands in which the capsule is much longer than the calyx.

The stem is erect and wiry, either unbranched in small specimens, or with many opposite branches. The leaves are 1/6 to 1/2 inch long and about 1/4 inch broad, opposite to one another on the lower portion of the stem, alternate above, more often lance-shaped, though sometimes, as already stated, much broader, and with four to five teeth on each side.

The flowers, white, or lilac and purpleveined, are in terminal spikes, with leafy bracts interspersed. The structure of the flower places the plant in the family of the Foxglove and the Speedwell - Scrophulariaceae. The corolla is two-lipped, its lower, tube-like portion being enclosed in a green calyx, tipped with four teeth. The upper lip is two-lobed and arches over the stamens, forming a shelter from the rain. The lower lip is spreading and three-lobed, each lobe being notched. A yellow patch emphasizes the central lobe and purple 'honey guides' on both upper and lower lips - marked streaks of color - point the way down the throat. Four stamens, with brown, downy anthers lie under the upper lip, in pairs, one behind the other; on the underside of each anther is a stiff spur, the two lowest spurs longer than the others and projecting over the throat of the flower. The upper spurs end in miniature brushes which are intended to prevent the pollen being scattered at the side and wasted.

When a bee visitor comes in search of the honey lying round the ovary at the bottom of the petal tube, it knocks against the projecting anther spurs, which sets free the pollen, so that it falls on the insect's head. On visiting the next flower, the bee will then rub its dusty head against the outstanding stigma which terminates the style, or long thread placed on the ovary and projects beyond the stamens, and thus cross-fertilization is effected. But though this is the normal arrangement, other and smaller flowers are sometimes found, which suggests that self- fertilization is aimed at. In these, the corolla elongates after opening, and as the stamens are attached to it, their heads are gradually brought almost up to the stigma and eventually their pollen will fertilize it.

The seeds in all kinds of the flowers are produced in tiny, flattened capsules, and are numerous and ribbed.

The Eyebright will not grow readily in a garden if transplanted, unless 'protected' apparently, by grass. The reason for this is that it is a semi-parasite, relying for part of its nourishment on the roots of other plants. Above ground, it appears to be a perfectly normal plant, with normal flowers and bright green leaves - the leaves of fully parasitic plants are almost devoid of green coloring matter - but below the surface, suckers from its roots spread round and lie on the rootlets of the grassplants among which it grows. Where they are in contact, tiny nodules form and send absorption cells into the grass rootlets. The grass preyed upon does not, however, suffer very much, as the cells penetrate but a slight distance, moreover the Eyebright being an annual, renewing itself from year to year, the suckers on the grass roots to which it is attached also wither in the autumn, so there is no permanent drain of strength from the grass.

History

The name Euphrasia is of Greek origin, derived from Euphrosyne (gladness), the name of one of the three graces who was distinguished for her joy and mirth, and it is thought to have been given the plant from the valuable properties attributed to it as an eye medicine preserving eyesight and so bringing gladness into the life of the sufferer. The same Greek word is also given to the linnet, whence another old tradition says that it was the linnet who first made use of the leaf for clearing the sight of its young and who then passed on the knowledge to mankind, who named the plant in its honour.

Although always known under a name of Greek origin, the herb seems to have been unnoticed by the ancients and no mention of it is made by Dioscorides, Pliny, Galen or even by the Arabian physicians. In the fourteenth century, however, it was supposed to cure 'all evils of the eye' and is described as the source of 'a precious water to clear a man's sight." Matthaeus Sylvaticus, a physician of Mantua, who lived about the year 1329, recommended this plant in disorders of the eyes and Arnoldus Villanovanus, who died in 1313, was the author of a treatise on its virtues, Vini Euphrasiati tantopere celebrati. How long before Euphrasia was in repute for eye diseases it is impossible to say, but in Gordon's Liticium Medicina, 1305, among the medicines for the eyes, Euphragia is named 'and is recommended both outwardly in a compound distilled water and inwardly as a syrup." Euphragia is not, however, mentioned in the Schola Salernitana, compiled about 1100.

Markham (Countrie Farm, 1616) says: 'Drinke everie morning a small draught of Eyebright wine." In the eighteenth century Eyebright tea was used, and in Queen Elizabeth's time there was a kind of ale called 'Eyebright Ale."

Eyebright, says Salmon (Syn. Med., 1671), strengthens the head, eyes and memory and clears the sight.

Euphrasia was regarded as a specific in diseases of the eyes by the great herbalists of the sixteenth century, Tragus, Fuchsius, Dodoens, etc., and has been a popular remedy in most countries.

The French call it Casse-lunette, the Germans Augentröst (consolation of the eyes).

It was the Euphrasy of Spenser, Milton and other

poets. Milton relates how the Archangel Michael ministered to Adam after the Fall:

" . . . to nobler sights

Michael from Adam's eyes the film removed,

Then purged with euphrasine and rue

His visual orbs, for he had much to see."

It is probable that the belief in its value as an eye medicine originated in the old Doctrine of Signatures, for as an old writer points out-

'the purple and yellow spots and stripeswhich are upon the flowers of the Eyebright doth very much resemble the diseases of the eye, as bloodshot, etc., by which signature it hath been found out that this herb is effectual for the curing of the same."

Part Used

A fluid extract is prepared from the plant in the fresh state, gathered when in flower, and cut off just above the root.

Euphrasia is best collected in July and August, when in full flower and the foliage in the best condition.

Constituents

The precise chemical constituents of the herb have not yet been recorded; it is known to contain a peculiar tannin, termed Euphrasia-Tannin acid (which gives a dark-green precipitate with ferric salts and is only obtainable by combination with lead) and also Mannite and Glucose, but the volatile oil and acrid and bitter principle have not yet been chemically analysed.

Medicinal Action and Uses

Slightly tonic and astringent.

Although neglected nowadays by the faculty, modern herbalists still retain faith in this herb and recommend its use in diseases of the sight, weakness of the eyes, ophthalmia, etc., combining it often with Golden Seal in a lotion stated to be excellent for general disorders of the eyes. The juice obtained by expression from the plant in the fresh state is sometimes employed, or an infusion in milk, but the simple infusion in water is the more usual form in which it is applied. An infusion of 1 OZ. of the herb to a pint of boiling water should be used and the eyes bathed three or four times a day. When there is much pain, it is considered desirable to use a warm infusion rather more frequently for inflamed eyes till the pain is removed. In ordinary cases, the cold application is found sufficient.

In Iceland, the expressed juice is used for most ailments of the eye, and in Scotland the Highlanders make an infusion of the herb in milk and anoint weak or inflamed eyes with a feather dipped in it.

The dried herb is an ingredient in British Herbal Tobacco, which is smoked most usefully for chronic bronchial colds.

Homoeopathists hold that Eyebright belongs to the order of scrofula-curing plants, and Dr. Fernie tells us that it has recently been found by experiment:

'to possess a distinct sphere of curative operation, within which it manifests virtues which are as unvarying as they are potential. It acts specifically on the mucous lining of the eyes and nose and the upper part of the throat to the top of the windpipe, causing when given so largely as to be injurious, a profuse secretion from these parts; if given of reduced strength, it cures the troublesome symptoms due to catarrh. Hay Fever, and acute attacks of cold in the head may be checked by an immediate dose of the infusion repeated every two hours. A medicinal tincture is prepared from the whole plant with spirits of wine, of which a lotion is made with rose-water, for simple inflammation of the eyes. Thirty drops of the tincture should be mixed with a wine glassful of rose-water for making this lotion, which may be used several times a day."

Preparation

Fluid extract, 1/2 to 1 drachm.

'A Marvelous Water to Preserve the Sight.

'Take the leaves of red roses, mints, sage, maidenhaire (or leave out sage and mint and take eyebright and vervin), bittony, such of the mountain, and endive, of each 6 handfuls: steep them in Whitewine 24 hours: then distill them in Alimpeck; the first water is like silver, the second like gold, the third like balme; keep it close in glasses.

'It helps all diseases of the eye." (A Plain Plantain.)

Gerard said that the powder of the Eyebright herb, mixed with mace, 'comforteth the memorie," and Culpepper says:

'If the herb was but as much used as it is neglected, it would half spoil the spectacle maker's trade and a man would think that reason should teach people to prefer the preservation of their natural before artificial spectacles, which that they may be instructed how to do, take the virtues of Eyebright as followeth: The juice or distilled water of the Eyebright taken inwardly in white wine, or broth, or dropped into the eyes for several days together helpeth all infirmities of the eye that cause dimness of sight. Some make conserve of the flowers to the same effect. Being used any of the ways, it strengthens the week brain or memory. This tunned with strong beer that it may work together and drunk, or the powder of the dried herb mixed with sugar, a little mace, fennel seed and drunk, or eaten in broth; or the said powder made into an electuary with sugar and taken, hath the same powerful effect to help and restore the sight decayed through age and Arnoldus de Villa Nova saith it hath restored sight to them that have been blind a long time."

This is another eye lotion of Culpepper:

'An Excellent Water to Clear the Sight.

'Take of Fennel, Eyebright, Roses, white Celandine, Vervain and Rue, of each a handful, the liver of a Goat chopt small, infuse them well in Eyebright Water, then distil them in an alembic, and you shall have a water will clear the sight beyond comparison."

Hildamus also firmly believed that Eyebright would restore the sight of many persons at the age of seventy or eighty years!

Many of the older herbalists describe a 'Red-flowered Eyebright," which, however, is no longer considered another species of Euphrasia, but regarded as a very closely allied plant. Linnaeus himself, though he afterwards made a new genus, Bartsia, for it, called it Euphrasia, both in his Flora Suecia, his monograph on the flora of Sweden, that appeared in 1755, and in his great work, Systema Vegetabilium, published in 1784. Later, however, he named it after his friend Dr. Johann Bartsch of Königsberg.

F

FENNEL

Botanical: Foeniculum vulgare (GÆRT.)
Family: N.O. Umbelliferae
Synonyms: Fenkel. Sweet Fennel. Wild Fennel.
Parts Used: Seeds, leaves, roots.

HABITAT

Fennel, a hardy, perennial, umbelliferous herb, with yellow flowers and feathery leaves, grows wild in most parts of temperate Europe, but is generally considered indigenous to the shores of the Mediterranean, whence it spreads eastwards to India. It has followed civilization, especially where Italians have colonized, and may be found growing wild in many parts of the world upon dry soils near the sea-coast and upon river-banks. It flourishes particularly on limestone soils and is now naturalized in some parts of this country, being found from North Wales southward and eastward to Kent, being most frequent in Devon and Cornwall and on chalk cliffs near the sea. It is often found in chalky districts inland in a semi-wild state.

For the medicinal use of its fruits, commonly called seeds, Fennel is largely cultivated in the south of France, Saxony, Galicia, and Russia, as well as in India and Persia.

This plant was attached by Linnaeus to the genus Anethum, but was separated from it by De Candolle and placed with three or four others in a new genus styled Foeniculum, which has been generally adopted by botanists. (Foeniculum was the name given to this plant by the Romans, and is derived from the Latin word, foenum = hay).

This was corrupted in the Middle Ages into Fanculum, and this gave birth to its alternative popular name, 'fenkel."

The Anethum Foeniculum of Linnaeus embraced two varieties, the Common or Wild Fennel and the Sweet Fennel. These are considered by De Candolle as distinct species named respectively F. vulgare (Gaertn.) - the garden form of which is often named F. Capillaceum (Gilibert) - and F. dulce.

HISTORY

Fennel was well known to the Ancients and was cultivated by the ancient Romans for its aromatic fruits and succulent, edible shoots. Pliny had much faith in its medicinal properties, according no less than twenty-two remedies to it, observing also that serpents eat it 'when they cast their old skins, and they sharpen their sight with the juice by rubbing against the plant." A very old English rhyming Herbal, preserved at Stockholm, gives the following description of the virtue of the plant:

'Whaune the heddere (adder) is hurt in eye
Ye red fenel is hys prey,
And yif he mowe it fynde
Wonderly he doth hys kynde.
He schall it chow wonderly,
And leyn it to hys eye kindlely,
Ye jows shall sang and hely ye eye
Yat beforn was sicke et feye."

Many of the older herbalists uphold this theory of the peculiarly strengthening effect of this herb on the sight.

Longfellow alludes to this virtue in the plant:

'Above the lower plants it towers,
The Fennel with its yellow flowers;
And in an earlier age than ours
Was gifted with the wondrous powers
Lost vision to restore."

In mediaeval times, Fennel was employed, together with St. John's Wort and other herbs, as a preventative of witchcraft and other evil influences, being hung over doors on Midsummer's Eve to warn off evil spirits. It was likewise eaten as a condiment to the salt fish so much consumed by our forefathers during Lent. Like several other umbelliferae, it is carminative.

Though the Romans valued the young shoots as a

vegetable, it is not certain whether it was cultivated in northern Europe at that time, but it is frequently mentioned in Anglo-Saxon cookery and medical recipes prior to the Norman Conquest. Fennel shoots, Fennel water and Fennel seed are all mentioned in an ancient record of Spanish agriculture dating A.D. 961. The diffusion of the plant in Central Europe was stimulated by Charlemagne, who enjoined its cultivation on the imperial farms.

It is mentioned in Gerard (1597), and Parkinson (Theatricum Botanicum, 1640) tells us that its culinary use was derived from Italy, for he says:

'The leaves, seede and rootes are both for meate and medicine; the Italians especially doe much delight in the use thereof, and therefore transplant and whiten it, to make it more tender to please the taste, which being sweete and somewhat hot helpeth to digest the crude qualitie of fish and other viscous meats. We use it to lay upon fish or to boyle it therewith and with divers other things, as also the seeds in bread and other things."

William Coles, in Nature's Paradise (1650) affirms that -

'both the seeds, leaves and root of ourGarden Fennel are much used in drinks and broths for those that are grown fat, to abate their unwieldiness and cause them to grow more gaunt and lank."

The ancient Greek name of the herb, Marathron, from maraino, to grow thin, probably refers to this property.

It was said to convey longevity, and to give strength and courage.

There are many references to Fennel in poetry. Milton, in Paradise Lost alludes to the aroma of the plant:

'A savoury odor blown,
Grateful to appetite, more pleased my sense
Than smell of sweetest Fennel."

Description

Fennel is a beautiful plant. It has a thick, perennial root-stock, stout stems, 4 to 5 feet or more in height, erect and cylindrical, bright green and so smooth as to seem polished, much branched bearing leaves cut into the very finest of segments. The bright golden flowers, produced in large, flat terminal umbels, with from thirteen to twenty rays, are in bloom in July and August.

In the kitchen garden this naturally ornamental, graceful plant, generally has its stems cut down to secure a constant crop of green leaves for flavoring and garnishing, so that the plant is seldom seen in the same perfection as in the wild state. In the original wild condition, it is variable as to size, habit, shape and color of leaf, number of rays in the flower-head or umbel, and shape of fruit, but it has been under cultivation for so long that there are now several well-marked species. The Common Garden Fennel (F. Capillaceum or officinale) is distinguished from its wild relative (F. vulgare) by having much stouter, taller, tubular and larger stems, and less divided leaves, but the chief distinction is that the leaf-stalks form a curved sheath around the stem, often even as far as the base of the leaf above. The flower-stalks, or pedicels, of the umbels are also sturdier, and the fruits, 1/4 to 1/2 inch long, are double the size of the wild ones.

Cultivation

Fennel will thrive anywhere, and a plantation will last for years. It is easily propagated by seeds, sown early in April in ordinary soil. It likes plenty of sun and is adapted to dry and sunny situations, not needing heavily manured ground, though it will yield more on rich stiff soil. From 4 1/2 to 5 lb. of seed are sown per acre, either in drills, 15 inches apart, lightly, just covered with soil and the plants afterwards thinned to a similar distance, or sewn thinly in a bed and transplanted when large enough. The fruit is heavy and a crop of 15 cwt. per acre is an average yield.

The roots of Fennel were formerly employed in medicine, but are generally inferior in virtues to the fruit, which is now the only portion recognized by any of the Pharmacopoeias.

The cessation of the supply of Fennel fruits from the Continent during the War led to its being grown more extensively here, any crop produced being almost certain to sell well.

There are several varieties of Fennel fruit known in commerce - sweet or Roman Fennel, German or Saxon Fennel, wild or bitter Fennel, Galician Russian and Roumanian Fennel, Indian, Persian and Japanese. The fruits vary very much in length, breadth, taste and other characters, and are of very different commercial value.

The most esteemed Fennel fruit vary from three to five lines in length, are elliptical, slightly curved, somewhat obtuse at the ends and pale greyish green in color. Wild fruits are short, dark coloured and blunt at their ends, and have a less agreeable flavor and odor than those of sweet Fennel - they are not official.

Fennel fruits are frequently distinguished into 'shorts' and 'longs' in commerce, the latter being the most valued.

The odor of Fennel seed is fragrant, its taste, warm, sweet and agreeably aromatic. It yields its virtues to hot water, but more freely to alcohol. The essential oil may be separated by distillation with water.

For medicinal use, the fruits of the cultivated Fennel, especially those grown in Saxony, are alone official, as they yield the most volatile oil. Saxon fruits are greenish to yellowish-brown in color, oblong, smaller and straighter than the French or Sweet Fennel (F. dulce). This French Fennel, known also as Roman Fennel, is distinguished by its greater length, more oblong form, yellowish-green color and sweet taste; its anise-like odor is also stronger. It is cultivated in the neighborhood of Nimes, in the south of France, but yields comparatively little oil, which has no value medicinally.

Indian Fennel is brownish, usually smaller, straighter and not quite so rounded at the ends with a sweet anise taste. Persian and Japanese fennel, pale greenish brown in color, are the smallest and have a sweeter, still more strongly anise taste and an odor intermediate between that of French and Saxon.

The Saxon, Galician, Roumanian and Russian varieties all yield 4 to 5 per cent of volatile oil, and these varieties are alone suitable for pharmaceutical use. In the ordinary way they furnish some of the best Fennel crops, and from their fruit a large portion of the oil of commerce is derived.

For family use, 1/2 oz. of seed will produce an ample supply of plants and for several years, either from the established roots, or by re-seeding. Unless seed is needed for household or sowing purposes, the flower stems should be cut as soon as they appear.

Adulteration

Commercial Fennel varies greatly in quality, this being either due to lack of care in harvesting, or deliberate adulteration. It may contain so much sand, dirt, stem tissues, weed seeds or other material, that it amounts to adulteration and is unfit for medicinal use, or it may have had some of its oil removed by distillation.

Fruits exhausted by water or steam are darker, contain less oil and sink at once in water, but those exhausted by alcohol still retain 1 to 2 per cent, and are but little altered in appearance, they acquire, however, a peculiar fusel oil odor.

Exhausted, or otherwise inferior fennel is occasionally improved in appearance by the use of a factitious coloring, but old exhausted fruits that have been re-coloured may be detected by rubbing the fruit between the hands, when the color will come off.

Constituents

As found in commerce, oil Fennel is not uniform.

The best varieties of Fennel yield from 4 to 5 per cent of volatile oil (sp. gr. 0.960 to 0.930), the principal constituents of which are Anethol (50 to 60 per cent) and Fenchone (18 to 22 per cent). Anethol is also the chief constituent of Anise oil.

Fenchone is a colorless liquid possessing a pungent, camphoraceous odor and taste, and when present gives the disagreeable bitter taste to many of the commercial oils. It probably contributes materially to the medicinal properties of the oil, hence only such varieties of Fennel as contain a good proportion of fenchone are suitable for medicinal use.

There are also present in oil of Fennel, d-pinene, phellandrine, anisic acid and anisic aldehyde. Schimmel mentions limonene as also at times present as a constituent.

There is reason to believe that much of the commercial oil is adulterated with oil from which the anethol or crystalline constituent has been separated. Good oil will contain as much as 60 per cent.

Saxon Fennel yields 4.7 per cent of volatile oil, containing 22 per cent of fenchone.

Russian, Galician and Roumanian, which closely resembles one another, yield 4 to 5 per cent of volatile oil, of which about 18 per cent is fenchone. They have a camphoraceous taste.

French sweet or Roman Fennel yields only 2.1 per cent. of oil, containing much less anethol and with a milder and sweeter taste, probably due to the entire absence of the bitter fenchone.

French bitter Fennel oil differs considerably, anethol being only present in traces. The oil (Essence de Fenouil amer) is distilled from the entire herb, collected in the south of France, where the plant grows without cultivation.

Indian Fennel yields only 0.72 per cent of oil, containing only 6.7 per cent of fenchone.

Japanese Fennel yields 2.7 per cent of oil, containing 10.2 of fenchone and 75 per cent of anethol.

Sicilian Fennel oil is yielded from F. piperitum.

It was formerly the practice to boil Fennel with all fish, and it was mainly cultivated in kitchen gardens for this purpose. Its leaves are served nowadays with salmon, to correct its oily indigestibility, and are also put into sauce, in the same way as parsley, to be eaten with boiled mackerel.

The seeds are also used for flavoring and the carminative oil that is distilled from them, which has a sweetish aromatic odor and flavor, is employed in the making of cordials and liqueurs, and is also used in perfumery and for scenting soaps. A pound of oil is the usual yield of 500 lb. of the seed.

Medicinal Action and Uses

On account of its aromatic and carminative properties, Fennel fruit is chiefly used medicinally with purgatives to allay their tendency to griping and for this purpose forms one of the ingredients of the well-known compound Liquorice Powder. Fennel water has properties similar to those of anise and dill water: mixed with sodium bicarbonate and syrup, these waters constitute the domestic 'Gripe Water," used to correct the flatulence of infants. Volatile oil of Fennel has these properties in concentration.

Fennel tea, formerly also employed as a carminative, is made by pouring half a pint of boiling water on a teaspoonful of bruised Fennel seeds.

Syrup prepared from Fennel juice was formerly given for chronic coughs.

Fennel is also largely used for cattle condiments.

It is one of the plants which is said to be disliked by fleas, and powdered Fennel has the effect of driving away fleas from kennels and stables. The plant gives off ozone most readily.

Culpepper says:

'One good old custom is not yet left off, viz., to boil fennel with fish, for it consumes the phlegmatic humour which fish most plentifully afford and annoy the body with, though few that use it know wherefore they do it. It benefits this way, because it is a herb of Mercury, and under Virgo, and therefore bears antipathy to Pisces. Fennel expels wind, provokes urine, and eases the pains of the stone, and helps to break it.

The leaves or seed boiled in barley water and drunk, are good for nurses, to increase their milk and make it more wholesome for the child. The leaves, or rather the seeds, boiled in water, stayeth the hiccup and taketh away nausea or inclination to sickness. The seed and the roots much more help to open obstructions of the liver, spleen, and gall, and thereby relieve the painful and windy swellings of the spleen, and the yellow jaundice, as also the gout and cramp. The seed is of good use in medicines for shortness of breath and wheezing, by stoppings of the lungs. The roots are of most use in physic, drinks and broths, that are taken to cleanse the blood, to open obstructions of the liver, to provoke urine, and amend the ill color of the face after sickness, and to cause a good habit through the body; both leaves, seeds, and roots thereof, are much used in drink, or broth, to make people more lean that are too fat. A decoction of the leaves and root is good for serpent bites, and to neutralize vegetable poison, as mushrooms, etc."

'In warm climates," says Mattiolus, 'the stems are cut and there exudes a resinous liquid, which is collected under the name of Fennel Gum."

In Italy and France, the tender leaves areoften used for garnishes and to add flavor to salads, and are also added, finely chopped, to sauces served with puddings. Roman bakers are said to put the herb under their loaves in the oven to make the bread taste agreeably.

The tender stems are employed in soups in Italy, though are more frequently eaten raw as a salad. John Evelyn, in his Acetaria (1680), held that the peeled stalks, soft and white, of the cultivated garden Fennel, when dressed like celery exercised a pleasant action conducive to sleep. The Italians eat these peeled stems, which they call 'Cartucci' as a salad, cutting them when the plant is about to bloom and serving with a dressing of vinegar and pepper.

Formerly poor people used to eat Fennel to satisfy the cravings of hunger on fast days and make unsavoury food palatable; it was also used in large quantities in the households of the rich, as may be seen by the record in the accounts of Edward I.'s household, 8 1/2 lb. of Fennel were bought for one month's supply.

Preparations

Fluid extract, 5 to 30 drops. Oil, 1 to 5 drops. Water, B.P. and U.S.P., 4 drachms.

FENNEL, FLORENCE

Botanical: Foeniculum dulce
Family: N.O. Umbelliferae
Synonyms: Finnochio.
Parts Used: Seeds, herb.

Finnochio or Florence Fennel is a native of Italy, and bears a general resemblance to Foeniculum vulgare, but is an annual and a much smaller plant, being as a rule little more than a foot high. It is a very thick-set plant, the stem joints are very close together and their bases much swollen. The large, finely-cut leaves are borne on very broad, pale green, or almost whitish stalks, which overlap at their bases somewhat like celery, swelling at maturity to form a sort of head or irregular ball - often as big as a man's head and resembling a tuber. The flowers appear earlier than those of common Fennel, and the number of flowers in the umbel is only six to eight.

Cultivation

The cultivation is much the same as for common Fennel though it requires richer soil, and owing to the dwarf nature of the plant, the rows and the plants may be placed closer together, the seedlings only 6 to 8 inches apart. They are very thirsty and require watering frequently in dry weather. When the 'tubers' swell and attain the size of an egg, draw the soil slightly around them, half covering them. Cutting may begin about ten days later. The flowerheads should be removed as they appear.

Florence Fennel should be cooked in vegetarian or meat stock and served with either a rich butter sauce or cream dressing. It suggests celery in flavor, but is sweeter, and very pleasantly fragrant. In ordinary times, it can be bought from Italian greengrocers in London. In Italy it is one of the commonest and most popular of vegetables.

It is grown in this country at Hitchin.

FENNEL FLOWER

Botanical: Nigella sativa (LINN.)
Family: N.O. Ranunculaceae
Synonyms: Roman Coriander. Nutmeg Flower.
(French) Faux cumin. (Quatre épices. Toute épice.
(German) Schwarzkummel.
Parts Used: Seeds, herb.

Fennel Flower, or Nutmeg Flower, is a small Asiatic annual, native to Syria, not in any way related to the Fennel, but belonging to the buttercup order of plants and grown to a limited extent in southern Europe and occasionally in other parts of the world.

Among the Romans it was esteemed in cooking, hence one of its common names, Roman Coriander.

French cooks employ the seeds of this plant under the name of quatre épices or toute épice. They were formerly used as a substitute for pepper.

Description

The plant has a rather stiff, erect, branching stem, bears deeply-cut greyish-green leaves and terminal greyishblue flowers, followed by odd, toothed seed-vessels, filled with small somewhat compressed seeds, usually three-cornered, with two sides flat and one convex, black or brown externally, white and oleaginous within, of a strong, agreeable aromatic odor, like that of nutmegs, and a spicy, pungent taste.

Cultivation

The seed is sown in spring, after the ground gets warm. The drills may be 15 to 18 inches apart and the plants thinned to 10 to 12 inches asunder. No special attention is necessary until mid-summer when the seeds ripen. They are easily threshed and cleaned. After drying, they should be carefully stored in a cool, dry place.

Constituents

The chief constituents of the seeds are a volatile oil and a fixed oil (1.3 per cent of the former and 35 per cent of the latter), and an amorphous, glucoside Melanthin, which is decomposed by diluted hydrochloric acid into Melanthigenin and sugar. Rochebrune, Toxicol Africaine, has found a powerful paralysing alkaloid, to which he gives the name of Nigelline. Melanthin is stated to exhibit the typical physiological action of the most poisonous saponines.

Medicinal Action and Uses

In India, the seeds are considered as stimulant, diaphoretic and emmenagogue, and are believed to increase the secretion of milk. They are also used as a condiment and as a corrigent or adjuvant of purgative and tonic medicines.

In Eastern countries they are commonly used for seasoning curries and other dishes, and the Egyptians spread them on bread or put them on cakes like comfits, believing them to be fattening. They are also used in India for putting among linen to keep away insects- and the native doctors employ them medicinally as a carminative in indigestion and bowel complaints.

FENNEL, HOG'S

Botanical: Peucedanum palustre (LINN.), Peucedanum officinale (LINN.)
Family: N.O. Compositae
Synonyms: Sow Fennel. Sulphurwort. Chucklusa.
Hoar Strange. Hoar Strong. Brimstonewort. Milk Parsley. Marsh Parsley. Marsh Smallage.
(French) Persil des Marais.
(German) Sumpfsilge.
Part Used: Herb.

The Hog's Fennel, a native of Great Britain, though not commonly met with, is more closely allied to the dill than to the true Fennel, belonging to the same genus as the former.

The ordinary Hog's Fennel (Peucedanum officinale, Linn.) occurs, though somewhat rarely, in salt marshes on the eastern coast of England. It seems to have been less rare in the days of Culpepper, who states that it grows plentifully in the salt marshes near Faversham.

Description

It grows to a height of 3 or 4 feet, and is remarkable for its large umbels of yellow flowers, which are in bloom from July to September. Its leaves are cut into long narrow segments, hence perhaps its popular name of Hog's Fennel.

The thick root has a strong odor of sulphur - hence one of the other popular names of the plant, Sulphurwort, and when wounded in the spring, yields a considerable quantity of a yellowish-green juice, which dries into a gummy resin and retains the strong scent of the root.

This plant is now naturalized in North America, where in addition to the name of Sulphurwort, it is called Chucklusa.

Constituents

The active constituent of the root is Peucedanin, a very active crystalline principle, stated to be diuretic and emmenagogue.

Medicinal Action and Uses

Culpepper gives Hog's Fennel the name of Hoar Strange, Hoar Strong, Brimstonewort and Sulphurwort, and tells us, on the authority of Dioscorides and Galen, that -

'the juice used with vinegar and rose-water, or with a little Euphorbium put to the nose benefits those that are troubled with the lethargy, frenzy or giddiness of the head, the falling sickness, long and inveterate headache, the palsy, sciatica and the cramp, and generally all the diseases of the sinews, used with oil and vinegar. The juice dissolved in wine and put into an egg is good for a cough or shortness of breath, and for those that are troubled with wind. It also purgeth gently and softens hardness of the spleen.... A little of the juice dissolved in wine and dropped into the ears or into a hollow tooth easeth the pains thereof. The root is less effectual to all the aforesaid disorders, yet the powder of the root cleanseth foul ulcers, and taketh out splinters of broken bones or other things in the flesh and healeth them perfectly; it is of admirable virtue in all green wounds and prevents gangrene."

P. palustre, the Marsh Hog's Fennel, is also a rare plant, found in marshes in Yorks and Lincoln and a few other districts.

Its grooved stem grows 4 to 5 feet high, bears white flowers and abounds in a milky juice which dries to a brown resin. The root is, when dried, of a brown color externally, having a strong aromatic odor and an acrid, pungent, aromatic taste.

The resin in it has been found, by Peschier, to contain a volatile oil, a fixed oil and a peculiar acid which he named Selinic. It has been used as a substitute for ginger in Russia and has been employed in that country as a remedy for epilepsy, having the same stimulating qualities as the former species, the dose given being from 20 to 30 grains thrice daily, rapidly increased to four times the amount.

FENUGREEK

Botanical: Foenum-graecum (LINN.)
Family: N.O. Leguminosae
Synonyms: Bird's Foot. Greek Hay-seed.
Part Used: Seeds.

Habitat

Indigenous to the countries on the eastern shores of the Mediterranean. Cultivated in India, Africa, Egypt, Morocco, and occasionally in England.

Description

The name comes from Foenum-graecum, meaning Greek Hay, the plant being used to scent inferior hay. The name of the genus, Trigonella, is derived from the old Greek name, denoting 'three-angled," from the form of its corolla. The seeds of Fenugreek have been used medicinally all through the ages and were held in high repute among the Egyptians, Greeks and Romans for medicinal and culinary purposes.

Fenugreek is an erect annual herb, growing about 2 feet high, similar in habit to Lucerne. The seeds are brownish, about 1/8 inch long, oblong, rhomboidal, with a deep furrow dividing them into two unequal lobes. They are contained, ten to twenty together, in long, narrow, sickle-like pods.

Taste, bitter and peculiar, not unlike lovage or celery. Odor, similar.

Constituents

About 28 per cent mucilage; 5 per cent of a stronger-smelling, bitter fixed oil, which can be extracted by ether; 22 per cent proteids; a volatile oil; two alkaloids, Trigonelline and Choline, and a yellow coloring substance. The chemical composition resembles that of cod-liver oil, as it is rich in phosphates, lecithin and nucleoalbumin, containing also considerable quantities of iron in an organic form, which can be readily absorbed. Reutter has noted the presence of trimethylamine, neurin and betain; like the alkaloids in cod-liver oil, these substances stimulate the appetite by their action on the nervous system, or produce a diuretic or ureo-poietic effect.

Medicinal Action and Uses

In Cairo it is used under the name of Helba. This is an Egyptian preparation, made by soaking the seeds in water till they swell into a thick paste. Said to be equal to quinine in preventing fevers; is comforting to the stomach and has been utilized for diabetes. The seeds are soaked in water, then allowed to sprout, and when grown about 2 or 3 inches high, the green eaten raw with the seeds.

The seeds yield the whole of their odor and taste to alcohol and are employed in the preparation of emollient cataplasms, ointments and plasters.

They give a strong mucilage, which is emollient and a decoction of 1 OZ. seeds to 1 pint water is used internally in inflamed conditions of the stomach and intestines. Externally it is used as a poultice for abscesses, boils, carbuncles, etc. It can be employed as a substitute for cod-liver oil in scrofula, rickets, anaemia, debility following infectious diseases. For neurasthenia, gout and diabetes it can be combined with insulin. It possesses the advantage of being cheap and readily taken by children, if its bitter taste is disguised: 1 or 2 teaspoonful of the powder is taken daily in jam, etc.

The ground seeds are used also to give a maple-flavoring to confectionery and nearly all cattle like the flavor of Fenugreek in their forage. The powder is also employed as a spice in curry. At the present day, the ground seeds are utilized to an enormous extent in the manufactures of condition powders for horses and cattle; Funugreek is the principal ingredient in most of the quack nostrums which find so much favour among grooms and horsekeepers. It has a powerful odor of coumarin and is largely used for flavoring cattle foods and to make damaged hay palatable.

In India the fresh plant is employed as an esculent.

Other Species

Trigonella purpurascens, a British species,with small pinky-white flowers, one to three together, and straight, six- to eight-seeded pods, twice as long as the calyx.

FERNS

Family: N.O. Filices

Ferns are herbs, with a perennial (rarely annual) short, tufted or creeping root-stock. The British genera comprise about forty-five species, only one of which, a small Jersey species, is annual.

The leaves of Ferns are mostly radical, partaking of the nature of branches and distinguished by the name of fronds. When divided laterally (as is generally the case) the leaflets are termed pinnae, and their subdivisions pinnules.

The classification of the order Filices is according to fructification. The dust-like and almost invisible seeds or spores of Ferns are contained in little cases or thecae, of a roundish shape, which are themselves encircled (except in some groups) by a jointed ring, the elasticity of which eventually bursts open the thecae and scatters the spores when mature. These thecae are in the majority of the genera arranged on the back of the pinnules in linear, oblong or circular clusters, called sori mostly having above the mass a thin membrane called the Indusium, though in some genera the sori are naked. In some instances, as in the Maidenhairs, the sori are arranged on the margins of the fronds, the indusium being a continuation of the bleached, recurved margin of the pinnule itself. In a few genera, as in the Osmunda and Adder's Tongue, the plant is divided into barren and fertile fronds, either of a distinctly different or of the same form, the fructification rising at the top of the fertile fronds in spikes or panicles. The spores when sown develop minute green leafy expansions, called Prothalli. On each prothallus are produced tiny bodies which have been compared to stamens and pistils, from whence the young Fern is subsequently developed.

As regards culture, Ferns prefer a northern aspect, shade and shelter is not indispensable, but tends to their finer and most perfect condition and growth. They flourish best in asoil that is a mixture of peat, earth and sand, pebbles being intermixed for the roots in many instances to cling to. The only manure needed is that from dried leaves or other vegetable matter. They should not be set too deep and are best kept rather moist. In all the wall species, the roots are best placed under the protection of the stones among which they are to grow. Attention should be paid in cultivation to the natural habits of the species. Ferns may be raised from the spores if carefully potted and looked after.

MALE FERN

Botanical: Dryopteris Felix-mas (LINN.), Aspidium Filix-mas (SCHWARZ)
Family: N.O. Filices
Synonym: Male Shield Fern.
Part Used: Root.

The common Male Fern, often known as Dryopteris Filix-mas (Linn.), and assigned by other botanists to the genera Lastrea, Nephrodium and Polypodium, is one of the commonest and hardiest of British Ferns and, after the Bracken, the species most frequently met with, growing luxuriantly in woods and shady situations, and along moist banks and hedgerows. In sheltered spots it will sometimes remain green all the winter.

This Fern grows in all parts of Europe, temperate Asia, North India, North and South Africa, the temperate parts of the United States and the Andes of South America. It is very variable, some of its forms in this country markedly differing and described under the names of sub-species, the chief being affine, Borreri, pumilum, abbreviatum, and elongatum.

Description

The root-stock or rhizome is short, stumpy and creeping, lying along the surface of the ground or just below it. From its under surface spring the slender, matted roots. The crown of the rhizome is a brown, tangled mass, with the hairy bases of the leaves, and in it is contained the mass of undeveloped fronds which, as they unroll, grow in a large circular tuft and attain a length of from 2 to 4 feet. Each frond is wide and spreading, stiff, erect, broadly lanceolate or lance-shaped, the stalk covered with brown scaly hairs. The pinnae are arranged alternately on the mid-rib (which is also hairy), the lower ones decreasing in size, and each pinna divided again almost to its own mid-rib, the pinnules being oblong and rounded, with their edges slightly notched and their surface somewhat furrowed. The sori are on the upper half of the frond, at the back of the pinnules, in round masses towards the base of the segments, covered with a conspicuous, kidney-shaped indusium.

The name of this genus, Aspidium, is derived from aspis (a shield), because the spores are thus enclosed in bosses, resembling the shape of the round shields of ancient days.

Parts Used Medicinally

An oil is extracted from the rhizome of this Fern, which, as far back as the times of Theophrastus and Dioscorides, was known as a valuable vermifuge, and its use has in modern times been widely revived.

Gerard writes:

'The roots of the Male Fern, being taken in the weight of half an ounce, driveth forth long flat worms, as Dioscorides writeth, being drunke in mede or honied water, and more effectually if it be given with two scruples, or two third parts of a dram of scammonie, or of black hellebore: they that will use it, must first eat garlicke."

The famous remedy of Madame Nouffer, for expelling tapeworms, contained this plant as its basis.

Comparatively little Male Fern has so far been collected in this country, Germany until the War having supplied nearly all our requirements.

It may be collected in late autumn, winter or early spring, from the time the fronds die down, till February, late autumn being considered the best time. Only old rhizomes should be taken.

The rhizome varies in length and thickness according to its age. For medicinal purposes it should be from 3 to 6 inches or more long and from 1 1/2 to 2 inches or more broad. When removed from the ground, it is cylindrical and covered with the closelyarranged, overlapping remains of the leafstalks of the decayed fronds. These stalks are from I to 2 inches long, somewhat curved, angular, brown-coloured, and surrounded at the base with thin, silky scales, of a light brown color. From between these remains of the leaf stalks, the black, wiry, branched roots may be seen. Internally in the fresh state, the rhizome is fleshy and of a light yellowish-green color. It has very little odor, but a sweetish, astringent and subsequently nauseous and bitter taste.

Before drying, it is divested of its scales, roots and all dead portions, leaving the lower swollen portion attached to the rhizome, and is carefully cleansed from adhering soil. It is then sliced in half longitudinally. For pharmaceutical use, it is reduced to a coarse powder and at once exhausted with ether. Extract obtained in this way is more efficacious than that which has been obtained from rhizome that has been kept for some time. It should never be more than a year old.

There is also a market for Male Fern Fingers which are the bases of the fronds, collected in late summer, scraped when fresh (not peeled), cut up into pieces 2 to 3 inches long and then dried, when they present a wrinkled appearance externally and internally and should have the color of pistachio nuts.

Substitutes

English oil of Male Fern has always proved more reliable than that imported from the Continent, which is often extracted from an admixture of other species. The rhizomes of Asplenium Filix-foemina (Bernh.), Aspidium Oreopteris (Sw.), and A. spinulosum (Sw.), resemble those of the Male Fern and have often been found mixed with it when imported. They are best distinguished by examining the transverse section of their leaf bases with a magnifying lens: in Filix-mas, the section exhibits eight wood bundles, forming an irregular circle, whilst in the three other ferns named only two are observed. The presence of secreting cells in the hard tissue, the number of bundles at the base of the leaf-stalk, and the absence of glandular hairs from the margin of the scales, readily distinguish Male Fern from the other species. The margin of the scales borne by the leaf-stalk has in the Male Fern merely hair-like projections, whereas in A. spinulosum, the hairs are glandular. Felixfoemina has no glandular hairs, and has only two large bundles in the base of the leafstalk in distinction to the eight of Filix-mas. The United States Pharmacopoeia includes the rhizome of a Canadian species, A. marginale, which in transverse section shows only six wood bundles.

This fern appears to have some qualities in common with the Bracken. The ashes of both have been used in soap and glassmaking, and the young curled fronds have been boiled and eaten like Asparagus. In times of great scarcity the Norwegians (over a century ago) used the fronds to mix with bread and also made them into beer. The leaves, cut green and dried, make an excellent bitter, and when infused in hot water make good fodder for sheep and goats.

The Scottish roots of Male Fern (according to an account published in the Chemist and Druggist of February 26, 1921) yield an oleoresin which contains 30 per cent of filicin, whereas the British Pharmacopoeia only requires 20 per cent.

Constituents

By extraction with ether, Male Fern yields a dark green, oily liquid extract, Oil of Male Fern, containing the more important constituents of the drug. The chief constituents are about 5 per cent of Filmaron - an amorphous acid, and from 5 to 8 per cent of Filicic acid, which is also amorphous and tends to degenerate into its inactive crystalline anhydride, Filicin. The Filicic acid is regarded as the chief, though not the only active principle. Tannin, resin, coloring matter and sugar are also present in the rhizome. The drug has a disagreeable, bitter taste and an unpleasant odor

Medicinal Action and Uses

The liquid extract is one of the best anthelmintics against tapeworm, which it kills and expels. It is usual to administer this worm medicine last thing at night, after several hours of fasting, and to give a purgative, such as castor oil, first thing in the morning. A single sufficient dose will often cure at once. The powder, or the fluid extract, may be taken, but the ethereal extract, or oleoresin, if given in pill form, is the more pleasant way of taking it.

The drug is much employed for similar purposes by veterinary practitioners. In the powdered form, the dose varies from 60 to 180 grains, taken in honey or syrup, or infused in half a teacupful of boiling water. The dose often given is too small, and failure is then due to the smallness of the dose. In too large doses, however, it is an irritant poison, causing muscular weakness and coma, and has been proved particularly injurious to the eyesight, even causing blindness.

The older herbalists considered that 'the roots, bruised and boiled in oil or lard, made a good ointment for healing wounds, and that the powdered roots cured rickets in children."

Preparations and Dosages

Powdered root, 1 to 4 drachms. Fluid extract, 1 to 4 drachms. Oleoresin, 5 to 20 drops. Ethereal extract, B.P., 45 to 90 drops.

SHEILD FERN, PRICKLY-TOOTHED

Botanical: Aspidium spinulosum
Family: N.O. Filices
Part Used:Root.

The Prickly-toothed Shield Fern is allied to the Male Shield Fern, but is not so tall, about 8 to 14 inches, and has very much broader leaves. The rootstock is similar to Male Fern, but there are differences in the number of wood bundles in the stems, also in the hairs on the margins of the leaf-stalk scales. The fronds are more divided - twice or thrice pinnate - and are spinous, the pinnae generally opposite and the lowest pair much shorter than the others. The sori are circular, with kidney-shaped indusium, much smaller than in Filix-mas.

The Prickly-toothed Shield Fern is moderately erect and firm and grows in masses, being common in sheltered places on moist banks and in open woods.

The medicinal uses are as in Male Fern, with the rhizome of which, as imported from the Continent, it has always been much mixed.

LADY FERN

Botanical: Asplenium Felix-foemina (BERNH.)
Family: N.O. Filices
Synonym: Athyrium Filix-foemina.

The Lady Fern is similar in size and general appearance to the Male Fern. It grows abundantly in Britain, in masses, in moist, sheltered woods, on hedgebanks and in ravines. The rootstock is short and woody; the fronds 2 to 3 feet high, grow in circular tufts and are light, feathery and succulent, generally drooping, and while young and tender, not infrequently soon shrivelling up after being gathered. The leaf base - as already stated - has only two large bundles, and the stalks are less scaly than in the Male Fern. The pinnae are alternate, the lowest decreasing much in size at the bottom, and are divided into numerous long, narrow, deeply-divided and toothed pinnules, with abundant sori on their undersides, the indusium attached along one side, in shape rather like an elongated and rather straightened kidney. The Lady Fern is very variable in form, tint and flexibility: it is more graceful and somewhat more delicate than the Male Fern, and is early cut down by autumn frosts. It is easy of cultivation.

The medicinal uses are as in Male Fern, but it is

less powerful in action.

SPLEENWORT COMMON

Botanical: Asplenium ceterach (LINN.)
Family: N.O. Filices
Synonyms: Scaly Fern. Finger Fern. Miltwaste. Ceterach (Arabian).

The Common Spleenwort grows on old walls and in the clefts of moist rocks. The fronds are 4 to 6 inches long, leathery, light green above, beneath densely covered with rusty, toothed scales, the sori hidden under the scales.

This Fern used also to be called 'Miltwaste," because it was said to cure disorders of the milt or spleen, for which it was much recommended by the Ancients. Probably this virtue has been attributed to the plant because the lobular milt-like shape of its leaf resembles the form of the spleen. The name of the genus, Asplenium, is derived from the Greek word for the spleen, for which the various species originally assigned to the genus were thought to have curative powers. This particular species was used to cure an enlarged spleen. It was also used as a pectoral and as an aperient in obstructions of the viscera, and an infusion of the leaves was prescribed for gravel. Meyrick considered that a decoction of the whole plant was efficacious, if persevered in, for removing all obstructions of the liver and spleen. Pliny considered that it caused barrenness.

SPLEENWORT, BLACK

Botanical: Asplenium Adiantum nigrum (LINN.)
Family: N.O. Filices
Synonym: Black Maidenhair.
Part Used: Herb.

The Black Spleenwort is a small fern growing in rather circular masses, either on walls, where its fronds are only from 3 to 6 inches long, or on shady hedgebanks, where its oblong-triangular, evergreen fronds may attain as much as 20 inches in length. The pinnae are alternate, slanting upwards; the pinnules thick, leathery, shiny, irregularly wedge-shaped. It is rather variable in form; when on exposed walls, it is more rigid and pointed and yellowish-green, instead of dark green. The sori are abundant, swelling over the edges of the pinnules. This is a very hardy and ornamental fern. Its stalks are polished and dark chestnut-brown in color.

It is sometimes called Black Maidenhair, and has medicinal virtues similar to other Maidenhairs, a decoction of it relieving a troublesome cough and proving also a good hair wash.

Dosage of Infusion

3 tablespoonfuls.

WALL RUE

Botanical: Asplenium Ruta-muraria (LINN.)
Family: N.O. Filices
Synonyms: White Maidenhair. Tentwort.
Part Used: Herb.

The Wall Rue, named by some old writers Salvis vitae, also White Maidenhair, is a small fern, only 2 to 3 inches high, growing in tufts and embedded in the crevices and joints of walls. It is much the color of Garden Rue, its wedge-shaped pinnules being like those of the Rue, and also its slender stalks of a pale-green color.

It was considered good for coughs and ruptures in children. One of its old names, 'Tentwort," refers to its use as a specific for the cure of rickets, a disease once known as 'the taint." It was also used to prevent hair from falling out.

Culpepper says:

'This is used in pectoral decoction. The decoction being drunk helps those that are troubled with coughs, shortness of breath, yellow jaundice, diseases of the spleen, stoppings of the urine, and helps to break the stone in the kidneys.... It cleanses the lungs, and by rectifying the blood causes a good color to the whole body. The herb boiled in oil of camomile dissolves knots, allays swellings and drys up moist ulcers. The lye made thereof is singularly good to cleanse the head from scurf and from dry and running sores, stays the shedding or falling of the hair, and causes it to grow thick, fair and well-coloured, for which purpose boil it in wine, putting some smallage-seed thereto and afterwards some oil."

MAIDENHAIR, COMMON

Botanical: Asplenium trichomanes (LINN.)
Family: N.O. Filices

A tea derived from our Common Maidenhair, a simple little fern, common on old walls, with long, simply pinnate fronds, their sori arranged on the back in oblique lines, has also demulcent effect. The fronds are sweet, mucilaginous, and expectorant, causing the tea to have been considered useful in pulmonary disorders. In Arran, the fronds have been dried and used as a substitute for tea; it acts as a laxative.

Other Species

The 'Golden Maidenhair," which Culpepper also mentions is not a Fern, but a Moss. He describes it as 'rarely used, but very good to prevent the falling off of the hair and to make it grow thick, being boiled in water or lye and the head washed with it."

The above three species are the doradilles of France, sometimes used as rather unsatisfactory substitutes for the Maidenhair of Montpellier and Canada and Mexico.

MAIDENHAIR, TRUE

Botanical: Adiantum Capillus-veneris
Family: N.O. Filices
Synonyms: Capillaire commun, or de Montpellier. Hair of Venus.
Part Used: The herb.
Habitat: Southern Europe. Southern and Central Britain.

History

Several varieties of Maidenhair Fern are used in medicine, the most common being the present species, when grown in France, and the Canadian Adiantum pedatum.

Habitat

A. Capillus-veneris, called the True Maidenhair, is a dainty little evergreen fern found in the milder parts of the West of England - in Dorset, Devon and Cornwall - and in mild parts of the west of Ireland, growing in moist caves and on rocks near the sea, on damp walls and in wells.

Description

The rootstock is tufted and creeping. The fern grows in masses, the fronds, however, separating and arching apart, giving the appearance of a perfect miniature tree. The stems are slender, of a shining, brownish black, the fronds themselves usually twice or three times pinnate, 6 inches to a foot long, the delicate pinnules fan-shaped, indented and notched. The sori are conspicuous, occupying the extremities of most of the lobes of the pinnules, in oval spots on the inner surface of the indusium, which is formed of the reflexed edge of the pinnule. The pinnules are very smooth: 'in vain," said Pliny, 'do you plunge the Adiantum into water, it always remains dry."

Constituents

Tannin and mucilage. It has not been very fully investigated.

Medicinal Action and Uses

Has been used from ancient times medicinally, being mentioned by Dioscorides. Its chief use has been as a remedy in pectoral complaints. A pleasant syrup is made in France from its fronds and rhizomes, called Sirop de Capillaire, which is given as a favorite medicine in pulmonary catarrhs. It is flavoured with orange flowers and acts as a demulcent with slightly stimulating effects. Narbonne Honey is generally added to the syrup.

Culpepper tells us:

'This and all other Maiden Hairs is a good remedy for coughs, asthmas, pleurisy, etc., and on account of its being a gentle diuretic also in jaundice, gravel and other impurities of the kidneys. All the Maidenhairs should be used green and in conjunction with other ingredients because their virtues are weak."

Gerard writes of it:

'It consumeth and wasteth away the King's Evil and other hard swellings, and it maketh the haire of the head or beard to grow that is fallen and pulled off."

It also enters into the composition of Elixir de Garus. It is employed on the Continent as an emmenagogue under the names of polytrichi, polytrichon, or kalliphyllon, administered as a sweetened infusion of 1 OZ. to a pint of boiling water.

A. pedatum is a perennial fern of the United States and Canada, a little larger than the European variety, used in similar ways and more highly valued by many.

A. lunulatum of India is similarly employed.

A. trapeziforme of Mexico is more aromatic but less valuable medicinally.

A. radiatum and A. fragile of Jamaica and A. Æthiopicum of Ethiopia are both used in medicine.

HART'S TONGUE

Botanical: Scolopendrium vulgare; Asplenium scolopendrium (LINN.)
Family: N.O. Filices
Synonyms: Hind's Tongue. Buttonhole. Horse Tongue. God's-hair. Lingua cervina.
Part Used: Fronds.

The Hart's Tongue, a fern of common growth in England in shady copses and on moist banks and walls, is the Lingua cervina of the old apothecaries, and its name refers to the shape of its fronds.

Description

Its broad, long, undivided dark-green fronds distinguish it from all other native ferns, and render it a conspicuous object in the situations where it abounds, as it grows in masses. It receives its name of Scolopendrium because its fructification is supposed to resemble the feet of Scolopendra, a genus of Mydrapods. The sori are in twin oblique lines, on each side of the midrib, covered by what looks like a single indusium, but really is two, one arranged partially over the other. In the early stages of its growth, the folding over of the indusium can be clearly seen through a lens. The fronds are stalked and the root, tufted, short and stout. This fern is evergreen and easy of cultivation.

Medicinal Action and Uses

In common with Maidenhair, this fern was formerly considered one of the five great capillary herbs.

The older physicians esteemed it a very valuable medicine, and Galen gave it in infusion for diarrhea and dysentery, for which its astringent quality made it a useful remedy. In country districts, especially in Wales and the Highlands, an ointment is made of its fronds for burns and scalds and for piles, and it has been taken internally for Bright's Disease, in a decoction made of 2 oz. to a pint of water, in wine glassful doses. In homeopathy, it is administered in combination with Golden Seal, for diabetes. It is specially recommended for removing obstructions from the liver and spleen, also for removing gravelly deposits in the bladder. Culpepper tells us:

'It is a good remedy for the liver, both to strengthen it when weak and ease it when afflicted.... It is commended for hardness and stoppings of the spleen and liver, and the heat of the stomach. The distilled water is very good against the passion of the heart, to stay hiccough, to help the falling of the palate and to stay bleeding of the gums by gargling with it."

BRACKEN

Botanical: Pteris aquilina (LINN.)
Family: N.O. Filices
Synonyms: Brake Fern. Female Fern.
Parts Used: Fronds. root.

The Bracken or Brake Fern, often called by old writers the Female Fern, is found in almost every part of the globe, except the extreme north and south; it grows more freely than any other of the Fern tribe throughout Britain, flourishing luxuriantly on heaths and moors.

Description

The rootstock is long and fibrous (creeping horizontally), very thick and succulent, throwing up solitary fronds at intervals, which soon cover large patches of ground. The stems are erect and treelike, velvety at the base, very brittle at first, afterwards tough and wiry, ordinarily 2 to 3 feet high, though in favourable soil and situations attaining a height of 8 to 10 feet. They bear branched fronds, twice or thrice pinnate, the pinnae more or less opposite, the pinnules long, narrow, smooth-edged, roundpointed and leathery. The sori on the back of the frond form a continuous line along the margin, being covered by an indusium attached to the slightly recurved edge of the pinnule.

The lower portion of the stem, when cut obliquely at the base, shows a pattern or figure formed of the wood bundles, which was supposed by Linnaeus to represent a spread eagle, hence he gave the species the name of Aquilina. The name of the genus, Pteris, is derived from pteron (a feather), from the feathery appearance of the fronds, in the same way that the English name Fern is a contraction of the Anglo-Saxon fepern (a feather). In some parts of England it is called 'King Charles in the Oak Tree." In Scotland, it is said to be an impression of the Devil's Foot, and yet witches were reputed to detest this fern, for the reason that it bears on its cut stem the Greek letter X, which is the initial of Christos. In Ireland, it is called the Fern of God, because if the stem is cut into three sections, on the first of these will be seen the letter G, on the second O, and on the third D.

The spores of this and other Ferns are too minute to be visible to the naked eye. Before the structure of Ferns was understood, their reproduction was thought to be due to unknown agencies - whence various superstitions arose.

'This kind of Ferne," writes Lyte in 1587, 'beareth neither flowers nor sede, except we shall take for sede the black spots growing on the backsides of the leaves, the whiche some do gather thinking to worke wonders, but to say the truth, it is nothing els but trumperi and superstition."

The minute spores were reputed to confer invisibility on their possessor if gathered at the only time when they were said to be visible, i.e. on St. John's Eve, at the precise moment at which the saint was born. Shakespeare says, I Henry IV:

'We have the receipt of Fern seed - we walk invisible."

and Ben Jonson:

'I had no medicine, Sir, to walk invisible

No fern seed in my pocket."

The Fern was also said to confer perpetual youth.

Medicinal Action and Uses

The Ancients used both the fronds and stems of the Bracken in diet-drinks and medicine for many disorders. Culpepper gives several uses for it:

'The roots being bruised and boiled in mead and honeyed water, and drunk kills both the broad and long worms in the body, and abates the swelling and hardness of the spleen. The leaves eaten, purge the belly and expel choleric and waterish humours that trouble the stomach. The roots bruised and boiled in oil or hog's grease make a very profitable ointment to heal the wounds or pricks gotten in the flesh. The powder of them used in foul ulcers causes their speedier healing.

'Fern, being burned, the smoke thereof drives away serpents, gnats, and other noisome creatures, which in fenny countries do, in the night-time, trouble and molest people lying in their beds with their faces uncovered."

Gerard says that 'the root of Ferne cast into an hogshead of wine keepeth it from souring." 'For thigh aches' (sciatica), says another old writer, 'smoke the legs thoroughly with Fern Bracken."

Use as Food

The rhizome is astringent and also contains much starch, and has been considered recently as a possible source of starch for food and industry. There seems, however, to be some doubt as to whether its astringent properties do not render the Bracken unsuitable for human food. Humboldt reported that the inhabitants of Palmaand Gomera - islands of the Canary Group use Bracken as food, grinding the rhizome to powder and mixing it with a small quantity of barley-meal, the composition being termed goflo - the use of such food being, however, a sign of the extreme poverty of the inhabitants. The rootstock of the Esculent Brake (Pteris esculenta) was much used by the aborigines of New Zealand as food, when the British first settled there, and is also eaten much by the natives of the Society Islands and Australia.

The young fronds used sometimes to be used as a vegetable, being sold in bundles like Asparagus, but although considered a delicacy in Japan, they are somewhat flavourless and insipid to our modern Western taste, though they are not indigestible, and in the absence of all other fresh vegetables might prove useful. In Japan, before cooking, the tender shoots are first washed carefully in fresh water, then plunged into boiling water for two minutes or so, and then immersed again in cold water for a couple of hours. After this preparation they may be used for cooking, either being prepared as a pur,e, like spinach, or like asparagus heads, being served with melted butter or some similar sauce.

In Siberia and in Norway, the uncoiled fronds have been employed with about twothirds of their weight of malt for brewing a kind of beer.

Other Uses

The astringent properties of the rhizome have caused a decoction to be recommended for the dressing and preparation of kid and chamois leather.

Before the introduction of soda from seasalt and other sources, the large amount of alkali obtained from the ashes of Bracken was found serviceable for glassmaking, both in the northern parts of this Island and in other countries, and was used freely for the purpose. The ash contains enough potash to be used as a substitute for soap. The ashes are mixed with water and formed into balls; these made hot in the fire are used to make lye for the scouring of linen. In the East, tallow boiled with Bracken ash is made into soap.

The potash yield of Bracken ash is so considerable that in view of the present scarcity of fertilizers, this source of supply is well worth attention. Potash is a particularly valuable fertilizer for potato and sugar-beet land, especially for light loams and gravels and sandy soils. It should be borne in mind by persons having access to quantities of Bracken, that they have a usable supply of this almost indispensable manure at hand, either for cultivating flowers or crops, at the expense of a little trouble.

The best time for cutting Bracken for burning is from June to the end of October, but the ash from green Bracken is much more valuable than from the old and withered plant. In the month of June, the fronds and stems hold as much as 20 per cent of potash, but in August that amount is reduced to 5 per cent, a large proportion having been given back to the rhizome or soil. Experiments have been contemplated by the Board of Agriculture to determine whether the cutting and incineration of Bracken in June, with a view to obtaining its potash content, would be economically feasible.

Where Bracken flourishes unchecked, it becomes injurious to sheep-farming by its encroachments on the grass on the runs, this being especially the case in the Lake District, and it would be of double advantage to cut it down and use it to supplement the reduced stocks of manures. Potash from Bracken is very soluble and should not be exposed to rain. The ashes as soon as cool should be collected and kept dry until required for use. It is stated that 50 tons of the dried fern produces 1 ton of potash. Instructions for dealing with Bracken are given by the Board of Agriculture for Scotland in Leaflets 18, 25, 39 and 42.

Formerly in both the green and the dried state, Bracken was used as fodder for cattle. When dry, it makes excellent litter for both horses and cattle, and forms also a very durable thatch. The young tops of the Fern are boiled in Hampshire for pigs' food, and the peculiar flavor of Hampshire bacon has sometimes been attributed to this custom. The fronds are much used as packing material for fruit, keeping it fresh and cool and imparting neither color nor flavor. The dried fronds may be used in the garden for protecting tender plants.

In early spring, when dormant, large clumps may be lifted from moors or commons to serve as screens in the wilder parts of the garden, though the Fern is somewhat difficult to transplant and afterwards preserve with success, and is often destroyed by spring frosts. While growing in its natural habitats, Bracken is of value as cover and shelter for game.

In the seventeenth century it was customary to set growing Bracken on fire, believing that this would produce rain. A like custom of 'firing the Bracken' still prevails to-day on the Devonshire moors.

POLYPODY, COMMON

Botanical: Polypodiurn vulgare (LINN.)
Family: N.O. Filices
Synonyms: Polypody of the Oak. Wall Fern. Brake Root. Rock Brake. Rock of Polypody. Oak Fern.
Parts Used: Root, leaves.

The Common Polypody is a common Fern in sheltered places, on shady hedge-banks, and on roots and stumps of trees, moist rocks and old walls.

Description

It has a creeping rhizome, which runs along the surface of the ground, or substance on which it grows, and is thick and woody, covered with yellowish scales. At intervals it throws up fronds, from a few inches to a foot in length, which hang down in tresses and have plain, long, narrow, smooth pinnae, placed alternately on the stalk and joined together at the base. The stalk has no scales. The sori are rather large and prominent, white at first, ripening into a golden yellow, and in round masses, placed in two rows along the underside of the upper segments, equally distant from the centre and the margin. Unlike all the preceding species described, they are not covered with an indusium. The young fronds come out in May, but in sheltered places the plant is nearly evergreen.

The name is derived from poly (many) and pous, podos (a foot), from the many foot-like divisions of the caudex.

Part Used Medicinally

The root, which is in perfection in October and November, though it may be collected until February. It is used both fresh and dried, and the leaves are also sometimes used.

This Fern was employed by the Ancients as a purgative: it is the Oak Fern of the older herbalists - not that of the modern botanists, Polypodium dryopteris. It was held that such Fern plants as grew upon the roots of an oak, which this Fern frequently does, owned special medicinal powers. In the same way the mistletoe that grew on the oak was esteemed by the Druids to have special powers of which that growing on other trees was devoid. The True Oak Fern is a much more delicate Fern and grows chiefly in mountainous districts, among the mossy roots of old oak-trees and sometimes in marshy places.

Medicinal Actions and Uses

Alterative, tonic, pectoral and expectorant. Its principal use has been as a mild laxative. It serves as a tonic in dyspepsia and loss of appetite, and as an alterative in skin diseases is found perfectly safe and reliable. It is also used in hepatic complaints.

It proves useful in coughs and catarrhal affection, particularly in dry coughs: it promotes a free expectoration, and the infusion, prepared from 1/2 oz. of crushed root to a pint of boiling water and sweetened, is taken in teacupful doses frequently, proving valuable in the early stages of consumption. The powder is stated to have been used with success for some kinds of worms.

It sometimes produces a rash, but this disappears in a short time and causes no further inconvenience.

Preparation

Fluid extract: dose, one drachm.

A mucilaginous decoction of the fronds was formerly, and probably still is, used in country places as a cure for whooping-cough in children, for this purpose the matured, fruitful fronds, gathered in the autumn, are dried, and when required for use are slowly boiled with coarse sugar. It is still used as a demulcent by the Italians.

The fresh root used to be employed in decoction, or powdered, for melancholia and also for rheumatic swelling of the joints. It is efficacious in jaundice, dropsy and scurvy, and combined with mallows removes hardness of the spleen, stitches in the side and colic. The distilled water of the roots and leaves was considered by the old herbalists good for ague, and the fresh or dried roots, mixed with honey and applied to the nose, were used in the cure of polypus.

Gerard tells us:

'Johannes Mesues reckoneth up Polypodie among those things that do especially dry and make thin: preadventure he had respect to a certain kind of arthritis or ache in the joints: in which not one part but many together most commonly are touched: for which it is very much commended by the Brabanders and other inhabitants about the river Rhene and the Maze. Furthermore Dioscorides saith that the root of Polypodie is very good for members out of joint and for chaps between the fingers."

Culpepper considers Polypody 'a mild and useful purge, but being very slow, it is generally mixed by infusion or decoction with other ingredients, or in broths with beets, parsley, mallow, cummin, ginger, fennel or anise. The best form to take it for a complaint in the intestines is as follows: To an ounce of the fresh root bruised add an ounce and a half of the fresh roots of white beets and a quart of water, boiling hot and let it stand till next day, then drain it off. A quarter of a pint of this liquor contains the infusion of 2 drams of this root. It should be sweetened with cane sugar or honey."

The leaves of Polypody when burnt furnish a large proportion of carbonate of potash.

ROYAL FERN

Botanical: Osmunda regalis (LINN.)
Family: N.O. Filices
Synonyms: Osmund the Waterman. Heart of Osmund. Water Fern. Bog Onion.
Part Used: Root.

The Royal Fern grows abundantly in some parts of Great Britain, chiefly in the western counties of England and Scotland, and in Wales and the west of Ireland. It needs a soil of bog earth and is incorrectly styled the 'Flowering Fern," from the handsome spikes of fructification. One of its old English names is Osmund the Waterman, and the white centres of its roots have been called the 'Heart of Osmund."

There is a legend that the wife and daughter of Osmund, a waterman of Loch Tyne, took refuge among Osmundes during an invasion of the Danes.

Osmund is a Saxon word for domestic peace, from os (hoise) and mund (peace).

By some the name Osmunda is said to be derived from the god Thor (Osmunda). Others have traced its derivation from os (a bone) and mundare (to cleanse), in reference to the medicinal uses of the Fern.

The Fern is dedicated to St. Christopher.

Description

The rootstock is tuberous, large and lobed, densely clothed with matted fibres, often forming a trunk rising perceptibly from the ground, sometimes to the height of a foot or more. It is many headed and sends up tufts of fronds, the brown stems of which are cane-like, very tough and wiry, varying from 2 to 3 feet in drier situations, to from 8 to 10 feet in damp, sheltered places when very luxuriant. It is the tallest of our British ferns.

The fronds are twice pinnate, the pinnae far apart, mostly opposite, the pinnules undivided, narrow and oblong, slightly tapering to their apex, smooth, very short-stalked. When young, they are of a very delicate texture and of a reddish color, changing afterwards to a dull green. The fronds are divided into fertile and barren. The barren fronds are entirely leafy, the fertile fronds are terminated by long, branched spikes of fructification, composed of bunches of clustered thecae or spore cases, green when young and ripening into brown, not covered by an indusium. These fertile fronds are developed in April.

This handsome Fern is easy of cultivation and hardy, and is best transplanted when large.

Part Used Medicinally

The root, or rhizome, which has a mucilaginous and slightly bitter taste. The actual curative virtues of this Fern have been said to be due to the salts of lime, potash and other earths which it derives in solution from the bog soil and from the water in which it grows.

Medicinal Action and Uses

A decoction of the root is of good effect in the cure of jaundice, when taken in its early stages, and for removing obstructions of the viscera. The roots may also be made into an ointment for application to wounds, bruises and dislocations, the young fronds being likewise thought 'good to be put into balms, oils and healing plasters." A conserve of the root was used for rickets. Gerard says, drawing his information from Dodonaeus and other older herbalists:

'The root and especially the heart or middle thereof, boiled or else stamped and taken with some kind of liquor, is thought to be good for those that are wounded, dry beaten and bruised, that have fallen from some high place."

And Culpepper says:

'This has all the virtues mentioned in the former Ferns, and is much more effectual than they, both for inward and outward griefs: and is accounted singularly good in wounds, bruises or the like: the decoction to be drunk or boiled into an ointment of oil, as a balsam or balm, and so it is singularly good against bruises and bones broken or out of joint, and gives much ease to the colic and splenetic diseases: as also for ruptures and burstings."

It has been recommended for lumbago.

ADDER'S TONGUE, ENGLISH

Botanical: Ophioglossum vulgatum (LINN.)
Family: N.O. Filices
Synonym: Christ's Spear.
Parts Used: Root, leaves.

The Adder's Tongue, known also in some parts of England as Christ's Spear, has no resemblance to any other Fern. The stems which grow up solitarily from the small root - formed merely of a few stout, yellow fibres - are round, hollow and succulent, bearing on the upper part a simple spike, issuing from the sheath of a smooth, oblong-oval, tapering, concave, undivided, leafy frond. Embedded on each side of the stalk - at the top is a single row of yellow thecae, not covered by any indusium. The whole has much the appearance of the Arum flower.

The name is derived from ophios (a serpent) and glossa (a tongue).

This strange little Fern, growing only from 3 to 9 inches in height, is generally distributed over Great Britain, being not uncommon, buried in the grass in moist pastures and meadows. It is tolerably easy of cultivation.

Medicinal Action and Uses

This Fern has long had a reputation as a vulnerary. A preparation of it, known as the 'Green Oil of Charity," is still in request as a remedy for wounds.

The older herbalists called it 'a fine cooling herb." The expressed juice of the leaves, drunk either alone, or with distilled water of Horse Tail, used much to be employed by country people for internal wounds and bruises, vomiting or bleeding at the mouth or nose. The distilled water was also considered good for sore eyes. An efficacious ointment for wounds was made as follows:

'Put 2 lb. of leaves chopped very fine into 1/2 pint of oil and 1 1/2 lb. suet melted together. Boil the whole till the herb is crisp, then strain off from the leaves."

This is a very ancient recipe for wounds.

MOONWORT

Botanical: Botrychium lunaria (LINN.)
Family: N.O. Filices
Part Used: Fronds.

The Moonwort is said to possess similar vulnerary virtues to Adder's Tongue. The Ancients regarded it as a plant of magical power, if gathered by moonlight, and it was employed by witches and necromancers in their incantations.

Parkinson says that it was used by the alchemists, who thought it had power to condensate or to convert quicksilver into pure silver.

Culpepper says: 'Moonwort (they absurdly say) will open locks and unshoe such horses as tread upon it; but some country people call it unshoe the horse."

Description

It is a very singular-looking plant, the stem hollow and succulent, throwing off a single, barren pinna, having on each side very peculiar stalked pinnules, occasionally deeply notched throughout to their base. The stem itself, continuing upwards, has near the top other very short, alternate, branched offshoots, on which, or on the spike itself, are arranged the thecae in regular lines - like the Osmunda and Ophioglossum, uncovered by any indusium. This fructification appears in April.

The Moonwort is not uncommon on open heaths and pastures, where the soil is peaty, but not very wet.

This and Ophioglossum, alone among the Ferns, grow up straight, not with their fronds curled inward, crosier-fashion.

FEVER BUSH

Botanical: Garrya fremonti (TORR.)
Family: N.O. Cornaceae
Synonyms: Skunk Bush. Californian Feverbush.
Part Used: Leaves.
Habitat: California, Oregon, Mexico, Cuba, Jamaica.

Description

This is a small evergreen bush. The leaves are broad, leathery, grey green on the upperside; on the underside mealy and lighter grey green. It has grown in the Author's garden, but needs care in the winter. The leaves are intensely bitter, and are largely used in California as an antiperiodic and tonic. A new alkaloid has been found in it called garryine. It is best administered as a fluid extract.

Dosages

Powder, 10 to 30 grains - leaves. Fluid extract, 10 to 30 minims - leaves.

FEVERFEW

Botanical: Chrysanthemum Parthenium (BERNH.)
Family: N.O. Compositae
Synonyms: Pyrethrum Parthenium (Sm.). Featherfew. Featherfoil. Flirtwort. Bachelor's Buttons.
Part Used: Herb.

Description

Feverfew (a corruption of Febrifuge, from its tonic and fever-dispelling properties) is a composite plant growing in every hedgerow, with numerous, small, daisy-like heads of yellow flowers with outer white rays, the central yellow florets being arranged on a nearly flat receptacle, not conical as in the chamomiles. The stem is finely furrowed and hairy, about 2 feet high; the leaves alternate, downy with short hairs, or nearly smooth-about 4 1/2 inches long and 2 inches broad - bipinnatifid, with serrate margins, the leaf-stalk being flattened above and convex beneath. It is not to be confounded with other wild chamomile-like allied species, which mostly have more feathery leaves and somewhat large flowers; the stem also is upright, whereas that of the true garden Chamomile is procumbent. The delicate green leaves are conspicuous even in mild winter. The whole plant has a strong and bitter smell, and is particularly disliked by bees. A double variety is cultivated in gardens for ornamental purposes, and its flower-heads are sometimes substituted for the double Chamomile.

Country people have long been accustomed to make curative uses of this herb, which grows abundantly throughout England. Gerard tells us that it may be used both in drinks, and bound on the wrists is of singular virtue against the ague.

Pyrethrum is derived from the Greek pur (fire), in allusion to the hot taste of the root.

Cultivation

Feverfew is a perennial, and herbaceous in habit. When once planted it gives year after year an abundant supply of blossoms with only the merest degree of attention. Planting may be done in autumn, but the best time is about the end of April. Any ordinary good soil is suitable, but better results are obtained when well-drained, and of a stiff, loamy character, enriched with good manure. Weeding should be done by hand, the plants when first put out being small might be injured by hoeing.

There are three methods of propagation: by seed, by division of roots and by cuttings. If grown by seed, it should be sown in February or March, thinned out to 2 to 3 inches between the plants, and planted out early in June to permanent quarters, allowing a foot or more between the plants and 2 feet between the rows, selecting, if possible, a showery day for the operation. They will establish themselves quickly. To propagate by division, lift the plants in March, or whenever the roots are in an active condition, and with a sharp spade, divide them into three or five fairly large pieces. Cuttings should be made from the young shoots that start from the base of the plant, and should be taken with a heel of the old plant attached, which will greatly assist their rooting. They may be inserted at any time from October to May. The foliage must be shortened to about 3 inches, when the cuttings will be ready for insertion in a bed of light, sandy soil, in the open. Plant very firmly, surface the bed with sand, and water in well. Shade is necessary while the cuttings are rooting.

Keep a good watch at all times for snails, slugs and black fly. For the latter pest, try peppering the plants; for the others use soot, ashes or lime. Toads will keep a garden free of slugs.

'A few pots placed on their sides may be dotted about the garden, and it will be found that the toads will sit in these when they are not hunting around for their prey. The creatures are not at all likely to leave the garden, seeing that if the supply of slugs runs short they will turn their attention to all kinds of insects." (S. L. B.)

Medicinal Action and Uses

Aperient, carminative, bitter. As a stimulant it is useful as an emmenagogue. Is also employed in hysterical complaints, nervousness and lowness of spirits, and is a general tonic. The cold infusion is made from 1 OZ. of the herb to a pint of boiling water, allowed to cool, and taken frequently in doses of half a teacupful.

A decoction with sugar or honey is said to be good for coughs, wheezing and difficult breathing. The herb, bruised and heated, or fried with a little wine and oil, has been employed as a warm external application for wind and colic.

A tincture made from Feverfew and applied locally immediately relieves the pain and swelling caused by bites of insects and vermin. It is said that if two teaspoonfuls of tincture are mixed with 1/2 pint of cold water, and all parts of the body likely to be exposed to the bites of insects are freely sponged with it, they will remain unassailable. A tincture of the leaves of the true Chamomile and of the German Chamomile will have the same effect.

Planted round dwellings, it is said to purify the atmosphere and ward off disease.

An infusion of the flowers, made with boiling water and allowed to become cold, will allay any distressing sensitiveness to pain in a highly nervous subject, and will afford relief to the face-ache or earache of a dyspeptic or rheumatic person.

Preparations

Fluid extract: dose, 1 to 2 drachms.

Other Species

SWEET FEVERFEW

(Chrysanthemum Suaveolens) and C. maritima, found by the seashore, especially in the north, with leaves broader, more fleshy, succulent and smaller flower heads than the Common Feverfew.

FIG, COMMON

Botanical: Ficus Carica (LINN.)
Family: N.O. Urticaceae
Part Used: Fruit.

Habitat

The Common Fig-tree provides the succulent fruit that in its fresh and dried state has been valued from the earliest days. It is indigenous to Persia, Asia Minor and Syria, but now is wild in most of the Mediterranean countries. It is cultivated in most warm and temperate climates and has been celebrated from the earliest times for the beauty of its foliage and for its 'sweetness and good fruit' (Judges ix. 2), there being frequent allusions to it in the Scriptures. The Greeks are said to have received it from Caria in Asia Minor - hence the specific name. Under Hellenic culture it was improved and Attic figs became celebrated in the East. It was one of the principal articles of sustenance among the Greeks, being largely used by the Spartans at their public table; and athletes fed almost entirely on figs, considering that they increased their strength and swiftness. To such an extent, indeed, were figs a part of the staple food of the people in ancient Greece that there was a law forbidding the exportation of the best fruit from their trees.

Figs were early introduced into Italy. Pliny gives details of no less than twentynine kinds known in his day, and specially praises those of Tarant and Caria and also those of Herculaneum. Dried Figs have been found in Pompeii in our days and in the wall-paintings of the buried city Figs are represented together with other fruits. Pliny states that homegrown Figs formed a large portion of the food of slaves, especially in the fresh state for agricultural workers.

The Fig plays an important part in Latin mythology. It was dedicated to Bacchus and employed in religious ceremonies. The wolf that suckled Romulus and Remus rested under a Fig tree, which was therefore held sacred by the Romans, and Ovid states that among the celebrations of the first day of the year by Romans, Figs were offered as presents. The inhabitants of Cyrene crowned themselves with wreaths of Figs when sacrificing to Saturn, holding him to be the discoverer of the fruit. Pliny speaks also of the Wild Fig, which is mentioned also in Homer, and further classical references to the Fig are to be found in Theophrastus, Dioscorides, Varro and Columella.

Description

Ficus Carica is a bush or small tree, rarely more than 18 to 20 feet high, with broad, rough, deciduous, deeply-lobed leaves in the cultivated varieties, though in wild forms the leaves are often almost entire.

Considered botanically, the Fig, as we eat it, is a very remarkable form of fruit. It is actually neither fruit nor flower, though partaking of both, being really a hollow, fleshy receptacle, enclosing a multitude of flowers, which never see the light, yet come to full perfection and ripen their seeds - a contrary method from the strawberry, in which the minute pistils are scattered over the exterior of the enlarged succulent receptacle. In the Fig, the inflorescence, or position of the flowers is concealed within the body of the 'fruit." The Fig stands alone in this peculiar arrangement of its flowers. The edge of the pear-shaped receptacle curves inwards, so as to form a nearlyclosed cavity, bearing the numerous fertile and sterile flowers mingled on its surface, the male flowers mostly in the upper part of the cavity and generally few in number. As it ripens, the receptacle enlarges greatly and the numerous one-seeded fruits become embedded in it. The fruit of the wild kind never attains the succulence of the cultivated kinds. The Figs are borne in the axils of the leaves, singly.

Cultivation

The Fig is grown for its fresh fruit in all the milder parts of Europe, being cultivated in the Mediterranean countries, and in the United States of America. With protection in winter, it succeeds as far north as Pennsylvania. (Prof. Nancy Traill, York University, Toronto, Ontario, Canada points out.. "In some parts of Pennsylvania, people bury the trees. In Philadelphia, a mulch is necessary, and the fig is a "die-back" shrub. Ficus carica varieties have been grown in Southern Ontario for many years. Though by no means very much north of Pennsylvania, it is still further north. The figs need mulching, as in Philadelphia, and are die-back shrubs but they do produce very sweet fruit. Some that I have seen will grow back to about 10 or more feet in height, others about 6 or 7 feet, in a season. Some years the crop is quite heavy. People who bury their trees, as some still do, or give them the shelter of a house wall and some insulation, often have small trees, and these bear quite heavily.") It is said to have been introduced into England by the Romans, but was probably introduced from Italy early in the sixteenth century, when the Fig tree still growing in Lambeth Palace garden is said to have been planted.

The trees live to a great age, and along the southern coast of England bear fruit abundantly as standard trees, though in Scotland and many parts of England a south wall is indispensable for their successful cultivation out of doors. Old quarries are good situations for them. The roots are free from stagnant water and they are sheltered from cold, while exposed to a hot sun, which ripens the fruit perfectly. The trees also succeed well planted in a paved court against a building with a south aspect.

The best soil for a Fig border is a friable loam, not too rich, but well-drained; a chalky subsoil is congenial to the tree. To correct the tendency to over-luxuriance of growth, the roots should be confined within spaces surrounded by a wall enclosing an area of about a square yard. Grown as a standard, the tree needs very little pruning. When against a wall, a single stem should be trained to a height of a foot and a shoot be trained to either side - one to the right and the other to the left.

The principal part needing protection in the winter is the main stem, which is more tender than the young wood.

Fig trees are propagated by cuttings, which should be put into pots and placed in a gentle hot-bed. They may be obtained more speedily from layers, and these when rooted will form plants ready to bear fruit the first or second year after planting.

There are numerous varieties of Fig in cultivation, bearing fruit of various colors, from deep purple to yellow or nearly white.

The Fig produces naturally two sets of shoots and two crops of fruit in the season. The first shoots generally show young Figs in July and August but those in England rarely ripen and should therefore be rubbed off. The late midsummer shoots also put forth fruit buds which, however, do not develop till the following spring, ripening in late September and October, and these form the only crop of Figs on which the English gardener can depend.

There is sometimes a failure in the Fig crop, many immature receptacles dropping off in consequence of the pistils of the florets not having been duly fertilized by the pollen of the stamens. It is supposed that fertilization is caused naturally by the entry of insects through the very small orifice which remains open in the flowering Fig. Fig growers therefore adopt an artificial means of ensuring fertilization: a small feather is inserted and turned round in the internal cavity, the pollen thus being brushed against the pistils. This process is called 'Caprification," from the Latin caprificus (a wild Fig), as the same result was originally obtained in the countries where the Fig grows wild, by placing branches of the Wild Fig in flower over the cultivated bushes, so that the pollen might be shaken out over the orifices of their receptacles, thus ensuring the development of the young fruit.

Most of our supplies of dried Figs come from Asia Minor, Spain, Malta and the South of France. When the fruits are ripe, they are collected and dried in the sun. 'Natural' Figs are those which are packed loose and retain to some extent their original shape. 'Pulled' Figs have been kneaded and pulled to make them supple; they are usually packed for exportation in small square or circular boxes the latter being termed 'drums' - and are considered to be the best variety. A few bay leaves are put upon the top of each box, to keep the fruit from being injured by a gnat which feeds on it and is very destructive. 'Pressed' Figs have been closely packed into boxes so that they are compressed into discs. Maltese Figs are very good, but those from Smyrna, which are thin-skinned and soft (the best kind known as 'Elemi'), are most valued. Greek Figs are thicker skinned, tougher and have less pulp.

Constituents

The chief constituent of Figs is dextrose, of which they contain about 50 per cent.

Uses

Figs have long been employed for their nutritive value and in both their fresh and dried state form a large part of the food of the natives of both Western Asia and Southern Europe.

A sort of cake made by mashing up inferior Figs serves in parts of the Greek Archipelago as a substitute for bread.

Alcohol is obtained from fermented Figs in some southern countries, and a kind of wine, still made from the ripe fruit, was known to the Ancients and is mentioned by Pliny under the name of Sycites.

Medicinal Action and Uses

Figs are used for their mild, laxative action, and are employed in the preparation of laxative confections and syrups, usually with senna and carminatives. It is considered that the laxative property resides in the saccharine juice of the fresh fruit and in the dried fruit is probably due to the indigestible seeds and skin. The three preparations of Fig of the British Pharmacopoeia are Syrup of Figs, a mild laxative, suitable for administration to children; Aromatie Syrup of Figs, Elixir of Figs, or Sweet Essence of Figs, an excellent laxative for children and delicate persons, is compounded of compound tincture of rhubarb, liquid extract of senna, compound spirit of orange, liquid extract of cascara and Syrup of Figs. The Compound Syrup of Figs is a stronger preparation, composed of liquid extract of senna, syrup of rhubarb and Syrup of Figs, and is more suitable for adults.

Figs are demulcent as well as nutritive. Demulcent decoctions are prepared from them and employed in the treatment of catarrhal affections of the nose and throat.

Roasted and split into two portions, the soft pulpy interior of Figs may be applied as emolient poultices to gumboils, dental abscesses and other circumscribed maturating tumors. They were used by Hezekiah as a remedy for boils 2,400 years ago (Isaiah xxxviii. 21).

The milky juice of the freshly-broken stalk of a Fig has been found to remove warts on the body. When applied, a slightly inflamed area appears round the wart, which then shrivels and falls off. The milky juice of the stems and leaves is very acrid and has been used in some countries for raising blisters.

The wood of the tree is porous and of little value, though a piece, saturated with oil and spread with emery, is in France a common substitute for a hone.

Green Fig Jam is excellent. Choose very juicy Figs. Take off the stalks, but do not peel them. Make a syrup of 1/2 lb. of sugar and a glass of water (1/2 pint) for each pound of fruit. Put the Figs into it and cook them till the syrup pearls. Boil a stick of cinnamon with them and remove it before pouring the jam into pots.

The Sycamore Fig (Ficus Sycamorus) is a tree of large size, with heart-shaped, somewhat mulberry-like leaves. It is a favorite tree in Egypt and Syria, being often planted along roads, deep shade being cast by its spreading branches. It bears a sweet, edible fruit, somewhat like that of the Common Fig, but produced in racemes, on the older branches. The Ancients, after soaking it in water, preserved it like the Common Fig. The porous wood is only fit for fuel.

Our northern Sycamore tree is in no way related to this Sycamore Fig, but has wrongly acquired its name, Prior says, through a mistake of the botanist Ruellius, who transferred the Greek name, Sycamoros, properly the name of the Wild Fig, to the great Maple.

'This mistake," says Prior, 'arose perhaps from this tree, the great maple, being on account of the density of its foliage, used in the sacred dramas of the Middle

Ages to represent the Fig tree into which Zaccheus climbed and that in which the Virgin Mary on her journey into Egypt had hidden herself and the infant Jesus to avoid the fury of Herod; a legend quoted by Stapel on Theophrastus and by Thevenot in his Voyage de Levant: "At Mathave is a large sycamore or Pharaoh's Fig, very old, but which bears fruit every year. They say that upon the Virgin passing that way with her son Jesus and being pursued by the people, this Fig tree opened to receive her and closed her in again, until the people had passed by and then opened again. The tree is still shown to travellers." " (See Cowper's Apocryphal Gospels.)

FIGWORT, KNOTTED

Botanical: Scrophularia nodosa
Family: N.O. Scrophulariaceae
Synonyms: Throatwort. Carpenter's Square. Kernelwort.
(Welsh) Deilen Ddu.
(Irish) Rose Noble.
(French) Herbe du Siège.
Part Used: Herb.

The Knotted Figwort, common throughout England, is similar in general habit to the Water Figwort, but differs both in the form of its root and in having more acutely heartshaped leaves. The stem, too, is without the projections or wings at its angles, and the lobes of the calyx have only a very narrow membraneous margin. The plant, also, though found in rather moist, bushy places, either in cultivated or waste ground, and in damp woods, is not distinctly an aquatic, like the Water Figwort.

The flowers, which resemble in appearance and character the Water Figwort, are in bloom during July and are specially visited by wasps.

During the thirteen months' siege of Rochelle by the army of Richelieu in 1628, the tuberous roots of this Figwort yielded support to the garrison for a considerable period, from which circumstance the French still call it Herbe du siège. The taste and smell of the tubers are unpleasant, and they would never be resorted to for food except in times of famine.

Medicinal Action and Uses

It has been called the Scrofula Plant, on account of its value in all cutaneous eruptions, abscesses, wounds, etc., the name of the genus being derived from that of the disease for which it was formerly considered a specific.

It has diuretic and anodyne properties.

The whole herb is used, collected in June and July and dried. A decoction is made of it for external use and the fresh leaves are also made into an ointment.

Of the different kinds of Figwort used, this species is most employed, principally as a fomentation for sprains, swellings, inflammations, wounds and diseased parts, especially in scrofulous sores and gangrene.

The leaves simply bruised are employed by the peasantry in some districts as an application to burns and swellings.

The Welsh so highly esteem the plant that they call it Deilen Ddu ('good leaf'). In Ireland, it is known as Rose Noble and as Kernelwort. Gerard tells us, referring to what he evidently considered an exaggerated estimate of its worth: 'Divers do rashly teach that if it be hanged about the necke or else carried about one, it keepeth a man in health."

The herb was said to be curative of hydrophobia, by taking

"every morning while fasting a slice of bread and butter on which the powdered knots of the roots had been spread and eating it up with two tumblers of fresh spring water. Then let the patient be well clad in woollen garments and made to take a long, fast walk until in a profuse perspiration, the treatment being continued for seven days."

A decoction of the herb has been successfully used as a cure for the scab in swine. Cattle, as a rule, will refuse to eat the leaves, as they are bitter, acrid and nauseating, producing purging and vomiting if chewed.

Preparation and Dosage

Fluid extract, 1/2 to 1 drachm.

Other Species

BALM-LEAVED FIGWORT (Scrophularia Scorodoma), found only in Cornwall, and at Tralee, in Ireland; it is distinguished by its downy, wrinkled leaves.

YELLOW FIGWORT (S. vernalis) is a plant of local occurrence and is well distinguished by its remarkably bright green foliage and yellow flowers. It appears early in spring and is the only British species which can be called ornamental.

Gerard speaks of the 'yellow-flowered Figwort' as growing in his time 'in the moist medowes as you go from London to Hornsey." He also speaks of the 'rare whiteflowered Betony."

FIGWORT, WATER

Botanical: Scrophularia aquatica (LINN.)
Family: N.O. Scrophulariaceae
Synonyms: Water Betony. Fiddlewood. Fiddler. Crowdy Kit. Brownwort. Bishops' Leaves.
Part Used: Leaves.

The Water Figwort has obtained the name of Water Betony from a certain resemblance of its leaves to those of the Wood Betony, but it differs entirely from that plant in every other respect, not being even closely related to it, and nowadays is more generally called the Water Figwort, the name Figwort being derived from the form of the root in another member of the genus Scrophularia, the Knotted Figwort (S. nodosa), a fairly common plant.

Description

The root of the Water Figwort is perennial and throws out numerouslarge fibres. The plant is to be found only in damp ground, generally by the banks of rivers and ponds. It varies much in size, but on an average, the stems grow to a height of 5 feet. The general character of the stem is upright, though small lateral branches are thrown out from the rigid, straight, main stem, which is smooth and quadrangular, the angles being winged. The stems are often more or less reddish-purple in color; though hollow and succulent, they become rigid when dead, and prove very troublesome to anglers owing to their lines becoming tangled in the withered capsules. The Figwort is named in Somersetshire, 'Crowdy Kit' (the word kit meaning a fiddle), or 'Fiddlewood," because if two of the stalks are rubbed together, they make a noise like the scraping of the bow on violin strings, owing no doubt to the winged angles. In Devonshire, also, the plant is known as 'Fiddler."

The leaves are placed in pairs on the stem, each pair at right angles to the pair below it; all are on footstalks, the pairs generally rather distant from one another on the stem. The leaves are oblong and somewhat heartshaped; smooth, with very conspicuous veining. The flowers grow at the top of the stems, arranged in loose panicles, under each little branch of which is a little floral leaf, or bract. They are in bloom during July and August. The calyx has five conspicuous lobes, fringed by a somewhat ragged-looking, brown, membraneous border. The dark, greenish-purple, sometimes almost brown corolla is almost globular; the lobes at its mouth are very short and broad, the two upper ones stand boldly out from the flower, the two side ones taking the same direction, but are much shorter, and the fifth lobe turned sharply downward. The result is that the flowers look like so many little helmets. There are four anther-bearing stamens, and generally a fifth barren one beneath the upper lip of the corolla. The seed vessel when ripe is a roundish capsule opening with two valves, the edges of which are turned in, and contains numerous small brown seeds.

Wasps and bees are very fond of the flowers, from which they collect much honey.

The leaves are used, collected in June and July, when in best condition, just coming into flower, and used both fresh and dried.

Medicinal Action and Uses

This plant has vulnerary and detergent properties, and has enjoyed some fame as a vulnerary, both when used externally and when taken in decoction.

In modern herbal medicine, the leaves are employed externally as a poultice, or boiled in lard as an ointment for ulcers, piles, scrofulous glands in the neck, sores and wounds. It is said to have been one of the ingredients in Count Matthei's noted remedy, 'AntiScrofuloso."

In former days this herb was relied on for the cure of toothache and for expelling nightmare. It has also a reputation as a cosmetic, old herbalists telling us that:

'the juice or distilled water of the leaves is good for bruises, whether inward or outward, as also to bathe the face and hands spotted or blemished or discoloured by sun burning."

FIREWEED

Botanical: Erechtites hieracifolia (LINN. and RAFIN.), Cineraria Canadensis (WALTER.)
Family: N.O. Compositae
Synonyms: Senecio hieracifolius (Linn.).
Parts Used: Herb, oil.
Habitat: Newfoundland and Canada, southward to South America.

Description

This coarse, homely American weed is an annual and derives its name from its habit of growing freely in moist open woods and clearings, and in greatest luxuriance on newly-burnt fallows. It has composite flowers, blooming from July to September.

Lactuca Canadensis, the wild Lettuce or Trumpet Weed, and Hieracium Canadense, are also given the designation of 'Fireweed' in America from their habit of growing on newly-burnt fallow, but Erechtites hieracifolia (Rafin.) may be called the true Fireweed, as it is the plant which commonly goes by that name.

Senecio is derived from Senex (an old man), in reference to the hoary pappus, which in this order represents the calyx; Erechtites comes from the ancient name of some troublesome Groundsel.

Fireweed is a rank, slightly hairy plant, growing from 1 to 7 feet high. The thick, somewhat fleshy stem is virgate, sulcate, leafy to the top, branching above, the branches erect. The leaves are alternate, delicate and thin, very variable in size and form, lanceovate to linear, apex-pointed, margins irregular, sharply toothed, or divided right down to the midrib into leaflets, which are sometimes then bipinnatifid, the lower, very short-stalked and becoming sessile as they grow up the stem. The flowers are white or yellow, a corymbose panicle. The little fruits are oblong, slender, tapering at the end, striate and crowned with a very fine copious silky pappus, white or violet. The whole plant is succulent, the odor rank and slightly aromatic, with a bitterish and somewhat acrid and disagreeable taste.

In the United States Fireweed is a very troublesome weed; the fields often get infested with it, and when growing among Peppermint, it is definitely destructive, as it gets mingled with the plant in distilling and causes great deterioration of the oil.

Constituents

A peculiar volatile oil - oil of Erechtites - transparent and yellow, obtained by distilling the plant with water, taste bitter and burning, odor foetid, slightly aromatic, somewhat resembling oil of Erigeron, but not soluble as that is in an equal volume of alcohol. The specific gravity of the oil is variously given as 0.927 and 0.838-0.855, and its rotation 1 to 2. According to Bielstein and Wiegand, it consists almost wholly of terpenes boiling between 175 and 310 degrees F.

Medicinal Action and Uses

Astringent, alterative, tonic, cathartic, emetic. Much used among the aborigines of North America in various forms of eczema, muco-sanguineous diarrhea, and hemorrhages, also for relaxed throat and sore throat, and in the United States Eclectic Dispensatory in the form of oil and as an infusion, both herb and oil being beneficial for piles and dysentery. For its anti-spasmodic properties, it has been found useful for colic, spasms and hiccough. Applied externally, it gives great relief in the pains of gout, rheumatism and sciatica.

Dosage

(Internally) 5 to 10 drops on sugar, in capsules or in emulsion.

The homeopathic tincture is made from the whole fresh flowering plant. It is chopped, pounded to a pulp and weighed. Then two parts by weight of alcohol are taken, the pulp mixed thoroughly with one-sixth part of it and the rest of the alcohol added. After having stirred the whole, it is poured into a well-stoppered bottle and allowed to stand for eight days in a dark, cool place.

The resulting tincture has a clear, beautiful, reddish-orange color by transmitted light; a sourish odor, resembling that of claret, a taste at first sourish, then astringent and bitter, and an acid reaction.

FIVE-LEAF GRASS

Botanical: Potentilla reptans (LINN.)
Family: N.O. Rosaceae
Synonyms: Cinquefoil. Five Fingers. Five-Finger Blossom. Sunkfield. Synkefoyle.
Parts Used: Herb, root.

Five-leaf Grass is a creeping plant with large yellow flowers like the Silverweed, each one growing on its own long stalk, which springs from the point at which the leaf joins the stem.

Description

The rootstock branches at the top from several crowns, from which arise the long-stalked root-leaves and thread-like, creeping stems, which bear stalked leaves and solitary flowers. These stem-runners root at intervals and as they often attain a length of 5 feet, the plant is rapidly propagated, spreading over a wide area. It grows freely in meadows, pastures and by the wayside.

The name Five-leaved or Five Fingers refers to the leaves being divided into five leaflets. Each of these is about 1 1/2 inch long, with scattered hairs on the veins and margin, the veins being prominent below. The margins of the leaflets are much serrated. In rich soils the leaflets are often six or seven. Out of a hundred blossoms once picked as a test, eighty had the parts of the corolla, calyx and epicalyx in fives, and the remaining twenty were in sixes.

Although the flowers much resemble those of the Silverweed, the two plants can readily be distinguished by the difference in their leaves. The flowers secrete honey on a ringlike ridge surrounding the base of the stamens. Insects alighting on the petals dust themselves with the pollen, but do not touch the stigmas, as the honey ring extends beyond. If they alight in the middle of the next flower, they dust the pollen against the stigma and cross-pollinate it. But the flower is often self-pollinated. The flowers close up in part in dull weather and completely at night, and it is then that the anthers touch the stigmas.

Bacon says that frogs have a predilection for sitting on this herb: 'The toad will be much under Sage, frogs will be in Cinquefoil."

It was an ingredient in many spells in the Middle Ages, and was particularly used as a magic herb in love divinations. It was one of the ingredients of a special bait for fishing nets, which was held to ensure a heavy catch. This concoction consisted of corn boiled in thyme and marjoram water, mixed with nettles, cinquefoil and the juice of houseleek.

In an old recipe called 'Witches' Ointment' the juice of Five-leaf Grass, smallage and wolfsbane is mixed with the fat of children dug up from their graves and added to fine wheat flour.

Medicinal Action and Uses

stringent, febrifuge. The roots have a bitterish, styptic, slightly sweetish taste and have been employed medicinally since the time of Hippocrates and Dioscorides.

They were used to cure the intermittent fevers which prevailed in marshy, ill-drained lands, and especially ague.

Dioscorides stated that one leaf cured a quotidian, three a tertian, and four a quarten ague.

Culpepper says:

'It is an especial herb used in all inflammations and fevers, whether infectious or pestilential or, among other herbs, to cool and temper the blood and humours in the body; as also for all lotions, gargles and infections; for sore mouths, ulcers, cancers, fistulas and other foul or running sores.

'The juice drank, about four ounces at a time, for certain days together, cureth the quinsey and yellow jaundice, and taken for 30 days cureth the falling sickness. The roots boiled in vinegar and the decoction held in the mouth easeth toothache.

'The juice or decoction taken with a little honey removes hoarseness and is very good for coughs.

'The root boiled in vinegar, being applied, heals inflammations, painful sores and the shingles. The same also, boiled in wine, and applied to any joint full of pain, ache or the gout in the hands, or feet or the hip-joint, called the sciatica, and the decoction thereof drank the while, doth cure them and easeth much pain in the bowels.

'The roots are also effectual to reduce ruptures, being used with other things available to that purpose, taken either inwardly or outwardly, or both; as also bruises or hurts by blows, falls or the like, and to stay the bleeding of wounds in any part, inward or outward."

Robinson's Herbal directs that the roots are to be dug up in April and the outer bark taken off and dried, the rest not being used.

To make the decoction, it is directed that 1 1/2 OZ. of the root be boiled in a quart of water down to a pint. This decoction is recommended not only as a remedy for diarrhea, and of avail to stop bleeding of the lungs or bronchial tubes and bleeding at the nose, but as a good eyewash, as well as a gargle in relaxed sore throat.

The juice of the root, mixed with wheat bread, boiled first, is recommended as a good styptic.

A scruple of the powder in wine is the dose prescribed to cure the ague.

In modern Herbal Medicine, the dried herb is more generally now employed, for its astringent and febrifuge properties.

An infusion of 1 OZ. of the herb to a pint of boiling water is used in wine glassful doses for diarrhea and looseness of the bowels, and for other complaints for which astringents are usually prescribed, and it is employed externally as an astringent lotion and as a gargle for sore throat.

Preparation and Dosage

Fluid extract, 1/2 to 2 drachms.

FLAX

Botanical: Linum usitatissimum (LINN.)
Family: N.O. Linaceae
Synonym: Linseed.
Part Used: Seed.

History

Flax is one of the English-grown medicinal herbs, the products of which are included in the British Pharmacopoeia, its seed known as Linseed, being much employed in medicine.

Its cultivation reaches back to the remotest periods of history, Flax seeds as well as the woven cloth having been found in Egyptian tombs. It has been cultivated in all temperate and tropical regions for so many centuries that its geographical origin cannot be identified, for it readily escapes from cultivation and is found in a semi-wild condition in all the countries where it is grown.

The 'fine linen' mentioned in the Bible has been satisfactorily proved to have been spun from Flax; it was the plant to which the plague of hail proved so disastrous (Exodus ix. 31). Joseph was arrayed in this product (Genesis xii. 42), and it also furnished the garments of the Jewish High-Priests (Exodus xxviii.) as well as the curtains of the Tabernacle (Exodus xxvi. 1). We learn that the knowledge of spinning this linen was known to the Canaanites (see Joshua

ii. 6), and in New Testament times it formed the clothing of the Saviour in the tomb where Joseph of Arimathaea laid Him.

It was used for cord and sail-cloth ('white sails' are mentioned by Homer in the Odyssey), and it was used for lamp-wicks (Isaiah xlii. 3).

The seed-vessels with their five-celled capsules are referred to in the Bible as 'bolls," and the expression 'the flax was bolled' (Exodus ix. 31) means that it had arrived at a state of maturity. When the bolls are ripe, the Flax is pulled and tied in bundles, and in order to assist the separation of the fibre from the stalks, the bundles are placed in water for several weeks, and then spread out to dry. This custom is alluded to in Joshua ii. 6.

Pliny writes:

'What department is there to be found of active life in which flax is not employed? And in what production of the Earth are there greater marvels to us than in this? To think that here is a plant which brings Egypt to close proximity to Italy! - so much so, in fact, that Galerius and Balbillus, both of them prefects of Egypt, made the passage to Alexandria from the Straits of Sicily, the one in six days, the other in five! . . . What audacity in man! What criminal perverseness! Thus to sow a thing in the ground for the purpose of catching the winds and tempests; it being not enough for him, forsooth, to be borne upon the waves alone!"

Bartholomew the mediaeval herbalist, refers to the making of linen from the soaking of Flax in water till it is dried and turned in the sun and then bound in 'praty bundels' and afterwards 'knockyd, beten and brayd and carflyd, rodded and gnodded; ribbyd and heklyd, and at the last sponne'; of the bleaching, and finally of its many uses for making clothing, and for sails, and fish-nets, and thread and ropes, and strings ('for bows'), and measuring lines, and sheets ('to reste in'), and 'sackes and bagges, and purses (to put and to kepe thynges in').

Of the making of tow 'uneven and full of knobs' used for stuffing into the cracks in ships, and 'for bonds and byndynges and matches for candelles, for it is full drye and taketh sone fyre and brenneth."'And so," he concludes somewhat breathlessly, 'none herbe is so needfull to so many dyurrse uses to mankynde as is the flexe."

Darwin studied several species of Linum, and found that some like the primrose had flowers with two forms of stamens and pistil. His object was to test the relative degrees of fertility of the long and short-styled pistils. L. perenne, for instance, is dimorphic:

'Of the flowers on the long-styled plants he found that twelve were fertilized with their own form pollen, but from a different plant. A seed capsule was only set when pollinated from anthers of the same height as the stigmas."

So Darwin concluded:

'We have the clearest evidence that the stigmas of each form require for full fertility that pollen from the stamens of a corresponding height, belonging to the opposite form, should be brought to them." (Forms of Flowers, p. 92.)

This plant is visited by bees, who perform the function Darwin describes.

The Flax is a graceful little plant with turquoise blue blossoms, a tall, erect annual, 1 to 2 feet high, the stems usually solitary quite smooth, with alternate, linear, sessile leaves, 3/4 to 1 inch long.

Many traditions are associated with this useful plant. Flax flowers were believed in the Middle Ages to be a protection against sorcery. The Bohemians have a belief that if seven-year-old children dance among Flax, they will become beautiful, and the whole plant was supposed to be under the protection of the goddess Hulda, who, in Teuton mythology, was held to have first taught mortals the art of growing Flax, of spinning, and of weaving it.

Cultivation and Preparation for Market

Linseed requires ground as rich as for wheat, and if cultivated for seed is not of much use for Flax.

Its cultivation in this country could only pay on a large scale. The very exhausting nature of the crop has prevented its extensive cultivation in England, and the area under cultivation has declined in consequence. This peculiarity was well known to the Ancients, and Pliny asserted that it scorched the ground. Its culture requires care and suitable soil to secure a good crop. It has been grown in large quantities in the alluvial soils of Lincolnshire and in the eastern counties, and flourishes well in Ireland. It succeeds best in deep, moist loams such as contain a large proportion of vegetable matter, in good condition, firm, not loose. Strong clays do not answer well, nor poor soils, nor such as are of a gravelly or sandy nature, nor should the soil be freshly manured.

It is best treated as a farm crop. Being quickly grown and quickly harvested, it can be grown after a winter root crop, being over and reaped in time to secure a catch crop for the following season. The seed, which must be kept dry, as damp injures it, is sown in March or April, in drills, 70 lb. to the acre, on land carefully prepared and freed from weeds by ploughing. The crop itself must be handweeded, or the roots, being surface rooted, will be injured. It should be reaped in August, before the seed is fully ripe. The fibres of the plant, when grown for Flax, are found to be softer and stronger when the blossom has just fallen and the stalk begins to turn yellow before the leaves fall, than if left standing till the seeds are quite mature. The seeds, however, will ripen after the plant is gathered, if they be allowed to remain on the plant for a time. The Dutch avail themselves of this fact with regard to their Flax crops. After pulling the plants they stack them. The seeds by this means ripen, while the fibres are collected at the most favourable period of their growth. They thus obtain both of the valuable products of the plant.

Parts Used Medicinally

The fruit is a globular capsule, about the size of a small pea, containing in separate cells ten seeds, which are brown (white within), oval-oblong and flattened, pointed at one end, shining and polished on the surface, 1/6 to 1/4 inch long. They are inodorous except when powdered, but the taste is mucilaginous and slightly unpleasant.

Linseed varies much in size and tint - a yellowish variety occurring in India. Holland, Russia, the United States, Canada, the Argentine and India furnish the principal supplies. The Russian seed or Dutch-grown of Russian origin, though small, is preferred for Flax-growing, as it is hardier than the large southern seed from the Mediterranean and India. For medicinal purposes, English and Dutch seeds are preferred, on account of their freedom from weedseeds and dirt. If containing more than 4 per cent of weedseeds, linseed may be said to be adulterated. Of English and Dutch seeds about twelve weigh 1 grain, but some of the Indian and Mediterranean varieties are twice as large and heavy.

Constituents

The envelope or testa of the seed contains about 15 per cent of mucilage. The seeds themselves contain in the cotyledons and endosperm from 30 to 40 per cent of a fixed oil, of a light yellow color, and about 25 per cent proteids, together with wax, resin, sugar, phosphates, acetic acid, and a small quantity of the glucoside Linamarin. On incineration, linseed should not yield more than 5 per cent of ash.

The oil is obtained by expression, with little or no heat. The cake which remains after expressing the oil, and which contains the farinaceous and mucilaginous part of the seed, is familiarly known as oil-cake, and is largely used as a fattening food for cattle. It is also used as a manure. When ground up, it is known as linseed meal, which is employed for making poultices. The meal is sold in two forms, crushed linseed and linseed meal. Formerly linseed meal was always obtained by grinding English oil-cake to powder and contained little oil, but now the crushed seeds, containing all the oil, are official. Crushed linseed of good quality usually contains from 30 to 35 per cent of oil.

Linseed oil rapidly absorbs oxygen from the air and forms, when laid on in thin layers, a hard, transparent varnish. It is largely used in the arts for its properties as a drying oil. It is a viscid, yellow liquid, its chief constituent being Linolein. It also contains palmitin, stearin and myristin, with glyceride of linoleic acid. Boiled oil, produced by heating raw linseed oil to a temperature of 150 degrees C., together with a small proportion of a metallic drier, possesses the drying properties of linseed oil to an enhanced degree. It becomes of a brown color and dries much more rapidly, and in this state is used in the manufacture of printer's ink.

Medicinal Action and Uses

Emollient, demulcent, pectoral. The crushed seeds or linseed meal make a very useful poultice, either alone or with mustard. In ulceration and superficial or deep-seated inflammation a linseed poultice allays irritation and pain and promotes suppuration. The addition of a little lobelia seed makes it of greater value in cases of boils. It is commonly used for abscesses and other local affections.

Linseed is largely employed as an addition to cough medicines. As a domestic remedy for colds, coughs and irritation of the urinary organs, linseed tea is most valuable. A little honey and lemon juice makes it very agreeable and more efficacious. This demulcent infusion contains a large quantity of mucilage, and is made from 1 OZ. of the ground or entire seeds to 1 pint of boiling water. It is taken in wine glassful doses, which may be repeated ad libitum.

Linseed oil, mixed with an equal quantity of lime water, known then as Carron Oil, is an excellent application for burns and scalds.

Internally, the oil is sometimes given as a laxative; in cases of gravel and stone it is excellent, and has been administered in pleurisy with great success. It may also be used as an injection in constipation. Mixed with honey, linseed oil has been used as a cosmetic for removing spots from the face.

The oil enters into veterinary pharmacy as a purgative for sheep and horses, and a jelly formed by boiling the seeds is often given to calves.

Linseed is often employed, with other seeds, as food for small birds.

Plantain seeds, also a favorite food of small birds, can, it is said, be used instead of linseed in making poultices, as they contain much mucilage, though not so much oil.

Linseed has occasionally been employed as human food - we hear of the seeds being mixed with corn by the ancient Greeks and Romans for making bread - but it affords little actual nourishment and is apparently unwholesome, being difficult of digestion and provoking flatulence.

The meal has sometimes been used fraudulently for adulterating pepper.

FLAX, MOUNTAIN

Botanical: Linum catharticum (LINN.)
Family: N.O. Linaceae
Synonyms: Purging Flax. Dwarf Flax. Fairy Flax. Mill Mountain.
Part Used: Whole Herb.

Mountain Flax is a pretty little herb, which grows profusely in hilly pastures.

Description

It is an annual, with a small, thready root, which sends up several slender, smooth, straight stems, which rise to a height of 6 to 8 inches, and are sometimes branched towards the upper part. The leaves are small, linear-oblong and obtuse, the lower ones opposite, and the upper alternate. The flowers, 1/3 to 1/4 of an inch in diameter, are white. The plant at first glance much resembles chickweed, being glaucous and glabrous.

Part Used

The whole herb is used mediinally, both fresh and dried, collected in July, when in flower, in the wild state.

Constituents

A green, bitter resin and a neutral, colorless, crystalline principle of a persistently bitter taste, called Linin, to which the herb owes its activity.

Medicinal Action and Uses

This herb was highly extolled by Gerard as a purgative. It operates chiefly as a gentle cathartic, and is useful in all cases where a brisk purgative is required. As a laxative, it is preferred to senna, though the action is very similar. It is generally taken combined with a carminative, such as peppermint.

The dried herb has been found very useful in muscular rheumatism and catarrhal affections, the infusion of 1 oz. in a pint of boiling water being taken in wine glassful doses. In liver complaints and jaundice, it has been employed with benefit.

FLAX, PERENNIAL

Botanical: Linum perenne
Family: N.O. Linaceae
Part Used: Seeds.

Preparations and Dosage

Fluid extract, 10 to 30 drops.

A tincture is also made from the entire fresh plant, 2 or 3 drops in water being given every hour or two for diarrhea.

Country people boil the fresh herb and take it for rheumatic pains, colds, coughs and dropsy.

The Perennial Flax is a native plant not uncommon in some parts of the country upon calcareous soils. It grows about 2 feet in height and is readily distinguished from the annual kind by its paler flowers and narrower leaves. The rootstock usually throws up many stems. It flowers in July.

This species has been recommended for cultivation as a fibre plant, but it has been little adopted, the fibre being coarser and the seeds smaller than those of the Common Flax.

As the plant will last several years and yields an abundant crop of stems, it might be advantageously grown for paper making.

The seeds contain the same kind of oil as the ordinary species.

The All-Seed or Flax-Seed (Radiola linoides) belongs to the Flax family also; it is a minute annual with very fine, repeatedly forked branches. The leaves are opposite. Flowers in clusters very small, and seeding abundantly. It occurs inland on gravelly and sandy places, but is not common, from the Orkneys to Cornwall, e.g., near St. Ives, on the hills, and in the New Forest, near Lyndhurst.

Culpepper mentions remedies which include 'Linseed," more than once - usually in the form of 'mussilage of Lin-seed'; in one he mentions 'the seeds of Flax' and (later in the same prescription) 'Linseed." He says it 'heats and moistens, helps pains of the breast, coming cold and pleurises, old aches, and stitches, and softens hard swellings."

FLEABANE, CANADIAN

Botanical: Erigeron Canadense (LINN.)
Family: N.O. Compositae
Synonyms: Fleawort. Coltstail. Prideweed.
Parts Used: Herb, seeds.

Habitat

This species of Fleabane is an American annual, common in Northern and Middle States as well as in Canada, growing in fields and meadows and by roadsides, and closely allied to the Common Fleabane.

History

It was introduced into Europe in the seventeenth century. Parkinson, in his Theatrum Botanicum (1640), mentions it as having been brought to Europe, but describes it as an American species, not yet growing in England. In 1653 we hear of it growing in the Botanic Gardens of Paris, and soon after it had become a weed about Paris. We first hear of it in England in 1669, and since its introduction it has often been found in the neighborhood of London and in the Thames Valley, where it appears to have naturalized itself here and there, though it is very rare in the rest of England. Green (Universal Herbal, 1832) stated that it was to be found on cultivated ground in

Glamorganshire and also on rubbish heaps.

The name Erigeron denotes 'soon becoming old," and is most appropriate, for in many of the species the plant, even when in flower, has a worn-out appearance, giving the idea of a weed which has passed its prime.

Parkinson says Fleabane 'bound to the forehead is a great helpe to cure one of the frensie."

Culpepper says 'Flea-wort' (Fleabane) obtained its name 'because the seeds are so like Fleas'!

Description

It has an unbranched stem, with lance-shaped leaves, the lower ones with short stalks and with five teeth, the upper ones with uncut edges and narrower, 1 to 2 inches long. The stem is bristly and grows several feet high, bearing composite heads of flowers, small, white and very numerous, blossoming from June to September.

Part Used

The whole herb is gathered when in bloom and dried in bunches. The seeds are also used.

Constituents

The herb contains a bitter extractive, tannic and gallic acids and a volatile oil, to which its virtues are due

Medicinal Action and Uses

Astringent, diuretic, tonic. It is considered useful in gravel, diabetes, dropsy and many kidney diseases, and is employed in diarrhea and dysentery.

Oil of Erigeron resembles in its action Oil of Turpentine, but is less irritating. It has been used to arrest hemorrhage from the lungs or alimentary tract, but this property is not assigned to it in modern medicine.

It is said to be a valuable remedy for inflamed tonsils and ulceration and inflammation of the throat generally.

The drug has a feeble odor and an astringent, aromatic and bitter taste. It is given in infusion (dose, wine glassful to a teacupful), oil (dose, 2 to 5 drops) on sugar. Fluid extract, 1/2 to 1 drachm.

FLEABANE, COMMON

Botanial: Inula dysenterica (LINN.)
Family: N.O. Compositae
Synonyms: Pulicaria dysenterica (Gaertn.). Middle Fleabane.
(Arabian) Rarajeub.
Parts Used: Herb, root.

Habitat

This species is a native of most parts of Europe, in moist meadows, watery places, by the sides of ditches, brooks and rivers, growing in masses and frequently overrunning large tracts of land on account of its creeping underground stems. In Scotland, however, it is rare, though common in Ireland.

The Common Fleabane is nearly related to elecampane and other species of Inula, and by Linnaeus, whom Hooker follows, is assigned to the same genus, although placed, with a smaller variety, in a separate genus, Pulicaria, by the botanist Gaertner.

This plant has medicinal properties, and though in England it has never had much reputation as a curative agent it has ranked high in the estimation of herbalists abroad. It was formerly used in dysentery, and on this account received its specific name from Linnaeus, who in his Flora Suecia says that he had been informed by General Keit, of the Russian Army, that his soldiers, in one of their expeditions against Persia, were cured of dysentery by means of this plant. Our old authors call it 'Middle Fleabane' - Ploughman's Spikenard being the Great Fleabane; both names being derived from the fact that, if burnt, the smoke from them drives away fleas and other insects. The generic name, Pulicaria, refers to this property, the Latin name for the flea being Pulex.

By the Arabians, it is called Rarajeub, or Job's Tears, from a tradition that Job used a decoction of this herb to cure his ulcers. It was formerly recommended for the itch and other cutaneous disorders.

Description

It is a rough-looking plant, well marked by its soft, hoary foliage, and large terminal flat heads of bright yellow flowers, single, or one or two together, about an inch across, large in proportion to the size of the plant, the ray florets very numerous, long and narrow, somewhat paler than the florets in the centre or disk.

The creeping rootstock is perennial, and sends up at intervals stems reaching a height of 1 to 2 feet. These stems are woolly, branched above and very leafy, the leaves oblong, 1 1/2 to 2 1/2 inches long, heart or arrowshaped at the base, embracing the stem, irregularly waved and toothed. Like the stem, the leaves are more or less covered with a woolly substance, varying a good deal in different plants. The under surface is ordinarily more woolly than the upper, and though the general effect of the foliage varies according to its degree of woolliness, it is at best a somewhat dull and greyish green.

The plant is in bloom from the latter part of July to September. The fruit is silky and crowned by a few short, unequal hairs of a dirty-white, with an outer ring of very short bristles or scales, a characteristic which distinguishes it from Elecampane and other members of the genus Inula, whose pappus consists of a single row of hairs this being the differing point which has led to its being assigned to a distinct genus, Pulicaria.

Another English plant bears the name of Fleabane (Erigeron acris), a member of the same order. For the sake of distinction, it is commonly known as the Blue Fleabane, its flowerheads having a yellow centre, and being surrounded by purplish rays. It is a smaller, far less striking plant, growing in dry situations.

Medicinal Action and Uses

The leaves when bruised have a somewhat soap-like smell. The sap that lies in the tissues is bitter, astringent and saltish, so that animals will not eat the plant, and this astringent character, to which no doubt the medicinal properties are to be ascribed, is imparted to decoctions and infusions of the dried herb.

FOXGLOVE

POISON
Botanical: Digitalis purpurea (LINN.)
Family: N.O. Scrophulariaceae
Synonyms: Witches' Gloves. Dead Men's Bells. Fairy's Glove. Gloves of Our Lady. Bloody Fingers. Virgin's Glove. Fairy Caps. Folk's Glove. Fairy Thimbles.
(Norwegian) Revbielde.
(German) Fingerhut.
Part Used: Leaves.

Habitat

The Common Foxglove of the woods (Digitalis purpurea), perhaps the handsomest of our indigenous plants, is widely distributed throughout Europe and is common as a wild-flower in Great Britain, growing freely in woods and lanes, particularly in South Devon, ranging from Cornwall and Kent to Orkney, but not occurring in Shetland, or in some of the eastern counties of England. It flourishes best in siliceous soil and grows well in loam, but is entirely absent from some calcareous districts, such as the chain of the Jura, and is also not found in the Swiss Alps. It occurs in Madeira and the Azores, but is, perhaps, introduced there. The genus contains only this one indigenous species, though several are found on the Continent.

Needing little soil, it is found often in the crevices of granite walls, as well as in dry hilly pastures, rocky places and by roadsides. Seedling Foxgloves spring up rapidly from recently-turned earth. Turner (1548), says that it grows round rabbitholes freely.

Description

The normal life of a Foxglove plant is two seasons, but sometimes the roots, which are formed of numerous, long, thick fibres, persist and throw up flowers for several seasons.

In the first year a rosette of leaves, but no stem, is sent up. In the second year, one or more flowering stems are thrown up, which are from 3 to 4 feet high, though even sometimes more, and bear long spikes of drooping flowers, which bloom in the early summer, though the time of flowering differs much, according to the locality. As a rule the flowers are in perfection in July. As the blossoms on the main stem gradually fall away, smaller lateral shoots are often thrown out from its lower parts, which remain in flower after the principal stem has shed its blossoms. These are also promptly developed if by mischance the central stem sustains any serious injury.

The radical leaves are often a foot or more long, contracted at the base into a long, winged footstalk, the wings formed by the lower veins running down into it some distance. They have slightly indented margins and sloping lateral veins, which are a very prominent feature. The flowering stems give off a few leaves, that gradually diminish in size from below upwards. All the leaves are covered with small, simple, unbranched hairs.

The flowers are bell-shaped and tubular, 1 1/2 to 2 1/2 inches long, flattened above, inflated beneath, crimson outside above and paler beneath, the lower lip furnished with long hairs inside and marked with numerous dark crimson spots, each surrounded with a white border. The shade of the flowers varies much, especially under cultivation, sometimes the corollas being found perfectly white.

In cultivated plants there frequently occurs a malformation, whereby one or two of the uppermost flowers become united, and form an erect, regular, cup-shaped flower, through the centre of which the upper extremity of the stem is more or less prolonged.

The Foxglove is a favorite flower of the honey-bee, and is entirely developed by the visits of this insect. For that reason, its tall and stately spikes of flowers are at their best in those sunny, midsummer days when the bees are busiest. The projecting lower lip of the corolla forms an alighting platform for the bee, and as he pushes his way up the bell, to get at the honey which lies in a ring round the seed vessel at the top of the flower, the anthers of the stamens which lie flat on the corolla above him, are rubbed against his back. Going from flower to flower up the spike, he rubs pollen thus from one blossom on to the cleft stigma of another blossom, and thus the flower is fertilized and seeds are able to be produced. The life of each flower, from the time the bud opens till the time it slips off its corolla, is about six days. An almost incredible number of seeds are produced, a single Foxglove plant providing from one to two million seeds to ensure its propagation.

It is noteworthy that although the flower is such a favorite with bees and is much visited by other smaller insects, who may be seen taking refuge from cold and wet in its drooping blossoms on chilly evenings, yet no animals will browse upon the plant, perhaps instinctively recognizing its poisonous character.

The Foxglove derives its common name from the shape of the flowers resembling the finger of a glove. It was originally Folksglove - the glove of the 'good folk' or fairies, whose favorite haunts were supposed to be in the deep hollows and woody dells, where the Foxglove delights to grow. Folksglove is one of its oldest names, and is mentioned in a list of plants in the time of Edward III. Its Norwegian name, Revbielde (Foxbell), is the only foreign one that alludes to the Fox, though there is a northern legend that bad fairies gave these blossoms to the fox that he might put them on his toes to soften his tread when he prowled among the roosts.

The earliest known form of the word is the Anglo-Saxon foxes glofa (the glove of the fox).

The mottlings of the blossoms of the Foxglove and the Cowslip, like the spots on butterfly wings and on the tails of peacocks and pheasants, were said to mark where the elves had placed their fingers, and one legend ran that the marks on the Foxglove were a warning sign of the baneful juices secreted by the plant, which in Ireland gain it the popular name of 'Dead Man's Thimbles." In Scotland, it forms the badge of the Farquharsons, as the Thistle does of the Stuarts. The German name Fingerhut (thimble) suggested to Leonhard Fuchs (the well-known German herbalist of the sixteenth century, after whom the Fuchsia has been named) the employment of the Latin adjective Digitalis (from Digitabulum, a thimble) as a designation for the plant, which, as he remarked, up to the time when he thus named it, in 1542, had had no name in either Greek or Latin.

The Foxglove was employed by the old herbalists for various purposes in medicine, most of them wholly without reference to those valuable properties which render it useful as a remedy in the hands of modern physicians. Gerard recommends it to those 'who have fallen from high places," and Parkinson speaks highly of the bruised herb or of its expressed juice for scrofulous swellings, when applied outwardly in the form of an ointment, and the bruised leaves for cleansing for old sores and ulcers. Dodoens (1554) prescribed it boiled in wine as an expectorant, and it seems to have been in frequent use in cases in which the practitioners of the present day would consider it highly dangerous. Culpepper says it is of: 'a gentle, cleansing nature and withal very friendly to nature. The Herb is familiarly and frequently used by the Italians to heal any fresh or green wound, the leaves being but bruised and bound thereon and the juice thereof is also used in old sores, to cleanse, dry and heal them. It has been found by experience to be available for the King's evil, the herb bruised and applied, or an ointment made with the juice thereof, and so used.... I am confident that an ointment of it is one of the best remedies for a scabby head that is." Strangely enough, the Foxglove, so handsome and striking in our landscape, is not mentioned by Shakespeare, or by any of the old English poets. The earliest known descriptions of it are those given about the middle of the sixteenth century by Fuchs and Tragus in their Herbals. According to an old manuscript, the Welsh physicians of the thirteenth century appear to have frequently made use of it in the preparation of external medicines. Gerard and Parkinson advocate its use for a number of complaints, and later Salmon, in the New London Dispensatory, praised the plant. It was introduced into the London Pharmacopoeia in 1650, though it did not come into frequent use until a century later, and was first brought prominently under the notice of the medical profession by Dr. W. Withering, who in his Acount of the Foxglove, 1785, gave details of upwards of 200 cases, chiefly dropsical, in which it was used.

A domestic use of the Foxglove was general throughout North Wales at one time, when the leaves were used to darken the lines engraved on the stone floors which were fashionable then. This gave them a mosaiclike appearance.

The plant is both cultivated and collected in quantities for commercial purposes in the Harz Mountains and the Thuringian Forest.

Cultivation

The Foxglove is cultivated by a few growers in this country in order to provide a drug of uniform activity from a true type of Digitalis purpurea. It is absolutely necessary to have the true medicinal seeds to supply the drug market: crops must be obtained from carefully selected wild seed and all variations from the new type struck out.

The plant will flourish best in welldrained loose soil, preferably of siliceous origin, with some slight shade. The plants growing in sunny situations possess the active qualities of the herb in a much greater degree than those shaded by trees, and it has been proved that those grown on a hot, sunny bank, protected by a wood, give the best results.

It grows best when allowed to seed itself, but if it is desired to raise it by sown seed, 2 lb. of seed to the acre are required. As the seeds are so small and light, they should be mixed with fine sand in order to ensure even distribution. They should be thinly covered with soil. The seeds are uncertain in germination, but the seedlings may be readily and safely transplanted in damp weather, and should be pricked out to 6 to 9 inches apart. Sown in spring, the plant will not blossom till the following year. Seeds must be gathered as soon as ripe. The flowers of the true medicinal type must be pure, dull pink or magenta, not pale-coloured, white or spotted externally.

It is estimated that one acre of good soil will grow at least two tons of the Foxglove foliage, producing about 1/2 ton of the dried leaves.

Preparation for Market

The leaves alone are now used for the extraction of the drug, although formerly the seeds were also official.

No leaves are to be used for medicinal purposes that are not taken from the twoyear-old plants, picked when the bloom spike has run up and about two-thirds of the flowers are expanded, because at this time, before the ripening of the seeds, the leaves are in the most active state. They may be collected as long as they are in good condition: only green, perfect leaves being picked, all those that are insect-eaten or diseased, or tinged with purple or otherwise discoloured, must be discarded. Leaves from seedlings are valueless, and they must also not be collected in the spring, before the plant flowers, or in the autumn, when it has seeded, as the activity of the alkaloids is in each case too low.

If the fresh leaves are sent to the manufacturing druggists for Extract-making, they should be in 1/2 cwt. bundles, packed in aircovered railway cattle-trucks, or if in an open truck, must be covered with tarpaulin. The fresh crop should, if possible, be delivered to the wholesale buyer the same day as cut, but if this is impossible, on account of distance, they should be picked before the dew falls in the late afternoon and despatched the same evening, packed loosely in wicker baskets, lined with an open kind of muslin. Consignments by rail should be labelled: 'Urgent, Medicinal Herbs," to ensure quick delivery. The weather for picking must be absolutely dry - no damp or rain in the air and the leaves must be kept out of the sun and not packed too closely, or they may heat and turn yellow.

The odor of the fresh leaves is unpleasant, and the taste of both fresh and dried leaves is disagreeably bitter.

Foxglove leaves have in some places been recklessly gathered by over-zealous and thoughtless collectors without due regard to the future supply of the plants. The plant should not be roughly treated and never cut off just above the root, but the bottom leaves should in all cases be left to nourish the flower-spikes, in order that the seed may be ripened. In patches where Foxgloves grow thickly, the collection and redistribution of seed in likely places is much to be recommended.

The dried leaves as imported have occasionally been found adulterated with the leaves of various other plants. The chief of these are Inula Conyza (Ploughman's Spikenard), which may be distinguished by their greater roughness, the less-divided margins, the teeth of which have horny points, and odor when rubbed; I. Helenium (Elecampane), the leaves of which resemble Foxglove leaves, though they are less pointed, and the lower lateral veins do not form a 'wing' as in the Foxglove, the leaves of Symphytum officinale (Comfrey), which, however, may be recognized by the isolated stiff hairs they bear, and Verbascum Thapsus (Great Mullein), the leaves of which, unlike those of the Foxglove, have woolly upper and under surfaces, and the hairs of which, examined under a lens, are seen to be branched. Primrose leaves are also sometimes mingled with the drug, though they are much smaller than the average Foxglove leaf, and may be readily distinguished by the straight, lateral veins, which divide near the margins of the leaves. Foxglove leaves are easy to distinguish by their veins running down the leaf.

There is no reason why Foxglove leaves, properly prepared, should not become a national export.

Digitalis has lately been grown in Government Cinchona plantations in the Nilgiris, Madras, India. The leaves are coarser and rather darker in color than British or German-grown leaves, wild or cultivated, but tests show that the tincture prepared from them contains glucosides of more than average value.

Constituents

Digitalis contains four important glucosides of which three arecardiac stimulants. The most powerful is Digitoxin, an extremely poisonous and cumulative drug, insoluble in water, Digitalin, which is crystalline and also insoluble in water; Digitalein, amorphous, but readily soluble in water, rendering it, therefore, capable of being administered subcutaneously, in doses so minute as rarely to exceed of a grain; Digitonin, which is a cardiac depressant, containing none of the physiological action peculiar to Digitalis, and is identical with Saponin, the chief constituent of Senega root. Other constituents are volatile oil, fatty matter, starch, gum, sugar, etc.

The amount and character of the active constituents vary according to season and soil: 100 parts of dried leaves yield about 1.25 of Digitalin, which is generally found in a larger proportion in the wild than in the cultivated plants.

The active constituents of Digitalis are not yet sufficiently explored to render a chemical assay effective in standardizing for therapeutic activity. The different glucosides contained varying from each other in their physiological action, it is impossible to assay the leaves by determining one only of these, such as Digitoxin. No method of determining Digitalin is known. Hence the chemical means of assay fail, and the drug is usually standardized by a physiological test. One of our oldest firms of manufacturing druggists standardizes preparations of this extremely powerful and important drug by testing their action upon frogs.

Preparations

The preparations of Foxglove on the market vary considerably in composition and strength. Powdered Digitalis leaf is administered in pill form. The pharmacopoeial tincture, which is the preparation in commonest use, is given in doses of 5.15 minims, and the infusion is the unusually small dose of 2 to 4 drachms, the dose of other infusions being an ounce or more. The tincture contains a fair proportion of both Digitalin and Digitoxin.

The following note from the Chemist and Druggist (December 30, 1922) is of interest here:

Cultivation of Digitalis

'As is well known, for many years prior to the War digitalis was successfully cultivated on a large scale in various parts of the former Austro-Hungarian monarchy, and indeed the Government actively promoted the cultivation of this as well as of other medicinal plants. B. Pater, of Klausenburg, gives a résumé of his experiences in this direction (Pharmazeutische Monatshefte, 7, 1922), dealing not only with the best methods for cultivating digitalis from the seeds of this plant, but also with his investigations into certain differences and abnormalities peculiar to Digitalis purpurea. Apart from the fact that, occasionally, some plants bear flowers already in the first year of growth, the observation was made that the color of the flowers showed a wide scale of variation, ranging from the well-known distinctive purple shade through dark rose, light rose, to white. These variations in color of the flowers of cultivated digitalis plants induced the author to undertake a study of the activity of the several varieties, based on the digitoxin content of the stem leaves collected from flowering plants. In the case of Digitalis purpurea with normal purple flowers, the content of purified digitoxin, ascertained by Keller's method, averaged 0.17 per cent, while the leaves of plants bearing white flowers showed a slightly lower content, i.e. an average of 0.155 per cent of purified digitoxin. On the other hand, the plants with rose-coloured flowers were found to possess a very low content of digitoxin, averaging only 0.059 per cent. In the course of these investigations the fact was confirmed that the upper stem leaves are more active than the lower leaves."

Medicinal Action and Uses

Digitalis has been used from early times in heart cases. It increases the activity of all forms of muscle tissue, but more especially that of the heart and arterioles, the all-important property of the drug being its action on the circulation. The first consequence of its absorption is a contraction of the heart and arteries, causing a very high rise in the blood pressure.

After the taking of a moderate dose, the pulse is markedly slowed. Digitalis also causes an irregular pulse to become regular. Added to the greater force of cardiac contraction is a permanent tonic contraction of the organ, so that its internal capacity is reduced, which is a beneficial effect in cases of cardiac dilatation, and it improves the nutrition of the heart by increasing the amount of blood.

In ordinary conditions it takes about twelve hours or more before its effects on the heart muscle is appreciated, and it must thus always be combined with other remedies to tide the patient over this period and never prescribed in large doses at first, as some patients are unable to take it, the drug being apt to cause considerable digestive disturbances, varying in different cases. This action is probably due to the Digitonin, an undesirable constituent.

The action of the drug on the kidneys is of importance only second to its action on the circulation. In small or moderate doses, it is a powerful diuretic and a valuable remedy in dropsy, especially when this is connected with affections of the heart.

It has also been employed in the treatment of internal hemorrhage, in inflammatory diseases, in delirium tremens, in epilepsy, in acute mania and various other diseases, with real or supposed benefits.

The action of Digitalis in all the forms in which it is administered should be carefully watched, and when given over a prolonged period it should be employed with caution, as it is liable to accumulate in the system and to manifest its presence all at once by its poisonous action, indicated by the pulse becoming irregular, the blood-pressure low and gastro-intestinal irritation setting in. The constant use of Digitalis, also, by increasing the activity of the heart, leads to hypertrophy of that organ.

Digitalis is an excellent antidote in Aconite poisoning, given as a hypodermic injection.

When Digitalis fails to act on the heart as desired, Lily-of-the-Valley may be substituted and will often be found of service.

In large doses, the action of Digitalis on the circulation will cause various cerebral symptoms, such as seeing all objects blue, and various other disturbances of the special senses. In cases of poisoning by Digitalis, with a very slow and irregular pulse, the administration of Atropine is generally all that is necessary. In the more severe cases, with the very rapid heartbeat, the stomach pump must be used, and drugs may be used which depress and diminish the irritability of the heart, such as chloral and chloroform.

Preparations of Digitalis come under Table II of the Poison Schedule.

Preparations and Dosages

Tincture, B.P., 5 to 15 drops. Infusion, B.P., 2 to 4 drachms. Powdered leaves, 1/2 to 2 grains. Fluid extract, 1 to 3 drops. Solid extract, U.S.P., 1/8 grain.

A method of preparing the drug in a noninJurious manner is given in the Chemist and Druggist (December 30, 1922):

Digitalis Maceration

'On preparing an infusion of digitalis leaves in the usual manner, one of the active principles, gitalin, is destroyed by the action of the boiling water. To obviate the possibility of destroying any of the active principles in the leaves, Th. Koch (Süddeutsche Apotheker-Zeitung, 63, 1922) has for some years past adopted the following procedure: 20 gm. powdered standardized digitalis leaves, 1000 gm. chloroform water (7.1000) and 40 drops of 10 per cent. Solution of Sodium Carbonate are shaken for four hours. The liquid is then passed through a flannel cloth, and, after standing for some time, filtered in the ordinary way, taking the precaution to cover the filter with a glass plate. The use of chloroform water as the solvent serves a threefold purpose: It promotes the solution of the gitalin present in the leaves, ensures the stability and keeping properties of the maceration, and prevents the occurrence of gastric troubles. The presence of Sodium Carbonate prevents the plant acid from reacting with the chloroform to produce hydrochloric acid. In this maceration no digitoxin is present, the principle which is assumed to exert a deleterious action on the heart as well as a cumulative effect."

FRANKINCENSE

Botanical: Boswellia Thurifera
Family: N.O Burseraceae
Synonym: Olibanum.
Part Used: The gum resin.
Habitat: Arabia, Somaliland

Description

Obtained from the leafy forest tree Boswellia Thurifera, with leaves deciduous, alternate towards the tops of branches, unequally pinnated; leaflets in about ten pairs with an odd one opposite, oblong, obtuse, serrated, pubescent, sometimes alternate; petioles short. Flowers, white or pale rose on short pedicels in single axillary racemes shorter than the leaves. Calyx, small five-toothed, persistent; corolla with five obovate-oblong, very patent petals, acute at the base, inserted under the margin of the disk, acstivation slightly imbricative. Stamens, ten, inserted under the disk, alternately shorter; filaments subulate, persistent. Anthers, caducous, oblong. Torus a cupshaped disk, fleshy, larger than calyx, crenulated margin. Ovary, oblong, sessile. Style, one caducous, the length of the stamens; stigma capitate, three-lobed. Fruit capsular, three-angled three-celled, three-valved, septicidal, valves hard. Seeds, solitary in each cell surrounded by a broad membranaceous wing. Cotyledons intricately folded multifid.

The trees on the Somali coast grow, without soil, out of polished marble rocks, to which they are attached by a thick oval mass of substances resembling a mixture of lime and mortar. The young trees furnish the most valuable gum, the older yielding merely a clear, glutinous fluid, resembling coral varnish.

To obtain the Frankincense, a deep, longitudinal incision is made in the trunk of the tree and below it a narrow strip of bark 5 inches in length is peeled off. When the milk-like juice which exudes has hardened by exposure to the air, the incision is deepened. In about three months the resin has attained the required degree of consistency, hardening into yellowish 'tears." The large, clear globules are scraped off into baskets and the inferior quality that has run down the tree is collected separately. The season for gathering lasts from May till the middle of September, when the first shower of rain puts a close to the gathering for that year.

The coast of Southern Arabia is yearly visited by parties of Somalis, who pay the Arabs for the privilege of collecting Frankincense, and in the interior of the country, about the plain of Dhofar, during the southwest Monsoon, Frankincense and other gums are gathered by the Bedouins. (The incense of Dhofar is alluded to by the Portuguese poet, Camoens.)

Constituents

Resins 65 per cent, volatile oil 6 per cent, water-soluble gum 20 per cent, bassorin 6 to 8 per cent, plant residue 2 to 4 per cent; the resins are composed of boswellic acid and alibanoresin.

Medicinal Action and Uses

It is stimulant, but seldom used now internally, though formerly was in great repute . Pliny mentions it as an antidote to hemlock. Avicenna (tenth century) recommends it for tumors, ulcers, vomiting, dysentery and fevers. In China it is used for leprosy.

Its principal use now is in the manufacture of incense and pastilles. It is also used in plasters and might be substituted for Balsam of Peru or Balsam or Tolu. The inhalation of steam laden with the volatile portion of the drug is said to relieve bronchitis and laryngitis.

The ceremonial incense of the Jews was compounded of four 'sweet scents," of which pure Frankincense was one, pounded together in equal proportion. It is frequently mentioned in the Pentateuch. Pure Frankincense formed part of the meet offering and was also presented with the shew-bread every Sabbath day. With other spices, it was stored in a great chamber of the House of God at Jerusalem.

According to Herodotus, Frankincense to the amount of 1,000 talents weight was offered every year, during the feast of Bel, on the great altar of his temple in Babylon. The religious use of incense was as common in ancient Persia as in Babylon and Assyria. Herodotus states that the Arabs brought every year to Darius as tribute 1,000 talents of Frankincense, and the modern Parsis of Western India still preserve the ritual of incense.

Frankincense, though the most common, never became the only kind of incense offered to the gods among the Greeks. According to Pliny, it was not sacrificially employed in Trojan times. Among the Romans, the use of Frankincense (alluded to as mascula thura by Virgil in the Eclogues) was not confined to religious ceremonials. It was also used on state occasions, and in domestic life.

The kohl, or black powder with which the Egyptian women paint their eyelids, is made of charred Frankincense, or other odoriferous resin mixed with Frankincense. Frankincense is also melted to make a depilatory, and it is made into a paste with other ingredients to perfume the hands. A similar practice is described by Herodotus as having been practiced by the women of Scythia and is alluded to in Judith x. 3 and 4. In cold weather, the Egyptians warm their rooms with a brazier whereon incense is burnt, Frankincense, Benzoin and Aloe wood being chiefly used for the purpose.

The word 'incense," meaning originally the aroma given off with the smoke of any odoriferous substance when burnt, has been gradually restricted almost exclusively to Frankincense, which has always been obtainable in Europe in greater quantity than any other of the aromatics imported from the East.

There is no fixed formula for the incense now used in the Christian churches of Europe, but it is recommended that Frankincense should enter as largely as possible intoits composition. In Rome, Olibanum alone is employed: in the Russian church, Benzoin is chiefly employed.

The following is a formula for an incense used in the Roman Church: Olibanum, 10 OZ. Benzoin, 4 oz. Storax, 1 OZ. Break into small pieces and mix.

FRINGE TREE

Botanical: Chionanthus virginica (LINN.)
Family: N.O. Oleaceae
Synonyms: Old Man's Beard. Fringe Tree Bark. Chionathus. Snowdrop Tree. Poison Ash.
Part Used: The dried bark of the root.
Habitat: The United States, from Pennsylvania to Tennessee.

Description

A small tree, bearing in June white flowers like snowdrops, and with large leaves like those of Magnolia, it presents a charming appearance. The root-bark is found in single, transversely-curved pieces, often heavy enough (though small) to sink in water. The outside is reddish or greyish-brown, with root scars and whiter patches. The inner surface is a yellowish brown. The fracture is short, coarsely granular, and yellowish-white. It is almost odourless, but very bitter in taste. The powder is light brown in color.

Constituents

It is said that both saponin and a glucoside have been found, but neither appears to have been officially confirmed.

Medicinal Action and Uses

Aperient, diuretic. Some authorities regard it as tonic and slightly narcotic. It is used in typhoid, intermittent, or bilious fevers, and externally, as a poultice, for inflammations or wounds. Is useful in liver complaints.

Dosage

Of fluid extract, 1/2 to 1 fluid drachm two or three times a day. Of infusion, 1/2 to 2 fluid ounces two or three times a day. Chiomanthin, 1 to 3 grains.

FRITILLARY, COMMON

Botanical: Fritillaria Meleagris (LINN.)
Family: N.O. Liliaceae
Synonyms: Lilium variegatum. Chequered Daffodil. Narcissus Caparonius. Turkey Hen. Ginny Flower.

Fritillaria Meleagris (Linn.), the Snake's Head Fritillary, is a native of Great Britain, found in meadows and pastures in the southern and eastern counties of England, chiefly in Oxfordshire. It is not common and does not occur farther north than Norfolk, or farther west than Somerset.

It has a tiny, solid bulb, not larger than a good-sized black currant, with two or three long, narrow leaves, on a stem about a foot high, which bears a single, drooping flower of a dull red color, marked curiously with pink and dark purple, in quaint squares and blotches. The petals are only overlapping and not joined together in any way, although the flowers look bell-like. Though the open flower is pendulous the bud stands erect, and so does the capsule. The plant is in bloom in April and May, in mild seasons in March.

The botanical name, meleagris, is derived from a Greek term applied to a guinea-hen, and many of the popular English names have a similar allusion to the markings of the flower, viz. Guinea-hen flower, Turkey-hen flower, Pheasant Lily, Leopards Lily, Chequered Lily, Chequered Daffodil and Lazarus Bell.

Bees visit the flower for the nectar secreted largely at the base of the perianth.

Many garden varieties are now cultivated. The best mode of propagation is by offsets, but also by seed, which ripens readily. Rabbits are very fond of this plant and will destroy it wholesale.

The bulb is poisonous and very distasteful to the palate and is said to have no medicinal value, though from its presence on the elaborate allegorical frontispiece of the old Herbal of Clusius, Rariorum Plantarum Historia, published in 1601, it bore at that time a reputation as a herb of healing.

FROSTWORT

Botanical: Helianthemum Canadense (MISCH.)
Family: N.O. Cistaceae
Synonyms: Cistus. Frostweed. Frostplant. Rock Rose. Canadisches Sonnenroschen. Helianthemum Ramultoflorum. Helianthemum Rosmarinifolium. Helianthemum michauxii. Helianthemum Corymbosum. Cistus Canadensis. Lechea Major. Heterameris Canadensis.
Part Used: The dried herb.
Habitat: Eastern United States.

Description

The official name comes from the Greek helios (the sun) and anthemon (a flower). The genus differs from the Cistus in having imperfectly three-celled instead of five or ten-celled capsules. Two distinct varieties of the species are known, the early and late flowering forms. They grow in sandy soil, from 6 to 12 inches high, with upright stems, branching or almost without branches, leaves light or dark green, small and lanceolate, and flat, yellow flowers, solitary or in terminal clusters. The popular names spring from the peculiarity of thin, curved, ice-crystals projecting in early winter from fissures in the bark near the root. The taste is astringent, slightly aromatic and bitter. It has no odor.

Constituents

A volatile oil, wax, tannin, fatty oil, and a glucoside that will crystallize into white needles. Chlorophyll, gum and inorganic salts were also found in Helianthemum Corymbosum.

Medicinal Action and Uses

Antiscro fulous, astringent, alterative and tonic. It has for long been used in secondary syphilis, diarrhea, ulcerations, ophthalmia, and any conditions arising from a scrofulous constitution. Locally it is useful as a wash in prurigo and as a gargle in scarlatina, and in poultice form for scrofulous tumors and ulcers.

It is said that an oil helpful in cancer has been obtained from it.

It may be combined with Corydalis Formosa and Stillingia, in secondary syphilis, and the infusion may be used in chronic diarrhea and dysentery.

An overdose may produce nausea and vomiting.

Dosage

Of extract, 2 grains. Of fluid extract, 1 fluid drachm as an alternative and astringent.

Other Species

H. Corymbosum may be used indiscriminately as officinal.

Cistus Creticus, or European Rock Rose, the only other plant of the order used in medicine, yields the gum resin Ladanum or Labdanum, a natural exudation valued as a stimulant expectorant and emmenagogue. It has been used in plasters, and formerly in catarrh and dysentery. An oil with the odor of ambergris has been obtained from the resin.

Labdanum is found in masses weighing up to several pounds, enclosed in bladders. It softens in the hand when broken, becoming adhesive and balsamic. It burns with a clear flame. An adulterated kind is in contorted, hard pieces, mixed with sand and earth.

C. Landaniferous, C. Ledon and C. Laurifolius are said to yield the same substance, most of which comes from the Grecian Islands.

All these Cistus and Helianthenums grow in the author's garden at Chalfont St. Peters.

G

GALANGAL

Botanical: Alpinia officinarum (HANCE.)
Family: N.O. Zingaberaceae or Scilaminae
Synonyms: Galanga. China Root. India Root. East India Catarrh Root. Lesser Galangal. Rhizoma Galangae. Gargaut. Colic Root. Kaempferia Galanga.
Part Used: Dried rhizome.
Habitat: China (Hainan Island), Java.

Description

The genus Alpinia was named by Plumier after Prospero Alpino, a famous Italian botanist of the early seventeenth century. The name Galangal is derived from theArabic Khalanjan, perhaps a perversion of a Chinese word meaning 'mild ginger.'

The drug has been known in Europe for seven centuries longer than its botanical origin, for it was only recognized in 1870, when specimens were examined that had been found near Tung-sai, in the extreme south of China, and later, on the island of Hainan, just opposite. The name of Alpinia officinarum was given to the herb, as the source of Lesser Galangal. The Greater Galangal is a native of Java (A. Galanga or Maranta Galanga), and is much larger, of an orange-brown color, with a feebler taste and odor. It is occasionally seen at London drug sales, but is scarcely ever used. There is also a resemblance to A. calcarata. The herb grows to a height of about 5 feet, the leaves being long, rather narrow blades, and the flowers, of curious formation, growing in a simple, terminal spike, the petals white, with deep-red veining distinguishing the lippetal.

The branched pieces of rhizome are from 1 1/2 to 3 inches in length, and seldom more than 3/4 inch thick. They are cut while fresh, and the pieces are usually cylindrical, marked at short intervals by narrow, whitish, somewhat raised rings, which are the scars left by former leaves. They are dark reddish-brown externally, and the section shows a dark centre surrounded by a wider, paler layer which becomes darker in drying. Their odor is aromatic, and their taste pungent and spicy. They are tough and difficult to break, the fracture being granular, with small, ligneous fibres interspersed throughout one side. The drug is exported, chiefly from Shanghai, in bales made of split cane, plaited, and bound round with cane. The root has been used in Europe as a spice for over a thousand years, having probably been introduced by Arabian or Greek physicians, but it has now largely gone out of use except in Russia and India. Closely resembling ginger, it is used in Russia for flavouring vinegar and the liqueur 'nastoika': it is a favorite spice and medicine in Lithuania and Esthonia. Tartars prepare a kind of tea that contains it, and it is used by brewers. The reddishbrown powder is used as snuff, and in India the oil is valued in perfumery.

Constituents

The root contains a volatile oil, resin, galangol, kaempferid, galangin and alpinin, starch, etc. The active principles are the volatile oil and acrid resin. Galangin is dioxyflavanol, and has been obtained synthetically. Alcohol freely extracts all the properties, and for the fluid extract there should be no admixture of water or glycerin.

Medicinal Action and Uses

Stimulant and carminative. It is especially useful in flatulence, dyspepsia, vomiting and sickness at stomach, being recommended as a remedy for sea-sickness. It tones up the tissues and is sometimes prescribed in fever. Homoeopaths use it as a stimulant. Galangal is used in cattle medicine, and the Arabs use it to make their horses fiery. It is included in several compound preparations, but is not now often employed alone.

The powder is used as a snuff for catarrh.

Dosage

From 15 to 30 grains in substance, and double in infusion. Fluid extract, 30 to 60 minims.

GALBANUM

Botanical: Ferula galbaniflua (BOISS. ET BUHSE)
Family: N.O. Umbelliferae

Part Used: Gum resin.
Habitat: Persia; also Cape of Good Hope.

Description

There are two kinds of Galbanum in commerce, viz. Levant Galbanurn and the Persian Galbanum. The latter is softer than the Levant, has a more terebinthic odor, has the smell and consistency of Venice turpentine, and contains fruit and fragments of stalks in place of bits of sliced roots. Several species of Ferula are used as a source for commercial Galbanum, but the official plant is Ferula galbaniflua, a perennial, with smooth stem, and shining leaflets, ovate, wedge-shaped, acute and finely serrated on the edges. The umbels of flowers are few, the seeds shiny.

The whole plant abounds with a milky juice, which oozes from the joints of old plants, and exudes and hardens from the base of the stem after it has been cut down, then is finally obtained by incisions made in the root. The juice from the root soon hardens and forms the tears of the Galbanum of Commerce. The best tears are palish externally and about the size of a hazel nut and when broken open are composed of clear white tears. The taste is unpleasant, bitterish, acrid, with a strong, peculiar, somewhat aromatic smell. The common kind is an agglutinated mass, showing reddish and white tears, this is of the consistency of firm wax, and can easily be torn to pieces and softened by heat; when cold it is brittle, and mixed with seeds and leaves, when imported in lumps it is often considered preferable to the tears as it contains more volatile oil. Distilled with water it yields a quantity of essential oil, about 6 drachms, to 1 lb. of gum. It was well known to the ancients and Pliny called it 'bubonion.' Galbanum under dry distillation yields a thick oil of a bluish color, which after purification becomes the blue color of the oil obtained from the flowers of Matricaria Chamomilla.

Constituents

Gum resin, mineral constituents, volatile oil, umbelliferine, galbaresino-tannol.

Medicinal Action and Uses

Stimulant, expectorant in chronic bronchitis. Antispasmodic and considered an intermediate between ammoniac and asafoetida for relieving the air passages, in pill form it is specially good, in some forms of hysteria, and used externally as a plaster for inflammatory swellings.

Preparations and Dosage

In pill form 10 to 20 grains, or as an emulsion, mixed with gum, sugar and water.

Other species

In Beyrout the people use the root of F. Hermonic, commonly known as Zalou root, as an aphrodisiac.

GALE, SWEET

Botanical: Myrica gale (LINN.)
Family: N.O. Myricaceae
Synonyms: Bayberry. English Bog Myrtle. Dutch Myrtle. Herba Myrti Rabanitini. Gale palustris (Chevalier).
Parts Used: Leaves, branches.

Habitat

Higher latitudes of Northern Hemisphere; Great Britain, especially in the north; abundant on the Scottish moors and bogs.

Description

The badge of the Campbells. A deciduous, bushy shrub, growing to 4 feet high. The wood and leaves fragrant when bruised. The leaves, not unlike a willow or myrtle, are oblanceolate, tapering entire at the base, toothed and broadest at the apex, the upper side dark glossy green, the underside paler and slightly downy, under which are a few shining glands. The male plant produces flowers in May and June in crowded, stalkless catkins. The fruit catkins about the same size, but thicker, are closely-set, resinous nutlets, the flowers being borne on the bare wood of one year's growth. The sexes are on different plants. The leaves are often dried to perfume linen, etc., their odor being very fragrant, but the taste bitter and astringent. The branches have been used as a substitute for hops in Yorkshire and put into a beer called there 'Gale Beer.' It is extremely good to allay thirst. The catkins, or cones, boiled in water, give a scum beeswax, which is utilized to make candles. The bark is used to tan calfskins; if gathered in autumn, it will dye wool a good yellow color and is used for this purpose both in Sweden and Wales. The Swedes use it in strong decoction to kill insects, vermin and to cure the itch. The dried berries are put into broth and used as spice. In China, the leaves are infused like tea, and used as a stomachic and cordial.

Constituents

Said to contain a poisonous volatile oil and to have properties similar to those of Myrica cerifera.

Medicinal Action and Uses

The leaves have been used in France as an emmenagogue and abortifacient.

Other Species

M. Gale, var. tomentosa. The young wood and leaves on both sides are very downy and specially so on the underside.

GAMBOGE

Botanical: Garcinia hanburyii (HOOK)
Family: N.O. Guttiferae
Synonyms: Gutta gamba. Gummigutta. Tom Rong. Gambodia. Garcinia Morella.
Part Used: Gum resin.
Habitat: Siam, Southern Cochin-China, Cambodia, Ceylon.

Description

The commercial Gamboge is obtained from several varieties, though Garcinia Hanburyii is the official plant, an almost similar gum is obtained from Hypericum (St. Johnswort). The Gamboge tree grows to a height of 50 feet, with a diameter of 12 inches, and the gum resin is extracted by incisions or by breaking off the leaves and shoots of the trees, the juice which is a milky yellow resinous gum, resides in the ducts of the bark and is gatheredin vessels, and left to thicken and become hardened. Pipe Gamboge is obtained by letting the juice run into hollowed bamboos, and when congealed the bamboo is broken away from it. The trees must be ten years old before they are tapped, and the gum is collected in the rainy season from June to October. The term 'Gummi Gutta,' by which Gamboge is generally known, is derived from the method of extracting it indrops. Gamboge was first introduced into England by the Dutch about the middle of the seventeenth century; it is highly esteemed as a pigment, owing to the brilliancy of its orange color. It has no odor, and little taste, but if held in the mouth a short time it gives an acrid sensation. The medicinal properties of Gamboge are thought to be contained in the resin. It is official in the United States Pharmacopoeia.

Constituents

Resin gum, vegetable waste, garonolic acids; the gum is analogous to gum acacia.

Medicinal Action and Uses

A very powerful drastic hydragogue, cathartic, very useful in dropsical conditions and to lower blood pressure, where there is cerebral congestion. A full dose is rarely given alone, as it causes vomiting, nausea and griping, and a dose of 1 drachm has been known to cause death. It is usually combined with other purgatives which it strengthens. A safe dose is from 2 to 6 grains, but in the treatment of tapeworm the dose is often as much as 10 grains. It provides copious watery evacuations with little pain, but must be used with caution. Dose, 2 to 5 grains in an emulsion or in an alkaline solution.

Other Species

The tree G. Morella is the Indian Gamboge; a gum resin is obtained from it; it has a similar action to Gamboge and is used as its equivalent in India and Eastern Colonies. Dose, 1/2 to 2 grains.

GARLIC

Botanical: Allium sativum (LINN.)
Family: N.O. Liliaceae
Synonym: Poor Man's Treacle.
Part Used: Bulb.

The Common Garlic a member of the same group of plants as the Onion, is of such antiquity as a cultivated plant, that it is difficult with any certainty to trace the country of its origin. De Candolle, in his treatise on the Origin of Cultivated Plants, considered that it was apparently indigenous to the southwest of Siberia, whence it spread to southern Europe, where it has become naturalized, and is said to be found wild in Sicily. It is widely cultivated in the Latin countries bordering on the Mediterranean. Dumas has described the air of Provence as being 'particularly perfumed by the refined essence of this mystically attractive bulb.'

Description

The leaves are long, narrow and flat like grass. The bulb (the only part eaten) is of a compound nature, consisting of numerous bulblets, known technically as 'cloves,' grouped together between the membraneous scales and enclosed within a whitish skin, which holds them as in a sac.

The flowers are placed at the end of a stalk rising direct from the bulb and are whitish, grouped together in a globular head, or umbel, with an enclosing kind of leaf or spathae, and among them are small bulbils.

To prevent the plant running to leaf, Pliny (Natural History, XIX, 34) advised bending the stalk downward and covering it with earth, seeding, he observed, may be prevented by twisting the stalk.

In England, Garlic, apart from medicinal purposes, is seldom used except as a seasoning, but in the southern counties of Europe it is a common ingredient in dishes, and is largely consumed by the agricultural population. From the earliest times, indeed, Garlichas been used as an article of diet.

History

Garlic was placed by the ancient Greeks (Theophrastus relates) on the piles of stones at cross-roads as a supper for Hecate, and according to Pliny garlic and onion were invocated as deities by the Egyptians at the taking of oaths.

It was largely consumed by the ancient Greeks and Romans, as we may read in Virgil's Eclogues. Horace, however, records his detestation of Garlic, the smell of which, even in his days (as much later in Shakespeare's time), was accounted a sign of vulgarity. He calls it 'more poisonous than hemlock,' and relates how he was made ill by eating it at the table of Maecenas. Among the ancient Greeks, persons who partook of it were not allowed to enter the temples of Cybele. Homer, however, tells us that it was to the virtues of the 'Yellow Garlic' that Ulysses owed his escape from being changed by Circe into a pig, like each of his companions.

Homer also makes Garlic part of the entertainment which Nestor served up to his guest Machaon.

There is a Mohammedan legend that:

'when Satan stepped out from the Garden of Eden after the fall of man, Garlick sprang up from the spot where he placed his left foot, and Onion from that where his right foot touched.'

There is a curious superstition in some parts of Europe, that if a morsel of the bulb be chewed by a man running a race it will prevent his competitors from getting ahead of him, and Hungarian jockeys will sometimes fasten a clove of Garlic to the bits of their horses in the belief that any other racers running close to those thus baited, will fall back the instant they smell the offensive odor.

Many of the old writers praise Garlic as a medicine, though others, including Gerard, are sceptical as to its powers. Pliny gives an exceedingly long list of complaints, in which it was considered beneficial, and Galen eulogizes it as the rustics' Theriac, or Heal-All. One of its older popular names in this country was 'Poor Man's Treacle,' meaning theriac, in which sense we find it in Chaucer and many old writers.

A writer in the twelfth century - Alexander Neckam - recommends it as a palliative for the heat of the sun in field labour, and in a book of travel, written by Mountstuart Elphinstone about 100 years ago, he says that-

'the people in places where the Simoon is frequent eat Garlic and rub their lips and noses with it when they go out in the heat of the summer to prevent their suffering from the Simoon.'

Garlic is mentioned in several Old English vocabularies of plants from the tenth to the fifteenth centuries, and is described by the herbalists of the sixteenth century from Turner (1548) onwards. It is stated to have been grown in England before the year 1540. In Cole's Art of Simpling we are told that cocks which have been fed on Garlic are 'most stout to fight, and 50 are Horses': and that if a garden is infested with moles, Garlic or leeks will make them 'leap out of the ground presently.'

The name is of Anglo-Saxon origin, being derived from gar (a spear) and lac (a plant), in reference to the shape of its leaves.

Cultivation

The ground should be prepared in a similar manner as for the closelyallied onion.

The soil may be sandy, loam or clay, though Garlic flourishes best in a rich, moist, sandy soil. Dig over well, freeing the ground from all lumps and dig some lime into it. Tread firmly. Divide the bulbs into their component 'cloves' - each fair-sized bulb will divide into ten or twelve cloves - and with a dibber put in the cloves separately, about 2 inches deep and about 6 inches apart, leaving about 1 foot between the rows. It is well to give a dressing of soot.

Garlic beds should be in a sunny spot. They must be kept thoroughly free from weeds and the soil gathered up round the roots with a Dutch hoe from time to time.

When planted early in the spring, in February or March, the bulbs should be ready for lifting in August, when the leaves will be beginning to wither. Should the summer have been wet and cold, they may probably not be ready till nearly the middle of September.

The use of Garlic as an antiseptic was in great demand during the past war. In 1916 the Government asked for tons of the bulbs, offering 1s. per lb. for as much as could be produced. Each pound generally represents about 20 bulbs, and 5 lb. divided up into cloves and planted, will yield about 38 lb. at the end of the growing season, so it will prove a remunerative crop.

The following appeared in the Morning Post of December 12, 1922:

'A Dog's Recovery

'Mr. W. H. Butlin, Tiptree, records the following experience: A fox-terrier, aged 14 years, appeared to be developing rapidly a pitiable condition, with a swollen neck and an ugly intractable sore at the root of the tail, and dull, coarse coat shedding abundantly. I administered "Yadil Antiseptic" in his drinking water and in less than a month the dog became perfectly sound and well, a mirabile dictu, his coat became firm, soft, and glossy.' (Yadil is a patent medicine said to contain Garlic.)

'In cases of arterial tension, MM. Chailley-Bert, Cooper, and Debrey, at the Society of Biology, recommended about 30 drops of alcoholic extract as a remedy. To be administered by the mouth or intravenously.'

Although only the cultivated Garlic is utilized medicinally, all of the other species have similar properties in a greater or less degree. Several of the species of Allium are natives of this country.

The CROW GARLIC (A. vineale) is widely distributed and fairly common in many districts, but the bulbs are very small and the labour of digging them would be great. It is frequent in pastures and communicates its rank taste to mike and butter, when eaten by cows.

NOTE.--Professor Henslow calls A. vineale the Field Garlic, and A. oleraceum the Crow Garlic.

RAMSONS (A. ursinum) grows in woods and has a very acrid taste and smell, but it also has very small bulbs, which would hardly render it of practical use.

Ransoms is also very generally known as 'Broad-leaved Garlic.'

The FIELD GARLIC (A. oleraceum) is rather a rare plant. Both this and the Crow Garlic have, however, occasionally been employed as potherbs or for flavouring. It is an old country notion that if crows eat Crow Garlic, itstupefies them.

Ramsons, the wild Wood Garlic, but for its evil smell would rank among the most beautiful of our British plants. Its broad leaves are very similar to those of the Lily-of-the-Valley, and its star-like flowers are a dazzling white, but its odor is too strong to admit of it being picked for its beauty, and many woods, especially in the Cotswold Hills, are spots to be avoided when it is in flower, being so closely carpeted with the plants that every step taken brings out the offensive odor.

There are many species of Allium grown in the garden, the flowers of some of which are even sweet-smelling (as A. odorum and A. fragrans), but they are the exceptions, and even these have the Garlic scent in their leaves and roots.

Constituents

The active properties of Garlic depend on a pungent, volatile, essentialoil, which may readily be obtained by distillation with water. It is a sulphide of the radical Allyl, present in all the onion family. This oil is rich in sulphur, but contains no oxygen. The pecular penetrating odor of Garlic is due to this intensely smelling sulphuret of allyl, and is so diffusive that even when the bulb is applied to the soles of the feet, its odor is exhaled by the lungs.

Medicinal Action and Uses

Diaphoretic, diuretic, expectorant, stimulant. Many marvellous effects and healing powers have been ascribed to Garlic. It possesses stimulant and stomachic properties in addition to its other virtues.

As an antiseptic, its use has long been recognized. In the late war it was widely employed in the control of suppuration in wounds. The raw juice is expressed, diluted with water, and put on swabs of sterilized Sphagnum moss, which are applied to the wound. Where this treatment has been given, it has been proved that there have been no septic results, and the lives of thousands of men have been saved by its use.

It is sometimes externally applied in ointments and lotions, and as an antiseptic, to disperse hard swellings, also pounded and employed as a poultice for scrofulous sores. It is said to prevent anthrax in cattle, being largely used for the purpose.

In olden days, Garlic was employed as a specific for leprosy. It was also believed that it had most beneficial results in cases of smallpox, if cut small and applied to the soles of the feet in a linen cloth, renewed daily.

It formed the principal ingredient in the 'Four Thieves' Vinegar,' which was adapted so successfully at Marseilles for protection against the plague when it prevailed there in 1722. This originated, it is said, with four thieves who confessed, that whilst protected by the liberal use of aromatic vinegar during the plague, they plundered the dead bodies of its victims with complete security.

It is stated that during an outbreak of infectious fever in certain poor quarters of London, early last century, the French priests who constantly used Garlic in all their dishes, visited the worst cases with impunity, whilst the English clergy caught the infection, and in many instances fell victims to the disease.

Syrup of Garlic is an invaluable medicine for asthma, hoarseness, coughs, difficulty of breathing, and most other disorders of the lungs, being of particular virtue in chronic bronchitis, on account of its powers of promoting expectoration. It is made by pouring a quart of water, boiled hot, upon a pound of the fresh root, cut into slices, and allowed to stand in a closed vessel for twelve hours, sugar then being added to make it of the consistency of syrup. Vinegar and honey greatly improve this syrup as a medicine. A little caraway and sweet fennel seed bruised and boiled for a short time in the vinegar before it is added to the Garlic, will cover the pungent smell of the latter.

A remedy for asthma, that was formerly most popular, is a syrup of Garlic, made by boiling the bulbs till soft and adding an equal quantity of vinegar to the water in which they have been boiled, and then sugared and boiled down to a syrup. The syrup is then poured over the boiled bulbs, which have been allowed to dry meanwhile, and kept in a jar. Each morning a bulb or two is to be taken, with a spoonful of the syrup.

Syrup made by melting 1 1/2 OZ. of lump sugar in 1 OZ. of the raw expressed juice may be given to children in cases of coughs without inflammation.

The successful treatment of tubercular consumption by Garlic has been recorded, the freshly expressed juice, diluted with equal quantities of water, or dilute spirit of wine, being inhaled antiseptically.

Bruised and mixed with lard, it has been proved to relieve whooping-cough if rubbed on the chest and between the shoulder-blades.

An infusion of the bruised bulbs, given before and after every meal, has been considered of good effect in epilepsy.

A clove or two of Garlic, pounded with honey and taken two or three nights successively, is good in rheumatism.

Garlic has also been employed with advantage in dropsy, removing the water which may already have collected and preventing its future accumulation. It is stated that some dropsies have been cured by it alone.

If sniffed into the nostrils, it will revive a hysterical sufferer. Amongst physiological results, it is reported that Garlic makes the eye retina more sensitive and less able to bear strong light.

The juice of Garlic, and milk of Garlic made by boiling the bruised bulbs in milk is used as a vermifuge.

Preparations

Juice, 10 to 30 drops. Syrup, 1 drachm. Tincture, 1/2 to 1 drachm.

Wine of Garlic - made by macerating three or four bulbs in a quart of proof spirit is a good stimulant lotion for baldness of the head.

Used in cookery it is a great aid to digestion, and keeps the coats of the stomach healthy. For this reason, essential oil is made from it and is used in the form of pills.

If a very small piece is chopped fine and put into chicken's food daily, it is a sure preventative of the gapes. Pullets will lay finer eggs by having garlic in their food before they start laying, but when they commence to lay it must be stopped, otherwise it will flavor the eggs.

Mrs. Beeton (in an old edition of her Household Management, 1866) gives the following recipe for making 'Bengal MangoChutney,' which she states was given by a native to an English lady who had long been a resident in India, and who since her return to England had become quite celebrated amongst her friends for the excellence of this Eastern relish.

Ingredients. 1 1/2 lb. moist sugar, 3/4 lb. salt, 1/4 lb. Garlic, 1/4 lb. onions, 3/4 lb. powdered ginger, 1/4 lb. dried chillies, 3/4 lb. dried mustard-seed, 3/4 lb. stoned raisins, 2 bottles of best vinegar, 30 large, unripe, sour apples.

Mode. The sugar must be made into syrup; the Garlic, onions and ginger be finely pounded in a mortar; the mustard-seed be washed in cold vinegar and dried in the sun; the apples be peeled, cored and sliced, and boiled in a bottle and a half of the vinegar. When all this is done, and the apples are quite cold, put them into a large pan and gradually mix the whole of the rest of the ingredients, including the remaining half-bottle of vinegar. It must be well stirred until the whole is thoroughly blended, and then put into bottles for use. Tie a piece of wet bladder over the mouths of the bottles, after which they are well corked. This chutney is very superior to any which can be bought, and one trial will prove it to be delicious.

GELSEMIUM

POISON
Steadman Shorter's Medical Dictionary, Poisons & Antidotes: Gelsemium
Botanical: Gelsemium nitidum (MICH.)
Family: N.O. Loganiaceae
Synonyms: Yellow Jasmine. Gelsemium Sempervirens (Pers.). False Jasmine. Wild Woodbine. Carolina Jasmine.
Part Used: Root.

Habitat

Gelsemium is one of the most beautiful native plants of North America, occurring in rich, moist soils, by the sides of streams, along the seacoast from Virginia to the south of Florida. extending into Mexico.

The important drug Gelsemium, official in the principal Pharmacopoeias, is composed of the dried rhizome and root of Gelsemium nitidum (Michaux), a climbing plant growing in the southern States of North America and there known as Yellow Jasmine, though it is in no way related to the Jasmines, and is best distinguished as Caroline Jasmine, as it belongs to the Loganiaceae, an order that forms a connecting link between the orders Gentianaceae, Apocynaceae, Scrophulariaceae and Rubiaceae. The plant is not to be confounded with the true Yellow Jasmine (Jasminum odoratissimum), of Madeira, which is often planted in the southern States for the sake of its fragrant flowers and has also been known there under the name of Gelseminum; this has only two stamens, while Gelsemium has five.

Description

Its woody, twining stem often attains great height, its growth depending upon its chosen support, ascending lofty trees and forming festoons from one tree to another. It contains a milky juice and bears opposite, shining and evergreen lanceolate leaves and axillary clusters of from one to five large, funnel-shaped, very fragrant yellow flowers, which during its flowering season, in early spring, scent the atmosphere with their delicious odor. The fruit is composed of two separable, jointed pods containing numerous, flat-winged seeds.

The stem often runs underground for a considerable distance, and these portions (the rhizome) are used indiscriminately with the roots in medicine, and exported from the United States in bales.

The plant was first described in 1640 by John Parkinson, who grew it in his garden from seed sent by Tradescant from Virginia; at the present time it is but rarely seen, even in botanic gardens, in Great Britain, and specimens grown at Kew have not flowered.

Description of the Drug

The drug in commerce mostly consists of the undergroundstem or rhizome, with occasional pieces of the root. The rhizome is easily distinguished by occurring in nearly straight pieces, about 6 to 8 inches long, and 1/4 to 3/4 inch in diameter, having a small dark pith and a purplish-brown, longitudinally fissured bark. The root is smaller, tortuous, and of a uniform yellowish-brown color, finely wrinkled on the surface.

Both rhizome and root in transverse section exhibit a distinctly radiate appearance, the thin cortex or bark enclosing a large, pale, yellowish-white wood, which consists of narrow bundles with small pores, alternating with straight, whitish, medullary rays about six or eight cells in thickness. In the case of the rhizome, a small pith, frequently divided into four nearly equal parts, is also present, particularly in smaller and younger pieces.

The drug is hard and woody, breaking with an irregular splintery fracture, and frequently exhibits silky fibres in the bast, which are isolated, or occur in groups of two or three and form an interrupted ring, whereas in the aerial stem, they are grouped in bundles.

The drug has a bitter taste, due to the presence of alkaloids, which occur chiefly in the bark. The slight aromatic odor is probably due to the resin in the drug.

Collection

Adulterations. The drug is commonly collected

in the autumn and dried.Though consisting usually of the dried rhizomes with only the larger roots attached, sometimes smaller roots are present, and it is often adulterated with the aerial portions of the stem, which can be easily detected by the thinness and dark-purplish color of the latter. It is stated to be destitute of alkaloid and therefore of no medicinal value.

Similar roots of Jasmine, especially those of Jasminum fruticans, are sometimes intermixed, and can be distinguished by the absence of indurated pith cells, which occur in Gelsemium, by the abundance of thin-walled starch cells in the pith and in the medullary ray cells (those of Gelsemium being thickwalled and destitute of starch), and by the bast fibres round the sieve tubes.

Constituents

Gelsemium contains two potent alkaloids, Gelseminine and Gelsemine.

Gelseminine is a yellowish, bitter andpoisonous amorphous alkaloid, readily soluble in ether and alcohol, forming amorphous salts.

The alkaloid Gelsemine is colourless, odourless, intensely bitter and forms crystalline salts. It is only sparingly soluble inwater, but readily forms a hydrochloride, which is completely so. This alkaloid is not to be confounded with the resinoid known as 'Gelsemin,' an eclectic remedy, a mixture of substances obtained by evaporating an alcoholic extract of Gelsemium to dryness.

The rhizome also contains Gelsemic acid a crystalline substance which exhibits an intense bluish-green fluorescence in alkaline solution; it is probably identical with methylaesculatin or chrysatropic acid found in Belladonna root.

There are also present in the root 6 per cent of a volatile oil, 4 per cent of resin and starch.

Poisoning by Gelsemium

The drug is a powerful spinal depressant; its most marked action being on the anterior cornus of grey matter in the spinal cord.

The drug kills by its action on the respiratory centre of the medulla oblongata. Shortly after the administration of even a moderate dose, the respiration is slowed and is ultimately arrested, this being the cause of death.

Poisonous doses of Gelsemium produce a sensation of languor, relaxation and muscular weakness, which may be followed by paralysis if the dose is sufficiently large. The face becomes anxious, the temperature subnormal, the skin cold and clammy and the pulse rapid and feeble. Dropping of the upper eyelid and lower jaw, internal squint, double vision and dilatation of the pupil are prominent symptoms. The respiration becomes slow and feeble, shallow and irregular, and death occurs from centric respiratory failure, the heart stopping almost simultaneously. Consciousness is usually preserved until late in the poisoning, but may be lost soon after the ingestion of a fatal dose. The effects usually begin in half an hour, but sometimes almost immediately. Death has occurred at periods varying from 1 to 7 1/2 hours.

The treatment of Gelsemium poisoning consists in the prompt evacuation of the stomach by an emetic, if the patient's condition permits; and secondly, and equally important, artificial respiration, aided by the early administration, subcutaneously, of ammonia, strychnine, atropine or digitalis.

An allied species, G. elegans (Benth.) of Upper Burma, is used in China as a criminal poison, its effects are very rapid.

Medicinal Action and Uses

Antispasmodic, sedative, febrifuge, diaphoretic.

The medical history of the plant is quite modern. It is stated to have been brought into notice by a Mississippi planter, for whom, in his illness, the root was gathered in mistake for that of another plant. After partaking of an infusion, serious symptoms arose, but when, contrary to expectations, he recovered, it was clear that the attack of bilious fever from which he had been suffering had disappeared. This accidental error led to the preparation from the plant of a proprietary nostrum called the 'Electric Febrifuge.' Later, in 1849, Dr. Porcher, of South Carolina, brought Gelsemium to the notice of the American Medical Association. Dr. Henry, in 1852, and after him many others, made provings of it the chief being that of Dr. E. M. Hale, whose Monograph on Gelsemium was an efficient help to the true knowledge of the new American drug.

In America, it was formerly extensively used as an arterial sedative and febrifuge in various fevers, more especially those of an intermittent character, but now it is considered probably of little use for this purpose, for it has no action on the skin and no marked action on the alimentary or circulatory system.

It has been recommended and found useful in the treatment of spasmodic disorders, such as asthma and whooping cough, spasmodic croup and other conditions depending upon localized muscular spasm. In convulsions, its effects have been very satisfactory.

It is, at present, mainly used in the treatment of neuralgic pains, especially those involving the facial nerves, particularly when arising from decaying teeth.

It is said it will suspend and hold in check muscular irritability and nervous excitement with more force and power than any known remedy. While it relaxes all the muscles, it relieves, by its action on the general system, all sense of pain.

The drug is also said to be most useful in the headache and sleeplessness of the drunkard and in sick headache.

It has been used in dysmenorrhoea, hysteria, chorea and epilepsy, and the tincture has been found efficacious in cases of retention of urine.

Some recommend its use in acute rheumatism and pleurisy, in pneumonia and in bronchitis, and it has been advocated, though not accepted by all authorities, as of avail in the early stages of typhoid fever.

GENTIANS

Family: N.O. Gentianaceae

The Gentians are an extensive group of plants, numbering about 180 species, distributed throughout all climates, though mostly in temperate regions and high mountains, being rare in the Arctic. In South America and New Zealand, the prevailing color of the flower is red, in Europe blue (yellow and white being of rarer occurrence).

The name of the genus is derived from Gentius, an ancient King of Illyria (180-167 B.C.), who, according to Pliny and Dioscorides, discovered the medicinal value of these plants. During the Middle Ages, Gentian was commonly employed as an antidote to poison. Tragus, in 1552, mentions it as a means of diluting wounds.

GENTIAN, YELLOW

Botanical: Gentiana lutea (LINN.)
Part Used: Root.

HABITAT

The Yellow Gentian is a native of the Alpine and sub-alpine pastures of central and southern Europe, frequent in the mountains of Spain and Portugal, the Pyrenees, Sardinia and Corsica, the Apennines, the Mountains of Auvergne, the Jura, the lower slopes of the Vosges, the Black Forest and throughout the chain of the Alps as far as Bosnia and the Balkan States. It does not reach the northern countries of the Continent, nor the British Isles. At an elevation of from 3,000 to 4,500 feet, it is a characteristic species of many parts of France and Switzerland, where, even when not in flower, the numerous barren shoots form conspicuous objects: the leaves are at first sight very similar to Veratrum album, the White Hellebore, which is its frequent companion. Out of Europe, the plant occurs in the mountains of Lydia. In some parts it occupies large tracts of country, being untouched by any kind of cattle.

All the known species are remarkable for the intensely bitter properties residing in the root and every part of the herbage, hence they are valuable tonic medicines. That most commonly used in Europe is

Gentiana lutea, the Yellow Gentian. The root of this species is the principal vegetable bitter employed in medicine, though the roots of several other species, including our native ones, are said to be equally efficacious. Before the introduction of hops, Gentian, with many other bitterherbs, was used occasionally in brewing.

Gentian roots are collected and dried in central and southern Europe, much of the supply for this country having formerly come from Germany, though it is also imported from Switzerland, France and Spain, and French Gentian is considered of special excellence.

Yellow Gentian is one of the many herbs so far not cultivated in England for medicinal use, though preparations of the root are in constant use in every dispensary, and it is much prescribed also by veterinary surgeons. Though the plant is indigenous in central Europe, it can readily be grown from seed in England, and could quite easily be cultivated as a garden or field crop in this country. Though not often met with, it has been grown in gardens since the time of Gerard, who tells us that a learned French physician sent him from Burgundy plants of this species for his garden on Holborn Hill. It is a highly ornamental plant, forming one of the most stately hardy herbaceous perennials for the garden border, and when successfully treated will grow luxuriantly, even if in the neighborhood of London.

Description

The root is long and thick, generally about a foot long and an inch in diameter, but sometimes even a yard or more long and 2 inches in diameter, of a yellowish-brown color and a very bitter taste. The stem grows 3 or 4 feet high or more, with a pair of leaves opposite to one another, at each joint. The lowest leaves have short foot-stalks, but the upper ones are stalkless, their bases almost embracing the stem. They are yellowish-green in color, oblong in shape and pointed, rather stiff, with five prominent veins on the underside, and diminish gradually in size as they grow up the stem. The large flowers are in whorls in the axils of the uppermost few pairs of leaves, forming big orange-yellow clusters. The corollas are wheel-shaped, usually five-cleft, 2 inches across, sometimes marked with rows of small brown spots, giving a red tinge to the otherwise deep yellow. Seeds in abundance are produced by strong plants, and stock is easily raised from them.

Cultivation

For the successful cultivation of G. lutea, a strong, loamy soil is most suitable, the deeper the better, as the stout roots descend a long way down into the soil. Plenty of moisture is also desirable and a position where there is shelter from cold winds and exposure to sunshine. Old plants have large crowns, which may be divided for the purpose of propagation, but growing it on a large scale, seeds would be the best method. They could be sown in a frame, or in a nursery bed in a sheltered part of the garden and the young seedlings transplanted. They take about three years to grow to flowering size. It is, however, likely that the roots are richest in medicinal properties before the plants have flowered. A big clump of G. lutea is worthy of a conspicuous position in any large flower garden, quite apart from its medicinal value.

Part Used

The rhizome and roots collected in autumn and dried. When fresh, they are yellowish-white externally, but gradually become darker by slow drying. Slow drying is employed to prevent deterioration in color and to improve the aroma. Occasionally the roots are longitudinally sliced and quickly dried, the drug being then pale in color and unusually bitter in taste, but this variety is not official.

The dried root as it occurs in commerce is brown and cylindrical, 1 foot or more in length, or broken up into shorter pieces, usually 1/2 inch to 1 inch in diameter, rather soft and spongy, with a thick reddish bark, tough and flexible, and of an orange-brown color internally. The upper portion is marked with numerous rings, the lower longitudinally wrinkled. The root has a strong, disagreeable odor, and the taste is slightly sweet at first, but afterwards very bitter.

Substitutes

G. purpurea, G. pannonica, G. punctata and G. acaulis are European gentians having similar medicinal properties to G. lutea and are used indiscriminately with each other and the official root, from which they differ but little in appearance, though are somewhat smaller.

American Gentian root is derived from G. puberula, G. saponaria and G. Andrewsii. This drug is said to have properties practically identical with those of European varieties.

Belladonna and Aconite roots, and the rhizomes of Orris and White Hellebore have been found mixed with the genuine root, and the powdered root of commerce is frequently adulterated, ground almond shells and olive stones having been used for this purpose.

Constituents

The dried Gentian root of commerce contains Gentiin and Gentiamarin, bitter glucosides, together with Gentianic acid (gentisin), the latter being physiologically inactive. Gentiopicrin, another bitter glucoside, a pale yellow crystalline substance, occurs in the fresh root, and may be isolated from it by treatment with boiling alcohol. The saccharine constituents of Gentian are dextrose, laevulose, sucrose and gentianose, a crystallizable, fermentable sugar. It is free from starch and yields from 3 to 4 per cent ash.

Medicinal Action and Uses

Gentian is one of the most useful of our bitter vegetable tonics. It is specially useful in states of exhaustion from chronic disease and in all cases of general debility, weakness of the digestive organs and want of appetite. It is one of the best strengtheners of the human system, and is an excellent tonic to combine with a purgative to prevent its debilitating effects. Many dyspeptic complaints are more effectually relieved by Gentian bitters than by Peruvian Bark. It is of extreme value in jaundice and is prescribed extensively.

Besides being unrivalled as a stomachic tonic, Gentian possesses febrifuge, emmenagogue, anthelmintic and antiseptic properties, and is also useful in hysteria, female weakness, etc. Gentian with equal parts of Tormentil or galls has been used with success for curing intermittent fever.

As a simple bitter, Gentian is considered more palatable combined with an aromatic, and for this purpose orange peel is frequently used. A tincture made with 2 OZ. of the root, 1 OZ. of dried orange peel, and 1/2 oz. bruised cardamom seeds in a quart of brandy is an excellent stomachic tonic, and is efficacious in restoring appetite and promoting digestion. A favorite form in which Gentian has been administered in country remedies is as an ingredient in the so-called Stockton bitters, in which Gentian and the root of Sweet Flag play the principal part.

The dose of the fluid extract is 1/2 to 1 teaspoonful in water, three times daily.

Fresh Gentian root is largely used in Germany and Switzerland for the production of an alcoholic beverage. The roots are cut, macerated with water, fermented and distilled; the distillate contains alcohol and a trace of volatile oil, which imparts to it a characteristic odor and taste.

Preparations and Dosages

Fluid extract, 1/2 to 1 drachm. Compound infusion, B.P. 1/2 to 1 OZ. Compound tincture, B.P. and U.S.P., 1/2 to 1 drachm. Solid extract, B.P., 2 to 8 grains.

Culpepper states that our native Gentians 'have been proved by the experience of divers physicians not to be a whit inferior in virtue to that which comes from beyond sea.'

'comforts the heart and preserves it against faintings and swoonings: The powder of the dry roots helps the biting of mad dogs and venomous beasts.... The herb steeped in wine, and the wine drank, refreshes such as be over-weary with traveling, and grow lame in their joints, either by cold or evil lodgings: it helps stitches, and griping pains in the sides: is an excellent remedy for such as are bruised by falls . . . when Kine are bitten on the udder by any venomous beast, do but stroke the place with the decoction of any of these and it will instantly heal them.'

In the eighteenth century Gentian wine was drunk as an aperitif before dinner.

GENTIAN, JAPANESE

Botanical: Gentiana scabrae
Synonym: Ryntem Root.
Part Used: Root.

Description

The rhizome is dark greyish brown, attaining about 10 cm. in length and 5 mm. in diameter. It is irregularly annulate, and bears on the top stem-bases occasionally stem-remnants, and on the lateral and lower sides numerous roots. The crosssection of the rhizome is dark brown, and shows in the wood fibro-vascular bundles, running irregularly. The roots are brownishyellow, attaining about 20 cm. in length and 3 mm. in diameter, and longitudinally wrinkled. The cross-section of the root is brown, having a darker coloured wood, which shows radially arranged trachea at the periphery. It does not contain sclerenchymatous cells; the parenchymatous cells contain many oxalate crystals, but no starch grains. It has a very bitter taste. It may be used as a substitute for radix gentianae. (From The Chemist and Druggist of August 19, 1922.)

Other Species

The two most frequently found nativeGentians are Gentiana amarella, the Autumn Gentian, and G. campestris, the Field Gentian, which were formerly pronounced by both Linnaeus and Scopoli to be merely variations of the same species, but are now universally described as separate species.

Both have been used for their bitterness instead of hops, and also as a medicine, in common with others of the same genus, and the dried root and dried herb of the Field Gentian are still sold by herbalists for use as a bitter tonic, having the same properties as the foreign Gentian. The old English names for these Gentians - Bitterwort and Felwort (Fel being an old word for the gall) testify to their bitter qualities being popularly known.

GENTIAN, AUTUMN

Botanical: Gentiana amarella (LINN.)
Synonyms: Bitterwort. Felwort. Baldmoney.
Part Used: Root.

The Autumn Gentian (Gentiana amarella, Linn.) is not uncommon in calcareous soils and in dry pastures, in most parts of Europe, flowering from July to September. It has an annual root, twisted and yellowish, somewhat thready. The stem is square, erect, bearing several pairs of stalkless, dark green leaves, each with three prominent veins, and clothed from top to bottom with flowers on short stalks in the axils of the leaves, one flower terminating the stem. The calyx is pale, with green ribs, divided half-way down into five lance-shaped, nearly equal segments. The corolla is salver-shaped, blue-purple in color, the tube quite as long as the calyx, and five-cleft, the lobes being nearly equal; the mouth of the tube is provided with a purple, upright fringe, which conceals the stamens. In sunshine, the lobes of the corolla are spread wide horizontally, forming conspicuous blue stars.

GENTIAN, FIELD

Botanical: Gentiana campestris (LINN.)
Synonyms: Bitterroot. Felwort.
Part Used: Root.

The Field Gentian (Gentiana campestris, Linn.) resembles the Autumn Gentian in general character, though the plant is as a rule smaller, 4 to 12 inches high. Its stems are erect and much branched, the branches long with leaves and flowers scattered the whole length, whereas G. amarella, when branched, has the branches short, even the lower ones not exceeding the length of the leaves from which they spring, and the upper ones mostly much shorter. The flowers are fewer in number than those of amarella, though larger and on longer flower-stalks. The essential difference between the species, however, is that both calyx and corolla are four-cleft in G. campestris, the two outer, oval lobes of the calyx being also much larger, completely enfolding and concealing the two smaller ones, which are not a fifth part as broad. The salver-shaped corolla is of a dull purplish color, fringed in the throat, as in G. amarella. The roots are small, but penetrate some distance into the soil. This species grows in pastures, particularly near the sea, but is not so much confined to a calcareous soil as G. amarella. It is an annual, and flowers in August and September. This is the principal species used by the peasantry in Sweden in lieu of hops in brewing beer.

GENTIAN, MARSH

Botanical: Gentiana Pneumonanthe (LINN.)
Part Used: Root.

The Marsh Gentian (Gentiana Pneumonanthe, Linn.), though occasionally found on moist, boggy heaths, is a plant of much more local occurrence in Great Britain than the two previous species. Its stems are 3 to 18 inches high, the leaves 1 to 2 inches long. The flowers, 1 1/2 to 2 inches long are rather few in number, pale blue externally, with five paler stripes and dark, vivid blue within, variegated with white in the throat. Gerard tells us of this pretty little plant, which is quite worthy of cultivation, that 'the gallant flowers hereof bee in their bravery about the end of August,' and goes on to say that 'the later physicians hold it to be effectual against pestilent diseases and the bitings and stingings of venomous beasts.' It has the bitterness and other qualities of the preceding species.

This variety grows in moist places on heaths near Swanage, Dorset.

GENTIAN, SPRING

Botanical: Gentiana verna
Part Used: Root.

The flowers are of such a startling blue that A. C. Benson has described it as 'the pure radiance of the untroubled heaven.'

The flowers grow singly on exceedingly short stalks, and only open if the sun is shining when they stretch their blue petals wide and face the blue above them. There is a narrow, green calyx-cup and a blue tube issuing therefrom which opens out into five lobes star-wise. The leaves grow in pairs, stalkless, clasping the stem. They are not very numerous on the short flower-stalks, but form close rosettes of foliage near the soil. The flower-stems are rigidly erect, about 4 to 12 inches being their usual height. It flowers in April and May and is to be found in Westmorland, but is not so much at home in England as it is on Irish soil; it grows in profusion, too, on the Isle of Arran. It likes limestone and chalky ground.

We have only six varieties of Gentians in Great Britain, one of which (G. nivalis) is found on the Breadalbane and Clora Mountains. Another species (G. acaulis) most nearly resembles our G. Pneumonanthe. The flowers are bright blue and rather elongated, 1 to 2 inches in length.

GENTIAN, CROSS-LEAVED

Botanical: Gentiana cruciata
Part Used: Root.

Gentiana cruciata (Cross-leaved Gentian), so called because its leaves grow in the form of a cross, has been recommended in hydrophobia. In homeopathic medicine a tincture of the root is used in hoarseness and sore throat.

GENTIAN, FIVE-FLOWERED

Botanical: Gentiana quinqueflora
Part Used: Root.

A tincture is also made from the fresh flowering plant of Gentiana quinqueflora (Five-flowered Gentian) and used in homeopathy as a tonic and stomachic, and in intermittent fevers.

GERMANDER, SAGE-LEAVED

Botanical: Teucrium scorodonia (LINN.)
Family: N.O. Labiatae
Synonyms: Wood Sage. Large-leaved Germander. Hind Heal. Ambroise. Garlic Sage.
Part Used: Herb.

Habitat

Sage-leaved Germander (Teucrium scorodonia) is a common woodland plant in healthy districts. It is a native of Europe and Morocco, found in woody and hilly situations among bushes and under hedges, where the soil is dry and stony. It is frequent in such places in most parts of Great Britain, flowering from July to September.

Description

The roots are perennial and creeping, the stems square, a foot or two in height, of a shrubby character, with opposite greyish-green, sage-like leaves, in form somewhat oblong heart-shaped, the edges coarsely toothed, very much wrinkled in texture like those of the Sage, hence its familiar names, Wood Sage and Sage Germander.

The whole plant is softly hairy or pubescent. The small labiate flowers are in onesided spike-like clusters, the corollas greenish-yellow in color, with four stamens, which have yellow anthers, and very noticeable purple and hairy filaments. The terminal flowering spike is about as long again as those that spring laterally below it from the axils of the uppermost pair of leaves.

The generic name of Teucrium was bestowed by Linnaeus, it has been suggested, from a belief that this plant is identical with the plant that Dioscorides says was first used medicinally by an ancient king of Troy, named Teucer, but it is also said that Linnaeus named the genus after a Dr. Teucer, a medical botanist.

The specific name, scorodonia, is derived from the Greek word for Garlic, and does not appear to be particularly appropriate to this species.

It has been popularly called ' Hind Heal,' from a theory that the hind made use of it when sick or wounded, and was probably the same herb as Elaphoboscum, the Dittany taken by harts in Crete.

In taste and smell, the species resembles Hops. It is called 'Ambroise' in Jersey, and used there and in some other districts as a substitute for hops. It is said that when this herb is boiled in wort the beer becomes clear sooner than when hops are made use of, but that it is apt to give the liquor too much color.

The bitter taste is due to the presence of a peculiar tonic principle found in all the species of this genus.

There are about 100 species of Teucrium widely dispersed throughout the world, but chiefly abounding in the northern temperate and subtropical regions of the Eastern Hemisphere. Of the three other British species besides the Wood Sage, two have been used medicinally, T. Chamaedrys (Wall Germander), a famous old gout medicine, and T. Scordium (Water Germander).

Cultivation

Wood Sage is generally collected in the wild state, but will thrive in any moderately good soil, and in almost any situation.

It may be increased by seeds, by cuttings, inserted in sandy soil, under a glass, in spring and summer; or by division of roots in the autumn.

Part Used

The whole herb, collected in July.

Constituents

A volatile oil, some tannin and a bitter principle.

Medicinal Action and Uses

Alterative and diuretic, astringent tonic, emmenagogue. Much used in domestic herbal practice for skin affections and diseases of the blood, also in fevers, colds, inflammations, and as an emmenagogue.

Fluid extract, 1/2 to 1 drachm.

It is useful for quinsy, sore throat, and in kidney and bladder trouble.

In chronic rheumatism it has been used with benefit, and is considered a valuable tonic and restorer of the system after an attack of rheumatism, gout, etc.

The infusion (freshly prepared) is the proper mode of administration, made from 1 OZ. of the dried herb to 1 pint of boiling water, taken warm in wine glassful doses, three or four times a day.

Wood Sage is an appetizer of the first order, and as a tonic will be found equal to Gentian. It forms an excellent bitter combined with Comfrey and Ragwort, which freely influences the bladder.

It is also good to cleanse old sores. If used in the green state with Comfrey and Ragwort, the combination makes an excellent poultice for old wounds and inflammations in any part of the body. Culpepper tells us:

'The decoction of the green herb with wine is a safe and sure remedy for those who by falls, bruises or blows suspect some vein to be inwardly broken, to disperse and void the congealed blood and consolidate the veins. The drink used inwardly and the herb outwardly is good for such as are inwardly or outwardly bursten, and is found to be a sure remedy for the palsy. The juice of the herb or the powder dried is good for moist ulcers and sores. It is no less effectual also in green wounds to be used upon any occasion.'

A snuff has been made from its powdered leaves to cure nasal polypi.

GERMANDER, WALL

Botanical: Teucrium chamaedrys (LINN.)
Family: N.O. Labiatae
Synonyms: Petit Chêne. Chasse fièvre.
Part Used: Whole herb.

The Common or Wall Germander (Teucrium Chamaedrys) is a native of many parts of Europe, the Greek Islands and also of Syria, being found near Jerusalem, but in England is scarce and hardly indigenous being chiefly found on the ruins of old buildings and in other places where it has escaped from cultivation. It was formerly much cultivated in this country for medicinal purposes.

Description

The roots are perennial and creeping, the square stem, 6 to 18 inches high, erect, much branched, leafy. The opposite, dark green leaves are 1/2 to 1 1/2 inch long and indented, somewhat like an oak leaf, hence the name Chamaedrys, from chamai (ground) and drus (oak). The name Germander is considered also to be a corruption of Chamaedrys. The French term this plant Petit Chêne, from the shape of the leaves, as well as Chasse fièvre, from its use in medicine.

The rose-coloured, labiate flowers, which bloom in June and July, are in three to six flowered whorls, in the axils of leafy bracts, and in leafy, terminal spikes. The whole plant is almost roughly hairy.

The fresh leaves are bitter and pungent to the taste and when rubbed, emit a strong odor somewhat resembling garlic.

Cultivation

Germander will grow in almost any soil and is propagated by seeds,by cuttings taken in spring or summer, and by division of roots, in the autumn. Plant about a foot apart each way.

Part Used

The whole herb, collected in July and dried in the same manner as Wood Sage.

Medicinal Action and Uses

Stimulant, tonic, diaphoretic, diuretic. Germander acts as a slight aperient, as well as a tonic.

The reputation of Germander as a specific for gout is of very old date, the Emperor Charles V having been cured by a decoction of this herb taken for sixty days in succession.

It has been employed in various forms and combinations, of which the once celebrated Portland Powder is one of the chief instances.

It was also used as a tonic in intermittent fevers, and is recommended for uterine obstructions.

The expressed juice of the leaves, with the addition of white wine, is held to be good in obstruction of the viscera.

Possessing qualities nearly allied to those of Horehound, a decoction of the green herb, taken with honey, has been found useful in asthmatic affections and coughs, being recommended for this purpose by Dioscorides. The decoction has also been given to relieve dropsy in its early stages.

Culpepper tells us that it is:

'most effectual against the poison of all serpents, being drunk in wine and the bruised herb outwardly applied.... Used with honey it cleanseth ulcers and made into an oil and the eyes anointed therewith, taketh away dimness and moisture. It is also good for pains in the side and cramp.... The decoction taken for four days driveth away and cureth tertian and quartan agues. It is also good against diseases of the brain, as continual headache, falling sickness, melancholy, drowsiness and dulness of spirits, convulsions and palsies.'

He further states that the powdered seeds are good against jaundice. The tops, when in flower, steeped twenty-four hours in white wine will destroy worms.

GERMANDER, WATER

Botanical: Teucrium scordium (LINN.)
Family: N.O. Labiatae
Part Used: Herb.

The Water Germander (Teucrium Scordium) is a creeping plant growing in marshy places in various parts of Europe, but very rare in Great Britain except in the Isle of Ely. It was formerly cultivated in gardens for medicinal uses.

Description

The square, hairy stalks, are of a dirty green color and very weak. The leaves are short, broad, woolly and soft, and indented at the edges. The flowers are small, of a purplish-rose color, in whorls, in the axils of the leaves. It flowers in July and August.

The whole plant is bitter and slightly aromatic.

The fresh leaves, when rubbed, have a penetrating odor, like Garlic, and it is said that when cows eat it through hunger, it gives the flavor of Garlic to their milk.

Medicinal Action and Uses

It was once esteemed as an antidote for poisons and as an antiseptie and anthelmintic, but is now searcely used, though its tonic and aromatic bitter qualities and diaphoretic action make a decoction of it an excellent remedy in all inflammatory diseases, and it may be used with advantage in weak, relaxed constitutions.

The tincture in small doses is considered a good remedy for exhilarating and rousing torpid faculties.

For intermittent fever and scrofulous complaints the infusion of 1 OZ. of the dried herb to 1 pint of boiling water, taken in wine glassful doses, is recommended.

The dried leaves have been employed as a vermifuge, and decoction is said to be a good fomentation in gangrenous cases.

Preparation

Fluid extract, 1/2 to 1 drachm.

GINGER

Botanical: Zingiber officinale (ROSC.)
Family: N.O. Zingiberaceae
Part Used: Root.
Habitat: Said to be a native of Asia. Cultivated in West Indies, Jamaica, Africa.

Description

Naturalized in America after the discovery of that country by the Spaniards. Francisco de Mendosa transplanted it from the East Indies into Spain, where Spanish-Americans cultivated it vigorously, so that in 1547 they exported 22,053 cwt. into Europe.

It is now cultivated in great quantities in Jamaica and comes into this country dried and preserved. The root from the West Indies is considered the best. Also imported from Africa, there are several varieties known in commerce. Jamaica or White African is a light-brown color with short rhizome, very pungent. Cochin has a very short rhizome, coated red-grey color. 'Coated or Uncoated' is the trade term for peel on or skinned. Green Ginger is the immature undried rhizome. Preserved Ginger is made by steeping the root in hot syrup. Ratoon is uncultivated Ginger. Ginger is a perennial root which creeps and increases underground, in tuberous joints; in the spring it sends up from its roots a green reed, like a stalk, 2 feet high, with narrow lanceolate leaves; these die down annually. The flowering stalk rises directly from the root, ending in an oblong scallop spike; from each spike a white or yellow bloom grows. Commercial Ginger is called black or white, according to whether it is peeled or unpeeled; for both kinds the ripened roots are used, after the plant has died down. The black are scalded in boiling water, then dried in the sun. The white (best) are scraped clean and dried, without being scalded. For preserve young green roots are used-they are scalded and are washed in cold water and then peeled. The water is changed several times, so that the process takes three or four days. The tubers are then put into jars and covered with a weak syrup; this is changed after a few days' soaking for a stronger syrup, which is again changed for a still stronger one. The discarded syrups are fermented and made into a liquor called 'cool drink'; a few drops of chloroform or chloride are generally added to the preserve to prevent insects breeding in it. Ginger flowers have an aromatic smell and the bruised stem a characteristic fragrance, but the root is considered the most useful part of the plant, and must not be used under a year's growth. The peeling has to be done very thinly or the richest part of the resin and volatile oil is lost. It is sometimes soaked in lime-juice instead of plain water, and the color is improved by a final coating of chalk. The Chinese fresh Ginger is grated into powder. African and Cochin Ginger yield the most resin and volatile oil. The root must be kept in a dry place, or it will start growing and is then spoilt. The odor of Ginger is penetrating and aromatic, its taste spicy, hot and biting; these properties are lost by exposure. The most common adulterants are flour, curcuma, linseed, rapeseed, the hulls of cayenne pepper and waste ginger.

Constituents

Volatile oil, acrid soft resin, resin insoluble in ether and oil, gum, starch, lignin, vegeto matter, asmazone, acetic acid, acetate of potassa, sulphur.

Medicinal Action and Uses

Stimulant, carminative, given in dyspepsia and flatulent colic excellent to add to bitter infusions; specially valuable in alcoholic gastritis; of use for diarrhea from relaxed bowel where there is no inflammation. Ginger Tea is a hot infusion very useful for stoppage of the mensesdue to cold, externally it is a rubefacient. Essence of Ginger should be avoided, as it is often adulterated with harmful ingredients.

Dosage

Infusion: 1/2 oz. bruised or powdered root to 1 pint boiling water is taken in 1 fluid ounce. Dose, 10 to 20 grains.

Preparation

Fluid extract, 10 to 20 drops. Tincture, B.P., 1/2 to 1 drachm. Syrup, B.P. and U.S.P., 1/2 to 1 drachm. Oleoresin, U.S.P., 1/2 grain.

GINGER, WILD

Botanical: Asarum canadense (LINN.)
Family: N.O. Aristolochiaceae
Synonyms: Canada Snakeroot. Indian Ginger. Coltsfoot.
Parts Used: Rhizome dried and roots.
Habitat: North America, North Carolina, Kansas.

Description

An inconspicuous but fragrant little plant, not over 12 inches high, found growing in rich soil on roadsides and in woods. A stemless perennial, much resembling the European Asarum, but with larger leaves, provided with a short spine, leaves usually only two, kidney-shaped, borne on thin fine hairy stems, dark above and paler green under-surface, 4 to 8 inches broad, strongly veined. A solitary bell-shaped flower, dull brown or brownish purple, drooping between the two leaf stems, woolly, the inside darker than the outside and of a satiny texture, the fruit a leathery six-celled capsule. It has a yellowish creeping rootstock, slightly jointed, with thin rootlets from the joints. In commerce the rootstock is found in pieces 4 to 5 inches long, 1/8 inch thick, irregular quadrangular, brownish end wrinkled outside, whitish inside, showing a large centre pith hard and brittle, breaking with a short fracture. Odor fragrant, taste aromatic, spicy and slightly bitter--it is collected in the autumn.

Constituents

A volatile oil once largely used in perfumery, also resin, a bitter principle called asarin, mucilage, alkaloid, sugar and a substance like camphor.

The plant yields its properties to alcohol and to hot water.

Medicinal Action and Uses

Stimulant, carminative, diuretic, diaphoretic. Used in chronic chest complaints, dropsy with albuminaria, painful spasms of bowels and stomach.

Dosage

1/2 oz. of the powdered root in 1 pint of boiling water, taken hot, produces copious perspiration.

Dry powder, 20 to 30 grains.

As an adjuvant to tonic mixtures or infusions, 1/2 to 1 drachm.

Other Species

ASARUM EUROPAEUM

Synonyms: Hazlewort, Wild Nard, very similar in properties to above).
Part Used: Root and leaves dried.

Description

A European plant growing in most hilly woods, flowering from May till August. The root smells like pepper, with a spicy taste and gives an ash-coloured powder. The leaves give a green powder and have the same properties as the root.

Medicinal Action and Uses

Emetic, cathartic and errhine, for which latter purpose it is principally used in affections of the brain, eyes, throat, toothache and paralysis of the mouth. In France drunkards use it as an emetic, and it promotes sneezing and is therefore helpful for colds in the head.

Dosage

Powder, 10 to 12 grains. As anemetic, 1/2 to 1 drachm.

A. ARIFOLIUM yields an oil with the odor of sassafras.

GINSENG

Botanical: Panax quinquefolium (LINN.)
Family: N.O. Araliaceae
Synonyms: Aralia quinquefolia. Five Fingers. Tartar Root. Red Berry. Man's Health.
Part Used: Root.

Habitat

Ginseng is distinguished as Asiatic or Chinese Ginseng. It is a native of Manchuria, Chinese Tartary and other parts of eastern Asia, and is largely cultivated there as well as in Korea and Japan.

Panax, the generic name, is derived from the Greek Panakos (a panacea), in reference to the miraculous virtue ascribed to it by the Chinese, who consider it a sovereign remedy in almost all diseases.

It was formerly supposed to be confined to Chinese Tartary, but now is known to be also a native of North America, from whence Sarrasin transmitted specimens to Paris in 1704.

The word ginseng is said to mean 'the wonder of the world.'

Description

The plant grows in rich woods throughout eastern and central North America, especially along the mountains from Quebec and Ontario, south to Georgia. It was used by the North American Indians. It is a smooth perennial herb, with a large, fleshy, very slow-growing root, 2 to 3 inches in length (occasionally twice this size) and from 1/2 to 1 inch in thickness. Its main portion is spindle-shaped and heavily annulated (ringed growth), with a roundish summit, often with a slight terminal, projecting point. At the lower end of this straight portion, there is a narrower continuation, turned obliquely outward in the opposite direction and a very small branch is occasionally borne in the fork between the two.

Some small rootlets exist upon the lower portion. The color ranges from a pale yellow to a brownish color. It has a mucilaginous sweetness, approaching that of liquorice, accompanied with some degree of bitterness and a slight aromatic warmth, with little or no smell. The stem is simple and erect, about a foot high, bearing three leaves, each divided into five finely-toothed leaflets, and a single, terminal umbel, with a few small, yellowish flowers. The fruit is a cluster of bright red berrles.

The plant was first introduced into England in 1740 by the botanist Collinson.

Chinese Ginseng is a larger plant, but presents practically the same appearance and habits of growth. Its culture in the United States has never been attempted, though it would appear to be a promising field for experiment.

Father Jartoux, who had special privileges accorded him in the study of this plant, says that it is held in such esteem by the natives of China, that the physicians deem it a necessity in all their best prescriptions, and regard it as a remediable agency in fatigue and the infirmities of old age. Only the Emperor has the right to collect the roots. The prepared root is chewed by the sick to recover health, and by the healthy to increase their vitality; it is said to remove both mental and bodily fatigue, to cure pulmonary complaints, dissolves tumours and prolongs life to a ripe old age.

Father Jartoux was satisfied that its praise was justified, and he adds his own testimony to its efficacy in relieving fatigue and increasing vitality. The roots are called, by the natives of China, Jin-chen, meaning 'like a man,' in reference to their resemblance to the human form. The American Indian name for the plant, garantoquen, has the same meaning.

Owing to the enormous demand for the root in China recourse was had to the American species, Panax quinquefolium (Linn.), and in 1718 the Jesuits of Canada began shipping the roots to China, and the first shipment from North America to Canton yielded enormous profits. In 1748 the roots sold at a dollar a pound in America and nearly five in China. Afterwards, the price fluctuated, but the root is still eagerly purchased by Chinese traders for export to China, and at the present time commands a yet higher price in the American markets, though it is not an official medicine and has only a place in the eclectic Materia Medica. The American Consul at Amoy stated a few years ago that it is possible to market twenty million dollars worth of American Ginseng annually to China, if it could be produced; but since its collection for exportation, it has been so eagerly sought that it has become exterminated in many districts where it was formerly abundant.

This has led to its cultivation and to various devices for preserving the natural supply. In Canada a fine is imposed for collecting between January and the 1st of September. Among the Indians, it is customary to collect the root only after the maturity of the fruit and to bend down the stem before digging the root, thus providing for its propagation. Indian collectors assert that a large number of such seeds will germinate, and that they have been able to increase their area of collection by this method.

In 1876, 550,624 lb. were exported at an average price of 1 dollar 17 cents; the amount available for export since then has steadily decreased and the price has gone up in proportion, till in 1912 the export was only 155,308 lb., at an average price of 7 dollars 20 cents per pound.

Cultivation

On account of the growing scarcity of the American Ginseng plant, experiments have been made by the State of Pennsylvania to determine whether it can be grown profitably, resulting in the conclusion that in five years, starting with seeds and one year plants (or sooner if a start were made with older plants), an acre of ground would yield a profit of 1,500 dollars, without allowance for rental, but many precautions are necessary for success. The cultivated plants produced larger roots than those of the wild plant.

In 1912 it was estimated that the acreage of cultivated Ginseng in the United States was about 150 acres, and it is calculated that to supply China with twenty million dollars' worth of dry root would require the American growers to plant 1,000 acres annually for five years, before this estimated annual supply could be sold. The cultivation of Ginseng would therefore appear to offer a rich field to American agriculture. It presents, however, considerable difficulty, owing to the great care and special methods required and to the fact that it is a very slow-growing crop, so that rapid returns can hardly be anticipated, and it is doubtful if its cultivation can be carried on profitably except by specialists in the crop. None the less, the percentage returns for the industrious, patient and painstaking farmer are large, and the demand for a fine article for export is not at all likely to be exceeded by the supply.

For successful cultivation of Ginseng in America, it is stated that a loose, rich soil, with a heavy mulch of leaves and about 80 per cent shade - generally provided artificially is necessary.

It is difficult to cultivate it here with success. A rich compost is necessary. Most of the species of this genus need greenhouse treatment in this country. Propagation by cuttings of the roots is the most successful method, the cuttings being placed in sand, under a handglass. Seeds, generally obtained from abroad, are sown in pots in the early spring and require gentle heat. When the plants are a few inches high, they must be transplanted into beds or sheltered borders. They require a good, warm soil, but much shade. To grow on a commercial basis is not considered feasible in this country.

Harvesting, Preparation for Market

The root should be collected only in the autumn, in which case it retains its plump and handsome appearance after drying. It is much more highly prized when of a fine light color, which it is more apt to assume when grown in deep, black, fresh mould.

The best root is said to be that collected by the Sioux Indian women, who impart this white appearance by rotating it with water in a partly-filled barrel, through which rods are run in a longitudinal direction. In no other way, it is said, can the surface be so thoroughly and safely cleansed.

The structure of the root is fleshy and somewhat elastic and flexible, and it is of a firm, solid consistence if collected at the proper time and properly cured. The bark is very thick, yellowish-white, radially striate in old roots and contains brownishred resin cells. The wood is strongly and coarsely radiate, with yellowish wood wedges and whitish rays.

The best roots for the Chinese market are sometimes submitted before being dried to a process of clarification, which renders them yellow, semi-transparent and of a horny appearance and enhances their value. This condition is gained by first plunging them in hot water, brushing until thoroughly scoured and steaming over boiling seed. Its commercial value is determined in a high degree by its appearance. The roots are valued in accordance with their large size and light color, their plumpness and fine consistence, their unbroken and natural form, and above all by the perfectly developed condition of the branches.

Constituents

A large amount of starch and gum, some resin, a very small amount of volatile oil and the peculiar sweetish body, Panaquilon. This occurs as a yellow powder, precipitating with water a white, amorphous substance, which has been called Panacon.

Medicinal Action and Uses

Panax is not official in the British Pharmacopoeia, and it was dismissed from the United States Pharmacopceia at a late revision. It is cultivated almost entirely for export to China.

In China, both varieties are used particularly for dyspepsia, vomiting and nervous disorders. A decoction of 1/2 oz. of the root, boiled in tea or soup and taken every morning, is commonly held a remedy for consumption and other diseases.

In Western medicine, it is considered a mild stomachic tonic and stimulant, useful in loss of appetite and in digestive affections that arise from mental and nervous exhaustion.

A tincture has been prepared from the genuine Chinese or American root, dried and coarsely powdered, covered with five times its weight of alcohol and allowed to stand, well-stoppered, in a dark, cool place, being shaken twice a day. The tincture, poured off and filtered, has a clear, light-lemon color, an odor like the root and a taste at first bitter, then dulcamarous and an acid reaction.

Substitutes

A substitute for Ginseng, somewhat employed in China, is the root of Codonopsis Tangshen, a bell-flowered plant, used by the poor as a substitute for the costly Ginseng.

Ginseng is sometimes accidentally collected with Senega Root (Polygala Senega, Linn.) and with Virginian Snake Root (Aristolochia Serpentaria, Linn.), but is easily detected, being less wrinkled and twisted and yellower in color. It is occasionally found with the collected root of Cypripedium parviflorum (Salis) and Stylophorum diphyllum (Nuttall).

Blue Cohosh (Caulophyllum thalictroides, Linn.) is often called locally in the United States 'Blue' or 'Yellow Ginseng,' and Fever Root (Triosteum perfoliatum, Linn.) also is sometimes given the name of Ginseng.

GIPSYWEED, COMMON

Botanical: Lycopus Europaeus
Family: N.O. Labiatae
Synonyms: Water Horehound. Gipsy-wort. Egyptian's Herb.
Part Used: Herb.

Common Gipsyweed (Lycopus Europaeus), frequent throughout Europe, yields a black dye, stated to give a permanent color to wool and silk. As its name implies, it was formerly used by gipsies to stain their skins darker. It is common by the banks of streams, flowers from July to September, and is an erect plant with scarcely branched stems, about 2 feet high, with deeply-cut, pointed leaves and small, pale flesh-coloured flowers, growing in crowded whorls in the axils of the upper leaves.

Anne Pratt says it received its old name of Egyptian's Herb 'because of the rogues and runnegates which call themselves Egyptians, and doe color themselves black with this herbe.'

Medicinal Action and Uses

Astringent, sedative.

GLADWYN, STINKING

Botanical: Iris foetidissima (LINN.)
Family: N.O. Iridaceae
Synonyms: Gladwin. Spurge Plant. Roast Beef Plant.
Part Used: Root.

Stinking Gladwyn is found only locally in England, but is common in all the southwestern counties, growing in woods and shady places, on hedgebanks and sloping grounds.

Description

The creeping rhizomes are thick, tufted and fibrous. The leaves are firm, deep green, sword-shaped, shorter, narrower and less rigid and of a darker green than those of the Yellow Flag, and are evergreen in winter. When bruised or crushed, they emit a strong odor, at a distance not unlike that of hot, roast beef, hence its country name of 'Roast Beef Plant.' On closer acquaintance, the scent becomes disagreeable, hence the more usual common name 'Stinking Gladwyn,' and the Latin specific name.

It flowers from June to August, but sparingly, and the corollas, of a dull, livid purple color, rarely bluish or yellowish, are smaller than those of the other flags and not fragrant at night.

The flowers are followed by triangular seed-vessels, which, when ripe, open, disclosing beautiful orange-red coloured seeds.

Cultivation

Stinking Gladwyn flourishes in moist and partially-shaded places, in ordinary garden soil. Seeds scattered in semiwild places soon make good plants and plants may also be increased by division of the rhizomes. The brilliant seeds in their gaping capsules make it an effective garden plant in autumn.

Medicinal Action and Uses

Antispasmodic, cathartic, anodyne. Iris foetidissima has been employed for the same medicinal purposes as the Yellow Flag and is equally violent in its action. A decoction of the roots acts as a strong purge. It has also been used as an emmenagogue and for cleansing eruptions. The dried root, in powder or as an infusion, is good in hysterical disorders, fainting, nervous complaints and to relieve pains and cramps.

Taken inwardly and applied outwardly to the affected part, it is an excellent remedy for scrofula.

The use of this Iris was well known to the Ancients and is referred to by Theophrastus, in the fourth century before Christ.

GLASSWORTS

Botanical: Salicornia herbacea (LINN.)
Family: N.O. Chenopodiaceae
Synonym: Marsh Samphire.

Many species of the genera Salsola, Suaeda and Salicornia belonging to Chenopodiaceae are rich in soda and were formerly much employed in making both soap and glass, hence the name Glasswort. Large quantities of the ashes of these plants were formerly imported from southern Europe and northern Africa under the name of Barilla, the chief sources being Salsola Kali (Linn.) and Salsola Soda (Linn.), the Spanish Salsola sativa (Loft) and S. tragus (Linn.). On the introduction of Le Blanc's process of obtaining soda from common salt, the importance of Barilla as an article of commerce ceased.

Our native plant, the Jointed Glasswort (Salicornia herbacea, Linn.), was, as its name implies, also regarded as of value in the manufacture of glass.

Description

It is a low-growing, annual herb, common in salt marshes and on muddy seashores all round the British Islands and was much used for this purpose. It has no leaves, but is formed of cylindrical, jointed branches of a light green color, smooth, very succulent and full of a salt, bitterish juice, its minute flowers produced in threes in little pits in the axils of the branches.

The whole plant is greedily devoured by cattle for its saltish taste. Steeped in malted vinegar, the tender shoots make a good pickle and were often used as a substitute for Samphire in those parts of the coast where the latter did not abound, on which account the plant is also called Marsh Samphire. Sir Thomas More, enumerating the useful native plants that would improve 'many a poor knave's pottage' if he were skilled in their properties, says that 'Glasswort might afford him a pickle for his mouthful of salt meat.'

Parkinson relates a theory in connexion with Glasswort in his days:

'If the soap that is made of the lye of the ashes be spread upon a piece of thicke coarse brown paper cut into the forme of their shooe sole that are casually taken speechless and bound to the soles of their feete, it will bring again the speech and that within a little time after the applying thereof if there be any hope of being restored while they live: this hath been tried to be effectuall upon diverse persons.'

There are references in the Bible to the uses of Glasswort for soap and for glass.

GLASSWORT, PRICKLY

Botanical: Salsola Kali (LINN.)
Family: N.O. Chenopodiaceae

The Prickly Glasswort (Salsola Kali, Linn.) has a thick, round, brittle stem, with few, rigid leaves of a bluish-green color and small, yellow flowers.

Medicinal Action and Uses

The juice of the fresh plant was said to be an excellent diuretic, the twisted seed-vessels having the same virtue and being given in infusion.

The whole plant was likewise burnt for its fixed salt used in making glass.

GLEDITSCHIA

Botanical: Gleditschia triacanthos (LINN.)
Family: N.O. Leguminosae
Synonyms: Gleditschine. Honey Locust. Gleditschia Ferox. Three-(t)horned Acacia.
Parts Used: The twigs and leaves.
Habitat: Eastern and Central United States.

Description

A small, thorny tree, with pinnated leaves and greenish flowers growing in dense spikes. The younger and smaller branches have strong, triple tapering thorns. In the autumn they bear thin, flat pods resembling apple-parings. They contain seeds surrounded by a sweetish pulp from which it is stated that sugar has been extracted. The wood is chiefly used for fencing.

Constituents

An alkaloid, Gleditschine, has been abstracted, and another called Stenocarpine. It also contains cocaine, and probably atropine.

Medicinal Action and Uses

Stenocarpine was introduced as a local anaesthetic in 1887. Gleditschine was found to produce stupor and loss of reflex activity in a frog.

Other Species

G. Macracantha possesses similar properties, and is indigenous to China.

GLOBE FLOWER

Botanical: Trollius Europaeus
Family: N.O. Ranunculaceae
Synonyms: Globe Trollius. Boule d'Or. European Globe Flower. Globe Ranunculus. Globe Crowfoot. Lucken-Gowans.
Part Used: The whole plant, fresh.

Habitat

Northern and Central Europe, from the Caucasus and Siberia to Wales and sometimes Ireland. Found wild in northern counties of England and in Scotland.

Description

The plant grows usually in moist woods and mountain pastures, and is about 2 feet high, the stalk being hollow, smooth, and branching towards the top, each branch bearing one yellow flower without a calix, shaped like that of Crowfoot. The leaves are beautifully cut into five, indented sections. It is a favorite bloom for rustic festivals, and early in June collections of it are made by youths and maidens to decorate cottage doors.

It is often cultivated as a border flower, as are the other two species of the genus.

Constituents

The Swedish naturalist Peter Kalm affirms that these plants have medicinal properties, but lose the greater part of their active principles in drying. The irritant, acrid principle is not well defined, and appears to be destroyed by the action of heat.

Medicinal Action and Uses

It is stated that Trollius is used in Russia in certain obscure maladies, while another authority claims that it has cured a scorbutic case declared incurable by doctors. It is a plant to be investigated.

Other Species

T. Asiaticus, or Asiatic Globe Flower. The leaves of this species are larger than in the European plant, resembling those of Yellow Monk's Hood, although the stature of T. Asiaticus is less. The flowers are an orange tinged yellow. It is a native of Siberia, but can be grown in any garden with shade and a moist soil.

T. Laxus is yellow, and grows in shady, wet places on the mountains of New York and Pennsylvania.

GNAPHALIUMS

Family: N.O. Compositae

The Gnaphaliums are a group of plants, individual species of which are known as Life Everlasting, Eternal Flowers, etc. They are used by the aborigines of America, who taught the white settlers their medical properties.

The Antennaria dioica, known under the name of Life Everlasting or Catsfoot, is the only British species and must not be confused with Antennaria plantaginifolia, or White Plantain, which is also sometimes called Life Everlasting.

GNAPHALIUM ARENARIUM

Family: N.O. Compositae
Habitat: Scania, Denmark, Germany, Japan.

Medicinal Action and Uses

Formerly much recommended for dysentery. Said to preserve woollen cloths from moth. In Japan it is used for moxas and as tobacco.

Description

Leaves lanceolate, lower ones obtuse, flowers compound corymb, stalks simple. An annual hoary plant, stem upright, white, downy, about 1 foot high, with shiny yellow heads of flowers - the calicine scales ovate, blunt, lemon-coloured; also the corollets. Found in dry sandy pastures and hills. Blooming in Germany, Denmark and Scania July to December, in Japan December to April.

Other Species

Gnaphalium cymosum, or Branching Everlasting. The leaves when rubbed emit an odor like Southern Wood.

G. plantaginifolia. For a small fee the American Indians allow themselves to be bitten by a rattlesnake and immediately cure themselves with this herb.

GNAPHALIUM STOECHAS

Botanical: Helichrysum stoechas
Family: N.O. Compositae
Synonyms: Eternal Flower. Goldilocks. Stoechas Citrina. Gnaphalium citrinum. Common Shrubby Everlasting.
Parts Used: Tops and the flowers.
Habitat: Germany, France, Spain, Italy.

Medicinal Action and Uses

Expectorant, deobstruent, used for colds, flowers formerly used as attenuants, discutients, diaphoretics.

Description

Leaves linear; compound corymb; branches wandlike; stem 3 feet high, with long slender irregular branches, lower ones have blunt leaves, 2 1/2 inches long 1/8 inch broad at end; those on flower stalks very narrow, ending in acute points. Whole plant very woolly, calyces at first silvery, then turn a sulphur yellow. Taste warm, pungent, bitter, agreeable odor when rubbed.

GOAT'S BEARD

Botanical: Tragopogon pratensis (LINN.)
Family: N.O. Compositae
Synonyms: Noon Flower. Jack-go-to-bed-at-noon.

Habitat

Goat's Beard (Tragopogon pratensis), a rather close relation of the Hawkweeds, is a handsome plant fairly common throughout Britain in meadows and on the broad green strips that often border country roads, being very common in the north of England.

Description

It has an erect, slightly branching stem, rising to a height of 1 to 2 feet, from a perennial tap-root. The leaves are long, narrow and grass-like in character, without any indentations, broadening at the base and sheathing the stem, bluish-green in color, the lower ones 8 or 9 inches long, the upper ones much shorter.

The plant is in bloom during June and July. Each flower-stem has at its summit a single, large flower-head, the stem being slightly thickened just below it. The involucre or cup at the base of the flower-head is composed of a ring of about eight narrow lance-shaped, leaf-like bracts, which, when the flower is expanded, spread out in rays beyond the florets, which are golden-yellow in color, and all of the 'ligulate' or strapshaped type. After flowering, the green rays of the involucre elongate and the lower portion becomes thicker, till finally a big, round head of winged, long seeds - like the familiar clock of the Dandelion - develops, which becomes broken up by the wind. The pappus, or feathery down crowning each seed, is very beautiful, being raised on a long stalk and interlaced, so as to form a kind of shallow cup. By means of the pappus, the seeds are wafted by the wind and freely scattered.

The Goat's Beard opens its blossoms at daybreak and closes them before noon, except in cloudy weather, hence its old country name of 'Noon-flower' and 'Jack-go-to-bedat-noon,' a peculiarity noticed more than once by the poets and referred to in Cowley's lines:

'The goat's beard, which each morn abroad doth peep
But shuts its flowers at noon and goes to sleep.'

The name of the genus, Tragopogon, is formed from two Greek words, having the same signification as the popular English name, Goat's Beard, which is thought to have been suggested by the fluffy character of the seed-ball.

Gerard says:

'it shutteth itselfe at twelve of the clocke, and sheweth not his face open untill the next dayes Sun doth make it flower anew. Whereupon it was called go-to-bed-at-noone; when these flowers be come to their full maturitie and ripenesse they grow into a downy Blowball like those of Dandelion, which is carriedaway by the winde.'

Medicinal Action and Uses

In mediaeval times, the Goat's Beard had some reputation as a medicinal plant, though it has fallen out of use.

The tapering roots were formerly eaten as we now eat parsnips, and the young stalks, taken before the flowers appear, were cut up into lengths and boiled like asparagus, of which they have somewhat the flavor, and are said to be nearly as nutritious. The roots were dug up in the autumn and kept in dry sand for winter use.

The fresh juice of the young plant has been recommended as 'the best dissolvent of the bile, relieving the stomach without danger and without introducing into the blood an acrid, corrosive stimulant, as is frequently done by salts when employed for this purpose.'

Culpepper tells us:

'A large double handful of the entire plant, roots, flowers and all bruised and boiled an then strained with a little sweet oil, is an excellent clyster in most desperate cases of strangury or suppression of urine. A decoction of the roots is very good for the heartburn, loss of appetite, disorders of the breast and liver, expels sand and gravel, and even small stone. The roots dressed like parsnips with butter are good for cold, watery stomachs, boiled or cold, or eaten as a raw salad; they are grateful to the stomach strengthen the lean and consumptive, or the weak after long sickness. The distilled water gives relief to pleurisy, stitches or pains in the side.'

Another close relation of the above is the Bristly Ox-Tongue (Helmintha Echioides), a stout, much-branched plant, 2 to 3 feet high, well distinguished by its numerous prickles, each of which springs from a raised white spot, and by the large heart-shaped bracts at the base of the yellow flowers. The fruit, which is beaked and singularly corrugated, bears some resemblance to 'a little worm,' which is the meaning of the systematic name. The English name 'Ox-Tongue' has reference to the shape and roughness of the leaves. Not uncommon.

GOLD THREAD

Botanical: Coptis trifolia (SALIS.)
Family: N.O. Ranunculaceae
Synonyms: Helleborus triflius or trilobus. Helleborus pumilus. Coptis. Anemone grcenlandica. Coptide. Mouthroot. Vegetable Gold. Chrusa borealis.
Parts Used: The dried rhizome, with roots, stems, and leaves.
Habitat: Northern America and Asia. Greenland and Iceland.

Description

The name of the genus Coptis is suggested by the form of the leaflets, and means 'to cut.' The popular name is derived from the thin, creeping, gold-coloured rhizome, which yields a yellow dye. The solitary, yellowish flowers, and obovate, evergreen leaves grow in tufts with yellow scales surrounding the base. The herb is a small perennial, usually found creeping in swamps or damp, sandy places. In commerce, the dried herb is found in loose masses, odourless, and with a pure, bitter taste. The powder is yellowish-green. It resembles gentian and quassia in its properties.

The Coptis family is closely linked to that of the Hellebores.

Constituents

Its bitterness is imparted to both water and alcohol, but more readily to the latter. As there is neither tannic nor gallic acid, the activity is due to berberia or berberine, which is associated with another alkaloid called Coptine or Coptina, resembling hydrastia. It also contains albumen, fixed oil, colouring matter, lignin, extractive, and sugar. Authorities differ as to the presence of resin.

Medicinal Action and Uses

It may be used as other pure bitters. In New England it is valued as a local application in thrush, for children.

It is stated to be good for dyspepsia, and combined with other drugs is regarded as helpful in combating the drink habit.

Dosage

Of powder, 10 to 30 grains. Of tincture of 1 OZ. of root to a pint of diluted alcohol, 1 fluid drachm. Of fluid extract, 30 minims.

Other Species and Substitutes

Statice monopetala, used as an astringentin the United States, sometimes used to adulterate C. trifolia.

Coptis Teeta, or Coptidis Rhizoma, Coptidis Radix, Mahmira, Tita, Mishmi Bitter, Mishmi Tita, Hwang-lien, Honglane, Chuen-lien, Chonlin, Mulien, is official in the Pharmacopoeia of India. It grows in the Mishmi Mountains, East Assam, is imported into Bengal in little rattan bags, and is thus sold in the Indian bazaars. Large quantities have been sold in London. It contains a higher percentage of berberia than any other drug, and is much used as a tonic in India and China, especially for the stomach, and in Scind for inflammation of the eyes.

The Chinese and Japanese variations (var. chinensis and C. anemonaefolia) imported into Bombay are thinner and duller than the Assam rhizomes. In Japan, the last variety is used for intestinal catarrh.

GOLDEN ROD

Botanical: Solidago virgaurea (LINN.)
Family: N.O. Compositae
Synonyms: Verge d'Or. Solidago. Goldruthe. Woundwort. Aaron's Rod.
Part Used: Leaves.
Habitat: Europe, including Britain. Central Asia. North America.

Description

The generic name comes from solidare, for the plant is known as a vulnerary, or one that 'makes whole.' It grows from 2 to 3 feet in height, with alternate leaves, of a clear green, and terminal panicles of golden flowers, both ray and disk. It is the only one (of over eighty species) native to Great Britain.

The leaves and flowers yield a yellow dye.

When bruised, the herb smells like Wild Carrot.

Constituents

The plant contains tannin, with some bitter and astringent principles.

Medicinal Action and Uses

Aromatic, stimulant, carminative. Golden Rod is an ingredient in the Swiss Vulnerary, faltrank. It is astringent and diuretic and efficacious for stone in the bladder. It is recorded that in 1788 a boy of ten, after taking the infusion for some months, passed quantities of gravel, fifteen large stones weighing up to 1 1/4 OZ., and fifty over the size of a pea. It allays sickness due to weak digestion.

In powder it is used for cicatrization of old ulcers. It has been recommended in many maladies, as it is a good diaphoretic in warm infusion, and is in this form also helpful in dysmenorrhoea and amenorrhoea. As a spray and given internally, it is of great value in diphtheria.

Dosage

1/2 to 1 drachm of the fluid extract.

Other Species

S. Rigida, Hardleaf Goldenrod, and S.Gigantea, Smooth Three-Ribbed Golden Rod, have leaves and blossoms which are valuable for all forms of hemorrhage, being astringent and styptic. The oil is diuretic.

S. Odora or Sweet-scented, or Fragrantleaved Goldenrod, also of the United States, is used as an astringent in dysentery and ulceration of the intestines. The essence has been used as a diuretic for infants, as a local application in headache, and for flatulence and vomiting. The flowers are aperient, tonic, and astringent, and their infusion is beneficial in gravel, urinary obstructions, and simple dropsy.

S. Canadensis, or Gerbe d'Or, of Canada, and S. sempervirens of North America, are used as vulneraries.

RAYLESS GOLDEN ROD is an American name for Bigelovia.

GOLDEN ROD TREE is Bosea Yervamora.

GOLDEN ROD is also the common name of Leontice Chrysogonum.

GOLDEN SEAL

Botanical: Hydrastis Canadensis (LINN.)
Family: N.O. Ranunculaceae
Synonyms: Yellow Root. Orange Root. Yellow Puccoon. Ground Raspberry. Wild Curcuma. Turmeric Root. Indian Dye. Eye Root. Eye Balm. Indian Paint. Jaundice Root. Warnera.
Part Used: Root.

Habitat

The plant is a native of Canada and the eastern United States, the chief States producing it being Ohio, Kentucky, West Virginia, Indiana, New York and in Canada, Ontario. Most of the commercial supplies are obtained from the Ohio Valley, the chief market being Cincinnati. It is scarce east of the Alleghany Mountains, having become quite rare in New York State, where it has been almost exterminated by collectors. It is found in the rich soil of shady woods and moist places at the edge of wooded lands.

The North American plant Golden Seal produces a drug which is considered of great value in modern medicine. The generic name of the plant, Hydrastis, is derived from two Greek words, signifying water and to accomplish, probably given it from its effect on the mucous membrane.

Golden Seal belongs to the Buttercup family, Ranunculaceae, though its leaves and fruit somewhat resemble those of the Raspberry and the Rubus genus generally.

Description

It is a small perennial herb, with a horizontal, irregularly knotted, bright yellow root-stock, from 1/4 inch to 3/4 inch thick, giving off slender roots below and marked with scars of the flower-stems of previous years. The flowering stem, which is pushed up early in the spring, is from 6 to 12 inches high, erect, cylindrical, hairy, with downward-pointing hairs, especially above, surrounded at the base with a few short, brown scales. It bears two prominently-veined and wrinkled, dark green, hairy leaves, placed high up, the lower one stalked, the upper stalkless, roundish in outline, but palmately cut into 5 to 7 lobes, the margins irregularly and finely toothed. There is one solitary radical leaf on a long foot-stalk, similar in form to the stem leaves, but larger, when full-grown being about 9 inches across.

The flower, which is produced in April, is solitary, terminal, erect, small, with three small greenish-white sepals, falling away immediately after expansion, no petals and numerous stamens. The fruit is a head of small, fleshy, oblong, crimson berries, tipped with the persistent styles and containing one or two hard black, shining seeds. It is ripe in July and has much the appearance of a Raspberry (whence the name 'Ground Raspberry'), but is not edible.

Hydrastis Canadensis was first introduced into England by Miller in 1760, under the name of Warnera, after Richard Warner of Woodford, and later was grown at Kew, Edinburgh and Dublin. Having no claims to horticultural attractiveness, its cultivation has not been attempted in this country except in botanical gardens - and on a slight experimental scale - nor has it been cultivated on any scale in any other country until quite recently, when owing to its growing scarcity in the woods of Ohio, where it used to be abundant, plantations were started in a few parts of America, but the amount under cultivation there is still very small.

In 1905 the United States Department of Agriculture called attention to the increasing demand for Golden Seal for medicinal purposes in a Bulletin (No. 51). There it is stated that the early settlers learnt of the virtues of Golden Seal from the American Indians, who used the root as a medicine and its yellow juice as a stain for their faces and a dye for their clothing. It was not until about 1850 that the root became an article of commerce, and in 1905 the annual supply of it was estimated at from 200,000 lb. to 300,000 lb., about one-tenth of which was exported, with an ever-increasing demand. Thirty years ago it was plentiful in its wild haunts and sold for 8 cents per lb., but as its supply diminished, not only from overcollection, but from the forests in the central States being cut away, the price rose in proportion and is now almost prohibitive.

Cultivation

Experimental growing of the drug here has not been attended with much success, as it is of somewhat difficult culture.

The best conditions for the cultivation of Golden Seal are said to be a well-drained soil, rich in humus, in a partially shaded situation. Lath blinds (placed overhead on wires and light runners) are used by American cultivators - as with Ginseng - and these are considered to be preferable to the shade of trees, the roots of which interfere with operations. The plant requires from 60 to 75 per cent shade. The rootstocks are divided into small pieces and then planted about 8 inches apart in rows. Seeds are not considered reliable. Fresh plantations are made in autumn, after the plants have died down, or earlier, if they are lifted for a supply of marketable rhizomes. The strong fibrous roots sometimes develop buds which can be used as stock. Plantations thus formed take two or three years to grow to marketable size, the rhizomes deteriorating in their fourth year. According to an American grower, 32 sturdy plants set to each square yard, in three years' growth will produce 2 lb. of dry root. Experiments conducted by the United States Department of Agriculture recommend growing it only two years and marketing. It is stated that the plant may be transplanted at any time of the year with safety.

It has proved difficult to obtain a supply of living roots with which to start plantations in this country. The market is in the hands of American growers, collectors and dealers, and it may be that they are unwilling to spoil their monopoly by aiding other countries to grow their own Golden Seal, but the drug is growing in favour with medical practitioners, therefore its production on a commercial scale in this country would appear to be desirable, if it could be carried out with success.

The fresh rhizome is juicy and loses much of its weight in drying. When fresh, it has a well-marked, narcotic odor, which is lost in a great measure by age, when it acquires a peculiar sweetish smell, somewhat resembling liquorice root. It has a very bitter, feebly opiate taste, more especially when freshly dried.

The rhizome is irregular and tortuous, much knotted, with a yellowish-brown, thin bark and bright yellow interior, 1/2 inch to 1 1/2 inch long, and from 1/8 to 1/4 inch thick. The upper surface bears short ascending branches, which are usually terminated by cup-like scars, left by the aerial stems of previous years. From the lower surface and sides, numerous thin, wiry, brittle roots are given off, many of them breaking off, leaving small protuberances on the root.

The color of the rhizome, though yellow in the fresh root, becomes a dark, yellowishbrown by age; that of the rootlets and the interior of the root is yellow and that of the powder still more so.

When dry, the rhizome is hard and breaks with a clean, resinous fracture, the smooth, fractured surface is of a brownish-yellow, or greenish-yellow color, and exhibits a ring of bright yellow, somewhat distant narrow wood bundles surrounding a large pith.

Constituents

The chief constituents of Hydrastis rhizome are the alkaloids Berberine (3.5 to 4 per cent.), which constitutes the yellow colouring matter of the drug, Hydrastine (2 to 4 per cent.), a peculiar crystallizable substance and a third alkaloid, Canadine; resin, albumin, starch, fatty matter, sugar, lignin and a small quantity of volatile oil, to which its odor is due, are also present. The rhizome is stated to be much richer in alkaloid than the roots.

Hydrastis owes its virtues almost entirely to Hydrastine, the alkaloid Berberine, apart from some effect as a bitter being practically inert. The United States Pharmacopoeia requires Hydrastis to yield not less than 2.5 per cent of Hydrastine.

For many years the alkaloids and the powdered root were the chief forms administered, but now the fluid extract is the form most used. The tincture is also official in both the British and the United States Pharmacopoeias.

Medicinal Action and Uses

The American aborigines valued the root highly as a tonic, stomachic and application for sore eyes and general ulceration, as well as a yellow dye for their clothing and weapons.

It is official in most Pharmacopoeias, several of which refer to its yellowing the saliva when masticated.

The action is tonic, laxative, alterative and detergent. It is a valuable remedy in the disordered conditions of the digestion and has a special action on the mucous membrane, making it of value as a local remedyin various forms of catarrh. In chronic inflammation of the colon and rectum, injections of Hydrastine are often of great service, and it has been used in hemorrhoids with excellent results, the alkaloid Hydrastine having an astringent action. The powder has proved useful as a snuff for nasal catarrh.

It is employed in dyspepsia, gastric catarrh, loss of appetite and liver troubles. As a tonic, it is of extreme value in cases of habitual constipation, given as a powder, combined with any aromatic. It is an efficient remedy for sickness and vomiting.

Preparations

Powdered root, 10 grains. Fluid extract, 1/4 to 1 drachm. Tincture, B.P. and U.S.P., 1/2 to 1 drachm. Solid extract, 5 to 8 grains.

As an infusion, it has great influence in preventing and curing night-sweats. It is sometimes used as a wash for ulcerated mouth.

Externally, it is used as a lotion in treatment of eye affections and as a general cleansing application.

It is said to be a specific to prevent pitting by smallpox.

In large amounts the drug proves very poisonous.

The employment of Hydrastis as a dye by the Indians has led to investigations as to its possible commercial employment in this direction . Durand (Amer. Journ. Pharm., Vol. XXIII) states that 'it imparts to linen a rich and durable light yellow color, of great brilliancy, which might probably by proper mordants give all the shades of that color, from the pale yellow to the orange. The lake produced by the bichloride of tin might also prove a useful pigment in oil and water-color painting.' With indigo, it is said to impart a fine green to wool, silk and cotton.

Substitutes

Owing to the high price of Hydrastis, the quality

of the commercial article has steadily deteriorated, and in recent years, about every drug native to the soil which resembles this rhizome, either in fibre or in color, has been known to be mixed with it. The yellow color of Hydrastis rhizome, the appearance of a transverse section and the characteristic odor of the drug distinguish it readily from Blood Root, obtained from Sanguinaria Canadensis, which is usually of a dark reddish-brown color, while a transverse section exhibits a more or less pronounced red color and no evident wood bundles.

None of the substitutes can be reasonably mistaken for the drug in the entire condition.

GOOSEBERRY

Botanical: Ribes grossularia
Family: N.O. Grossulariaceae
Synonyms: Fea. Feverberry. Feabes. Carberry. Groseille. Grozet. Groser. Krusbaar. Deberries. Goosegogs. Honeyblobs. Feaberry.
Parts Used: Fruit, leaves.

Habitat

Central and Northern Europe, especially Britain. Ribes Uva Crispa, also, as far east as Nepal and south to Morocco.

Description

The well-known fruit grows on shrubs 3 to 4 feet high, with many branches, spreading prickles, and small, three- or five-lobed, hairy leaves. The flowers are green and hang singly or in pairs from little tufts of young leaves. The berries may be red, green, yellow, or white, hairy (Ribes grossularia) or smooth (R. uva crispa), over 200 varieties being recognized. It is especially cultivated in Lancashire and in the Lothians, in Scotland, the former district aiming at size, and the latter at flavor. The shrub may attain great age and size. In 1821, at Duffield, near Derby, a bush had been planted for at least forty-six years, and was 12 yards in circumference, while two, trained against a wall near Chesterfield, reached upwards of 50 feet in growth from end to end.

The yellow gooseberries have usually the richest flavor for dessert, and the best wine made from them very closely resembles champagne. The red are generally the most acid, supporting the fact that acids change vegetable blues to red.

The fruit does not appear to be highly valued in the South of Europe, but further North is very popular for tarts, pies, sauces, chutneys, jams, and dessert, also for preserving in bottles for winter use. The young and tender leaves are eaten in salads.

Constituents

Citric acid, pectuse, sugar, and mineral matters, the pectuse causing the fruit to be excellent for jellies.

Medicinal Action and Uses

The juice was formerly said to 'cure all inflammations.' In the green berries it is sub-acid and is corrective of putrescent foods, such as mackerel or goose. The light jelly made from the red berries is valuable for sedentary, plethoric, and bilious subjects.

As a spring medicine, gooseberry is more valuable than rhubarb. In one of the many books on the Plague, published in the sixteenth century, the patient is recommended to eat 'Goseberries.' Gerard, describing it under the name of 'Feaberry,' says:

'the fruit is much used in diners, sawces for meates and used in brothe instead of Verjuyce, which maketh the brothe not only pleasant to taste, but is greatly profitable to such as are troubled with a hot, burning ague.'

The leaves were formerly considered very wholesome and a corrective of gravel. An infusion taken before the monthly period will be found a useful tonic for growing girls.

Dosage

Of an infusion of 1 OZ. of dried leaves to 1 pint of water, 1 teacupful three times a day.

GOOSEFOOTS

Family: N.O. Chenopodiaceae
Botanical: Chenopodium Bonus Henricus

Synonyms: English Mercury. Mercury Goosefoot. Allgood. Tola Bona. Smearwort. Fat Hen. (German) Fette Henne.
Part Used: Herb.

Habitat

Good King Henry grows abundantly in waste places near villages, having formerly been cultivated as a garden pot-herb.

Description

It is a dark-green, succulent plant, about 2 feet, high, rising from a stout, fleshy, branching root-stock, with large, thickish, arrow-shaped leaves and tiny yellowish-green flowers in numerous close spikes, 1 to 2 inches long, both terminal and arising from the axils of the leaves. The fruit is bladder-like, containing a single seed.

The leaves used to be boiled in broth, but were principally gathered, when young and tender, and cooked as a pot-herb. In Lincolnshire, they are still eaten in place of spinach. Thirty years ago, this Goosefoot was regularly grown as a vegetable in Suffolk, Lincolnshire, and other eastern counties and was preferred to the Garden Spinach, its flavor being somewhat similar, but less pronounced. In common with several other closely allied plants, it was sometimes called 'Blite' (from the Greek, bliton, insipid), Evelyn says in his Acetaria, 'it is well-named being insipid enough.' Nevertheless, it is a very wholesome vegetable. If grown on rich soil, the young shoots, when as thick as a lead pencil, may be cut when 5 inches in height, peeled and boiled and eaten as Asparagus. They are gently laxative.

Cultivation

Good King Henry is well worth cultivating. Being a perennial, it will continue to produce for a number of years, being best grown on a deep loamy soil. The ground should be rich, well drained, and deeply dug. Plants should be put in about April, 1 foot apart each way, or seeds may be sown in drills at the same distance. During the first year, the plants should be allowed to establish themselves, but after that, both shoots and leaves may be cut or picked, always leaving enough to maintain the plant in health. Manure water is of great assistance in dry weather, or a dressing of 1 OZ. of nitrate of soda, or sulphate of ammonia may be given.

As with many of the wild plants, it does not always adapt itself to a change of soil when transplanted from its usual habitat and success is more often ensured when grown from seed.

Dodoens says the name Good King Henry, was given it to distinguish the plant from another, and poisonous one, called Malus Henricus ('Bad Henry'). The name Henricus in this case was stated by Grimm to refer to elves and kobolds ('Heinz' and 'Heinrich'), indicating magical powers of a malicious nature. The name has no connexion with our King Hal.

The plant is also known as Mercury Goosefoot, English Mercury and Marquery (to distinguish it from the French Mercury), because of its excellent remedial qualities in indigestion, hence the proverb: 'Be thou sick or whole, put Mercury in thy Koole.'

The name 'Smear-wort' refers to its use in ointment. Poultices made of the leaves were used to cleanse and heal chronic sores, which, Gerard states, 'they do scour and mundify.'

The roots were given to sheep as a remedy for cough and the seeds have found employment in the manufacture of shagreen.

The plant is said to have been used in Germany for fattening poultry and was called there Fette Henne, of which one of its popular names, Fat Hen, is the translation.

GOOSEFOOT, WHITE

Botanical: Chenopodium album (LINN.)
Family: N.O. Chenopodiaceae
Synonyms: Frost Blite. Mutton Tops. Dirtweed. Lamb's Quarters. Dirty Dick. Midden Myles. Pigweed (Canada). Baconweed. Fat Hen.
Part Used: Herb.

The White Goosefoot (Chenopodium album, Linn.), so called from its mealy leaves, rejoices in old manure heaps, and if the manure is stacked up on a farm ready for use at a later season, it is soon overrun by this weed, which has thus gained the popular names of 'Midden Myles,' 'Dirtweed' and 'Dirty Dick.'

It shares with its near relative Good King Henry the names of Allgood and Fat Hen from its usefulness as a pot-herb and its reputed value in feeding poultry. 'Boil Myles in water and chop them in butter and you will have a good dish,' is an old English saying. It is a very wholesome medicine, as well as a pleasant vegetable, and an excellent substitute for spinach.

Description

The stem is erect, from 1 to 3 feet high, the leaves oval, wedge-shaped, with wavy teeth, the flowers in dense spikes. The mealiness is most apparent in the flowers and undersides of the leaves, but has not the objectionable odor of that of the Stinking Goosefoot.

This nutritious plant is grown as food for pigs and sheep in Canada, where it is called 'Pigweed.'

The young and tender plants are collected by the Indians of New Mexico and Arizona, and boiled as herbs, alone or with other food; large quantities also are eaten in the raw state. The seeds of this species are gathered by many tribes, ground into flour after drying and made into bread. The flour resembles that of Buckwheat in color and taste and is regarded as equally nutritious. The small grey seeds are not unpleasant when eaten raw.

GOOSEFOOT, RED

Botanical: Chenopodium rubrum (LINN.)
Family: N.O. Chenopodiaceae
Synonyms: Sowbane. Pigweed.

The seeds of the Red Goosefoot (Chenopodium rubrum, Linn.) are a favorite food of birds and are also good for poultry. This species has a reddish stem, 1 to 3 feet high, usually upright, its leaves triangular to oval, with large blunt lobes and notches, but very variable in size and shape. It is very common about manure heaps. Its erect flowerspikes, intermixed with leaves, distantly resemble those of Dock.

Other Species

The leaves of another Goosefoot, C. hybridum, are sometimes found as an adulterant of Stramonium leaves, when these are imported in a broken condition, but they can be detected by their small epidermal cells, with nearly straight walls, and hairs terminated by a large, bladdery, waterstoring cell.

GORSE, GOLDEN

Botanical: Ulex europaeus (LINN.)
Family: N.O. Leguminosae
Synonyms: Furze. Broom. Whin. Prickly Broom. Ruffet. Frey. Goss.
Parts Used: Flowers, seed.

Habitat

It is found from Denmark to Italy, the Canaries and Azores, and in every part of Great Britain, though it is rarer in the north. There is probably hardly a heath in the country which lacks a patch, however small, of the dry-soil-loving Furze.

The Golden Gorse (Ulex Europaeus, Linn.) is conspicuous in waste places and on commons throughout Great Britain, from its spiny branches and bright yellow flowers, situated on the spines, either solitary or in pairs. It is thought to be the Scorpius of Theophrastus and the Ulex of Pliny. By botanists before Linnaeus, it was known as a Broom and called Genista spinosa. Linnaeus restored to it the name of Ulex, by which it has ever since been recognized.

Although it looks so sturdy, it is not very hardy. Severe frosts are liable to injure it, and during some exceptionally severe winters whole tracts of it on open commons have perished. Linnaeus, we are told in Johnson's Useful Plants of Great Britain:

'lamented that he could not keep Furze alive in Sweden, even in a greenhouse. It was one of his favorite plants, though the wellknown story of his falling on his knees when first seeing it in this country and thanking Heaven for having created a flower so beautiful is of rather doubtful authenticity as it is likewise related of Dillenius.'

Description

The plant is a dense, muchbranched, stunted shrub, rarely attaining a height of more than 6 feet. It is evergreen, but the leaves are very minute and fall off early, not being present in the older stages, when they take the form of long, thread-like spines, which are straight and furrowed, or branching. The stem is hairy and spreading.

The golden-yellow, papilionaceous flowers have a powerful scent, perfuming the air. They open from early spring right up to August, or even later, but the bushes are to be found in blossom, here and there practically all the year round, hence the old saying:

'When Gorse is out of bloom,
Kissing's out of season,'

and an old custom in some parts of the country of inserting a spray of Gorse in the bridal bouquet, is an allusion to this.

The following reference to its continuous flowering appeared in the Chemist and Druggist of January 15, 1921. The writer says:

'Sir, The impression that is prevalent concerning the perennial flowering of the common Furze is a very natural, although a mistaken one.

'The ordinary furze, U. Europaeus, begins to flower in December, is in full bloom in March and April, and continues sometimes in a desultory manner as late as June. Then the Dwarf Furze begins to flower, and is in lull bloom in August. When mixed with the heather - then in blossom - it forms gorgeous purple and gold carpets wherever, as in Jersey, it is abundant. U. Gallii then takes up the tale, and from August to November blossoms freely. U. Europaeus is rarely less than 2 ft. high when it begins to flower: the U. Nanus has a decumbent habit, and is rarely more than 1 1/2 ft. high, and the flowers are paler and do not expand the wings widely. U. Gallii is easily recognized by the larger lateral spines of the branches being decurved, and the flowers more of an orange tint. But an ordinary observer would discount these differences, if noticed at all, and merely regard the other species as more or less dwarf plants. U. Gallii is sometimes as short as U. nanus, and sometimes as tall as U. Europaeus, but may always be recognized by the stout spines curved backwards.

'Yours truly,

'SEMPERVIRENS.'

Its elastic seed-vessels, like those of the Broom, burst with a crackling noise in hot weather and scatter the seeds on all sides.

The Gorse has not as many uses as the Broom, nor is it of such importance medicinally.

'In France,' to quote Syme and Sowerby, British Botany, 1864, 'it is used for burning, being cut down every few years, in places where it grows naturally. In Surrey and other counties, it is used largely as fuel, especially by bakers in their ovens and is cultivated for that purpose and cut down every three years. When burned, it yields a quantity of ashes rich in alkali, which are sometimes used for washing, either in the form of a solution or lye, or mixed with clay and made into balls, as a substitute for soap. The ashes form an excellent manure and it is not uncommon where the ground is covered with Furze bushes to burn them down to improve the land and to secure a crop of young shoots, which are readily eaten by cattle. In some parts of England, it is usual to put the Furze bushes into a mill to crush the thorns and then to feed horses and cows with the branches. When finely cut or crushed, sheep will readily eat it.'

The bruised shoots form a very nutritious fodder and when well bruised are eaten with much relish by horses, and cows are said to give good milk upon this food alone. When crushed, it is necessary to use it quickly, as the mass soon ferments. The variety of Furze found in the west of England and in Ireland, called U. strictus, is the best for this purpose, its shoots being softer and more succulent. It has terminal bunches of flowers.

Professor Henslow (Uses of British Plants, 1905) states that Furze 'has also been used chopped up into small pieces and sown in drills with Peas, proving a good defence against the attack of birds and mice.'

The leaf-buds have been used as a substitute for tea and the flowers yield a beautiful yellow dye.

The seeds are said to be nutritious, but do not appear to have been used for cattle feeding, though in earlier days they were sometimes employed medicinally.

Goldsmith calls the Furze 'unprofitably gay,' but Furze is not 'unprofitable.' It is usually cut once in three years, and its ashes, after burning, yield a serviceable dressing for the land.

Gorse is frequently sown as a shelter to very young trees in plantations and as a cover for game and makes excellent hedges when kept closely cut, but is only to be recommended for this purpose in mild climates or sheltered situations, as it is always liable to be cut off by hard frost. Wherever sown, it requires to be kept free from weeds during the first year or two. Like Broom, it grows well near the sea.

The name Ulex was given it by Pliny, but its signification is unknown. He states that the plant was used in the collection of gold, being laid down in water to catch any golddust brought down by the water.

The word Furze is derived from the AngloSaxon name fyrs, while Gorse is also from the A.-S. gorst (a waste), a reference to the open moorlands on which it is found.

Medicinal Action and Uses

The plant has never played an important part in herbal medicine.

Parkinson tells us that 'some have used the flowers against the jaundice.' An infusion of the blossoms used to be given to children to drink in scarlet-fever.

Gerard states: 'the seeds are employed in medicines against the stone and staying of the laske' (laxness of the bowels). They have some astringent property, containing tannin.

Old writers also tell-us that 'sodden with honey, it clears the mouth' and that it 'is good against snakebite.'

It had an old reputation as an insecticide: 'Against fleas, take this same wort, with its seed, sodden; sprinkle it into the house; it killeth the fleas.'

In 1886 A. W. Gerrard discovered an alkaloid in the seeds, more powerful as a purgative than the Sparteine obtained from Cytisus scoparius (Link) (Pharm. Journal, Aug. 7, 1886). This was named Ulexine. In 1890 the German scientist Kobert, as the result of much investigation, came to the conclusion that Ulexine and Cytisine are identical. He also found indication of a second alkaloid. The suggestion gave rise to a considerable chemico-physiological discussion (see Pharm. Journal, Feb. 1891). Ulexine has been used in cardiac dropsy, the dose being from 1/15 to 1/20, of a grain.

GOUTWEED

Botanical: Ægopodium podagraria (LINN.)
Family: N.O. Umbelliferae
Synonyms: Jack-jump-about. Goatweed. Herb Gerard. Ashweed. Achweed. English Masterwort. Wild Masterwort. Pigweed. Eltroot. Ground Elder. Bishop's Elder. Weyl Ash. White Ash. Bishopsweed. Bishopswort. Ground Ash.
Parts Used: Herb, root.
Habitat: Europe (except Spain) and Russian Asia. Not really indigenous to England.

Description

The generic name is a corruption of the Greek aix, aigos (a goat) and pous, podos (a foot), from some fancied resemblance in the shape of the leaves to the foot of a goat. The specific name is derived from the Latin word for gout, podagra, because it was at one time a specific for gout.

It is a stout, erect plant, coarse and glabrous, a perennial; in height, 1 1/2 to 2 feet, sometimes more, the stem round, furrowed and hollow. It has a creeping root-stock and by this means it spreads rapidly and soon establishes itself, smothering all vegetation less rampant than its own. It is a common pest of orchards, shrubberies and ill-kept gardens, and is found on the outskirts of almost every village or town, being indeed rarely absent from a building of some description. It is possible that Buckwheat might drive it out if planted where Goutweed has gained a hold.

It was called Bishopsweed and Bishopswort, because so frequently found near old ecclesiastical ruins. It is said to have been introduced by the monks of the Middle Ages, who cultivated it as a herb of healing. It was called Herb Gerard, because it was dedicated to St. Gerard, who was formerly invoked to cure the gout, against which the herb was chiefly employed.

Its large leaves are alternate, the lobes ovate and sharply-toothed, 2 to 3 inches long. The radical leaves are on long stalks, bi- and tri-ternate. There are fewer stem-leaves; they are less divided, with smaller segments.

The umbels of flowers are rather large, with numerous, small white flowers, which are in bloom from June to August and are followed by flattened seed-vessels which when ripe are detached and jerked to a distance by the wind, hence its local name, 'Jack-jump-about.'

Gerard says:

'Herbe Gerard groweth of itself in gardens without setting or sowing and is so fruitful in its increase that when it hath once taken roote, it will hardly be gotten out againe, spoiling and getting every yeare more ground, to the annoying of better herbe.'

An Alpine species, which appears to possess all the bad properties of its congener, is found in Asia.

The plant is eaten by pigs, hence one of its names. The following charm is from an Anglo-Saxon Herbal:

'To preserve swine from sudden death take the worts lupin, bishopwort and others, drive the swine to the fold, hang the worts upon the four sides and upon the door' (Lacnunga, 82).

John Parkinson recommends cummin seed and bishopsweed 'for those who like to look pale.'

The white root-stock is pungent and aromatic, but the flavor of the leaves is strong and disagreeable.

Culpepper gives 'Bishop-weed' a separate description, and states it is also called 'Æthiopian Cummin-Seed,' and 'Cummin-Royal,' also 'Herb William' and 'Bull-Wort.' He also (like Parkinson) says that 'being drank or outwardly applied, it abates an high color, and makes pale.'

Linnaeus recommends the young leaves boiled and eaten as a green vegetable, as in Sweden and Switzerland, and it used also to be eaten as a spring salad.

Medicinal Action and Uses

Diuretic and sedative. Can be successfully employed internally for aches in the joints, gouty and sciatic pains, and externally as a fomentation for inflamed parts.

The roots and leaves boiled together, applied to the hip, and occasionally renewed,have a wonderful effect in some cases of sciatica.

Culpepper says:

'It is not to be supposed Goutwort hath its name for nothing, but upon experiment to heal the gout and sciatica; as also joint-aches and other cold griefs. The very bearing of it about one eases the pains of the gout and defends him that bears it from the disease.'

Gerard tells us that:

'with his roots stamped and laid upon members that are troubled or vexed with gout, swageth the paine, and taketh away the swelling and inflammation thereof, which occasioned the Germans to give it the name of Podagraria, because of his virtues in curing the gout.'

Other Species

Bishopsweed is also the common name of Ammi majus.

GRAPE, MOUNTAIN

Botanical: Berberis aquifolium (PURSH.)
Family: N.O. Berberidaceae
Synonyms: Mahonia aquifolia. Holly-leaved Barberry. Oregon Grape Root.
Part Used: Root.
Habitat: Western United States.

Description

Several varieties of the subgenus Mahonia contribute to the drug of commerce under the name of Berberis aquifolium. It is a quickly-growing shrub about 6 feet high: the oddly compound leaves have no spine at the base; they are evergreen and shining. The flowers grow in terminal racemes, are small and yellowish-green in color, and the purple berries are three- to nine-seeded. The bark is brown on the surface and yellow beneath. The root is from 1/2 inch in diameter to 3 inches at the base of the stem, odourless, and with a bitter taste. The shrub was introduced into England from North America in 1823. It was formerly known as Mahonia aquifolia and is very hardy.

Constituents

The principal constituent is a high proportion of berberin, and there is also oxycanthin.

Medicinal Action and Uses

Tonic and alterative, recommended in psoriasis, syphilis and impure blood-conditions. It may be used like colombo, berberis, etc., in dyspepsia and chronic mucous complaints. In constipation it is combined with Cascara Sagrada. It improves digestion and absorption.

Preparation

Fluid extract, 10 to 30 drops.

Other Species

B. nervosa and B. repens are frequently found in the drug.

GRASSES

Family: N.O. Graminaceae

The family of Grasses is, perhaps, of all groups in the plant world, the most important to mankind. The seeds of the valuable cereals, wheat, barley, oats, rye, etc., furnish us with indispensable farinaceous food and their stems with straw - the coarser kinds are useful for litter and fodder, also for thatching and other purposes, such as the making of mats, etc. - the finer varieties are widely employed in the making of hats, and our native Grasses furnish nutritious herbage, either as green pasture, or as hay, and some of them with mucilaginous roots possess distinctive medicinal virtues.

COUCH-GRASS

Botanical: Agropyrum repens (BEAUV.)
Synonyms: Twitch-grass. Scotch Quelch. Quick-grass. Dog-grass. Triticum repens (Linn.).
Part Used: Rhizome.

Habitat

Couch-grass is widely diffused, being not only abundant in fields and waste places in Britain and on the Continent of Europe, but also in Northern Asia, Australia and North and South America. It was formerly known as Triticum repens, though now assigned to the genus Agropyrum.

Among these the Couch-grass (Agropyrum repens) is pre-eminent, though anything but a favorite with the farmer, for it has a slender, creeping rhizome, or underground stem, which extends for a considerable distance just beneath the surface of the ground, giving off lateral branches occasionally, and marked at intervals of about an inch by nodes, from which leaf-buds and slender branching roots are produced. These long, creeping, subterranean stems increase with great rapidity, and the smallest piece left in the ground will vegetate and quickly extend itself, so that it is almost impossible to extirpate it when once established in the soil, while its exhaustive powers render it very injurious to the crops. Its very name, Couch, is supposed to be derived from the Anglo-Saxon, civice (vivacious), on account of its tenacity of life. It is said that the only way to extirpate it, is to lay the ground down in pasture for some years, when the Couch will soon be destroyed by the close-growing

Grasses, for it flourishes only in loose soil.

The name Agropyron is from the Greek agros (field), and puros (wheat).

On sandy seashores, the grass is often very abundant and assists in binding the sand and preventing the dunes from shifting, its long rhizome answering the purpose nearly as well as those of the Mat and Lyme Grasses.

Though commonly regarded in this country as a worthless and troublesome weed, its roots are, however, considered on the Continent to be wholesome food for cattle and horses. In Italy, especially, they are carefully gathered by the peasants and sold in the markets. The roots have a sweet taste, somewhat resembling liquorice, and Withering relates that, dried and ground into meal, bread has been made with them in time of scarcity.

Description

From its long creeping, pointed root-stock, it produces in July several round, hollow flower stems, 2 to 3 feet high, thickened at the joints, bearing five to seven leaves and terminated by long, denselyflowered, two-rowed spikes of flowers, somewhat resembling those of rye or beardless wheat, composed of eight or more oval spikelets on alternate sides of the spike, each containing four to eight florets, the awns, when present, being not more than half the length of the flower. The leaves are flat, with a long, cleft sheath, and are rough on the upper surface, having a row of hairs on each principal vein.

One of the names of this grass is Dog'sgrass, from its efficacy in relieving dogs when ill. They are often to be seen searching for its rough leaves, which they chew in order to procure vomiting. Culpepper closes his description of the grass by saying: 'If you know it not by this description, watch the dogs when they are sick and they will quickly lead you to it,' and concludes his account of its medicinal virtues with: 'and although a gardener be of another opinion, yet a physician holds half an acre of them to be worth five acres of carrots twice told over.'

Gerard wrote:

'Although that Couch-grasse be an unwelcome guest to fields and gardens, yet his physicke virtues do recompense those hurts; for it openeth the stoppings of the liver and reins without any manifest heat.' He says concerning a variety of Couch-grass that -

'the roots of this grass are knotty and tuberous in early spring, but in summer-time these bulbs lose all shape or form. . . . The learned Societie of London and the Physitions of the Colledge do hold this bulbous Couch grass in temperature agreeing with the common Couch Grass, but in vertues more effectual,' and mentions it as 'growing in the fields next to St. James' Wall, as ye go to Chelsea, and in the fields as ye go from the Tower Hill of London to Radcliffe.'

Culpepper greatly praises its virtues for diseases of the kidneys.

The juice of the roots drank freely is recommended by Boerhaave in obstruction of the viscera, particularly in cases of scirrhous liver and jaundice, and it is noteworthy that cattle having scirrhous livers in winter soon get cured when turned out to grass in spring. Sheep and goats eat the leaves as well as cows, horses eat them when young, but leave them untouched when fully grown.

The ancients were familiar with a grass under the names of Agrostis and Gramen - having a creeping root-stock like the Couchgrass. Dioscorides asserts that its root, taken in the form of decoction is a useful remedy in suppression of urine and stone in the bladder. The same statements are made by Pliny, and are found in the writings of Oribasius and Marcellus Empiricus in the fourth century and of Ætius in the sixth century, and figures of the plant may be found in Dodoens's herbal. The drug is also met with in the German pharmaceutical tariffs of the sixteenth century.

Formerly the decoction of Couch-grass roots was a popular drink taken to purify the blood in spring. The drug is still a domestic remedy in great repute in France, being taken as a demulcent and sudorific in the form of a tisane. Readers of Trilby will remember Little Billee being dosed with this, as most Parisians have been. The French also use the Cocksfoot-grass (Cynodon Dactylon), which they term Pied-de-poule, in a similar way and for a similar purpose.

Part Used

The rhizome, or underground stem, collected in the spring and freed from leaves and roots.

Couch-grass rhizome is long, stiff, pale yellow and smooth, about 1/10 inch in diameter, hollow except at the nodes and strongly furrowed longitudinally, with five or six longitudinal ridges. Where the nodes occur, traces of rootlets may be found on the under surfaces and the fibrous remains of sheathing leaf-bases on the upper surfaces, but all traces of rootlets and leaves must be removed before use.

As found in commerce, the rhizome is always free from rootlets, cut into short lengths of 1/8 to 1/4 inch and dried, being thus in the form of little shining, straw-coloured, many-edged tubular pieces, which are without odor, but have a sweet taste.

Constituents

Couch-grass rhizome contains about 7 to 8 per cent of Triticin (a carbohydrate resembling Inulin) and yielding levulose on hydrolysis. It appears to occur in the rhizome of other grasses, and possibly is widely diffused in the vegetable kingdom. Sugar, Inosite, Mucilage and acid malates are also constituents of the drug. Lactic acid and mannite may occur in an extract of the rhizome, but are understood to be fermentation products. Starch is not present and no definite active constituent has yet been discovered. The rhizome leaves about 4 1/2 per cent ash on incineration.

Medicinal Action and Uses

Diuretic demulcent. Much used in cystitis and thetreatment of catarrhal diseases of the bladder. It palliates irritation of the urinary passages and gives relief in cases of gravel.

It is also recommended in gout and rheumatism. It is supposed to owe its diuretic effect to its sugar, and is best given in the form of an infusion, made from 1 OZ. to a pint of boiling water, which may be freely used taken in wine glassful doses. A decoction is also made by putting 2 to 4 oz. in a quart of water and reducing down to a pint by boiling. Of the liquid extract 1/2 to 2 teaspoonsful are given in water.

Couch-grass is official in the Indian and Colonial Addendum of the British Pharmacopoeia for use in the Australasian, Eastern and North American Colonies, where it is much employed.

Substitutes

Agropyrum acutum (R. et S.) A. pungens (R. et S.) and A. junceum (Beauv.), by some botanists regarded as mere maritime varieties of A. repens, have rootstocks similar to the latter.

COUCH-GRASS, DOG'S TOOTH

Botanical: Cynodon dactylon (PERS.)
Synonyms: (French) Chien-dent. Pied-de-poule.
Part Used: Rhizome.

Cynodon dactylon (Pers.), a grass very common in the south of Europe and the warmer parts of Western Europe, also indigenous to Northern Africa as far as Abyssinia, affords the Gros Chien-dent or Chien-dent and Pied-de-poule of the French. It is a rhizome differing from that of Couch-grass, in being a little stouter and in containing much starch, of which there is no trace in Couch-grass. Under the microscope it displays an entirely different structure, inasmuch as it contains a large number of much stronger fibrovascular bundles and a cellular tissue loaded with starch, and is, therefore, in appearance much more woody. It thus approximates to the rhizome of Carex arenaria (Linn.) which is as much used in Germany as that of Cynodon in France and Southern Europe. The latter appears to contain Asparagin, or a substance similar in composition to it.

The herb of Hygrophila spinosa (Linn.) has been used for the same purpose as Couchgrass rhizome, and was formerly included in the Indian and Colonial Addendum to the British Pharmacopoeia. It contains much mucilage.

DARNEL, BEARDED

Botanical: Lolium temulentum (LINN.)
Synonyms: Ray-grass. Drake. Cheat.
Part Used: Seeds.

The Bearded Darnel, a common grass weed in English cornfields, is easily distinguished by its long glumes or awns and turgid, fruiting pales, containing the large grains, from the common Ray or Rye-grass (Lolium perenne), which is one of the best of the cultivated grasses, peculiarly adapted for both hay and pasture, especially in wet or uncertain climates. Both are often indiscriminately called Darnel or Ray-grass.

The seeds or grains of the Bearded Darnel were used medicinally by the ancient Greeks and Romans, but were never official in our Pharmacopoeia.

The admixture of the grain with those of the nutritious cereals amongst which it is often found growing should be guarded against, as its properties are generally regarded as deleterious. Gerard tells us: 'the new bread wherein Darnel is eaten hot causeth drunkenness.' When Darnel has been given medicinally in a harmful quantity, it is recorded to have produced all the symptoms of drunkenness: a general trembling, followed by inability to walk, hindered speech and vomiting. For this reason the French call Darnel: 'Ivraie,' from Ivre (drunkenness); the word Darnel is itself of French origin and testifies to its intoxicating qualities, being derived from an old French word Darne, signifying stupefied. The ancients supposed it to cause blindness, hence with the Romans, lolio victitare, to live on Darnel, was a phrase applied to a dim-sighted person.

The alleged poisonous properties of Darnel are now generally believed to be due to a fungus.

Darnel is in some provincial districts known as Cheat, and there is reason to suspect that the old custom of using Darnel to adulterate malt and distilled liquors has not been entirely abandoned.

Culpepper terms it 'a pestilent enemy among the corn,' and in olden days its name was so commonly used as a synonym for a pernicious weed that it has been said that the expression in Matthew xiii. 25, would have been better translated Darnel than tares.

The Arabs still give the name zirwan to a noxious grass (which is only too common in the cornfields of Palestine) simulating the wheat when undeveloped, though easily distinguishable at 'harvest' time.

In connection with this similarity, it may be of interest to relate an experiment made by a friend of the writer. She procured some ears of Palestine wheat and also some of Palestine 'Darnel' ('tares'), for the purpose of illustrating the truth of the Parable of the Tares to her Bible-class. After sowing both kinds in a patch of ground she asked her scholars to watch the appearance of the respective 'blades' as they appeared. They attached small strands of wool to distinguish each. In many cases wheat grew from the tare seeds, and tares from the wheat

It is said that the country people of Cheshire believed Darnel to be 'degenerated wheat.'

In the East it is a more serious enemy to the farmer, and in the low-lying districts of the Lebanon and other parts of Palestine it becomes alarmingly plentiful. If inadvertently eaten it produces sickness, dizziness, and diarrhrea. It would seem that the 'malice aforethought' of sowing this wild grass deliberately (as in our Lord's parable), was a not unusual practice. The following is a quotation from an old newspaper:

'The Country of Ill-Will is the by-name of a district hard by St. Arnaud, in the north of France. There tenants, when ejected by a landlord, or when they have ended their tenancy on uncomfortable terms, have been in the habit of spoiling the crop to come by vindictively sowing tares, and other coarse strangling weeds, among the wheat, whence has been derived the sinister name of the district. The practice has been made penal, and any man proved to have tampered with any other man's harvest will be dealt with as a criminal.'

Virgil speaks of 'unlucky darnel' (Georg., lib. i. 151-4) and groups it with thistles, thorns, and burs, among the enemies of the husbandman, and Shakespeare says:

'Darnel and all the idle weeds that grow
In our sustaining corn.'

In the Middle Ages it was sometimes called Cokil, as well as Ray, and in the fourteenth century we hear of it being used against 'festour and morsowe,' and of Cokkilmeal being thought good for freckles and to make the face white and soft. Culpepper, after calling it 'a malicious part of sullen Saturn,' adds: 'as it is not without some vices, hath it also many virtues . . . the meal of darnel is very good to stay gangrenes; it also cleanseth the skin of all scurvy, morphews, ringworms, if it be used with salt and reddish (Radish) roots.' Also: 'a decoction thereof made with water and honey, and the places bathed therewith cures the sciatica,' and finally: 'Darnel meal applied in a poultice draweth forth splinters and broken bones in the flesh.'

Medicinal Action and Uses

Darnel is usually regarded as possessing sedative and anodyne properties. It was not only employed medicinally by the Greeks and Romans and in the Middle Ages, but in more modern practice in the form of a powder or pill in headache, rheumatic meningitis, sciatica and other cases. Cases are on record of serious effects having resulted from the use of bread, containing by accidental admixture the flour of Darnel seeds. Chemically the seeds contain an acrid fixed oil and a yellow glucoside, but as far as microscopical appearances indicate, the Darnel contains nothing that is not contained in wheat, and analysis has not yet revealed its poisonous elements.

Of late years, it has been questioned whether the ill-effects of Darnel are inherent in the grain themselves, or whether they may not be ascribed to their having been ergotized. Lindley in his Vegetable Kingdom takes the latter view, stating moreover, 'this is the only authentic instance of unwholesome qualities in the order of grasses,' and Professor Henslow considers too that as the use of Darnel in the sixteenth century was similar to that of Ergot - a diseased condition of the grain of Rye - it is more probable that the injurious nature of Darnel has been due to an ergotized condition, especially as experiments have shown that perfectly healthy Darnel seeds have no injurious effects.

VERNAL GRASS, SWEET SCENTED

Botanical: Anthoxanthum odoratum (LINN.)
Part Used: Flowers.

The Sweet-scented Vernal Grass - with yellow anthers, not purple, as so many other grasses - gives its characteristic odor to newly-mown meadow hay, and has a pleasant aroma of Woodruff. It is, however, specially provocative of hay fever and hay asthma. The flowers contain Coumarin, the same substance that is present in the Melilot flowers, and the volatile pollen impregnates the atmosphere in early summer, causing much distress to hay-fever subjects. The sweet perfume is due chiefly to benzoic acid.

A medicinal tincture is made from this grass with spirit of wine, and it said that if poured into the open hand and sniffed well into the nose, almost immediate relief is afforded during an attack of hay fever. It is recommended that 3 or 4 drops of the tincture be at the same time taken as a dose with water, repeated if required, at intervals of twenty to thirty minutes.

The name Anthoxanthum is from the Greek anthos (flower) and xanthos (yellow).

Other Species

A. Puelii is a smaller species than A.odoratum, with many slender much-branched stems; lax panicles; long, slender awns, and a fainter perfume. It occurs occasionally as a modern introduction in sandy fields. Flowers from July to September.

The following British grasses have varying degrees of utility, though are not all medicinally valuable.

COMMON CORD-GRASS

Botanical: Spartina stricta

The generic name is from the Greek spartiné (a cord) from the use to which the leaves have been put. It grows on muddy saltmarshes in the south. It is cut at Southampton by the poorer classes for thatching.

Another variety grows on the mud-flats at Southampton, and is known as MANY-SPIKED CORD-GRASS (S. Towsendi) with shorter leaves; broader, larger spikelets, more lanceolate downy glumes, and a flexuous tip to the rachis; it also occurs on Southampton Water and in the Isle of Wight.

CANARY - GRASS

Botanical: Phalaris canariensis

Though probably an escape in England, it is much cultivated as 'canary-seed' in Central and Southern Europe for caged 'song birds.'

SOFT-GRASS

Botanical: Holcus

Name said to be from the Greek holkos, connected with helko (I draw), referring to a supposed power of drawing thorns out of the flesh. There are two British species, H. Mollis (Creeping Softgrass), abundant on light soil, and H. lanatus (Yorkshire Fog, Meadow Soft-grass) larger than the preceding.

DOG'S-TOOTH GRASS

Botanical: Fibichia umbellata

Of which the only British species is F. umbellata, a low prostrate grass, with long tough runners and short fat glaucous leaves, distinguished from all other British grasses (except Panicum sanguinale and P. glabrum) by the digitate arrangement of the three to five slender purplish spikes in the panicle, each of which is 1 to 1 1/2 inches long; and from those two species by having its awnless spikelets arranged singly, instead of in pairs, along the spikes. It is found in sandy pastures by the sea in the south-western counties, but is very rare. It is a good sand-binder, and one of the best pasture grasses of many dry climates. In India it is called Doorba or Doab-grass, and in Bermuda, Bermuda-grass. It was named after J. Fibich, a German botanist.

REED

Botanical: Phragmites communis

Of which P. communis (Common Reed) is the only species, is a stout grass, 5 to 10 feet high, with a long creeping root-stock. It is common all over the world, is very serviceable on river banks for binding the soil, and is used also for thatch (especially in Norfolk).

The runners are nutritious, containing much sugar, and might be used as fodder.

Name said to be from the Greek, phragma (a hedge).

CRESTED DOG'S-TAIL

Botanical: Cynosurus cristatus

Is a most useful grass, but the wiry stalks, when not eaten by sheep, remain in a dry state and are known as 'bents' or 'bennets.'

PURPLE MOLINIA

Botanical: Molinia varia

The only species, and a rather coarse, stiff plant, sometimes 3 feet high, with one node near the base of the stem. It grows in tussocks in company with Scabiosa succisa (Premorse, or Devil's-bit Scabious). The stems of this grass are sold in bundles by tobacconists for cleaning pipes. It was named after G. F. Molina, a Chilian botanist.

WATER WHORL-GRASS

Botanical: Catabrosa aquatica

The only species is a soft smooth pale-green plant, creeping or floating, sometimes muchbranched, 1 to 2 feet high. It grows in ditches and by the margins of ponds. Rather scarce, though distributed over the whole island. One of the sweet grasses; water-fowl and cattle are fond of it; but it is unsuitable for cultivation from the character of its habitat. Its name is derived from the Greek Katabrosis, an 'eating out,' alluding to the torn ends of the glumes.

REED MANNA-GRASS

Botanical: Glyceria aquatica

A conspicuous and imposing grass, 4 to 6 feet high, frequent in England and Ireland but rare in Scotland.

It is a fine covert for waterfowl.

SCENTED GRASSES

Among the Grasses may be included the SCENTED GRASSES, growing in tropical climates, largely cultivated in India, Ceylon and the Straits Settlements. They furnish very important essential oils for perfumery.

LEMONGRASS OIL is prepared from Cymbopogon citratus, formerly known as Andropogon Schoenanthus, a species growing abundantly in India and cultivated in Ceylon and Seychelles. It owes its scent almost entirely to its chief constituent, citral, and is one of the chief sources of the citral used in the manufacture of Tonone or artificial violet perfume. It is sometimes called Oil of Verbena from its similarity to the odor of the true Verbena Oil which is rarely found in commerce. It is frequently used to adulterate Lemon Oil. Samples of the oil produced experimentally in the West Indies, Uganda, and new districts of India were examined in the laboratories of the Imperial Institute in 1911, and as a result of the recommendations made, the production of Lemongrass has been taken up on a considerable scale in Uganda.

CITRONELLA OIL is derived from C. nardus, grown in Ceylon, Java and Burmah. The oil is distilled on an enormous scale and used for perfuming the cheapest household soaps and in the manufacture of coarse scents, and is also added as an adulterant to more expensive oils. Its scent is chiefly due to two substances, Geraniol and Citronellel.

PALMAROSA, Rosha or Indian Geranium Oil, is derived from C. martine. It is grown in India and was formerly known as 'Turkish Geranium Oil,' because it was imported into Europe via Turkey and Bulgaria as an adulterant to Otto of Roses. It has a strong geranium-like odor and is used in the commercial preparation of pure Geraniol, its chief constituent. The distillation of this oil was started in the eighteenth century.

GINGERGRASS OIL is also the product of the last-named grass, an oil of poorer quality, which is only suitable for cheap perfumes.

GRAVELROOT

Botanical: Eupatorium purpureum (LINN.)
Family: N.O. Compositae
Synonyms: Trumpet-weed. Gravelweed. Joe-pye Weed. Jopi Weed. Queen-of-the-Meadow Root. Purple Boneset. Eupatorium purpureum, trifoliatum, and maculatum. Eupatorium verticillatum. Eupatorium ternifolium. Hempweed.
Part Used: Fresh root.

Habitat

Is indigenous to North America, and common from Canada to Florida, growing in swampy and rich low grounds, where it blossoms throughout the summer months.

Description

This species varies greatly in form and foliage, the type being very tall and graceful.

The stem is rigidly erect, usually about 5 or 6 feet high, though sometimes even reaching a height of 12 feet, and is stout, unbranched and either hollow, or furnished with an incomplete pith. It is purple above the joints and often covered with elongated spots and lines (this variety having been called maculata by Linnaeus). The leaves, oblong and pointed, rough above, but downy beneath, are placed in whorls of four or five on the stem (mostly in fives) and are nearly destitute of resinous dots. The margins are coarsely and unequally toothed, the leafstalks either short or merely represented by the contracted bases of the leaves. The flowers are purple, in a dense terminal inflorescence, the heads very numerous, five to ten flowered, contained in an eight-leaved, fresh-coloured involucre.

It grows in low, swampy ground. There are over forty species of the genus, many of which are used medicinally. The name is derived from a king of Pontus, Mithridates Eupator, who first used the plant as a remedy, and the popular name of Jopi or Joe-pye is taken from an American Indian who cured the typhus with it.

The taste is aromatic, astringent, and bitter.

The roots should be collected in the autumn.

Constituents

The chief constituent is Euparin. It is yellow, neutral, and crystalline,and received the formula C12 = H11 = O3.

Eupurpurin, a so-called oleoresin, has been precipitated from a tincture of the drug.

A tincture and a fluid extract are prepared.

Medicinal Action and Uses

Diuretic, nervine. Formerly the use of this purple-flowered Boneset was very similar to that of the ordinary Boneset. It is especially valuable as a diuretic and stimulant as well as an astringent tonic, and is considered a valuable remedy in dropsy, strangury, gravel, hematuria, gout and rheumatism, exerting a special influence upon chronic renal and cystic troubles.

Preparations

Fluid extract, 1/2 to 1 drachm. Eupatorin, 3 to 5 grains.

GREENWEED (DYERS')

Botanical: Genista tinctoria (LINN.)
Family: N.O. Leguminosae
Synonyms: Greenweed. Greenwood. Woad or Wood-waxen, formerly Wede-wixen or Woud-wix. Base-broom. Genet des Teinturiers. F„rberginster. Dyers' Broom.
Part Used: Whole plant.
Habitat: Mediterranean countries. Canary Islands. Western Asia. Britain. Established in the United States.

Description

The name of the genus is derived from the Celtic Gen (a small bush). Genista tinctoria is a small, tufted shrub, bearing short racemes of yellow flowers. The bright, luxuriant growth of the latter has led to its cultivation in greenhouses in the United States.

The bright green, smooth stems, 1 to 2 feet high, are much branched, the branches erect, rather stiff, smooth or only slightly hairy and free from spines. The leaves are spear-shaped, placed alternately on the stem, smooth, with uncut margins, 1/2 to 1 inch in length, very smoothly stalked, the margins fringed with hairs.

The shoots terminate in spikes of brightyellow, pea-like flowers, opening in July. They are 1/2 to 3/4 inch long, on foot-stalks shorter than the calyx. Like those of the Broom, they 'explode' when visited by an insect. The 'claws' of the four lower petals are straight at first, but in a high state of tension, so that the moment they are touched, they curl downwards with a sudden action and the flower bursts open. The flowers are followed by smooth pods, 1 to 1 1/4 inch long, much compressed laterally, brown when ripe, containing five to ten seeds.

A dwarf kind grows in tufts in meadows in the greater part of England and is said to enrich poor soil.

Cows will sometimes eat the plant, and it communicates an unpleasant bitterness to their milk and even to the cheese and butter made from it.

All parts of the plant, but especially the flowering tops, yield a good yellow dye, and from the earliest times have been used by dyers for producing this color, especially for wool: combined with woad, an excellent green is yielded, the color being fixed with alum, cream of tartar and sulphate of lime. In some parts of England, the plant used to be collected in large quantities by the poor and sold to the dyers.

Tournefort (1708) describes the process of dyeing linen, woollen, cloth or leather by the use of this plant, which he saw in the island of Samos. It is still applied to the same purpose in some of the Grecian islands. The Romans employed if for dyeing and it is described by several of their writers.

In some countries the buds are prepared and

served as seasoning. As a dye the plant has largely been superseded by Reseda luteola.

The seeds have been suggested as a substitute for coffee.

In Spain and Italy strong cloths that take dyes well are woven from the fibres.

Constituents

The active principle, Scopnarine, is found as starry, yellow crystals, and is soluble in boiling water and in alcohol. From the liquid which remains another principle, Spartéine, is extracted, an organic base, liquid and volatile, with strong narcotic properties.

Medicinal Action and Uses

Diuretic, cathartic, emetic. Both flower tops and seedshave been used medicinally.

The powdered seeds operate as a mild purgative and a decoction of the plant has been used medicinally as a remedy in dropsy and is also stated to have proved effective in gout and rheumatism, being taken in wine glassful doses three or four times a day.

The ashes form an alkaline salt, which has also been used as a remedy in dropsy and other diseases.

In the fourteenth century it was used, as well as Broom, to make an ointment called Unguentum geneste, 'goud for alle could goutes,' etc. The seed was used in a plaister for broken limbs.

A decoction of the plant was regarded in the Ukraine as a remedy for hydrophobia, but its virtues in this respect do not seem to rest on very good evidence.

Dioscorides and Pliny speak of the purgative properties of the seeds and flowers, and the latter also regarded them as diuretic and good for sciatica. Cullen used a decoction of the young shoots for the same purpose. An infusion of the flowers has been found useful for albuminuria, and a combination of the tips with mustard, in dropsy. A poultice has benefited cold abscesses and scrofulous tumours. The infusion can be taken in wine glassful doses three or four times a day.

It has been stated that scoparine can replace all preparations, while one drop of spartéine dissolved in alcohol is a strong narcotic.

Other Species

G. scoparia, G. purgans, and G. griot havesimilar properties. The last two are employed by the peasants as purgatives.

The flowers of G. Hispanica have been used in dropsy combined with albuminaric.

Dyers' Woad or Dyers' Weed is also the common name of Isatis tinctoria, and Reseda Luteola, or Yellow Weed or Weld, used in dyeing and painting.

GRINDELIA

Botanical: Grindelia camporum (GREENE), Grindelia cuneifolia, Grindelia squarrosa
Family: N.O. Compositae
Synonyms: Hardy Grindelia. Gum Plant. California Gum Plant. Scaly Grindelia. Rosin Weed. Grindelia robusta (Nutt.).
Parts Used: Dried leaves and flowering tops.
Habitat: The western United States.

Description

Until the work of Perredes in 1906 the drug was supposed to be derived from Grindelia robusta, and the species now regarded as official were thought to be merely varieties. G. robusta, however, is rarely used.

There are about twenty-five species of the genus, seven or eight being found in South America. The early growth of most of them is covered with a glutinous varnish. They are perennial or biennial herbs or small shrubs, with stems up to half-a-yard long, round, yellow, and smooth, with alternate, light-green, coarsely-toothed leaves having a clasping base. They are easily broken off when dried, so are often found loose in packages. The solitary, terminal flower-heads are large and yellow, both disk and radiate. Taste and odor are slightly aromatic, the former bitter.

The distinctive mark of the genus is the limb of the calyx, consisting of two to eight rigid, narrow awns, which fall early.

The plant was only made widely known to the medical profession in the latter part of the nineteenth century, by Dr. C. A. Canfield, and Mr. J. G. Steele of San Francisco.

Constituents

Grindelia may contain as much as 21 per cent of amorphous resins. Two are dark-coloured, one being soluble in ether, and one soft and greenish, soluble in petroleum spirit. There is also found tannin, laevoglucose, and a little volatile oil. The presence of glucosides has not been confirmed.

Medicinal Action and Uses

Expectorant and sedative, with an action resembling atropine. It has been recommended in cystitis and catarrh of the bladder, but its principal use is in bronchial catarrh, especially when there is any asthmatic tendency. It relieves dyspnoea due to heart disease, has been successfully employed in whooping cough, and as a local application in rhus poisoning, burns, genito-urinary catarrh, etc. As its active principle is excreted from the kidneys, it sometimes produces signs of renal irritation; in chronic catarrh of the bladder it stimulates the mucous membrane.

A homeopathic tincture is prepared.

Dosage

Of fluid extract, 1/2 to 1 fluid drachm. Of Grindelia, 30 to 40 grains.

The Fluid extract is sometimes continued with liquorice in the proportion of 1/2 drachm of Grindelia to 1 draehm of the Fluid extract of Liquorice, mucilage to 1 oz.

Other Species

G. cuneifolia is a marsh plant, darker greenand less glutinous than G. camporum. It has a variety called paludosa.

G. squarrosa grows on prairies and dry banks. The bracts of the involucre are linear-lanceolate and spreading.

G. robusta var. latifolia is large, hardy, and a native of California.

These are all official varieties.

GROUNDSEL

Botanical: Senecio vulgaris (LINN.)
Family: N.O. Compositae
Synonyms: Scotch) Grundy Swallow, Ground Glutton.
(Norfolk) Simson, Sention.
Part Used: Whole herb.

Habitat

A very common weed throughout Europe and Russian Asia, not extending to the tropics. It is abundant in Britain, being found up to the height of I,600 feet in Northumberland. It grows almost everywhere, and is to be found as frequently on the tops of walls as among all kinds of rubbish and waste ground, but especially in gardens. Groundsel is one of those plants which follows civilized man wherever he settles, for there is hardly a European colony in the world in which it does not spring up upon the newly tilled land, the seeds probably having mingled with the grain which the European takes with him to the foreign country. Other home weeds, such as the thistle, have made their way across the seas in the same manner.

Groundsel, so well known as a troublesome weed, is connected in the minds of most of us with caged birds, and probably few people are aware that it has any other use except as a favorite food for the canary. And yet in former days, Groundsel was a popular herbal remedy, is still employed in some country districts, and still forms an item in the stock of the modern herbalist, though it is not given a place in the British Pharmacopoeia.

The name Groundsel is of old origin, being derived from the Anglo-Saxon groundeswelge, meaning literally, 'ground swallower,' referring to the rapid way the weed spreads. In Scotland and the north of England it is still in some localities called Grundy Swallow - only a slight corruption of the old form of the word - and is also there called Ground Glutton. In Norfolk it is often called Simson or Sention, which has by some been considered an abbreviation of 'Ascension Plant.' It seems more probable that 'Sention' is a corruption of the Latin, Senecio, derived from Senex (an old man), in reference to its downy head of seeds; 'the flower of this herb hath white hair and when the wind bloweth it away, then it appeareth like a bald-headed man.'

The genus Senecio, belonging to the large family Compositae, includes about 900 species, which are spread over all parts of the globe, but are found in greatest profusion in temperate regions. Nine are natives of this country. The essential character of the genus is an involucre (the enveloping outer leaves of the composite heads of flowers) consisting of a single series of scales of equal length. The florets of the flower-heads are either all tubular, or more commonly, the central tubular and the marginal strap-shaped. The prevailing color of the flowers in this genus is yellow purple (white or blue being comparatively rare).

Description

It is an annual, the root consisting of numerous white fibres and the round or slightly angular stem, erect, 6 inches to nearly 1 foot in height, often branching at the top, is frequently purple in color. It is juicy, not woody, and generally smooth, though some times bears a little loose, cottony wool. The leaves are oblong, wider and clasping at the base, a dull, deep green color, much cut into (pinnatifid), with irregular, blunt-toothed or jagged lobes, not unlike the shape of oak leaves. The cylindrical flower-heads, each about 1/4 inch long and 1/8 inch across, are in close terminal clusters or corymbs, the florets yellow and all tubular; the scales surrounding the head and forming the involucre are narrow and black-tipped, with a few small scales at their base. The flowers are succeeded by downy heads of seeds, each seed being crowned by little tufts of hairs, by means of which they are freely dispersed by the winds. Groundsel is in flower all the year round and scatters an enormous amount of seed in its one season of growth, one plant if allowed to seed producing one million others in one year.

A variety of Senecio vulgaris, named S. radiata (Koch), with minute rays to the outer florets, is found in the Channel Islands.

According to Linnaeus, goats and swine eat this common plant freely, cows being not partial to it and horses and sheep declining to touch it, but not only are caged birds fond of it, but its leaves and seeds afford food for many of our wild species. Groundsel, in common with many other common garden weeds, such as Chickweed, Dandelion, Bindweed, Plantain, etc., may be freely given to rabbits. It is said that Groundsel will at times entice a rabbit to eat when all other food has been refused. Rabbit-keeping is a very practical way of reducing the butcher's bill, and no means of feeding the rabbits economically should be neglected. Stores of both Groundsel and Chickweed might well be dried in the summer for giving to the rabbits in winter time with their hay.

Parts Used Medicinally

The whole herb, collected in May, when the leaves are in the best condition and dried. The fresh plant is also used for the expression of the juice.

Constituents

Chemically, Groundsel contains senecin and seniocine. The juice isslightly acrid, but emollient.

Medicinal Action and Uses

Diaphoretic, antiscorbutic, purgative, diuretic, anthelmintic.

It was formerly much used for poultices and reckoned good for sickness of the stomach. A weak infusion of the plant is now sometimes given as a simple and easy purgative, and a strong infusion as an emetic: it causes no irritation or pain, removes bilious trouble and is a great cooler, or as Culpepper puts it:

'This herb is Venus's mistress piece and is as gallant and universal a medicine for all diseases coming of heat, in what part of the body soever they be, as the sun shines upon: it is very safe and friendly to the body of man, yet causes vomiting if the stomach be afflicted, if not, purging. It doth it with more gentleness than can be expected: it is moist and something cold withal, thereby causing expulsion and repressing the heat caused by the motion of the internal parts in purges and vomits. The herb preserved in a syrup, in a distilled water, or in an ointment, is a remedy in all hot diseases, and will do it: first, safely; secondly, speedily.'

'The decoction of the herb, saith Dioscorides, made with wine and drunk helpeth the pains in the stomach proceeding from choler (bile). The juice thereof taken in drink, or the decoction of it in ale gently performeth the same. It is good against the jaundice and falling sickness (epilepsy), and taken in wine expelleth the gravel from the reins and kindeys. It also helpeth the sciatica, colic, and pains of the belly. The people in Lincolnshire use this externally against pains and swelling, and as they affirm with great success. The juice of the herb, or as Dioscorides saith, the leaves and flowers, with some Frankinsense in powder, used in wounds of the body, nerves or sinews, help to heal them. The distilled water of the herb performeth well all the aforesaid cures, but especially for inflammation or watering of the eye, by reason of rheum into them.'

Gerard says that 'the down of the flower mixed with vinegar' will also prove a good dressing for wounds, and recommends that when the juice is boiled in ale for the purpose of a purge, a little honey and vinegar be added, and that the efficacy is improved by the further addition of 'a few roots of Assarbace.' He states also that 'it helpeth the King's Evil, and the leaves stamped and strained into milk and drunk helpeth the red gums and frets in children.'

Another old herbalist tells us that the fresh roots smelled when first taken out of the ground are an immediate cure for many forms of headache. But the root must not be dug up with a tool that has any iron in its composition.

Some of the old authorities claimed that Groundsel was especially good for such wounds as had been caused by being struck by iron.

Groundsel in an old-fashioned remedy for chapped hands. If boiling water be poured on the fresh plant, the liquid forms a pleasant swab for the skin and will remove roughness.

For gout, it was recommended to 'pound it with lard, lay it to the feet and it will alleviate the disorder.'

A poultice of the leaves, applied to the pit of the stomach, is said to cause the same emetic effect as a dose of the strong infusion. A poultice made with salt is said to 'disperse knots and kernels in the flesh.'

In this country, farriers give Groundsel to horses as a cure for bot-worms, and in Germany it is said to be employed as a popular vermifuge for children.

A drachm of the juice is sufficient to take, internally.

GROUNDSEL, GOLDEN

Botanical: Senecio aureus (LINN.)
Family: N.O. Compositae
Synonyms: Life Root. Squaw Weed. Golden Senecio.
Part Used: Herb.

Senecio aureus, Golden Groundsel, an American species, native of Virginia and Canada, is considered a most useful plant, deserving of attention. The root and whole herb are employed medicinally for their emmenagogue, diuretic, pectoral, and astringent qualities. It has often been used in the first stage of consumption for the beneficial effects of its tonic properties, combined with its pectoral qualities, 1 teaspoonful of the fluid extract prepared from it being taken in water or combined with other pectorals. It is also of value in gravel, stone, diarrhrea, etc. The plant has slender, fluted, unbranched and cottony stems, 1 to 2 feet high. The rhizome is perennial, 1 to 2 inches long, the bark of the roots hard and blackish. The root-leaves are roundish and kidney-shaped, up to 6 inches long, on long leaf-stalks. The stem leaves decrease in size as they grow up the stem, and are cut into as far as the midrib, the upper ones being stalkless. The flower-heads are few in number, loosely arranged at the summit of the stem, the flowers two-thirds to nearly an inch broad, of a golden yellow, with the outer ray florets slightly reflexed. The plant has only a slight odor, but a bitter, astringent, slightly acrid taste.

Preparations

Senecin, 1 to 3 grains. Powdered root, 1/2 to 1 drachm. Fluid extract, 1/2 to 1 drachm. Solid extract, 5 to 10 grains.

GROUNDSEL, HOARY

Botanical: Senecio erucifolius (LINN.)
Family: N.O. Compositae

Senecio erucifolius, the Hoary Groundsel, which has similar properties to S. vulgaris, has been employed in poultices, ointments and plasters. It is a perennial, distributed over Europe and Siberia, growing not infrequently here on dry banks and by road-sides in limestone or chalky districts from Berwick southwards, but rarely in Ireland. It is a tall plant, in growth similar to S. Jacobae, but sending up several stems from its shortly creeping root. The whole plant is cottony, or softly hairy, with curled hairs, especially on the upper surfaces of the leaves, which have much narrower, regularly divided segments, slightly rolled back at theedges. The flower-heads are larger. It flowers from July to August.

All forms of this genus are not of such beneficial use, and one at least has lately been found to be distinctly harmful, for Molteno disease, a cattle and horse disease prevalent in certain parts of South Africa, has been definitely traced to the presence of a poisonous alkaloid in a plant eaten by the animals, this plant being Senecio latifolius, a near relative of the Common Groundsel of this country.

SENECIO MARITIMA

Botanical: Cineraria maritima (LINN.)
Family: N.O. Compositae

Senecio maritima, sometimes looked on as a variety of S. campestris (D.C.), and known by Linnaeus as Cineraria maritima, is found on maritime rocks at Holyhead. It is a shrubby plant, divided into many branches, which have a white, downy covering of hairs. The flowers bloom from June to August, and are about 3/8 inches across, arranged in a similar manner to Ragwort. The leaves are 5 to 8 inches long and about 2 to 2 1/4 inches wide, the segments broadly-toothed, about three-lobed and with soft hairs, which form a dense white covering. One or two drops of the fresh juice of the plant dropped into the eye is said to be of use in removing cataract.

GROUNDSEL, MOUNTAIN

Botanical: Senecio sylvaticus
Family: N.O. Compositae

Senecio sylvatica, Mountain Groundsel, is distinguished from Common Groundsel by its larger size, being 1 to 2 feet high, and by its having conical, rather than cylindrical heads of dull yellow flowers, with a few rays rolled back and often wanting. The stems are branched and the leaves pinnatifid, with narrower lobes, toothed. It is an annual, grows common on gravelly soil, on dry heaths and commons, growing in the Highlands up to 1,000 feet above sea-level and flowers from July to September. It has a somewhat unpleasant odor, and detergent and anti-scorbutic properties.

EGROUNDSEL, VISCID

Botanical: Senecio viscosus
Family: N.O. Compositae
Synonym: Stinking Groundsel.

Senecio viscosus, Viscid Groundsel, is near the last-named species in habit, though its erect stem is not so tall, and it is distinguished by being clothed with viscid down, causing the leaves, which are finely cut into, to be thick and clammy to the touch and lighter in color. The flower heads are less numerous, with the outer bracts of the involucre about half as long as the inner, and the flowers pale. It grows in similar situations, mostly on dry ditch banks and wastedry ground, from Forfar downwards, but is more local than S. sylvaticus, and is rare in Ireland. It, also, is an annual, flowering from July to September, and has a foetid odor, obtaining for it the popular name of Stinking Groundsel. The leaves are carminative: its emetic properties are slightly less than those of S. vulgaris.

GUAIACUM

Botanical: Guaiacum officinale (LINN.)
Family: N.O. Zygophyllaceae
Synonym: Lignum Vitae.
Parts Used: Resin, bark, wood.
Habitat: West Indian Islands. North Coast of South America.

Description

An ornamental evergreen tree with pretty rich blue flowers, the trunk is a greenish-brown color, the wood of slow growth but attains a height of 40 to 60 feet, stem almost always crooked, bark furrowed; the wood is extraordinarily heavy, solid and dense, fibres cross-grained; pinnate leaves, oval obtuse; fruit obcordate capsule; seeds solitary, hard, oblong. The old heart wood is dark green, the sap wood little in quantity and of a much lighter yellowish color; the wood is largely used by turners, where weight is not an obstacle; it is very hard and durable, suitable for making black sheaves, pestles, pulleys, rulers, skittle boards, etc.; it has a slight acrid taste and is odourless, unless heated, when it emits an agreeable scent. The bark yields 1 per cent volatile oil of delicious fragrance.

Guaiacum sanctum. Habitat, Bahamas and South Florida) is also used for the same purposes as G. officinale; it is easily distinguished from the latter, by its five-celled fruit, and its oblong leaflets, six to eight to each leaf. The leaves are sometimes used as a substitute for soap.

Guaiacum Resin. This is obtained from both the above trees and is procured by raising one end of the log and firing it; this melts the resin, which runs out of a hole cut in the other end, and is then caught into vessels. The resin is found in round or ovoid tears; some are imported the size of walnuts, but usually it is in large blocks; these break easily; the fracture is clean and glassy, in thin pieces, color yellow-reddish brown. The powder is grey, and must be kept in dark-coloured bottles, as exposure to the light and air soon turns it green.

Medicinal Action and Uses

The wood is very little used in medicine; it obtained a great reputation about the sixteenth century, when it was brought into notice as a cure for syphilis and other diseases; later on the resin obtained from the wood was introduced and now is greatly preferred, for medicinal use, to the wood. The wood is sometimes sold by chemists in the form of fine shavings, and as such called Lignum Vitae, which are turned green by exposure to the air, and bluish green by the action of nitric fumes. This test proves its genuiness.

It is a mild laxative and diuretic. For tonsilitis it is given in powdered form. Specially useful for rheumatoid arthritis, also in chronic rheumatism and gout, relieving the pain and inflammation between the attacks, and lessening their recurrence if doses are continued. It acts as an acrid stimulant, increasing heat of body and circulation; when the decoction is taken hot and the body is kept warm, it acts as a diaphoretic, and if cool as a diuretic. Also largely used for secondary syphilis, skin diseases and scrofula.

Dosage

Of the wood 30 to 60 grains, Decoction, 2 oz. to 4 oz. in a pint of water. Fluid extract, 1/2 to 1 drachm. Guaiacum tincture, B.P. and U.S.P., 1/2 to 1 drachm. Ammoniated tincture Guaiacum, B.P. and U.S.P., 1/2 to 1 drachm. Resin, 5 to 15 grains. Guaiacum mixture, B.P., 1/2 to 1 fluid ounce. Guaiacum Resin Lozenges, B.P., 1 to 6 may be taken.

GUARANA

Botanical: Paullinia Cupana, Kunth. (H. B. and K.)
Family: N.O. Sapindaceae
Synonyms: Paullinia. Guarana Bread. Brazilian Cocoa. Uabano. Uaranzeiro. Paullinia Sorbilis.
Part Used: Prepared seeds, crushed.
Habitat: Brazil, Uruguay. - NOTE: Dr Earle Sweet, Sayfer Botanicals, points out that this is incorrect, Guarana does NOT grow in Uruguay. - 12/16/96

Description

This climbing shrub took the name of its genus

from C. F. Paullini, a German medical botanist who died 1712. It has divided compound leaves, flowers yellow panicles, fruit pear shaped, three sided, three-celled capsules, with thin partitions, in each a seed like a small horse-chestnut half enclosed in an aril, flesh coloured and easily separated when dried. The seeds of Paullinia Sorbilis are often used or mixed with those of P. Cupana. Guarana is only made by the Guaranis, a tribe of South American Indians.

After the seeds are shelled and washed they are roasted for six hours, then put into sacks and shaken till their outside shell comes off, they are then pounded into a fine powder and made into a dough with water, and rolled into cylindrical pieces 8 inches long; these are then dried in the sun or over a slow fire, till they became very hard and are then a rough and reddish-brown color, marbled with the seeds and testa in the mass. They break with an irregular fracture, have little smell, taste astringent, and bitter like chocolate without its oiliness, and in color like chocolate powder; it swells up and partially dissolves in water.

Constituents

A crystallizable principle, called guaranine, identical with caffeine, which exists in the seeds, united with tannic acid, catechutannic acid starch, and a greenish fixed oil.

Medicinal Action and Uses

Nervine, tonic, slightly narcotic stimulant, aphrodisiac febrifuge. A beverage is made from the guaran sticks, by grating half a tablespoonful into sugar and water and drinking it like tea. The Brazilian miners drink this constantly and believe it to be a preventive of many diseases, as well as a most refreshing beverage. Their habit in travelling is to carry the stick or a lump of it in their pockets, with a palate bone or scale of a large fish with which to grate it. P. Cupana is also a favorite national diet drink, the seeds are mixed with Cassava and water, and left to ferment until almost putrid, and in this state it is the favorite drink of the Orinoco Indians. From the tannin it contains it is useful for mild forms of leucorrhoea, diarrhrea, etc., but its chief use in Europe and America is for headache, especially if of a rheumatic nature. It is a gentle excitant and serviceable where the brain is irritated or depressed by mental exertion, or where there is fatigue or exhaustion from hot weather. It has the same chemical composition as caffeine, theine and cocaine, and the same physiological action. Its benefit is for nervous headache or the distress that accompanies menstruation, or exhaustion following dissipation. It is not recommended for chronic headache or in cases where it is not desirable to increase the temperature, or excite the heart or increase arterial tension. Dysuria often follows its administration. It is used by the Indians for bowel complaints, but is not indicated in cases of constipation or blood pressure.

Dosage

Powder, 10 grains to 1/2 drachm. Fluid extract of Guarana, U.S.P., 30 minims sweetened with one teaspoonful of syrup in water three times a day.

As a strong diuretic 7 1/2 grains can be taken daily and in 24 hours it has been known to increase urine from 27 OZ. to 107 OZ.

Tincture of Guarana, B.P.C., for sick headaches, 1 to 2 fluid drachms in water.

GUELDER ROSE

Botanical: Viburnum opulus (LINN.)
Family: N.O. Caprifoliaceae
Synonyms: Cramp Bark. Snowball Tree. King's Crown. High Cranberry. Red Elder. Rose Elder. Water Elder. May Rose. Whitsun Rose. Dog Rowan Tree. Silver Bells. Whitsun Bosses. Gaitre Berries. Black Haw.
Part Used: Bark.

Habitat

The 'Gaitre-Beries' of which Chaucer makes mention among the plants that 'shal be for your hele' to 'picke hem right as they grow and ete hem in,' are the deep red clusters of berries of the Wild Guelder Rose (Viburnum Opulus, Linn.), a shrub growing 5 to 10 feet high, belonging to the same family as the Elder, found in copses and hedgerows throughout England, though rare in Scotland, and also indigenous to North America, where it is to be found in low grounds in the eastern United States.

Description

It resembles the Common Elder in habits of growth, hence in some districts we find it called Red Elder or Rose Elder. The conspicuous, large, nearly flattopped heads of snow-white flowers are 3 to 5 inches across, the inner ones very small, but with an outer ring of large, showy, sterile blossoms, containing undeveloped stamens with no pollen and an ovary without ovules. Only the inner, complete flowers provide the nectar for the attraction of insects who are to fertilize them. The resulting fruits, which ripen very quickly, form a drooping cluster of bright red berries, shining and translucent, perhaps the most ornamental of our wild fruits, the tree presenting a very beautiful appearance in August, when they are ripe, especially as the leaves assume a rich purple hue before falling. But although edible, the berries, in spite of Chaucer's recommendation, are too bitter to be palatable eaten fresh off the trees, and when crushed, smell somewhat disagreeable, though birds appreciate them and in Siberia the berries used to be, and probably still are, fermented with flour and a spirit distilled from them. They have been used in Norway and Sweden to flavor a paste of honey and flour.

In Canada, they are employed to a considerable extent as a substitute for Cranberries and are much used for making. a piquant jelly, their sourness gaining for them there the name of High Bush Cranberry, though the tree is, of course, quite unrelated to the true Cranberry.

The name Guelder comes from Gueldersland, a Dutch province, where the tree was first cultivated. It was introduced into England under the name of 'Gueldres Rose.' The garden variety, Viburnum sterile, with snowball flowers, does not produce the showy fruit of the wild species.

The berries have anti-scorbutic properties. They turn black in drying and have been used for making ink.

The wood, like that of the Spindle Tree and Dogwood, is used for making skewers.

Medicinal Action and Uses

The bark, known as Cramp Bark, is employed in herbal medicine. It used formerly to be included in the United States Pharmacopoeia, but is now omitted though it has been introduced into the National Formulary in the form of a Fluid Extract, Compound Tincture and Compound Elixir, for use as a nerve sedative and anti-spasmodic in asthma and hysteria.

In herbal practice in this country, its administration in decoction and infusion, as well as the fluid extract and compound tincture is recommended. It has been employed with benefit in all nervous complaints and debility and used with success in cramps and spasms of all kinds, in convulsions, fits and lockjaw, and also in palpitation, heart disease and rheumatism.

The decoction (1/2 oz. to a pint of water) is given in tablespoon doses.

The bark is collected chiefly in northern Europe and appears in commerce in thin strips, sometimes in quills, 1/20 to 1/12 inch thick, greyish-brown externally, with scattered brownish warts, faintly cracked longitudinally. It has a strong, characteristic odor and its taste is mildly astringent and decidedly bitter.

Constituents

The active principle of Cramp Bark is the bitter glucoside Viburnine; it also contains tannin, resin and valerianic acid.

Preparations and Dosages

Fluid extract, 1/2 to 2 drachms. Viburnin, 1 to 3 grains.

Its constituents are identical with the species of Viburnum that is more widely used and is an official drug in the United States, viz. Viburnum Prunifolium or Black Haw, though Cramp Bark contains 1/3 the resin contained in Black Haw and its similar properties are considered much weaker.

Fluid Extract of Cramp Bark has a reddishbrown color and the slight odor and somewhat astringent taste of the bark.

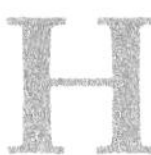

HARDHACK

Botanical: Spiraea tomentosa (LINN.)
Family: N.O. Rosaceae
Synonyms: Steeple Bush. White Cap. White Leaf. Silver Leaf.
Parts Used: Leaves, root, flowers.
Habitat: Canada. New Brunswick, Nova Scotia to the mountains of Georgia westward.

Description

Indigenous shrub, with leaves ovate, lanceolate, serrate, greenish-white and downy. The rose-coloured flowers are in panicles underneath.

Constituents

The root is said to contain gallic and tannic acid, and, when freshly dug, some volatile oils.

Medicinal Action and Uses

The flowers give feebly the medicinal action of salicylic acid and are used in decoction for their diuretic and tonic effect.

The root and leaves are astringent and useful in diarrhrea when there are no inflammatory symptoms.

Dose for diarrhrea, 30 to 60 minims of the fluid extract.

HAWKBIT, ROUGH

Botanical: Leontodon hispidus (LINN.)
Family: N.O. Compositae
Part Used: Herb.

Assigned also at one time to the genus Hieracium, but now placed by most botanists in the genus Leontodon, and sometimes in the genus Apargia, are the Hawkbits, of which there are two British species, the Autumnal Hawkbit and the Rough Hawkbit, both abundantly distributed throughout Britain, in meadowland, and on commons and waste ground.

The Rough Hawkbit has been used medicinally in the same manner as the Hawkweeds and the Dandelion, for its action on the kidneys and as a remedy for jaundice and dropsy, and is still used for its diuretic qualities in country districts in Ireland.

It is a plant somewhat resembling the Dandelion in appearance, the leaves all springing from the root, 3 to 4 inches long, jaggedly cut into, with the lobes pointing backwards, but instead of being smooth like the Dandelion, they are rough with forked bristles. The few flowers which the plant bears are borne singly on slender stems, 6 inches to a foot or more high, swollen at the top beneath the heads, which are 1 1/2 inches in diameter when expanded; when in bud, they droop.

The name of the genus, Leontodon, is formed from two Greek words, meaning Lion's tooth, referring to the toothed leaves. Apargia is derived from the name bestowed by the Greeks on this or some similar plant, and is taken from two Greek words, meaning 'From idleness,' the implication being that where these weeds are allowed to abound, the farmer has his own idleness to thank. The name of the genus, Hieracium, derived from the Greek, hieras (a hawk), refers to an ancient belief that hawks ate these plants to sharpen their sight, a belief also indicated in the popular English names, Hawkweed and Hawkbit.

All the Hawkweeds abound in honey and have a sweet honey-like smell when expanded in the full sunshine.

Other Species

Hieracium Aurantiacum, called also 'Grimthe-Collier,' from the black hairs which clothe the flower-stalk and involucre, is an ornamental plant with orange flowers.

HAWKWEED, WOOD

Botanical: Hieracium sylvaticum (LINN.)
Family: N.O. Compositae
Part Used: Herb.

The Hawkweeds, together with the Hawkbits, Goat's Beard and Salsify, belong to the Chicory group of the great order Compositae, which includes also the Dandelion and Sowthistles. All the plants of this group have milky juice, and the flowers - mostly yellow - have not two kinds of florets, like the daisy, but consist only of strap-shaped florets, each one of which is a complete flower in itself, not lacking stamens, as do the outer similarly shaped ray florets of the Daisy.

It is often a perplexing matter to distinguish the different members of the Hawkweed family. Some botanical authorities have recognized no less than thirty different species, but many of these are considered by other authorities to be merely variations or subspecies, and, as a rule, about ten species are regarded as distinct, of which the commonest among the taller species are the Wall Hawkweed (Hieracium murorum), and the Wood Hawkweed (H. sylvaticum), and the little Mouse-ear Hawkweed.

The older writers have often grouped together, as far as their medicinal qualities are concerned, the Hawkweeds, the Hawkbits and the Hawkbeards, all of which have yellow, dandelion-like flowers, and are much alike in appearance. Culpepper says:

'Saturn owns it. Hawkweed, saith Dioscorides, is cooling, somewhat drying and binding, and good for the heat of the stomach and gnawings therein, for inflammation and the bad fits of ague. The juice of it in wine helps digestion, dispels wind, hinders crudities abiding in the stomach; it is good against the biting of venomous serpents, if the herb be applied to the place, and is good against all other poisons. A scruple of the dried root given in wine and vinegar is profitable for dropsy. The decoction of the herb taken in honey digesteth the phlegm in the chest or lungs, and with hyssop helps the cough. The decoction of the herb and of wild succory made with wine, cures windy colic and hardness of the spleen, it procures rest and sleep, cools heat, purges the stomach, increases blood and helps diseases of the reins and bladder. Outwardly applied it is good for all the defects and diseases of the eyes, used with new milk- it is used with good success for healing spreading ulcers, especially in the beginning. The green leaves, bruised and with a little salt, applied to any place burnt with fire before blisters arise, help them: as also St. Anthony's fire (erysipelas) and all eruptions. Applied with meal and water as a poultice, it eases and helps cramps and convulsions. The distilled water cleanseth the skin and taketh away freckles, spots, or wrinkles in the face.'

The Wall Hawkweed, probably the commonest of the genus, grows freely in Great Britain in woods and on heaths, walls and rocks. It is a very variable plant, 1 to 2 feet high; the leaves, which are more or less hairy, mostly rise directly from the root and lie in a rosette on the ground. They are egg-shaped and toothed at the base and have slender footstalks. The stem is many-flowered and rarely bears more than one large leaf, sometimes none. The yellow flowers, which are in bloom in July and August, are from 3/4 to 1 inch in diameter, their stalks below the heads being covered with scattered, simple and gland-tipped black hairs.

The Wood Hawkweed is found on banks and in copses, flowering in August and September. It is also very variable, but is best distinguished from H. murorum by its more robust habit, rather larger heads of flowers and by the narrower leaves, less crowded in a rosette, the stem being as a rule more leafy, but some varieties of murorum would rank with this in form of foliage. The leaves are sometimes very slightly toothed, the teeth pointing upwards, at other times deeply so, and are often spotted with purple. The stems are 1 to 3 feet high and many flowered, the involucres of the heads being hoary with down.

HAWKWEED, MOUSE-EAR

Botanical: Hieracium Pilosella (LINN.)
Family: N.O. Compositae
Synonyms: Hawkweed. Pilosella. Mouse Ear.
Part Used: Herb.

None of the Hawkweeds are now much used in herbal treatment, though in many parts of Europe they were formerly employed as a constant medicine in diseases of the lungs, asthma and incipient consumption, but the small Mouse-ear Hawkweed, known commonly as Mouse-ear is still collected and used by herbalists for its medicinal properties. It is very common on sunny banks and walls, and in dry pastures, and is well distinguished from all other British plants of the order, by its creeping scions or runners, which are thrown out in the same manner as in the strawberry, by its small rosettes of hairy, undivided leaves, greyish green above and hoary beneath, with a dense white coat of stellately branched hairs, and by its bright lemon-coloured flowers, which are borne singly on the almost leafless stems, which are only a few inches high. The flower-heads, which are about an inch in diameter, are composed of about fifty florets, the outer having a broad, purple stripe on the under side. They open daily at 8 a.m. and close about 2 p.m. The plant is in bloom from May to September.

The Mouse-ear differs from all other milky plants of this class, in its juice being less bitter and more astringent, and on account of this astringency, it was much employed as a medicine in the Middle Ages under the name of Auricula muris, from which the popular name is taken. It has sudorific, tonic and expectorant properties, and is considered a good remedy for whooping cough (for which, indeed, it has been regarded as a specific) and all affections of the lungs.

The infusion of the whole herb is employed, made by pouring 1 pint of boiling water on 1 OZ. of the dried herb. This is well sweetened with honey and taken in wine glassful doses. A fluid extract is also prepared, the dose being 1/2 to 1 drachm. The powdered leaves prove an excellent astringent in hemorrhage, both external and internal, a strong decoction being good for hemorrhoids, and the leaves boiled in milk are a good external application for the same purpose.

Drayton has written:

'To him that hath a flux, of Shepherd's Purse he gives,
And Mouse-ear unto him whom some sharp rupture grieves.'

The name 'Mouse-ear' is also applied to 'Mouse-ear Chickweed,' a plant of the genus Cerastium, to a plant of the genus Myosotis, valued for its medicinal properties, and to various kinds of Woundworts.

Culpepper gives many uses for Mouse-ear Hawkweed. He tells us that:

'The juice taken in wine, or the decoction drunk, cures the jaundice, though of long continuance, to drink thereof morning and evening, and abstain from other drink two or three hours after. It is a special remedy for the stone and the tormenting pains thereof; and griping pains in the bowels. The decoction with Succory and Centaury is very effectual in dropsy and the diseases of the spleen. It stayeth fluxes of blood at the mouth or nose, and inward bleeding also, for it is a singular wound herb for wounds both inward and outward.... There is a syrup made of the juice and sugar by the apothecaries of Italy, which is highly esteemed and given to those that have a cough, and in phthisis, and for ruptures and burstings. The green herb bruised and bound to any cut or wound doth quickly close the lips thereof, and the decoction or powder of the dried herb wonderfully stays spreading and fretting cankers in the mouth and other parts. The distilled water of the plant is applicable for the diseases aforesaid and apply tents of cloths wet therein.'

The herb is collected in May and June, when in flower and is dried.

Parkinson states that if 'Mouseare' be given to any horse it 'will cause that he shall not be hurt by the smith that shooeth him.' Also that skilful shepherds are careful not to let their flocks feed in pastures where mouseare abounds 'lest they grow sicke and leane and die quickly after.'

HAWTHORN

Botanical: Crataegus oxyacantha (LINN.)
Family: N.O. Rosaceae
Synonyms: May. Mayblossom. Quick. Thorn. Whitethorn. Haw. Hazels. Gazels. Halves. Hagthorn. Ladies' Meat. Bread and Cheese Tree.
Part Used: Dried haws or fruits.
Habitat: Europe, North Africa, Western Asia.

Description

The Hawthorn is the badge of the Ogilvies and gets one of its commonest popular names from blooming in May. Many country villagers believe that Hawthorn flowers still bear the smell of the Great Plague of London. The tree was formerly regarded as sacred, probably from a tradition that it furnished the Crown of Thorns. The device of a Hawthorn bush was chosen by Henry VII because a small crown from the helmet of Richard III was discovered hanging on it after the battle of Bosworth, hence the saying, 'Cleve to thy Crown though it hangs on a bush.' The Hawthorn is called Crataegus Oxyacantha from the Greek kratos, meaning hardness (of the wood), oxcus (sharp), and akantha (a thorn). The German name of Hagedorn, meaning Hedgethorn, shows that from a very early period the Germans divided their land into plots by hedges; the word haw is also an old word for hedge. The name Whitethorn arises from the whiteness of its bark and Quickset from its growing as a quick or living hedge, in contrast to a paling of dead wood.

This familiar tree will attain a height of 30 feet and lives to a great age. It possesses a single seed-vessel to each blossom producing a separate fruit, which when ripe is a brilliant red and this is in miniature a stony apple. In some districts these mealy red fruits are called Pixie Pears, Cuckoo's Beads and Chucky Cheese. The flowers are mostly fertilized by carrion insects, the suggestion of decomposition in the perfume attracts those insects that lay their eggs and hatch out their larvae in decaying animal matter.

Constituents

In common with other members of the Prunus and Pyrus groups of theorder Rosaceae, the Hawthorn contains Amyddalin. The bark contains the alkaloid Crataegin, isolated in greyish-white crystals, bitter in taste, soluble in water, with difficulty in alcohol and not at all in ether.

Medicinal Action and Uses

Cardiac, diuretic, astringent, tonic. Mainly used as a cardiac tonic in organic and functional heart troubles. Both flowers and berries are astringent and useful in decoction to cure sore throats. A useful diuretic in dropsy and kidney troubles.

Preparation and dosage

Fluid Extract of Berries, 10 to 15 drops.

The leaves have been used as an adulterant for tea. An excellent liquer is made from Hawthorn berries with brandy.

Formerly the timber, when of sufficient size, was used for making small articles. The root-wood was also used for making boxes and combs; the wood has a fine grain and takes a beautiful polish. It makes excellent fuel, making the hottest wood-fire known and used to be considered more desirable than Oak for oven-heating. Charcoal made from it has been said to melt pig-iron without the aid of a blast.

The stock is employed not only for grafting varieties of its own species, but also for several of the garden fruits closely allied to it, such as the medlar and pear.

Other Species

C. Aronia is a bushy species giving larger fleshy fruit than C. Oxyacantha. It is indigenous to Southern Europe and Western Asia and is common about Jerusalem and the Mount of Olives, where its fruit is used for preserves.

C. odoratissima is very agreeable also as a fruit.

C. Azarole. Its fruit in the same way is highly esteemed in Southern Europe.

HEARTSEASE

Botanical: Viola tricolor (LINN.)
Family: N.O. Violaceae
Synonyms: Wild Pansy. Love-Lies-Bleeding. Love-in-Idleness. Live-in-Idleness. Loving Idol. Love Idol. Cull Me. Cuddle Me. Call-me-to-you. Jackjump-up-and-kiss-me. Meet-me-in-the-Entry. Kiss-her-in-the-Buttery. Three-Faces-under-a-Hood. Kit-run-in-the-Fields. Pink-o'-the-Eye. Kit-run-about. Godfathers and Godmothers. Stepmother. Herb Trinitatis. Herb Constancy. Pink-eyed-John. Bouncing Bet. Flower o'luce. Bird's Eye. Bullweed.
Part Used: Herb.

HABITAT

The Heartsease, or Wild Pansy, very different in habit from any other kind of Viola, is abundantly met with almost throughout Britain. Though found on hedgebanks and waste ground, it seems in an especial degree a weed of cultivation, found most freely in cornfields and garden ground. It blossoms almost throughout the entire floral season, expanding its attractive little flowers in the early days of summer and keeping up a succession of blossom until late in autumn.

DESCRIPTION

The Heartsease is as variable as any of the other members of the genus, but whatever modifications of form it may present, it may always be readily distinguished from the other Violets by the general form of its foliage, which is much more cut up than in any of the other species and by the very large leafy stipules at the base of the true leaves. The stem, too, branches more than is commonly found in the other members of the genus. Besides the free branching of the stem, which is mostly 4 to 8 inches in height, it is generally very angular. The leaves are deeply cut into rounded lobes, the terminal one being considerably the largest. In the other species of Viola the foliage is ordinarily very simple in outline, heartshaped, or kidney-shaped, having its edge finely toothed.

The flowers (1/4 to 1 1/4 inch across) vary a great deal in color and size, but are either purple, yellow or white, and most commonly there is a combination of all these colors in each blossom. The upper petals are generally most showy in color and purple in tint, while the lowest and broadest petal is usually a more or less deep tint of yellow. The base of the lowest petal is elongated into a spur, as in the Violet.

The flowers are in due course succeeded by the little capsules of seeds, which when ripe, open by three valves. Though a near relative of the Violet, it does not produce any of the curious bud-like flowers - cleistogamous flowers - characteristic of the Violet, as its ordinary showy flowers manage to come to fruition so that there is no necessity for any others. Darwin found that the humble bee was the commonest insect visitor of the Heartsease, though the moth Pluvia visited it largely - another observer mentions Thrips small wingless insects - as frequent visitors to the flowers. Darwin considered that the cultivated Pansy rarely set seed if there were no insect visitors, but that the little Field Pansy can certainly fertilize itself if necessary.

The flower protects itself from rain and dew by drooping its head both at night and in wet weather, and thus the back of the flower and not its face receives the moisture.

The wild species is an annual, but from it the countless varieties of the perennial garden pansies, with blossoms of large size and singular beauty, are supposed to have originated. It is a very widely distributed plant, found not only throughout Britain, but in such diverse places as Arctic Europe, North Africa, Siberia and N.W. India. Several of the varieties have been distinguished as subspecies: the most marked of these are V. arvensis, most common in cornfields, with white or yellowish flowers, with spreading petals; and lutea, which has a branched rootstock, short stems, with underground runners, and blue, purple or yellow flowers with spreading petals much longer than the sepals.

Miss Martineau tells us that many kinds are common in meadows in America, and says that as early as February the fields about Washington are quite gay with their flowers.

The Pansy is one of the oldest favorites in the English garden and the affection for it is shown in the many names that were given it. The Anglo-Saxon name was Banwort or Bonewort.

Miss Rohde is of opinion that Banwort was the old name for the daisy.

She says: 'It would be interesting to know if the daisy is still called banwurt in the north,' and she quotes from Turner's Herbal in support of this, 'The Northern men call thys herbe banwurt because it helpeth bones to knyt againe....'

Its common name of Pansy (older form 'Pawnce,'

as in Spenser) is derived from the French pensées, the name which is still used in France.

'Love in Idleness' is still in use in Warwickshire. In ancient days the plant was much used for its potency in love charms, hence perhaps its name of Heartsease. It is this flower that plays such an important part as a love-charm in the Midsummer Night's Dream.

The celebrated Quesnay, founder of the 'Economists,' physician to Louis XV, was called by the king his 'thinker,' and given, as an armorial bearing, three pansy flowers.

In many old Herbals the plant is called Herba Trinitatis, being dedicated by old writers to the Trinity, because it has in each flower three colors.

Stepmother is a familiar name for it in both France and Germany, from a fanciful reference to the different-shaped petals, supposed to represent a stepmother, her own daughters and her stepchildren.

Part Used Medicinally and Preparation for Market

The whole herb, collected in the wild state and dried.

The Wild Pansy may be collected any time from June to August, when the foliage is in the best condition.

Constituents

The herb contains an active chemical principle, Violine (a substance similar to Emetin, having an emeto-cathartic action), mucilage, resin, sugar, salicylic acid and a bitter principle. When bruised, the plant, and especially the root, smells like peach kernels or prussic acid. The seeds are considered to have the same therapeutic activity as the leaves and flowers.

Medicinal Action and Uses

The Pansy has very similar properties to the Violet.

It was formerly in much repute as a remedy for epilepsy, asthma and numerous other complaints, and the flowers were considered cordial and good in diseases of the heart, from which may have arisen its popular name of Heartsease as much as from belief in it as a love potion.

Gerard states:

'It is good as the later physicians write for such as are sick of ague, especially children and infants, whose convulsions and fits of the falling sickness it is thought to cure. It is commended against inflammation of the lungs and chest, and against scabs and itchings of the whole body and healeth ulcers.'

A strong decoction of syrup of the herb and flowers was recommended by the older herbalists for skin diseases and a homeopathic medicinal tincture is still made from it with spirits of wine, using the entire plant, and given in small diluted doses for the cure of cutaneous eruptions.

It was formerly official in the United States Pharmacopoeia, and is still employed in America in the form of an ointment and poultice in eczema and other skin troubles, and internally for bronchitis.

Some years ago attention was called to this herb by a writer in the Medical Journal as a valuable remedy for the cutaneous disorder called crusta lactes, or Scald head, in children. For this purpose, 1/2 drachm of dried leaves, or a handful of the fresh herb boiled in milk, was recommended to be given every morning and evening: poultices formed of the leaves were likewise applied with success. By several medical writers its use is said to have proved very efficacious in this complaint.

On the Continent, the herbaceous parts of the plant have been employed for their mucilaginous, demulcent and expectorant properties. The root and seeds are also emetic and purgative, which properties as well as the expectorant action of the plant are doubtless due to the presence of the violine.

Pansy leaves are used on the Continent in place of litmus in acid and alkali tests.

HELIOTROPE

Botanical: Heliotropium Peruviana
Family: N.O. Heliotropeae
Synonyms: Turnsole. Cherry Pie.

A sweet-scented plant which is called Heliotrope because it follows the course of the sun. After opening it gradually turns from the east to the west and during the night turns again to the east to meet the rising sun. The Ancients recognized this characteristic of the plant and applied it to mythology.

Medicinal Action and Uses

In homeopathic medicine a tincture of the whole fresh plant is used for clergyman's sore throat and uterine displacement.

HELLEBORE, BLACK

POISON
Botanical: Helleborus niger (LINN.)
Family: N.O. Ranunculaceae
Synonyms: Christe Herbe. Christmas Rose. Melampode.
Parts Used: Rhizome, root.

Habitat

It is a native of the mountainous regions of Central and Southern Europe, Greece and Asia Minor, and is cultivated largely in this country as a garden plant. Supplies of the dried rhizome, from which the drug is prepared, have hitherto come principally from Germany.

Two allied species are natives of this country, but this particular kind does not grow wild here.

The Black Hellebore - once known as Melampode - is a perennial, low-growing plant, with dark, shining, smooth leaves and flower-stalks rising directly from the root, its pure white blossoms appearing in the depth of winter and thereby earning for it the favorite name of Christmas Rose.

The generic name of this plant is derived from the Greek elein (to injure) and bora (food), and indicates its poisonous nature. The specific name refers to the darkcoloured rootstock.

The Black Hellebore used by the Greeks has been identified by Dr. Sibthorp as Helleborus officinalis, a handsome plant, with a branching stem, bearing numerous serrated bracts, and three to five whitish flowers. It is a native of Greece, Asia Minor, etc.

The two species found wild in many parts of England, especially on a limestone soil, are H. Foetidus, the Bearsfoot, and H. Viridis, the Green Hellebore; the latter has injurious effects on cattle if eaten by them.

Both these British species possess powerful medicinal effects and are at times substituted for the true H. niger.

History

According to Pliny, Black Hellebore was used as a purgative in mania byMelampus, a soothsayer and physician, 1,400 years before Christ, hence the name Melampodium applied to Hellebores. Spenser in the Shepheard's Calendar, 1579, alludes to the medicinal use of Melampode for animals. Parkinson, writing in 1641, tells us:

'a piece of the root being drawne through a hole made in the eare of a beast troubled with cough or having taken any poisonous thing cureth it, if it be taken out the next day at the same houre.'

Parkinson believed that White Hellebore would be equally efficacious in such a case, but Gerard recommends the Black Horehound only, as being good for beasts. He says the old farriers used to 'cut a slit in the dewlap, and put in a bit of Beare-foot, and leave it there for daies together.'

Gerard describes the plant in these words:

'It floureth about Christmas, if the winter be mild and warm . . . called Christ herbe. This plant hath thick and fat leaves of a deep green color, the upper part whereof is somewhat bluntly nicked or toothed, having sundry diversions or cuts, in some leaves many, in others fewer, like unto a female Peony. It beareth rose-coloured flowers upon slender stems, growing immediately out of the ground, an handbreadth high, sometimes very white, and ofttimes mixed with a little shew of purple, which being faded, there succeed small husks full of black seeds; the roots are many; with long, black strings coming from one end.'

Once, people blessed their cattle with this plant to keep them from evil spells, and for this purpose, it was dug up with certain mystic rites. In an old French romance, the sorcerer, to make himself invisible when passing through the enemy's camp, scatters powdered Hellebore in the air, as he goes.

The following is from Burton's Anatomy of Melancholy:

'Borage and hellebore fill two scenes,
Sovereign plants to purge the veins
Of melancholy, and cheer the heart
Of those black fumes which make it smart.'

Cultivation

All kinds of Hellebore will thrive in ordinary garden soil, but for some kinds prepared soil is preferable, consisting of equal parts of good fibry loam and welldecomposed manure, half fibry peat and half coarse sand. Thorough drainage is necessary, as stagnant moisture is very injurious. It prefers a moist, sheltered situation, with partial shade, such as the margins of shrubberies. If the soil is well trenched and manured, Hellebore will not require replanting for at least seven years, if grown for flowering, but a top dressing of well-decayed manure and a little liquid manure might be given during the growing season, when plants are making their foliage. Propagation is by seeds, or division of roots. Seedlings should be pricked off thickly into a shady border, in a light, rich soil. The second year they should be transplanted to permanent quarters, and will bloom in the third year. For division of roots, the plant is strongest in July, and the clumps to be divided must be well established, with rootstocks large enough to cut. The plants will be good flowering plants in two years, but four years are required to bring them to perfection.

Part Used

The rhizome, collected in autumn and dried.

The root has a slight odor, when cut or broken, somewhat resembling Senega root. The dry powder causes violent sneezing. It has a somewhat bittersweet and acrid taste.

Constituents

Two crystalline glucosides, Helleborin and helleborcin, both powerful poisons. Helleborin has a burning, acrid taste and is narcotic, helleborcin has a sweetish taste and is a highly active cardiac poison, similar in its effects to digitalis and a drastic purgative. Other constituents are resin, fat and starch. No tannin is present.

Medicinal Action and Uses

The drug possesses drastic purgative, emmenagogue and anthelmintic properties, but is violently narcotic. It was formerly much used in dropsy and amenorrhoea, and has proved of value in nervous disorders and hysteria. It is used in the form of a tincture, and must be administered with great care.

Applied locally, the fresh root is violently irritant.

Preparations and Dosages

Fluid extract, 2 to 10 drops. Solid extract, 1 to 2 grains. Powdered root, 10 to 20 grains as a drastic purge, 2 to 3 grains as an alterative. Decoction, 2 drachms to the pint, a fluid ounce every four hours till effective.

A tincture of the fresh root of H. foetidus is used in homeopathy.

HELLEBORE, FALSE

POISON
Botanical: Adonis autumnalis, Adonis vernalis
Family: N.O. Ranunculaceae
Synonyms: Red Chamomile. Pheasant's Eye. Adonis. Red Morocco. Rose-a-rubie. Red Mathes. Sweet Vernal.
Part Used: Herb.

The Pheasant's Eye (Adonis autumnalis), a plant very nearly allied to the Anemone, is sometimes found wild in England, mostly in cornfields in Kent, but is often regarded as a mere garden escape. Though generally only a cultivated species in this country, it is common enough on the Continent.

It is a graceful plant, growing about a foot high, with finely cut leaves and terminal flowers like small scarlet buttercups.

History

Its Latin name is derived from the ill-fated Adonis, from whose blood it sprang, according to the Greek legends. 'Red Morocco' was a somewhat strange old English name for this plant, also 'Rose-a-rubie' and 'Red Mathes,' 'by which name,' says Gerard, 'it is called of them that dwell where it groweth naturally and generally red camomill' - the latter on account of the finely-cut leaves. It is now aptly called Pheasant's Eye, on account of its brilliant little scarlet and black blossoms.

Although named A. autumnalis, it blossoms throughout the summer, commencing to flower in June, and the seeds ripen in August and September. It is an annual, propagated by its seeds, which may be sown at almost any season, but should always be sown where the plant is to grow, because it does not bear transplanting. Any soil will suit it: it blossoms more freely in the sunshine, but willalso flourish in shade.

In olden days it was considered to have some medicinal value, but is no longer used. Its near relative, A. vernalis (or 'Ox-eye'), though not officinal, is still regarded of medicinal value, and is a perennial species, not a native of this country, but common in central Europe, where its root is often used in the place of Black Hellebore.

'A. vernalis is one of the brightest and most effective of spring plants, known in many places as Sweet Vernal. It might be said of this, as of the Daffodil, that it "takes the winds of March with beauty," for often before the month is out it opens its rich, golden Anemone-like cups to the sun, and when planted in profusion, presents a glowing mass of color. The plant is only about 9 inches high, and its foliage is one of its beauties. It makes a good addition to the rockery. Another species, A. amurensis, which is among the earliest of all the flowers, for it comes into bloom in February and March, is rather taller, and the foliage is more finely cut. There is a double variety, flore pleno, with large, yellow flowers. These plants will grow in any good garden soil, well drained and not too heavy. They should have a sunny position, but should not be allowed to suffer from drought during summer. They are quite hardy, and if left undisturbed improve from year to year.'

Constituents

A. vernalis contains a glucoside Adonidin and has an action almost exactly like that of digitalin, but is much stronger and is said not to be cumulative. It appears to be about ten times as powerful as digitoxin. It has been prescribed instead of digitalis, and sometimes succeeds where digitalis fails, especially where there is kidney disease. It is, however, less certainly beneficial in valvular disease than digitalis, and should be used only where digitalis fails. It produces vomiting and diarrhrea more readily than digitalis. It is given in the form of an infusion.

Preparations and Dosages

Fluid extract, 1 to 2 drops. Glucoside adonidin, 1/4 to 1/2 grain.

The infusion is made with 1/4 oz. of the herb to a pint of boiling water and given in tablespoonful doses every three hours.

HELLEBORE, GREEN

POISON
Botanical: Veratrum viride
Family: N.O. Melanthaceae or Liliaceae
Synonyms: American Hellebore. Swamp Hellebore. Indian Poke. Itch-weed.
Parts Used: Dried rhizome and roots.
Habitat: Swamps, low grounds, and moist meadows of the United States.

Description

For commercial convenience, the roots are usually broken into small pieces or fragments, but are sometimes sliced, the cut surface being of a dingy white color, or whole, the outside dark brown, with characteristic markings. Often, portions of the dried stem or leafstalks remain attached, and these, being inert, should be rejected.

American Hellebore closely resembles the German Veratrum album, or White Hellebore, and the Mexican V. officinale, or Sabadilla (Cevadilla), N.O. Liliaceae. The name Veratrine is given to the mixture of bases obtained from Sabadilla by extracting with alcohol, distilling off the alcohol, and precipitating the mixed bases with ammonia. Official in the Pharmacopoeia of 1898. The British Pharmacopoeia Codex preparation is Oleinatum Veratrinae.

Constituents

It has been found that the alkaloids contained in V. viride are not the same as the veratrine contained in V. album and the seeds of Sabadilla. The principal alkaloids are Pseudojervine, Rubijervine, Jervine, Cevadine, Protoveratrine, and Protoveratridine. The last is probably a decomposition product, it is highly poisonous, and sternutatory. Starch and resin are also present.

Medicinal Action and Uses

Emetic, diaphoretic, sedative, highly poisonous. The German White Hellebore, resembling the American, but without its cevadine, is rarely given internally, but the powder has been used in preparing an ointment for itch.

Veratrine, a pale grey amorphous powder, is used externally as an analgesic, and also as a parasiticide. It is not known to affect the living blood but when the latter is drawn, veratrine kills the white corpuscles. Violent pain and irritation are caused if it is given internally or subcutaneously. It prolongs the contractions of heart and muscles. Its only justifiable use is as an anodyne counter irritant, especially for neuralgia. It was emphatically decided a few years ago that V. viride should whenever possible be used instead of the European V. album, which is more likely to upset the intestines. The various alkaloids present act in very different manners, and none in exactly the same way as the whole drug - jervine, for example, is less poisonous than the drug itself, while protoveratrine, although present in small quantity, is extremely toxic.

A moderate dose of veratrum produces a reduction in the rate of the pulse, with a fall in the arterial pressure. There may be slowing of respiration. It has been used in the treatment of pneumonia, peritonitis, and other sthenic fevers, but is chiefly useful in chronic diseases, such as arterio-sclerosis and interstitial nephritis. It differs from digitalis in that it diminishes cardiac tone, and has been used for threatened apoplexy and 'irritable heart'; also for puerperal eclampsia.

Sabadilla is the principal ingredient of the pulvis capocinorum, sometimes used in Europe for the destruction of vermin in the hair.

Dosages

V. viride, from 1 to 3 minims of the fluid extract every two or three hours until pulse rate is reduced. 1 to 2 grains. Of U.S. tincture, 10 to 30 minims.

V. album, 1 to 2 grains in powder. Rarely given internally.

Veratrine, 1/30 grain.

Poisons, if any, and Antidotes

Causes vomiting, with much nausea and retching. Pulse slow, later, rapid and irregular. Prostration, perspiration, pallor, with shallow and sometimes stertorous breathing.

If there is vomiting, two glasses of water should be given and 20 grains of tannic acid as an imperfect chemical antidote. Should vomiting not occur, it must be provoked, or a stomach pump employed. The patient must be kept in a horizontal position, not even being allowed to sit up to vomit. To stop the vomiting a counter-irritant must be used over the epigastrium and morphine employed very cautiously. In the early stages, when the pulse is low, atropine is very valuable, or active respiratory stimulants, such as hypodermic injections of ammonia and strychnine. If the bodily temperature is low, heat can be applied externally.

HELLEBORE, WHITE

POISON
Botanical: Veratrum album
Family: N.O. Lilaceae
Synonyms: Veratrum Lobelianium. Veratrum Californicum. Weiszer Germer. Weisze Nieszwurzel.
Parts Used: Rhizome, root.
Habitat: Europe, from Lapland to Italy. Does not occur in the British Isles.

Description

Veratrum album closely resembles the American species, but is distinguished by its yellowish-white flower.

The fresh rhizome has an alliaceous odor, but when dried it has no marked smell. Its taste is first sweet, then bitter and acrid, leaving the tongue tingling and numb. Its powder is ash-coloured. White Hellebore deteriorates by keeping. It is scarcely ever used internally owing to the severity of its action. It is stated to have been one of the principal poisons used in Europe for arrows, daggers, etc.

Constituents

Authorities differ as to the presence or absence of the veratria of cevadilla. It contains jervine, pseudo-jer-vine, rubijervine, veratralbine and veratrine. Cevadine is stated to be absent. There is fatty matter, composed of olein, stearin and a volatile acid, supergallate of Veratia, yellow colouring matter, starch ligneous matter, and gum; the ashes contain much phosphate and carbonate of lime, carbonate of potassa and some traces of silica, and sulphate of lime. There has been found in it a white, crystalline, fusible and inflammable substance called barytin, of which the properties have not been thoroughly investigated.

Medicinal Action and Uses

A violent, irritant poison. When snuffed up the nose it occasions profuse running of the nose; when swallowed, severe vomiting and profuse diarrhea. It was formerly used in cerebral affections, such as mania, epilepsy, etc., and for gout, as a substitute for colchicum or the Eau Mediciale of Husson, when 3 parts of the wine of White Hellebore added to 1 part of laudanum was given in doses of from 1/2 fluid drachm to 2 fluid drachms.

It is occasionally used in the form of an ointment or decoction in obstinate skin diseases such as scabies, or to kill lice, but even this use is not free from danger. It is also occasionally used as an errhine or sternutatory, diluted with starch or other mild powder, in cases of amaurosis and chronic affections of the brain.

The principal use of the plant is in veterinary medicine.

Dosages

Of the powder, 1 to 8 grains, gradually and cautiously increased, commencing with 1 grain. Of the vinous tincture, from 20 to 60 minims.

Poisons, if any, and Antidotes

Narcotic symptoms, such as stupor and convulsions, appear in addition to vomiting and diarrhea, when the dose is fatal. The poison may be treated by drinks and injections of coffee, stimulants to overcome the depressed condition of the heart and arteries, and opiates and demulcents to relieve internal inflammation.

Other Species

Helleborus orientalis (Lam.). A tincture ofthe root is used in homeopathy for indigestion and diarrhea.

HEMLOCK

POISON
Botanical: Conium maculatum (LINN.)
Family: N.O. Umbelliferae
Synonyms: Herb Bennet. Spotted Corobane. Musquash Root. Beaver Poison. Poison Hemlock. Poison Parsley. Spotted Hemlock. Kex. Kecksies.
Parts Used: Leaves, fruit, seeds.

Habitat

It is by no means an uncommon plant in this country, found on hedgebanks, in neglected meadows, on waste ground and by the borders of streams in most parts of England, occurring in similar places throughout Europe (except the extreme north) and also in temperate Asia and North Africa. It has been introduced into North and South America.

The Hemlock is a member of the great order Umbelliferae, the same family of plants to which the parsley, fennel, parsnip and carrot belong.

Many of the umbelliferous plants abound in an acrid, watery juice, which is more or less narcotic in its effects on the animal frame, and which, therefore, when properly administered in minute doses, is a valuable medicine. Among these the most important is Conium, or Hemlock. Every part of this plant, especially the fresh leaves and fruit, contains a volatile, oily alkaloid, which is so poisonous that a few drops prove fatal to a small animal.

History

The Ancients were familiar with the plant, which is mentioned in early Greek literature, and fully recognized its poisonous nature. The juice of hemlock was frequently administered to criminals, and this was the fatal poison which Socrates was condemned to drink.

The old Roman name of Conium was Cicuta, which prevails in the mediaeval Latin literature, but was applied about 1541 by Gesner and others to another umbelliferous plant, Cicuta virosa, the Water Hemlock, which does not grow in Greece and southern Europe. To avoid the confusion arising from the same name for these quite dissimilar plants, Linnaeus, in 1737, restored the classical Greek name and called the Hemlock (Conium maculatum), the generic name being derived from the Greek word Konas, meaning to whirl about, because the plant, when eaten, causes vertigo and death. The specific name is the Latin word, meaning 'spotted,' and refers to the stem-markings. According to an old English legend, these purple streaks on the stem represent the brand put on Cain's brow after he had committed murder.

Hemlock was used in Anglo-Saxon medicine, and is mentioned as early as the tenth century. The name Hemlock is derived from the Anglo-Saxon words hem (border, shore) and leác (leek or plant). Another authority derives the British name 'hemlock' from the Anglo-Saxon word healm (straw), from which the word 'haulm' is derived.

The use of Hemlock in modern medicine is due chiefly to the recommendation of Storch, of Vienna, since when (1760) the plant has been much employed, though it has lost some of its reputation owing to the uncertain action of the preparations made from it.

Description

Hemlock is a tall, much branched and gracefully growing plant, with elegantly-cut foliage and white flowers. Country people very generally call by the name of Hemlock many species of umbelliferous plants, but the real Hemlock may be distinguished by its slender growth, perfectly smooth stem which is marked with red, and its finely-divided leaves which are also smooth.

It is a biennial plant, usually growing from 2 to 4 feet high, but in sheltered situations sometimes attaining nearly double that height. The root is long, forked, pale yellow and 1/2 to 3/4 inch in diameter. The erect, smooth stem, stout below, much branched above and hollow, is bright green, but (as already stated) is distinctively mottled with small irregular stains or spots of a port-wine color and also covered with a white 'bloom' which is very easily rubbed off.

The leaves are numerous, those of the first year and the lower ones very large, even reaching 2 feet in length, alternate, longstalked, tripinnate (divided along the midrib into opposite pairs of leaflets and these again divided and subdivided in similar manner). The upper leaves are much smaller, nearly stalkless, with the short footstalk dilated and stem-clasping, often opposite or three together, more oblong in outline, dipinnate or pinnate, quite smooth, uniform dull green, segments toothed, each tooth being tipped with a minute, sharp white point.

The umbels are rather small, 1 1/4 to 2 inches broad, numerous, terminal, on rather short flower stalks, with 12 to 16 rays to the umbel. At the base of the main umbel there are 4 to 8 lance-shaped, deflexed bracts; at the base of the small umbels there are three or four spreading bractlets. The flowers are small, their petals white with an inflexed point, the stamens a little longer than the petals, with white anthers.

The fruit is small, about 1/8 inch long broad, ridged, compressed laterally and smooth. Both flowers and fruit bear a resemblance to caraway, but the prominent crenate (wavy) ridges and absence of vittae (oil cells between the ridges) are important characters for distinguishing this fruit from others of the same natural order of plants.

The entire plant has a bitter taste and possesses a disagreeable mousy odor, which is especially noticeable when bruised. When dry, the odor is still disagreeable, but not so pronounced as in the fresh plant. The seeds or fruits have very marked odor or taste, but when rubbed with a solution of potassium bi-oxide, the same disagreeable mouse-like odor is produced.

The poisonous property occurs in all parts of the plant, though it is stated to be less strong in the root. Poisoning has occurred from eating the leaves for parsley, the roots for parsnips and the seeds in mistake for anise seeds. Many children, too, have suffered by using whistles made from the hollow stems of the Hemlock, which should be extirpated from meadows and pastures since many domestic animals have been killed by eating it, though goats are said to eat it with impunity.

Parts Used, Harvesting and Drying

The leaves and fruit. The fresh green Hemlock is employed in the preparation of Juice of Conium, Conium Ointment, and the green Extract of Conium.

The British pharmacopoeia directs that the leaves and young branches should be gathered from wild British plants when the flowers are fully matured, and the fruits are just beginning to form, as they then possess their greatest medicinal activity. This is about the end of June. The smaller leaves are selected and the larger stalks picked out and discarded.

The leaves separated from the branches and dried are also official.

The dried ripe fruit is official in the British Pharmacopceia, and the Pharmacopceia of India, but in the Pharmacopceia of the United States the full-grown fruit, gathered before it turns from green to yellow and carefully dried, is directed to be used.

Hemlock fruits were introduced into British medicine in 1864 as a substitute for the dried leaf in making the tincture, but it has been shown that a tincture, whether of leaf or fruit, is far inferior to the preserved juice of the herb.

Constituents

By far the most important constituent of hemlock leaves is the alkaloid Coniine, of which they may contain, when collected at the proper time, as much as 2.77 per cent the average being 1.65 per cent. When pure, Coniine is a volatile, colourless, oily liquid, strongly alkaline, with poisonous properties and having a bitter taste and a disagreeable, penetrating, mouse-like odor.

There are also present the alkaloids, Methyl-coniine, Conhydrine, Pseudoconhydrine, Ethyl piperidine, mucilage, a fixed oil and 12 per cent of ash.

Hemlock fruits have essentially the same active constituents, but yield a greater portion of Coniine than the leaves.

Medicinal Action and Uses

As a medicine, Conium is sedative and antispasmodic, and in sufficient doses acts as a paralyser to the centres of motion. In its action it is, therefore, directly antagonistic to that of Strychnine, and hence it has been recommended as an antidote to Strychnine poisoning, and in other poisons of the same class, and in tetanus, hydrophobia, etc. (In mediaeval days, Hemlock mixed with betony and fennel seed was considered a cure for the bite of a mad dog.)

On account of its peculiar sedative action on the motor centres, Hemlock juice (Succus conii) is prescribed as a remedy in cases of undue nervous motor excitability, such as teething in children, epilepsy from dentition. cramp, in the early stages of paralysis agitans, in spasms of the larynx and gullet, in acute mania, etc. As an inhalation it is said to relieve cough in bronchitis, whooping-cough, asthma, etc.

The drug has to be administered with care, as narcotic poisoning may result from internal use, and overdoses produce paralysis. In poisonous doses it produces complete paralysis with loss of speech, the respiratory function is at first depressed and ultimately ceases altogether and death results from asphyxia. The mind remains unaffected to the last. In the account of the death of Socrates, reference is made to loss of sensation as one of the prominent symptoms of his poisoning, but the dominant action is on the motor system. It is placed in Table II of the Poison Schedule.

Hemlock was formerly believed to exercise an alterative effect in scrofulous disorders. Both the Greek and Arabian physicians were in the practice of using it for the cure of indolent tumours, swellings and pains of the joints, as well as for affections of the skin. Among the moderns Baron Storch was the first to call the attention of medical men to its use, both externally and internally, for the cure of cancerous and other ulcers, and in the form of a poultice or ointment it has been found a very valuable application to relieve pain in these cases.

In the case of poisoning by Hemlock, the antidotes are tannic acid, stimulants and coffee, emetics of zinc, or mustard and castor oil, and, if necessary, artificial respiration. It is essential to keep up the temperature of the body.

Like many other poisonous plants, when cut and dried, Hemlock loses much of its poisonous properties, which are volatile and easily dissipated. Cooking destroys it.

Its disagreeable odor has prevented its fatal use as a vegetable in the raw state.

Larks and quails are said to eat Hemlock with impunity, but their flesh becomes so impregnated with the poison that they are poisonous as food. Thrushes eat the fruits with impunity, but ducks have been poisoned by them.

Coles' Art of Simpling:

'If Asses chance to feed much upon Hemlock, they will fall so fast asleep that they will seeme to be dead, in so much that some thinking them to be dead indeed have flayed off their skins, yet after the Hemlock had done operating they have stirred and wakened out of their sleep, to the griefe and amazement of the owners.'

Adulteration

Commercial Conium occasionally contains the leaves of other umbelliferous plants somewhat like it in appearance, or it may even be almost wholly composed of such plants. Anise has been used as an adulterant of the fruit.

Among umbelliferous plants most frequently mistaken for the true Hemlock Anthriscus sylvestris (Wild Chervil) an Æthusa Cynapium (Fool's Parsley) have similar general characteristics, but are readily distinguished. A. sylvestris has hairy, not smooth leaves, its fruit is elongated, not broad, and the bracts of the partial involucre (or involucels) are not directed outwards, as in the Hemlock. The stem also is unspotted.

Preparations and Dosages

Powdered leaves 1 to 3 grains. Fluid extract of leaves, 5 to 10 drops. Fluid extract of seeds, 2 to 5 drops. Tincture seeds, B.P., 1/2 to 1 drachm. Juice of leaves, B.P., 1 to 2 drachms. Solid extract, 2 to 6 grains. Ointment, B.P.

HEMLOCK, WATER

POISON
Botanical: Cicuta virosa
Family: N.O. Umbelliferae
Synonym: Cowbane.
Part Used: Root.

The leaves of the Water Hemlock are sometimes found admixed with those of Conium. This is a semiaquatic plant growing in ditches and on the banks of pools and rivers, though not very common in England. It has similar properties to the true Hemlock.

Description

Water Hemlock is a perennial, with a short, thick, vertical, hollow rootstock, in shape somewhat like a parsnip, giving off whorls of slender, fibrous roots. The erect, very stout, hollow stem, rising 2 to 4 feet high or more, is smooth, branched and slightly furrowed. The lower leaves are large, 1 to 2 feet long and long-stalked; they are tripinnate, like the Hemlock. The upper leaves are divided into three leaflets, and each again into three (twice ternate). The flowers are pure white, arranged in rather large, longstalked umbels of 12 to 16 long, slender, curved rays. There is no general involucre.

The Water Hemlock may be distinguished from the true Hemlock as follows: (i) The pinnae of the leaves are larger and lanceshaped; (ii) the umbel of the flowers is denser and more compact; (iii) the stem is not spotted like the true Hemlock; (iv) the odor of the plant resembles that of smallage or parsley.

Both plants are poisonous; but while the root of the Water Hemlock is acrid and powerfully poisonous in its fresh state, though it loses its virulent qualities when dried, that of the true Hemlock possesses little or no active power.

The Water Hemlock produces tetanic convulsions, and is fatal to cattle. In April, 1857, two farmer's sons were found lying paralysed and speechless close to a ditch where they had been working. Assistance was soon rendered, but they shortly expired. A quantity of the Water Hemlock grew in the ditch, where they had been employed. A piece of the root was subsequently found with the marks of teeth in it, near to where the men lay, and another piece of the same root was discovered in the pocket of one of them.

Constituents

A resinous body has been obtained from Cicuta virosa named Cicutoxin, an amorphous substance of acid reaction, of slight odor, but disagreeable taste; the dry root yields 3 to 5 per cent. The presence of a volatile alkaloid termed Cicutine has also been traced.

Other Species

AMERICAN COWBEAN

Botanical: Circuta maculata
Family: N.O. Umbelliferae

The American Cowbane is closely analogous to the European species, and also possesses very poisonous properties. In several instances, children have been fatally poisoned by eating its roots. It is said to be the most poisonous plant native to the United States.

Although it has been recommended as a remedy in nervous and sick headaches, it is very rarely used.

No complete analysis of the plant has been published, but the alkaloid termed Cicutine, present in the European species, is said to exist in it. The seed is stated to contain an alkaloid identical with Coniine.

The root of this American variety is even more virulent than the English one.

HEMP, CANADIAN

Botanical: Apocynum Cannabinum (LINN.), Apocynum Androsaemum
Family: N.O. Apocynaceae
Synonyms: Black Indian Hemp. Dogsbane.
Parts Used: Dried rhizome, roots.
Habitat: United States of America, Canada.

Description

This plant must not be confused with Indian Hemp (Cannabis Indica). Both species have a milky juice and a tough fibrous bark, which when macerated affords a substitute for hemp, hence its common name. It is used in California for making twine, bags, cordage, fishing-nets, lines, and a coarse kind of linen. When the milky juice is properly dried it exhibits the properties of india-rubber. The corolla of this plant secretes a sweet liquid, which attracts flies and other insects to settle on them; the scales in the throat of the corolla are very sensitive, and as soon as the insects settle on them, they bend inwards and make them prisoners. None of these plants possess any great beauty, all are more or less poisonous and acrid. In Apocynum Cannabinum, a perennial herb, the stems and branches are upright, headed by erect many-flowered stems, leaves nearly sessile; it grows in gravelly or sandy soil, mostly near streams. While A. Androsaemifolium, or Dogsbane, has spreading forked branches, leaves slender petioled cymes, loose and spreading, grows in dry thickets and open woods, and is distinguished from A. Cannabinum by the root, thick-walled stone cells which are arranged in a broken circle, near middle of the bark, short fracture, with some pith occurring in pieces of the rhizome, very slight odor, taste starchy, afterwards bitter and acrid.

Constituents

The activity of the plants is due to a very bitter principle of a glucose nature to which is applied the name of Symarin. Apocynum belongs to the digitalis group of heart tonics, and acts very much in the same way, differing only from foxglove in the relative degree of its different effects. It is the most powerful of the group, often causing sickness and diarrhrea; it acts more irritantly on the mucous membrane than either strophanthus, or digitalis, and it may be this stimulating effect which is the cause of its violent diuretic action, though some authorities consider that this is caused by dilatation of the renal arteries. A. Docynum is the crystalline lactone cynotoxin, the crystalline substance. Apocynin is identical with acetovanillone. A. Androsaemifolium contains apocyanamarin, identical with cynotoxin, also apocynin and its glucoside, androsin ipuranil; the two phytosterols androsterol and homo-androsterol, and other fatty acids.

Medicinal Action and Uses

Diuretic, diaphoretic, expectorant. Should only be prescribed with the greatest caution. It is a very valuable heart tonic of great service in dropsy resulting from heart failure; it is also to be highly recommended in the ascites of hepatic cirrhosis, but care must be taken that it does not accumulate in the system. It causes violent vomiting.

Dosage

1 to 5 grains.

Preparations

Fluid extract of Apocynum, U.S.P., 15 minims. Tincture of Apocynum, 5 to 10 minims.

Other Species

HEMP, AFRICAN, or Bowstring (Sanseviera guineenesis, N.O. Liliaceae), native of tropical Africa, also S. Roxburghiana, a native of India, and S. Angolensis, native of western tropical Africa. The leaves contain much fibre for making ropes, the latter producing the best kind of fibre for deep-sea soundings and dredging lines.

HEMP, KENTUCKY (Urtica Canadensis and Cannabina, N. O. Urticaceae), natives of Canada and Northern U.S. These also contain a strong fibre and are known by the name given above.

HEMP, MANILLA, the fibre of Musitextilis (N.O. Musaceae), native of the Philippines, cultivated in India, and other countries, for its fibre, of which there are two qualities, the finer made into shawls and the coarser into ropes.

HEMP, SUNN, the Indian name for the fibre of Crotalaria Juncea (N.O. Leguminosae), native of India; it gives a very strong fibre, useful for ropes, canvas, etc.

HEMP, JUBBULPORE (Crotalaria tenuifolia), The plant closely resembles Sunn Hemp (C. Juncea).

HEMP, INDIAN

POISON
Botanical: Cannabis sativa (LINN.)
Family: N.O. Urticaceae
Synonyms: Cannabis Indica. Cannabis Chinense. Ganeb. Ganja. Kif. Hanf. Tekrouri. Chanvre.
Part Used: The dried, flowering tops of the female, or pistillate plants.
Habitat: India.

Habitat. In Britain, and formerly elsewhere, only

Hemp grown in India was recognized as official, but the heavy tax has resulted in the admission by the United States of any active Cannabis sativa, whether grown in the States or in Africa, Turkey, Turkestan, Asia Minor, Italy, or Spain.

Description

The plant is an annual, the erect stems growing from 3 to 10 feet or more high, very slightly branched, having greyish-green hairs. The leaves are palmate, with five to seven leaflets (three on the upper leaves), numerous, on long thin petioles with acute stipules at the base, linear-lanceolate, tapering at both ends, the margins sharply serrate, smooth and dark green on the upper surface, lighter and downy on the under one. The small flowers are unisexual, the male having five almost separate, downy, pale yellowish segments, and the female a single, hairy, glandular, five-veined leaf enclosing the ovary in a sheath. The ovary is smooth, one-celled, with one hanging ovule and two long, hairy thread-like stigmas extending beyond the flower for more than its own length. The fruit is small, smooth, light brownish-grey in color, and completely filled by the seed.

Hemp grows naturally in Persia, Northern India and Southern Siberia, and probably in China. It is largely cultivated in Central and Southern Russia. It is sometimes found as a weed in England, probably due to seeds from birdcages, as they are much used in feeding tame birds. The drug that is official in Europe comes from Bogra and Rajshabi, north of Calcutta, or sometimes from Guzerat and Madras. It is called Guaza by London merchants.

It is imported in parcels of small masses, with flowers, smaller leaves and a few ripe fruits pressed together by sticky, resinous matter. It is rough, brittle, dull-green in color and almost tasteless, with a peculiar, slightly narcotic odor. It should be freed from resin by macerating in spirit and then soaking in water. The leaves are said to be picked off to form bhang, and the little shoots which follow these are used as above, and called ganja. It is exported from Bombay in wooden cases. Two-year-old ganja is almost inert, and the law requires it to be burnt in the presence of excise officers. In the Calcutta areas the short tops are rolled under foot instead of being trodden, the weight of the workers being supported by a horizontal bamboo pole. This variety is very active, and is usually re-exported from England to the West Indies.

Hemp is prepared in various forms. Ganja is smoked like tobacco. Bhang, sidhee, or subjee is the dried, larger leaves, broken or mixed with a few fruits. It is pounded with water to make a drink, and is the chief ingredient of the sweetmeat majun. Churrus or charas is the resin which exudes spontaneously from the leaves, tops and stems. A usual way of collecting it is for men in leathern garments to rush through the bushes, the resin being afterwards scraped off the clothes. In Nepal the plant is squeezed between the palms of the hands, and in Baluchistan the resin is separated by rubbing the dried plant carefully between carpets. This is the hashish, haschisch, or hashash of the Arabians, the word 'assassin' being said to be derived from it, owing to the wild, fanatical courage given by its use. In Persia the woollen carpets, after scraping, are washed with water, and the evaporated extract is sold cheaply. Another way is to collect the dust after stirring dry bhang, this impure form of resin being only used for smoking.

Flat cakes called hashish by the Russians are a preparation made from Hemp in Central Asia, and also called nasha.

In Thibet momea or mimea is said to be made with Hemp and human fat.

Many electuaries and pastes are made with butter or other oily foundation, such as majun of Calcutta, mapouchari of Cairo, and the dawames of the Arabs.

The madjound of the Algerians is a mixture of honey and hashish powder.

Hemp Fibre is best produced by the plants in cooler latitudes, the best being obtained from Italy, but much from Russia. About one and a half million hundredweight are imported annually for cordage, sacking, and sail-cloths.

A varnish is made from the pressed seeds.

Two or three green twigs collected in spring and placed in beds will drive bedbugs from the room.

Constituents

Cannabinone or Hemp resin is soluble in alcohol and ether. Cannabinol is separated from it. It is fawn-coloured, in thin layers, and burns with a clear, white flame, leaving no ash. This is the active principle. There is a small amount of ambercoloured volatile oil, one of the linseed-oil group. It has been resolved into a colourless liquid called cannabene, and a solid hydride of this.

It is said that a volatile alkaloid has been found in the tops, resembling nicotine. It also contains alcoholic extract, ash, and the alkaloid Choline.

Medicinal Action and Uses

The principal use of Hemp in medicine is for easing pain and inducing sleep, and for a soothing influence in nervous disorders. It does not cause constipation nor affect the appetite like opium. It is useful in neuralgia, gout, rheumatism, delirium tremens, insanity, infantile convulsions, insomnia, etc.

The tincture helps parturition, and is used in senile catarrh, gonorrhoea, menorrhagia, chronic cystitis and all painful urinary affections. An infusion of the seed is useful in after pains and prolapsus uteri. The resin may be combined with ointments, oils or chloroform in inflammatory and neuralgic complaints.

The drug deteriorates rapidly and hence is very variable, so that it is best given in ascending quantities to produce its effect. The deterioration is due to the oxidation of cannabinol and it should be kept in hermetically-sealed containers.

The action is almost entirely on the higher nerve centres. It can produce an exhilarating intoxication, with hallucinations, and is widely used in Eastern countries as an intoxicant, hence its names 'leaf of delusion,' 'increaser of pleasure,' 'cementer of friendship,' etc. The nature of its effect depends much on the nationality and temperament of the individual. It is regarded as dangerous to sleep in a field of hemp owing to the aroma of the plants.

Dosage

Tincture, B.P. and U.S.P., 5 to 15 drops. Solid extract, B.P., 1/4 to 1 grain. Fluid extract, 1 to 3 drops. Of cannabis, 1 to 3 grains. Of best hashish, for smoking, 1/4 to 1 grain. Of tincture, 10 to 30 minims. Of tincture for menorrhagia, 5 to 10 minims. three to four times a day (i.e. 24 grains of resinous extract in a fluid ounce of rectified spirit).

Of extract, from 1 to 20 grains, according to quality.

The following is stated to be a certain cure for gonorrhcea. Take equal parts of tops of male and female hemp in blossom. Bruise in a mortar, express the juice, and add an equal portion of alcohol. Take 1 to 3 drops every two to three hours.

SLANG NAMES FOR MARIJUANA:

Devil Drug, Weed of Madness, Cannabis, Assassin of Youth, Mexican Ditch Weed, Hashish, Hay, Chronic, Blunts, Pot, Brick Weed, Ganja, joint, Acapulco Gold, dime Bag, Rope, Grass, Weed, "L", Jive Stick, Nickel Bag, MaryJane, Loco, Boom, Bhang, Ganja, Indo, Hydro, Stick

HENBANE

POISON
Botanical: Hyoscyamus niger (LINN.)
Family: N.O. Solanaceae
Synonyms: Common Henbane. Hyoscyamus. Hog's-bean. Jupiter's-bean. Symphonica. Cassilata. Cassilago. Deus Caballinus.
Parts Used: Fresh leaves, flowering tops and branches, seeds.

Habitat

It is found throughout Central and Southern Europe and in Western Asia, extending to India and Siberia. As a weed of cultivation it now grows also in North America and Brazil. It had become naturalized in North America prior to 1672, as we find it mentioned in a work published in that year among the plants 'sprung up since the English planted and kept cattle in New England.'

It is not considered truly indigenous to Great Britain, but occurs fairly frequently in parts of Scotland, England and Wales, and also in Ireland, and has been found wild in sixty British counties, chiefly in waste, sandy places, by road-sides, on rubbish heaps and near old buildings, having probably first escaped from the old herb gardens. It is frequently found on chalky ground and particularly near the sea. It appears to have been more common in Gerard's time (Queen Elizabeth's reign) than it is now.

Henbane (Hyoscyamus niger, Linn.) is a member of the important order Solanaceae, to which belong the Potato, Tobacco and Tomato, and also the valuable Belladonna.

There are about eleven species of the genus Hyoscyamus, distributed from the Canary Islands over Europe and Northern Africa to Asia. All those which have been investigated contain similar principles and possess similar properties.

The medicinal uses of Henbane date from remote ages; it was well known to the Ancients, being particularly commended by Dioscorides (first century A.D.), who used it to procure sleep and allay pains, and Celsus (same period) and others made use of it for the same purpose, internally and externally, though Pliny declared it to be 'of the nature of wine and therefore offensive to the understanding.' There is mention of it in a work by Benedictus Crispus (A.D. 681) under the names of Hyoscyamus and Symphonica. In the tenth century, we again find its virtues recorded under the name of Jusquiasmus (the modern French name is Jusquiame). There is frequent mention made of it in AngloSaxon works on medicine of the eleventh century, in which it is named 'Henbell,' and in the old glossaries of those days it also appears as Caniculata, Cassilago and Deus Caballinus.

Later it fell into disuse. It was omitted from the London Pharmacopoeia of 1746 and 1788, and only restored in 1809, its re-introduction being chiefly due to experiments and recommendations by Baron Storch, who gave it in the form of an extract, in cases of epilepsy and other nervous and convulsive diseases.

It is supposed that this is the noxious herb referred to by Shakespeare in Hamlet:

'Sleeping within mine orchard,
My custom always of the afternoon
Upon my secure hour thy uncle stole,
With juice of cursed hebenon in a vial,
And in the porches of mine ear did pour
The leprous distillment.'

Other authorities argue that the name used here is a varied form of that by which the Yew is known in at least five of the Gothic languages, and which appears in Marlowe and other Elizabethan writers as 'hebon.' There can be little doubt that Shakespeare took both the name and the use of this plant from Marlowe, who mentions 'juice of hebon' as a deadly poison. Hebenus, according to Gower, is a 'sleepy tree.' Spenser, too, makes 'heben' a tree, and speaks of 'the deadly heben bow,' a weapon that could hardly be made of Henbane. 'This tree,' wrote Lyte in his Herball, 1578, 'is altogether venomous and against man's nature; such as do only sleepe under the shadow thereof become sicke and sometimes they die,' whereas he recommends the juice of Henbane as an application for earache.

Speaking of Henbane, Gerard says:

'The leaves, the seeds and the juice, when taken internally cause an unquiet sleep, like unto the sleep of drunkenness, which continueth long and is deadly to the patient. To wash the feet in a decoction of Henbane, as also the often smelling of the flowers causeth sleep.'

Culpepper says:

'I wonder how astrologers could take on them to make this an herb of Jupiter: and yet Mizaldus, a man of penetrating brain, was of that opinion as well as the rest: the herb is indeed under the dominion of Saturn and I prove it by this argument: All the herbs which delight most to grow in saturnine places are saturnine herbs. Both Henbane delights most to grow in saturnine places, and whole cart loads of it may be found near the places where they empty the common Jakes, and scarce a ditch to be found without it growing by it. Ergo, it is a herb of Saturn. The leaves of Henbane do cool all hot inflammations in the eyes.... It also assuages the pain of the gout, the sciatica, and other pains in the joints which arise from a hot cause. And applied with vinegar to the forehead and temples, helps the headache and want of sleep in hot fevers.... The oil of the seed is helpful for deafness, noise and worms in the ears, being dropped therein; the juice of the herb or root doth the same. The decoction of the herb or seed, or both, kills lice in man or beast. The fume of the dried herb stalks and seeds, burned, quickly heals swellings, chilblains or kibes in the hands or feet, by holding them in the fume thereof. The remedy to help those that have taken Henbane is to drink goat's milk, honeyed water, or pine kernels, with sweet wine; or, in the absence of these, Fennel seed, Nettle seed, the seed of Cresses, Mustard or Radish; as also Onions or Garlic taken in wine, do all help to free them from danger and restore them to their due temper again. Take notice, that this herb must never be taken inwardly; outwardly, an oil, ointment, or plaister of it is most admirable for the gout . . . to stop the toothache, applied to the aching side....'

The leaves or roots eaten produce maniacal delirium, if nothing worse. Another old writer says:

'If it be used either in sallet or in pottage, then doth it bring frenzie, and whoso useth more than four leaves shall be in danger to sleepe without waking.'

It is poisonous in all its parts, and neither drying nor boiling destroys the toxic principle. The leaves are the most powerful portion, even the odor of them when fresh will produce giddiness and stupor. Accidental cases of poisoning by Henbane are, however, not very common, as the plant has too unpleasant a taste and smell to be readily mistaken for any esculent vegetable, but its roots, which are thick and somewhat like those of salsafy, have sometimes been gathered and eaten. In one case recorded, a woman pulled up a quantity of Henbane roots which she found in a field, supposing them to be parsnips. She boiled them in soup, which was eaten by the family. The whole of the nine persons who had partaken of them suffered severely, being soon seized with indistinctness of vision, giddiness and sleepiness, followed by delirium and convulsions.

It is also recorded that the whole of the inmates of a monastery were once poisoned by using the roots instead of chicory. The monks partaking of the roots for supper were all more or less affected during the night and following day, being attacked with a sort of delirious frenzy, accompanied in many cases by such hallucinations that the establishment resembled a lunatic asylum.

The herb was used in magic and diabolism, for its power of throwing its victims into convulsions. It was employed by witches in their midnight brews, and from the leaves was prepared a famous sorcerer's ointment.

Anodyne necklaces were made from the root and were hung about the necks of children as charms to prevent fits and to cause easy teething.

In mythology, we read that the dead in Hades were crowned with it as they wandered hopelessly beside the Styx.

The herb is also called Hog's-bean, and both its botanical name Hyoscyamus and the tenth-century Jusquiasmus are derived from the Greek words hyos and cyamos, signifying 'the bean of the hog,' which animal is supposed to eat it with impunity. An old AngloSaxon name for it was 'Belene,' probably from the bell-shaped flowers; then it became known as 'Hen-bell,' and from the time that its poisonous properties were recognized this name was changed to 'Henbane,' because the seeds were thought to be fatal to poultry. Dr. Prior is inclined to think that the name Henbane is derived from the Spanish hinna (a mule), e.g. 'henna bell,' referring to the similarity of its seed-vessel to the bell hung upon the neck of the mules.

Although swine are said to feed upon the leaves and suffer no ill effects, this plant should not be allowed to grow in places to which cattle have access, though they seldom touch it, and its effects seem less violent on most of the larger domestic animals than on man, sheep will sometimes eat it when young, and it has occasionally been noticed that no bad effects have followed. Cows, however, have been poisoned by having Henbane mixed with their forage, it is said for the purpose of fattening them. A small quantity of the seeds of the Stramonium or Thornapple, as well as those of Henbane, are also sometimes added, the idea appears to be that the tendency to stupor and repose caused by these plants is conducive to fattening. In some districts, horse-dealers mix the seeds of Henbane with their oats, in order to fatten their animals.

Description

H. niger is susceptible of considerable diversity of character, causing varieties which have by some been considered as distinct species. Thus the plant is sometimes annual, the stem almost unbranched, smaller and less downy than in the biennial form, the leaves shorter and less hairy and the flowers often yellow, without any purple markings. The annual plant also flowers in July or August, the biennial in May and June.

The annual and biennial form spring indifferently from the same crop of seed, the former growing during summer to a height of from 1 to 2 feet, and flowering and perfecting seed, the latter producing the first season only a tuft of radical leaves, which disappear in winter, leaving underground a thick, fleshy root, from the crown of which arises in spring a branched, flowering stem, usually much taller and more vigorous than the flowering stems of the annual plants. The annual form is apparently produced by the weaker and later developed seeds formed in the fruit at the ends of the shoots; it is considered to be less active than the typical species and differs in being of dwarfed growth and having rather paler flowers. The British drug of commerce consists of dense flowering shoots only, and of larger size.

Both varieties are used in medicine, but the biennial form is the one considered official. The leaves of this biennial plant spread out flat on all sides from the crown of the root like a rosette; they are oblong and egg-shaped, with acute points, stalked and more or less sharply toothed, often more than a foot in length, of a greyish-green color and covered with sticky hairs. These leaves perish at the appearance of winter. The flowering stem pushes up from the root-crown in the following spring, ultimately reaching from 3 to 4 feet in height, and as it grows, becoming branched and furnished with alternate, oblong, unequally lobed, stalkless leaves, which are stem-clasping and vary considerably in size, but seldom exceed 9 or 10 inches in length. These leaves are pale green in color, with a broad conspicuous mid-rib, and are furnished on both sides (but particularly on the veins on the under surface) with soft, glandular hairs, which secrete a resinous substance that causes the fresh leaves to feel unpleasantly clammy and sticky. Similar hairs occur on the sub-cylindrical branches. The flowers are shortly stalked, the lower ones growing in the fork of the branches, the upper ones stalkless, crowded together in onesided, leafy spikes, which are rolled back at the top before flowering, the hairy, leafy, coarsely-toothed bracts becoming smaller upwards. The flowers have a hairy, pitchershaped calyx, which remains round the fruit and is strongly veined, with five stiff, broad, almost prickly lobes. The corollas are obliquely funnel-shaped, upwards of an inch across, of a dingy yellow or buff, marked with a close network of lurid purple veins. A variety sometimes occurs in which the corolla is not marked with these purple veins. The seed-capsule opens transversely by a convex lid and contains numerous small seeds. Perhaps the most striking feature of the plant are these curious seed-vessels, a very detailed description of which is given in the works of Flavius Josephus, as it was upon this capsule that one of the ornaments of the Jewish High Priests' head-dress was modelled. The whole plant has a powerful, oppressive, nauseous odor.

Cultivation

Henbane is in such demand for medicinal purposes that it is necessary to cultivate it, the wild plants not yielding a sufficient supply. Both varieties were formerly cultivated in England, but at present the biennial is almost solely grown. Englishgrown Henbane has always been nearly sufficient to provide enough fresh leaves for the preparation of the juice, or green extract, but large quantities, chiefly of the annual kind, were imported before the War from Germany, Austria and Russia, in the form of dry leaves.

Henbane will grow on most soils, in sandy spots near the sea, on chalky slopes, and in cultivation flourishing in a good loam.

It is, however, very capricious in its growth, the seeds being prone to lie dormant for a season or more, refusing to germinate at all in some places, and the crop varying without any apparent reason, sometimes dying in patches. In some maritime localities it can be grown without any trouble. It requires a light, moderately rich and well-drained soil for successful growth and an open, sunny situation, but does not want much attention beyond keeping the ground free from weeds.

The seed should be sown in the open early in May or as soon as the ground is warm, as thinly as possible, in rows 2 to 2 1/2 feet apart, the seedlings thinned out to 2 feet apart in the rows, as they do not stand transplanting well. Only the larger seedlings should be reserved, especially those of a bluish tint. The soil where the crop is to be, must have been well manured, and must be kept moist until the seeds have germinated, and also during May and June of the first year. It is also recommended to sow seeds of biennial Henbane at their natural ripening time, August, in porous soil.

The ground must never be water-logged, especially in the first winter; it runs to stalk in a wet season. Drought and late frosts stunt the growth and cause it to blossom too early, and if the climatic conditions are unsuitable, especially in a dry spring and summer, the biennial Henbane will flower in its first year, while the growth is quite low, but wellmanured soil may prevent this.

Care must be taken in selecting the seed: commercial Henbane seed is often kiln-dried and useless for sowing. In order to more readily ensure germination, it is advisable to soak the seeds in water for twenty-four hours before planting: the unfertile seeds will then float on the top of the water and may thus be distinguished. Ripe seed should be grey, and yellowish or brown seeds should be rejected, as they are immature. Let the seeds dry and then sift out the smallest, keeping only the larger seeds.

Henbane seed being very small and light should be well mixed with fine dry soil as it is sown.

As seedlings often die off, a reserve should be kept in a box or bed to fill gaps, even though they do not always transplant success fully.

If it is desired to raise a crop of the annualvariety the plants, being smaller and not branching so freely, may be grown at a distance of 18 inches apart each way, but the annual is very little cultivated in this country.

If any annuals come up among the biennials sown, the flowers should be cut off until the leaves get larger and the stem branches.

There is usually some difficulty in growing Henbane owing to its destruction by insects: sometimes the whole of the foliage is destroyed by the larvae of a leaf-mining fly, Pegomyia Hyoscyami, and the crop is rendered worthless in a week. And when the large autumnal leaves of the first-year plants of the biennial variety decay, the large terminal bud is often destroyed by one of the various species of macro-lepidopterous caterpillars which hide themselves in the ground. The crown or bud should be covered as soon as the leaves have rotted away with soil mixed with soot or naphthaline, to prevent the depredations of these and other insects.

Floods may also rot the plants in winter, if grown on level ground. Potato pests are fond of the prickly leaves and will leave a potato patch to feed on the Henbane plant.

If mildew develops on the foliage in summer, dust the plants with powdered sulphur or spray with 1/2 oz. of liver of sulphur in 2 gallons of water.

When it is desired to preserve seed for propagation, it is well to cut off the top flowering shoots at an early stage of flowering (these may be dried and sold as flowering tops), and allow only about six seed-capsules to ripen. This will ensure strong seed to the capsules left, and this seed will probably produce biennial Henbane, weaker seeds being apt to produce the less robust and less valuable annual Henbane.

Seeds sown as soon as ripe in August may germinate in autumn, and thus constitute a biennial by growing on all through the winter and flowering the next summer.

Although the cultivation of Henbane in sandy ground near the sea, especially on the rich soil of estuaries, would probably pay well, it is hardly a profitable plant to grow in small gardens, more especially as the yield of dried leaf is very small. It is estimated that about 15 cwt. of dry herb are obtained from an acre of ground.

Parts Used, Preparation for Market

Henbane leaves are official in all pharmacopoeias. Some require that it be collected from uncultivated plants, others that it be not used after keeping for more than a year.

The official drug, according to the British Pharmacopoeia, consists of the fresh leaves, flowering tops and branches of the biennial variety of H. niger, and the same parts of the plant carefully dried.

The drug is preferably given in the form of the fluid extract or tincture. The smaller branches and leaves of the plant, with the leaves and flowers, is the drug from which the green extract and juice of Henbane are prepared, whilst the leaves and flowering tops are separated from the branches and dried and used for making tincture. The inspissated juice of the fresh leaves is considered exceedingly variable in its operation, and is not so much recommended.

The commercial drug presents three varieties, distinguished by the trade names 'Annual,' 'First Biennial' (the leaves from the biennial plant in its first year), and 'Biennial,' or 'Second Biennial,' the official drug, which is scarce and high-priced, the first two kinds commanding lower prices.

When grown in this country, the official Henbane plant, as already mentioned, is usually biennial. The leaves of the first year's growth are collected and sold under the name of 'First Biennial Henbane.' This variety consists of large, stalked leaves, attaining 10 inches or more in length, and is of course free from flower.

Under certain conditions the biennial plant will flower in the first year: this is also collected and sold as 'Annual (English) Henbane.' It closely resembles the biennial, but the flowering tops are usually less dense, and the drug often contains portions of the stem. Such plants are much stronger than the foreign imported annual, and being more carefully dried are richer in alkaloids.

Formerly the second year's growth of the biennial plant was thought to contain a considerably larger percentage of alkaloid than either the first year's growth of the same plant, or the annual plant, and only the actual flowering tops of such plants were official, but it is now held that leaves from the English-grown species of all the above are practically of equal alkaloidal value, though the imported drug is of much less value.

Much Henbane is imported from Germany and Russia; this is probably collected mostly from annual plants, and often arrives in very poor condition, sometimes mixed with other species of Henbane. In consequence, English Henbane has always commanded a much higher price. Foreign annual Henbane is usually a much more slender plant than the English, and as imported its alkaloidal value is lower than that of the English-grown varieties. This may be due to the large proportion of stem, sand, etc., that the drug contains, the whole plant being cut and dried. It is probable that the well-dried leaves alone of all the varieties are of approximately equal alkaloidal strength.

Harvesting

Much of the efficacy of Henbane depends upon the time at which itis gathered. The leaves should be collected when the plant is in full flower. In the biennial plant, those of the second year are preferred to those of the first; the latter are less clammy and foetid, yield less extractive, and are medicinally considered less efficient. Sometimes, however, the plant is destroyed by a severe winter in England, and then no leaves of the second year's growth are obtainable, and it has been suggested that this is, perhaps, one of the causes of the great uncertainty of the medicine as found in commerce.

The leaves of the biennial variety are collected in June or the first week of July and those of the annual in August.

The leaves and flowering tops which constitute the 'Second Biennial Henbane' are collected either with or without the smaller branches to which they are attached and carefully dried, unless they are required for the preparation of the juice or green extract, when they should be sent to the distillery at once on cutting.

The herb when required in the fresh state should be cut the first week in June, because in the second week the leaf-mining insect attacks the leaves, leaving only patches of white epidermis.

The herb requires very careful drying, as its properties are liable to be in great measure destroyed if kept too long in a damp state.

The fresh herb loses 80 to 86 per cent of its weight on drying, 100 lb. yielding 14 to 20 lb. of dry herb.

The fresh leaves have, when bruised, a strong, disagreeable narcotic odor, somewhat like that of tobacco: their taste is mucilaginous and very slightly acrid. The characteristic odor disappears to a large extent on drying, but the bitter taste then becomes more pronounced.

When the dried leaves are thrown upon the fire they burn with a crackling noise from the nitrate they contain, and at the same time they emit a strong odor.

The dried drug consists principally of the flowering tops. In commerce, it is commonly found in irregular rounded or flattened masses, in which the coarsely-toothed hairy bracts, the yellowish corolla with deep purple lines and two-celled ovary, with numerous ovules, can easily be identified.

The root is not employed in medicine, but experiments have shown that the seeds not only possess all the properties of the plant, but have ten times the strength of the leaves. They are also employed in pharmacy, having been much used in the Middle Ages. At the present time, they are much prescribed by the Mohammedan doctors of India.

The seed should be gathered in August; it may be kiln-dried for medicinal purposes, but the treatment renders it useless for culture, and if required for propagation seeds should be sun-dried. The capsules should be harvested before the lids split off, the seeds then being shaken out and dried in the sun.

Constituents

The chief constituent of Henbane leaves is the alkaloid Hyoscyamine, together with smaller quantities of Atropine and Hyoscine, also known as Scopolamine.

The proportion of alkaloid in the British Pharmacopoeia dried drug varies from 0.045 to 0.14 per cent. Higher yields are exceptional. The amount of Hyoscyamine is many times greater than that of Hyoscine.

Other constituents of Henbane are a glucosidal bitter principle called hyoscytricin, choline, mucilage, albumin, calcium oxalate and potassium nitrate. On incineration, the leaves yield about 12 per cent of ash. By destructive distillation, the leaves yield a very poisonous empyreumatic oil.

The chief constituent of the seeds is about 0.5 to 0.6 per cent of alkaloid, consisting of Hyoscyamine, with a small proportion of Hyoscine. The seeds also contain about 20 per cent of fixed oil.

Medicinal Action and Uses

Antispasmodic, hypnotic, mild diuretic. The leaves have long been employed as a narcoticmedicine. It is similar in action to belladonna and stramonium, though milder in its effects.

The drug combines the therapeutic actions of its two alkaloids, Hyoscyamine and Hyoscine. Because of the presence of the former, it tends to check secretion and to relax spasms of the involuntary muscles, while through the narcotic effects of its hyoscine it lessens pain and exercises a slight somnifacient action.

Its most important use is in relief of painful spasmodic affections of the unstriped muscles, as in lead colic and irritable bladder. It will also relieve pain in cystitis.

It is much employed to allay nervous irritation, in various forms of hysteria or irritable cough, the tincture or juice prepared from the bruised, fresh leaves and tops being given in mixtures as an antispasmodic in asthma.

Combined with silver nitrate, it is especially useful in the treatment of gastric ulcer and chronic gastric catarrh.

It is used to relieve the griping caused by drastic purgatives, and is a common ingredient of aperient pills, especially those containing aloes and colocynth.

In small repeated doses Henbane has been found to have a tranquillizing effect upon persons affected by severe nervous irritability, producing a tendency to sleep, not followed by the disorder of the digestive organs and headache, which too frequently result from the administration of repeated doses of opium, to which Henbane is often preferred when an anodyne or sedative is required. The comparatively small amount of atropine present does not give rise to the excitation and delirium occasioned by belladonna. It is, therefore, used in insomnia, especially when opium cannot be given. Except for this, it acts like atropine.

A watery solution of the extract applied to the eye has a similar effect to that of atropine, in dilating the pupil and thus preparing the eye for an operation, or assisting the cure of its internal inflammation. This dilution leaves no injurious effect afterwards.

In the form of extract or tincture, it is a valuable remedy, either as an anodyne, a hypnotic or a sedative, and will take effect when other drugs fail. When used for such a purpose, it is the active principle, Hyoscine, that is employed. This is very powerful - only a very small amount is used, from 1/200 to 1/70 of a grain of the Hydrobromate of Hyoscine. This drug comes under Table I of the Poisons Schedule. In poisonous doses Henbane in any form causes dimness of sight, faintness, delirium, and sometimes death.

Hyoscine, in combination with other drugs, has of late come into use in the treatment known as Twilight Sleep. This is on account of its sedative action on brain and spine, causing loss of recollection and insensibility. Hyoscine is also used to a considerable extent in asylum practice, for the treatment of acute mania and delirium tremens.

A sedative application for external use is prepared by macerating Henbane leaves in alcohol, mixing the strong tincture with olive oil and heating in a waterbath, until the alcohol is dissipated. A compound liniment of Henbane, when applied to the skin, is of great service for relieving obstinate rheumatic pains.

The fresh leaves, crushed and applied as a poultice, or fomentation, will similarly relieve local pains of gout or neuralgia. They have been employed also to allay pain in cancerous ulcers, irritable sores and swellings, but their use for this purpose is of doubtful real advantage, and seems only a palliative. The extract, in form of suppositories, is also frequently used to alleviate the pain of hemorrhoids.

Preparations and Dosages

Powdered leaves, 2 to 10 grains. Fluid extract, 2 to 10 drops. Tincture, B.P. and U.S.P., 1/2 to 1 drachm. Juice, B.P., 1/2 to 1 drachm. Solid extract, 2 to 8 grains. Hyoscyamine, 1/8 to 1 grain.

The seeds possess all the properties of the plant.

Their expressed oil was formerly used externally.

Henbane seeds are used in some parts of the country as a domestic remedy for toothache; the smoke obtained by heating the seeds on a hot plate is applied to the mouth by means of a funnel, or a poultice is sometimes made from the crushed drug. The seeds were a favorite remedy for toothache in the Middle Ages, but their use is dangerous, having caused convulsions and even insanity in some instances. Both leaves and seeds have also been smoked in a pipe as a remedy for neuralgia and rheumatism, but with equal risk, being too uncertain and violent in their effect to be safe.

Children have been known to eat the seeds with serious results.

Sir Hans Sloane records the case of four children who, having eaten some of the capsules in mistake for filberts, exhibited all the symptoms of narcotic poisoning, continuing for two days and nights in a profound sleep.

In the case of adults, twenty seeds have been proved insufficient to prove fatal, though they induced grave results, the effects being the same as in poisoning by atropine or belladonna, the remedies to be employed being an emetic of mustard, followed by large draughts of warm water, strong tea or coffee, with powdered charcoal; stimulants (whisky, etc.), if necessary; the patient to be roused if drowsy; heat and friction to be applied to the extremities and finally, in acute cases, artificial respiration.

Gerard writes with regard to the use of the seed of Henbane by mountebanks for obstinate toothache:

'Drawers of teeth who run about the country and pretend they cause worms to come forth from the teeth by burning the seed in a chafing dish of coals, the party holding his mouth over the fume thereof, do have some crafty companions who convey small lute strings into the water, persuading the patient that these little creepers came out of his mouth, or other parts which it was intended to ease.'

Another old writer says: 'These pretended worms are no more than an appearance of worms which is always seen in the smoak of Henbane seed.' As a matter of fact, the small white, cylindrical embryos of the seed are forced out of some of them by the heat (especially if the seed be put into a basin with boiling water), and these were mistaken by ignorant sufferers for 'worms' coming out of their teeth.

Other Species of Hyoscyamus

Henbane, except for the use of the unofficial forms, is scarcely subject to adulteration in the entire condition. It, however, frequently contains an excessive amount of stem, which reduces its alkaloidal percentage and value.

In the south of Europe, RUSSIAN HENBANE (H. albus) - a native of the region of the Mediterranean, and so called from the pale color of its flowers - is used as the official Henbane, and is regarded as equal in medicinal value. In France it is used indiscriminately with H. niger, though here it is not recognized as having identical properties. It is easily distinguished by the bracts, as well as the leaves being all stalked, and by the pale-yellow color of the flower. According to Pharmacographia, the Hyoscyamus of the Ancients was probably H. albus, and the white variety was preferred for internal use in the practice of more modern times. Both the black and the white occur in our first Pharmacopoeia, but the use of the former was confined to external applications, such as unguentum populeum, while the latter was an ingredient of the famous electuary, Philonium Romanum, the original of the Confection of Opium. In France, too, White Henbane had the preference, though it was held to be milder in operation: only the seeds were official, whereas in the black variety only the leaves were official.

The alkaloidal contents of H. muticus, EGYPTIAN HENBANE, from Egypt and the East Indies, often exceeds 1.25 per cent. This is mostly pure Hyoscyamine: its medicinal action is thus different, and its use as a substitute is dangerous.

The drug is readily distinguished, consisting chiefly of very light and light-coloured stems, often as thick as the finger, and capsules which are equally light-coloured and far more elongated than those of H. niger. The calyx limb is also further prolonged beyond the capsule. The leaves are much narrower; they are coarsely toothed or lobed at the summit, but lack the very large and sharp lateral lobe of the European Henbane.

The presence of H. muticus, as an admixture of the official imported drug, may be detected by the presence of characteristic branching non-glandular hairs, which are found on both the stems and leaves.

H. muticus is one of the most important medicinal herbs produced in Egypt, and is a valuable source of the alkaloids, Hyoscyamine, Hyoscine and Atropine, Hyoscyamine, practically pure, occurring in the drug in considerably greater proportion than in the European herb, the Egyptian-grown plant being much richer than the Indian, and being chiefly imported into this country for the manufacture of Hyoscyamine.

The drug occurs in three forms, as a mixture of broken stem, leaf and fruit, in which stem predominates - as leaves with little stem, and as seeds; the first named is the variety usually met with.

Although H. muticus is grown in Egypt, a British Protectorate before the War, the Germans had a monopoly of the supply. TheImperial Institute, during the War, investigated H. muticus as a source of atropine, and reported that if a sufficient supply of the drug could be imported, it would be an additional inducement to British manufacturers to take up the preparation of atropine. As a result, pressed bales have reached this country in fair supply, and the manufacture of atropine is now carried on here in increased quantities.

It has been grown in this country, but not to any great extent. In 1916 it was reported that it was proposed to experiment with the seed of this plant in certain districts in the West Indian islands.

In Egypt the drug is called Sakran, meaning 'the drunken.' In India it is considerably used as a narcotic.

Scopola carniolica, a common plant in Austria and Hungary, Bavaria and southwest Russia, which appears in our trade lists of plants recommended for our pleasure gardens, also yields the alkaloid Hyoscine (Scopolamine) and is worth attention. By selective cultivation, its yield of alkaloid might be raised.

In 1916 (reported in the Chemist and Druggist, Feb. 17, 1924) Wild Hyoscyamus was discovered growing in Montana, U.S.A., the plant growing to the height of about 6 feet near Bearmouth, also Big Timber and other nearby places. It is assumed that it was introduced by some foreigners who were working on a building at Big Timber, Montana. From here it spread and became such a pest that every property-owner was ordered to rid his place of it. The climate and soil seem to suit it and the plants yield the normal quantity of alkaloid.

HENNA

Botanical: Lawsonia alba (LANK.), Lawsonia inermis
Family: N.O. Lythraceae
Synonyms: Henne. Al-Khanna. Al-henna. Jamaica Mignonette. Mehndi. Mendee. Egyptian Privet. Smooth Lawsonia.
Parts Used: Flowers, powdered leaves, fruit.
Habitat: Egypt, India, Kurdistan, Levant, Persia, Syria.

Description

The small, white and yellow, heavy, sweet-smelling flowers are borne on dwarf shrubs 8 to 10 feet high. A distilled water prepared from them is used as a cosmetic, and the powdered leaves have been in use from the most ancient times in Eastern countries for dyeing the hair and the nails a reddish-yellow.

Since 1890 it has been widely used in Europe for tinting the hair, usually in the form of a shampoo, many shades being obtainable by mixing with the leaves of other plants, such as indigo. As a dye for the skin or nails the powder may be mixed with catechu or lucerne, made into a paste with hot water, and spread on the part to be dyed, being allowed to remain for one night.

Constituents

There has been found in it a brown substance of a resinoid fracture, having the chemical properties which characterize the tannins, and therefore named hennotannic acid.

Medicinal Action and Uses

It has been employed both internally and locally in jaundice, leprosy, smallpox, and affections of the skin. The fruit is thought to have emmenagogue properties.

The Egyptians are said to have prepared both an oil and an ointment from the flowers for making the limbs supple.

HOLLY

Botanical: Ilex aquifolium (LINN.)
Family: N.O. Aquifoliaceae
Synonyms: Hulver Bush. Holm. Hulm. Holme Chase. Holy Tree. Christ's Thorn.
Parts Used: Leaves, berries, bark.

Habitat

The Holly is a native of most of the central and southern parts of Europe. It grows very slowly: when planted among trees which are not more rapid in growth than itself, it is sometimes drawn up to a height of 50 feet, but more frequently its greatest height in this country is 30 to 40 feet, and it rarely exceeds 2 feet in diameter. In Italy and in the woods of France, especially in Brittany, it attains a much larger size than is common in these islands.

Holly, the most important of the English evergreens, forming one of the most striking objects in the wintry woodland, with its glossy leaves and clusters of brilliant scarlet berries, is in the general mind closely connected with the festivities of Christmas, having been from very early days in the history of these islands gathered in great quantities for Yuletide decorations, both of the Church and of the home. The old Christmas Carols are full of allusions to Holly:

.......'Christmastide
Comes in like a bride,
With Holly and Ivy clad.'

History

Christmas decorations are said to be derived from a custom observed by the Romans of sending boughs, accompanied by other gifts, to their friends during the festival of the Saturnalia, a custom the early Christians adopted. In confirmation of this opinion, a subsequent edict of the Church of Bracara has been quoted, forbidding Christians to decorate their houses at Christmas with green boughs at the same time as the pagans, the Saturnalia commencing about a week before Christmas. The origin has also been traced to the Druids, who decorated their huts with evergreens during winter as an abode for the sylvan spirits. In old church calendars we find Christmas Eve marked templa exornantur (churches are decked), and the custom is as deeply rooted in modern times as in either pagan or early Christian days.

An old legend declares that the Holly first sprang up under the footsteps of Christ, when He trod the earth, and its thorny leaves and scarlet berries, like drops of blood, have been thought symbolical of the Saviour's sufferings, for which reason the tree is called 'Christ's Thorn' in the languages of the northern countries of Europe. It is, perhaps, in connexion with these legends that the tree was called the Holy Tree, as it is generally named by our older writers. Turner, for instance, refers to it by this name in his Herbal published in 1568. Other popular names for it are Hulver and Holme, and it is still called Hulver in Norfolk, and Holme in Devon, and Holme Chase in one part of Dartmoor.

Pliny describes the Holly under the name of Aquifolius, needle leaf, and adds that it was the same tree called by Theophrastus Crataegus, but later commentators deny this. Pliny tells us that Holly if planted near a house or farm, repelled poison, and defended it from lightning and witchcraft, that the flowers cause water to freeze, and that the wood, if thrown at any animal, even without touching it, had the property of compelling the animal to return and lie down by it.

Description

It sometimes sends up a clean stem furnished with a bushy head, or it may form a perfect pyramid, leafy to the base. The trunk, like that of the Beech, frequently has small wood knots attached to it: these are composed of a smooth nodule of solid wood embedded in bark, and may be readily separated from the tree by a smart blow. The bark is of a remarkably light hue, smooth and grey, often touched with faint crimson, and is very liable to be infected with an exceedingly thin lichen, the fructification of which consists of numerous curved black lines, closely resembling Oriental writing.

The leaves are thick and glossy, about 2 inches long and 1 1/4 inch broad, and edged with stout prickles, whose direction is alternately upwards and downwards, and of which the terminal one alone is invariably in the same plane as the leaf. The upper leaves have mostly only a single prickle. The leaves have neither taste nor odor. They remain attached to the tree for several years, and when they fall, defy for a long time the action of air and moisture, owing to their leathery texture and durable fibres, which take a long time to decay.

Professor Henslow says:

'It has been gravely asserted that holly leaves are only prickly on trees as high as a beast can reach, but at the top it has no spines; that spiny processes of all sorts are a provision of Nature against browsing animals. The truth is that they are the result of drought. A vigorous shoot of Holly may have small leaves without spines at the base, when vigour was beginning; normal, large leaves in the middle when growth was most active; and later on small spineless leaves again appear as the annual energy is declining. Moreover, hollies of ten grow to twenty feet in height, with spiny leaves throughout, and if spineless ones do occur at the top, it is only the result of lessened energy. A cow has been known to be partial to some holly bushes within reach, which had to be protected, just as another would eat stinging-nettles: and the camel lives upon the "Camel-thorn." This animal has a hardened pad to the roof of its mouth, so feels no inconvenience in eating it.'

In May, the Holly bears in the axils of the leaves, crowded, small, whitish flowers, male and female flowers being usually borne on different trees. The fertile flowers are succeeded by the familiar, brilliant, coral-red berries. The same tree rarely produces abundant crops of flowers in consecutive seasons, and Hollies sometimes produce abundance of flowers, but never mature berries, this barrenness being caused by the male flowers alone being properly developed. Berries are rarely produced abundantly when the tree is much clipped, and are usually found in the greatest number on the upper part of the tree, where the leaves are less spiny.

The berries, though eaten by birds, are injurious to human beings, and children should be warned against them. Deer will eat the leaves in winter, and sheep thrive on them. They are infested with few insects.

The ease with which Holly can be kept trimmed renders it valuable as a hedge plant: it forms hedges of great thickness that are quite impenetrable.

It has been stated by M. J. Pierre, that the young stems are gathered in Morbihan by the peasants, and made use of as a cattle-food from the end of November until April, with great success. The stems are dried, and having been bruised are given as food to cows three times daily. They are found to be very wholesome and productive of good milk, and the butter made from it is excellent.

It is also well known to rabbit-breeders that a Holly-stick placed in a hutch for the rabbits to gnaw, will act as a tonic, and restore their appetite.

The wood of Holly is hard, compact and of a remarkable even substance throughout. Except towards the centre of very old trees, it is beautifully white, and being susceptible of a very high polish, is much prized for ornamental ware, being extensively used for inlaying, as in the so-called Tunbridge ware. The evenness of its grain makes it very valuable to the turner. When freshly cut, it is of a slightly greenish hue, but soon becomes perfectly white, and its hardness makes it superior to any other white wood. As it is very retentive of its sap and warps in consequence, it requires to be well dried and seasoned before being used. It is often stained blue, green, red or black; when of the latter color, its principal use is as a substitute for ebony, as in the handles of metal teapots. Mathematical instruments are made of it, also the blocks for calico printing, and it has been employed in wood engraving as a substitute for boxwood, to which, however, it is inferior. The wood of the silver-striped variety is said to be whiter than that of the common kind.

A straight Holly-stick is much prized for the stocks of light driving whips, also for walking-sticks.

The common Holly is the badge of the Drummonds.

Cultivation

The Holly will grow in almost any soil, provided it is not too wet, but attains the largest size in rich, sandy or gravelly loam, where there is good drainage, and a moderate amount of moisture at the roots, for in very dry localities it is usually stunted in its growth, but it will live in almost any earth not saturated with stagnant water. The most favourable situation seems to be a thin scattered wood of Oaks, in the intervals of which it grows up at once. It is rarely injured by even the most severe winters.

Holly is raised from seeds, which do not germinate until the second year, hence the berries are generally buried in a heap of earth for a year previously to being sown. The young plants are transplanted when about a foot or 18 inches high, autumn being the best time for the process. If intended for a hedge, the soil around should be previously well trenched and moderately manured if necessary. Holly exhausts the soil around it to a greater extent than most deciduous trees. At least two years will be needed to recover the check given by transplanting. Although always a slow grower, Holly grows more quickly after the first four or five years.

The cultivated varieties of Holly are very numerous: of these one is distinguished by the unusual color of its berries, which are yellow. Other forms are characterized by the variegated foliage, or by the presence of a larger or smaller number of prickles than ordinary.

In winter the garden and shrubbery are much indebted to the more showy varieties for the double contrast afforded by their leaves and berries. They are propagated by grafting on four- or five-year-old plants of the common sort and by cuttings.

The best time to cut down Holly is early in the spring, before the sap rises. A sloping cut is preferable to a straight one, as moisture is thus prevented from remaining on the cut portion, and as an additional precaution the wound should be covered with a coating of tar. The side growths should be left, as they will help to draw up the sap.

Part Used

The leaves and berries, also the bark. The leaves are used both fresh and dried, but usually in the dried condition, for which they are collected in May and June. They should be stripped off the tree on a dry day, the best time being about noon, when there is no longer any trace of dew on them. All stained or insect-eaten leaves must be rejected.

Medicinal Action and Uses

Holly leaves were formerly used as a diaphoretic and an infusion of them was given in catarrh, pleurisy and smallpox. They have also been used in intermittent fevers and rheumatism for their febrifugal and tonic properties, and powdered, or taken in infusion or decoction, have been employed with success where Cinchona has failed, their virtue being said to depend on a bitter principle, an alkaloid named Ilicin. The juice of the fresh leaves has been employed with advantage in jaundice.

The berries possess totally different qualities to the leaves, being violently emetic and purgative, a very few occasioning excessive vomiting soon after they are swallowed, though thrushes and blackbirds eat them with impunity. They have been employed in dropsy; also, in powder, as an astringent to check bleeding.

Culpepper says 'the bark and leaves are good used as fomentations for broken bones and such members as are out of joint.' He considered the berries to be curative of colic.

From the bark, stripped from the young shoots and suffered to ferment, birdlime is made. The bark is stripped off about midsummer and steeped in clean water; then boiled till it separates into layers, when the inner green portion is laid up in small heaps till fermentation ensues. After about a fortnight has elapsed, it becomes converted into a sticky, mucilaginous substance, and is pounded into a paste, washed and laid by again to ferment. It is then mixed with some oily matter, goosefat being preferred, and is ready for use. Very little, however, is now made in this country. In the north of England, Holly was formerly so abundant in the Lake District, that birdlime was made from it in large quantities and shipped to the East Indies for destroying insects.

The leaves of Holly have been employed in the Black Forest as a substitute for tea. Paraguay Tea, so extensively used in Brazil, is made from the dried leaves and young shoots of another species of Holly (Ilex Paraguayensis), growing in South America, an instance of the fact that similar properties are often found in more than one species of the same genus.

I. Gongonha and I. Theezans, also used in Brazil as tea, and like I. Paraguayensis are valuable diuretics and diaphoretics. The leaves of I. Paraguayensis and several others are used by dyers; the unripe fruits of I. Macoucoua abound in tannin, and bruised in a ferruginous mud, are used in dyeing cotton, acting something like galls.

HOLLY, SEA

Botanical: Eryngium maritinum, Eryngium campestre
Family: N.O. Umbelliferae
Synonyms: Eryngo. Sea Hulver. Sea Holme.
Part Used: Root.

Habitat

It abounds on most of our sandy seashores and is very plentiful on the East Coast, also on the sands of Mounts Bay, Cornwall, but is rare in Scotland.

Closely allied to the Wood Sanicle, not only belonging to the same order, Umbelliferae, but placed by Hooker in the same Tribe or subdivision of the order, Saniculae, is the Sea Holly (Eryngium maritinum).

This spiny plant, which at first sight might be taken rather for a thistle than a member of the umbelliferous order, is sometimes called by old English writers Sea Hulver and Sea Holme.

Description

The roots are perennial, large, fleshy and brittle, penetrating far into the sand, often reaching several feet in length.

The stems, 6 to 12 inches high, thick and solid, are branched at the summit. The radical leaves are on stalks, 2 to 7 inches long, the blades cut into three broad divisions at the apex, coarsely toothed, the teeth ending in spines and undulated. The margin of the leaf is thickened and cartilaginous. The lower stem-leaves are shortly stalked, resembling the radical ones, but the upper ones are sessile and half embracing the stem, which terminates in a shortly-stalked head, below which it gives off two or three spreading branches, all from one point, which is surrounded by a whorl of three leaves, spreading like the rays of the sun.

The heads of flowers appear in July and are at first round, afterwards egg-shaped, 3/4 to 1 inch across, the flowers stalkless, whitish-blue, 1/8 inch across. The calyx tube is thickly covered with soft, cartilaginous bristles; the calyx teeth end in a spine.

The plant is intensely glaucous tinged with blue towards the top, especially on the flowerheads and the leaves immediately below them.

The name of this genus has reference to its supposed efficacy in flatulent disorders, coming from the Greek word eruggarein (to eructate). Dioscorides recommended the roots for this purpose.

Another derivation is from the diminutive of eerungos (the beard of a goat), possibly from its appearance. Plutarch relates a curious story about the plant, saying:

'They report of the Sea Holly, if one goat taketh it into her mouth, it causeth her first to stand still and afterwards the whole flock, until such time as the shepherd takes it from her.'

According to Linnaeus, the young flowering-shoots, when boiled and eaten like asparagus, are palatable and nourishing. The leaves are sweetish, with a slight aromatic, warm pungency. The roots, boiled or roasted resemble chestnuts in taste, and are palatable and nutritious.

The roots are supposed to have the same aphrodisiac virtues as those of the Orchis tribe, and are still regarded by the Arabs as an excellent restorative. They are sold in some places in a candied form, and used to be obtainable in London shops as a sweetmeat. They are said to have been prepared in this manner by Robert Burton, an apothecary of Colchester, in the seventeenth century, who established a manufactory for the purpose, but the roots were in use long before, being considered both antiscorbutic and excellent for health, and we are told that the 'kissing comfits,' alluded to by Falstaff, were made of them. We read that once the town of Colchester presented royalty with a sample of their candied Sea Holly roots, whereon the sale of the article increased greatly, and many wonderful cures were supposed to be effected by the confection.

Gerard says:

'The roots if eaten are good for those that be liver sick, and they ease cramps, convulsions and the falling sickness. If condited, or preserved with sugar, they are exceeding good to be given to old and aged people that are consumed and withered with age, and who want natural moisture.'

He gives an elaborate recipe for 'conditing' the roots of Sea Holly or Eringos.

He also cultivated in his garden the Field Eryngo (E. campestre), a native of most parts of Europe, but not common in Britain, though a troublesome weed in the few spots where it does appear, as the roots run deep into the ground, and are not easily destroyed by the plough and spread greatly. The whole plant is very stiff and of a pale-green color, less glaucous and more branched than the Sea Holly; the corolla are blue, sometimes white or yellow. It is taller and more slender, also, than the Sea Holly. By many authorities it is considered a doubtful native of these islands.

Cultivation

The Sea Holly, in common with the ornamental varieties, Eryngo, now cultivated, will grow in a garden, if planted in a warm, well-drained and preferably a gravel soil, but the roots will not grow as large or as fleshy as those which are found upon the seashore within reach of salt water. Plenty of sun is essential for all varieties.

The best time to transplant the roots is in autumn, when the leaves decay; the young roots are much better to transplant than the old, because, being furnished with fibres, they will readily take root. They will require no further culture than to be kept free from weeds.

If propagated by seeds, they are more likely to succeed if the seeds are sown in the autumn, as the germination is very slow. They may be sown where intended to grow and thinned out to about a foot or more apart, to avoid transplanting, as the long roots may break in the process. The seedlings are, in any case, not ready for transplanting for a year, so that the mode of propagation generally preferred is by division of roots in spring.Cuttings of the roots will succeed in light soil, if planted about 2 inches deep.

Part Used

The root, dug in autumn, from plants at least two years old.

Culpepper says:

'The distilled water of the whole herb' (Sea Holly) 'when the leaves and stalks are young is profitably drank for all the purposes aforesaid, and helps the melancholy of the heart, and is available in quartan and quotidian agues; as also for them that have their necks drawn awry, and cannot turn them without turning their whole body.'

Eryngo roots when dry are in pieces from 2 to 4 inches long, or more, transversely wrinkled, blackish-brown, crowned with the bristly remains of leaf-stalks. The fracture is spongy and coarsely fibrous, with a small radiate, yellow centre.

The taste is sweetish and mucilaginous, but the root has no odor.

The roots of both the Common Sea Holly and of the Field Eryngo are both sold under the name of Eryngo Root.

Medicinal Action and Uses

Diaphoretic, diuretic, aromatic, stimulant, expectorant. Eryngo promotes a free expectoration and possessing an aromatic principle is very serviceable in debility attendant upon coughs of chronic standing in the advanced stages of pulmonary consumption, in which it has been used in the candied form with great benefit.

It is useful in paralysis and chronic nervous diseases, alike in simple nervousness and in delirium produced by diseases.

Boerhaave, the celebrated Danish physician, much recommended Eryngo, considering that a decoction of the roots, drunk freely, acted on the kidneys and is serviceable in scorbutic complaints. It is used with good results in cases of bladder disease.

The roots are also considered good in obstructions of the liver and in jaundice, operating as a diuretic and a good restorative.

They have been pronounced balsamic, as well as diuretic, old writers telling us that bruised and applied outwardly, they are good for King's Evil, and that when bruised and boiled in hog's fat and applied to broken bones, thorns in the flesh, etc., they draw the latter out and heal up the place again, 'gathering new flesh where it was consumed.'

Other Species

E. campestre was formerly abundant about Watling Street.

Of the foreign species, which are numerous, the most worthy of notice is E. amethystinum, so called from the brilliant blue tint not of its flowers only, but of the bracts and upper part of the stem; it is a native of Dalmatia and Croatia, but is frequently cultivated in English gardens; while E. Alpinum, a smaller plant of a still more brilliant color, is a native of the Swiss Alps.

E. aquaticum (Button Snake-root), a North American plant, is used in Homeopathy, a tincture being made from the root both fresh and dried.

HOLLYHOCK

Botanical: Althaea Rosea (LINN.)
Family: N.O. Malvaceae
Synonym: Garden Hollyhock.
Part Used: Flowers.

The Hollyhock, first brought to this country from China, was once eaten as a pot-herb, though it is not particularly palatable.

Its flowers are employed medicinally for their emollient, demulcent and diuretic properties, which make them useful in chest complaints. Their action is similar to Marshmallow.

The flowers are also used for colouring purposes. They are sold freed from the calyx and should be gathered in July and early August, when in full bloom, and dried in trays, in thin layers, in a current of warm air immediately after picking. When dry, they are a deep, purplish-black, about 2 1/2 inches in diameter, united with the stamens, which form a tube, the one-celled, reniform anthers remaining free.

HONEYSUCKLES

Botanical: Lonicera caprifolium (LINN.), Lonicera Periclymenum (LINN.)
Family: N.O. Caprifoliaceae

Synonyms: Dutch Honeysuckle. Goats' Leaf.
Parts Used: Flowers, seeds, leaves.

Caprifoliaceae, the order to which the Honeysuckles belong, includes about 300 species, chiefly shrubs, growing in the north temperate zone or extending into the higher cool tropical regions. Besides the Viburnums and Sambucus, a number have found more or less important uses in medicine, but they exhibit but little uniformity in composition or properties.

Medicinal Action and Uses

A dozen or more of the 100 species of Lonicera or Honeysuckle are used medicinally, the fruits generally having emiticocathartic properties. Several of these drugs have more than a local repute.

The herbage of L. caprifolium (Linn.), the smaller, or ITALIAN HONEYSUCKLE, of Mid- and Southern Europe, is used as a cutaneous and mucous tonic and vulnerary and the seeds as a diuretic.

L. Periclymenum (Linn.), our common ENGLISH WILD HONEYSUCKLE, is used similarly and the stems as a substitute or adulterant for Solanum Dulcamara, the Bittersweet.

Waller says: 'The leaves and flowers of Honeysuckle are possessed of diuretic and sudorific properties,' and adds:

'a decoction of the flowers has been celebrated as an excellent antispasmodic and recommended in asthma of the nervous kind. An elegant water may be distilled from these flowers, which has been recommended for nervous headache.'

Gerard says: 'The Honeysuckle is "neither cold nor binding, but hot and attenuating or making thin." ' He quotes Dioscorides as saying that:

'the ripe seed gathered and dried in theshadow and drunk for four days together, doth waste and consume away the hardness of the spleen and removeth wearisomeness, helpeth the shortness and difficulty of breathing, cureth the hicket (hiccough), etc. A syrup made of the flowers is good to be drunk against diseases of the lungs and spleen.'

He also recommends it for sores in various parts of the alimentary canal.

Salmon in his Herbal (1710) speaks only of the Meadow Honeysuckle, 'which was the name given by the agriculturists of his day to the Meadow Trefoil (Trifolium pratense).'

The herbage of the true Honeysuckles is a favorite food of goats, hence the Latin name Caprifolium (Goats' Leaf), the French Chèvre-feuille, German Geisblatt and Italian Capri-foglio, all signifying the same. The berries have been used as food for chickens. The name of the genus, Lonicera, was given by Linnaeus in honour of Adam Lonicer, a physician and naturalist, born at Marburg in 1528, who wrote, among other works, the Naturalis Historiae Opus novum, which contains much curious information about plants.

Our native Honeysuckle has expectorant and laxative properties. The flowers in the form of syrup have been used for diseases of the respiratory organs and in asthma and the leaves as decoction in diseases of the liver and spleen. It was also considered a good ingredient in gargles.

L. tartarica, a native of Siberia, an upright species, a shrub, not a climber, has berries which are nauseously bitter and purgative.

The wood of L. Xylosteum, native of Eastern Europe and Asia, but found naturalized in Sussex, also of shrub-like nature, is used by the Russians to prepare an empyrheumatic oil for 'cold tumours and chronic pains. ' It is sold in China as Jin-tung. Animals seldom touch the leaves of this species and birds eat its berries only in hard weather - they are reputed to be purgative and emetic.

L. brachypoda repens is used in Japan as a drastic purgative, and L. Japonica (Thunb.) is sold in China as Kin-yin-keva.

Diervilla, the Bush Honeysuckle, especially Diervilla Diervilla (L. Diervilla, Linn.), has a similar repute, especially as a diuretic and as an application to relieve itching.

Various species of Symphoricarpus, Snowberry, Wax-berry, Coral-berry, Indian Currant, Turkey-berry, Wolf-berry, to give a few of its names, of North America, are similarly employed. S. racemosa (Mich.) is often planted in hedges.

Culpepper says:

'Honeysuckles are cleansing, consuming and digesting, and therefore no way fit for inflammations. Take a leaf and chew it in your mouth and you will quickly find it likelier to cause a sore mouth and throat than cure it. If it be not good for this, what is it good for? It is good for something, for God and nature made nothing in vain. It is a herb of Mercury, and appropriated to the lungs; the celestial Crab claims dominion over it, neither is it a foe to the Lion; if the lungs be afflicted by Jupiter, this is your cure. It is fitting a conserve made of the flowers should be kept in every gentlewoman's house; I know no better cure for the asthma than this besides it takes away the evil of the spleen: provokes urine, procures speedy delivery of women in travail, relieves cramps, convulsions, and palsies, and whatsoever griefs come of cold or obstructed perspiration; if you make use of it as an ointment, it will clear the skin of morphew, freckles, and sunburnings, or whatever else discolours it, and then the maids will love it. Authors say, the flowers are of more effect than the leaves, and that is true: but they say the seeds are the least effectual of all. But there is a vital spirit in every seed to beget its like; there is a greater heat in the seed than any other part of the plant; and heat is the mother of action.'

HOPS

Botanical: Humulus Lupulus (LINN.)
Family: N.O. Urticaceae
Part Used: Flowers.

The Hop (Humulus Lupulus, Linn.) is a native British plant, having affinities, botanically speaking, with the group of plants to which the Stinging Nettles belong. The sole representative of its genus in these islands, it is found wild in hedges and copses from York southwards, being only considered an introduced species in Scotland, and rare and not indigenous in Ireland. It is found in most countries of the North temperate zone.

The root is stout and perennial. The stem that arises from it every year is of a twining nature, reaching a great length, flexible and very tough, angled and prickly, with a tenacious fibre, which has enabled it to be employed to some extent in Sweden in the manufacture of a coarse kind of cloth, white and durable, though the fibres are so difficult of separation, that the stems require to be steeped in water a whole winter. Paper has also been made from the stem, or bine, as it is termed.

The leaves are heart-shaped and lobed, on foot-stalks, and as a rule placed opposite one another on the stem, though sometimes the upper leaves are arranged singly on the stem, springing from altenate sides. They are of a dark-green color with their edges finely toothed.

The flowers spring from the axils of the leaves. The Hop is dioecious, i.e. male and female flowers are on separate plants. The male flowers are in loose bunches or panicles, 3 to 5 inches long. The female flowers are in leafy cone-like catkins, called strobiles. When fully developed, the strobiles are about 1 1/4 inch long, oblong in shape and rounded, consisting of a number of overlapping, yellowish-green bracts, attached to a separate axis. If these leafy organs are removed, the axis will be seen to be hairy and to have a little zigzag course. Each of the bracts enfolds at the base a small fruit (achene), both fruit and bract being sprinkled with yellow translucent glands, which appear as a granular substance. Much of the value of Hops depends on the abundance of this powdery substance, which contains 10 per cent of Lupulin, the bitter principle to which Hops owe much of their tonic properties.

As it is, these ripened cones of the female Hop plant that are used in brewing, female plants only are cultivated, since from these alone can the fruits be obtained. Those with undeveloped seeds are preferred to ensure which the staminate plants are excluded, only a few male plants being found scattered over a plantation of hops.

We find the Hop first mentioned by Pliny, who speaks of it as a garden plant among the Romans, who ate the young shoots in spring, in the same way as we do asparagus, and as country people frequently do in England at the present day. The young tops of Hop used formerly to be brought to market tied up in small bundles for table use. The tender first foliage, blanched, is a good potherb.

The leaves and flower-heads have been used also to produce a fine brown dye.

The origin of the name of the Hop genus, Humulus, is considered doubtful, though it has been assumed by some writers that it is derived from humus, the rich moist ground in which the plant grows. The specific name Lupulus, is derived from the Latin, lupus (a wolf), because, as Pliny explains, when produced among osiers, it strangles them by its light, climbing embraces, as the wolf does a sheep. The English name Hop comes from the Anglo-Saxon hoppan (to climb).

Hops appear to have been used in the breweries of the Netherlands in the beginning of the fourteenth century. In England they were not used in the composition of beer till nearly two centuries afterwards. The liquor prepared from fermented malt formed the favorite drink of our Saxon and Danish forefathers. The beverage went by the name of Ale (the word derived from the Scandinavian öl - the Viking's drink) and was brewed either from malt alone, or from a mixture of the latter with Honey and flavoured with Heath tops, Ground Ivy, and various other bitter and aromatic herbs, such as Marjoram, Buckbean, Wormwood, Yarrow, Woodsage or Germander and Broom. They knew not, however, the ale to which Hops give both flavor and preservation. For long after the introduction of Hops, the liquor flavoured in the old manner retained the name of Ale, while the word of German and Dutch origin, Bier or Beer, was given only to that made with the newly-introduced bitter catkins.

It has been stated that the planting of Hops in this country was forbidden in the reign of Henry VI, but half a century later the cultivation was introduced from Flanders, though only to a limited extent, and it did not become sufficient for the needs of the kingdom till the end of the seventeenth century. The prejudice against the use of Hops was at first great. Henry VIII forbade brewers to put hops and sulphur into ale, Parliament having been petitioned against the Hop as 'a wicked weed that would spoil the taste of the drink and endanger the people.' In the fifth year of Edward VI, however, privileges were granted to Hop growers, though in the reign of James I the plant was still not sufficiently cultivated to supply the consumption, as we find a statute of 1608 against the importation of spoiled Hops.

Hops were at first thought to engender melancholy.

'Hops,' says John Evelyn, in his Pomona (1670), 'transmuted our wholesome ale into beer, which doubtless much alters its constitution. This one ingredient, by some suspected not unworthily, preserves the drink indeed, but repays the pleasure in tormenting diseases and a shorter life.'

Cultivation

It has been estimated that in pre-war times 70 per cent of the Hops used in brewing was home produce and 30 per cent imported, chiefly from the United States and Germany.

Hops are also grown in France, South Russia, Australia and New Zealand.

The cultivation of Hops in the British Islands is restricted to England, where it is practically confined to half a dozen counties: four in the south-east (Kent, Surrey, Hants and Sussex) and two in the western Midland counties (Worcester and Hereford). As a rule, over 60 per cent of home-grown Hops are grown in Kent.

In the years 1898-1907, the average annual acreage of Hops under cultivation in this country was 48,841 acres (being 51,127 acres in 1901 and 33,763 acres in 1907). The average annual yield per acre for these ten years was 8.84 cwt., and the average annual home produce 434,567 cwt. In 1907 Kent had under cultivation 28,169 acres; Hereford, 6,143; Sussex, 4,243; Worcester, 3,622; Hants; 1,842, and Surrey, 744.

Hops require deep, rich soil, on dry bottom, with south or south-west aspect - free circulation of air is necessary. The ground is generally well pulverized and manured to considerable depth by plough or spade before planting. Hops in Kent are usually planted in October or November, the plants being placed 6 feet apart each way, thus giving 1,210 plant centres to the acre. The plants are usually set in 'stools' of from three to five, a few inches apart. They are obtained from cuttings or suckers taken from the healthiest old shoots, which are usually planted out closely in nursery lines a year before being planted permanently.

Very little growth takes place the first year. Some planters still grow potatoes or mangels between the rows of the first year, as the plants do not bear much till the second year, but this is considered a mistake, as it exhausts the ground.

As a rule, the plants are not full bearing till the third year, when four to six poles from 14 to 18 feet long are required for each stool. The most used timber for Hop poles is Spanish Chestnut, which is largely grown for this special purpose in coppices in hopgrowing districts. Ash is also used. The poles are set to the plants in spring, before growth commences, and removed when the latter are cut away in autumn. The plants are then dressed with manure, and the soil between the stools stirred lightly. Much of the Hop-land is ploughed between the rows, but it is better to dig Hop-land if possible, the tool used being the Kent spud.

Experiments in Hop manuring have been conducted in connexion with the South-East Agricultural College, Wye. The main results have been to demonstrate the necessity of a liberal supply of phosphates, if the full benefit is to be reaped from application of nitrogenous manures. Manuring is applied in the winter and dug or ploughed in. London manure from stables is used to an enormous extent. Rags, fur waste, sprats, wood waste and shoddy, are also put on in the winter. In the summer, rape dust, guano, nitrate of soda and various patent Hopmanures are chopped in with the Canterbury hoe. Fish guano, or desiccated fish, is largely used; it is very stimulating and more lasting than some of the forcing manures.

Hop-land is ploughed or dug between November and March. After this, the plants are trimmed or 'dressed,' i.e. all the old bine ends are cut off with a sharp curved Hop-knife and the plant centres kept level with the ground. Much attention is required to keep the bines in their places on the poles, strings or wire during the summer.

The Hop cones - or strobiles - are fit to gather when a brown-amber color and of a firm consistence. The stalks are then cut at the base and removed with the poles and laid horizontally on frames of wood, to each of which is attached a large sack into which the Hops fall as they are picked. When picked, the Hops are at once taken to the kiln or oast-house, and dried, as they are liable to become spoiled in a few hours, especially when picked moist. During the process of drying which is carried out in a similar manner to the drying of malt, great care is required to prevent overheating, by which the essential oil would become volatilized. The Hops are spread 8 to 12 inches deep, on hair-cloth, also being sometimes exposed to fumes of burning sulphur. When the ends of the stalks shrivel, they are removed from the kiln and laid on a woodenfloor till quite cool, when they are packed in bales, known as 'pockets.'

The difficulties attendant upon the cultivation of Hops have been aggravated and the expenses increased in recent years by the regularly recurring attacks of aphis blight, due to the insect Aphis humuli, which make it necessary to spray or syringe every Hop plant, every branch and leaf with insecticidal solutions three or four times and sometimes more often in each season. Quassia and soft soap solutions are usually employed: the soft soap serves as a vehicle to retain the bitterness of the quassia upon the bines and leaves, making them repulsive to the Aphides, which are thus starved out. The solution is made from 4 to 8 lb. of quassia chips to 100 gallons of water.

Another pest, the Red Spider (Tetranychus telarius) is most destructive in very hot summers. Congregating on the under surfaces of the leaves, the red spiders exhaust the sap and cause the leaves to fall. The Quassia and Soft Soap Hopwash is of little avail in the case of Red Spider. Some success has attended the use of a solution consisting of 8 to 10 lb. of soft soap to 100 gallons of water, with 3 pints of paraffin added. It must be applied with great force, to break through the webs with which the spiders protect themselves.

Hop washing is done by means of large garden engines worked by hand or by horseengines: even steam-engines have sometimes been employed.

Among fungoid parasites, Mould or Mildew is frequently the cause of loss to Hop planters. It is due to the action of the fungus Podosphaera castagnei, and the mischief is more especially that done to the cones. The remedy is sulphur, employed usually in the form of flowers of sulphur, from 40 to 60 lb. per acre being applied at each sulphuring, distributed by means of a blast pipe. The first sulphuring takes place when the plants are fairly up the poles and is repeated three or four weeks later, and even again if indications of mildew are present. Sulphur is also successfully employed in the form of an alkaline sulphur, such as a solution of liver of sulphur, a variety of potassium sulphide.

Parts Used Medicinally

(a) The strobiles, collected and dried as described. (b) The Lupulin, separated from the strobiles by sifting.

Chemical Constituents

The aromatic odor of the Hop strobiles is due to a volatile oil, of which they yield about 0.3 to 1.0 per cent. It appears to consist chiefly of the sesquiterpene Humulene. Petroleum spirit extracts 7 to 14 per cent of a powerfully antiseptic soft resin, and ether extracts a hard resin. The petroleum spirit extract contains the two crystalline bitter principles (a) Lupamaric acid (Humulone), (b) Lupamaric acid (Lupulinic acid). These bodies are chiefly contained in the glands at the base of the bracts. The leafy organs contain about 5 per cent of tannin which is not a constituent of the glands. Hops yield about 7 per cent Ash.

The oil and the bitter principle combine to make Hops more useful than Chamomile, Gentian or any other bitter in the manufacture of beer: hence the medicinal value of extra-hopped or bitter beer. The tannic acid contained in the strobiles adds to the value of Hops by causing precipitation of vegetable mucilage and consequently the cleansing of beer.

Fresh Hops possess a bitter aromatic taste and a strong characteristic odor. The latter, however, changes and becomes distinctly unpleasant as the Hops are kept. This change is ascribed to oxidation of the soft resin with production of Valerianic acid. On account of the rapid change in the odor of Hops, the recently dried fruits should alone be used: these may be recognized by the characteristic odor and distinctly green color. Those which have been subjected to the treatment of sulphuring are not to be used in pharmacy. This process is conducted with a view of improving the color and odor of the Hops, since sulphuric acid is found to retard the production of the Valerianic odor and to both preserve and improve the color of the Hops.

Lupulin, which consists of the glandular powder present on the seeds and surface of the scales, may be separated by shaking the strobiles. The drug occurs in a granular, brownish-yellow powder, with the strong odor and bitter aromatic taste characteristic of Hops. The glands readily burst on the application of slight pressure and discharge their granular oleo-resinous contents. Commercial Lupulin is often of a very inferior quality, and consists of the sifted sweepings from the floors of hop-kilns. It should contain not more than 40 per cent of matter insoluble in ether and not yield more than 12 per cent of ash on incineration. A dark color and disagreeable odor indicates an old drug.

The chief constituent of Lupulin is about 3 per cent of volatile oil, which consists chiefly of Humulene, together with various oxygenated bodies to which the oil owes its peculiar odor. Other constituents are the two Lupamaric acids, cholene and resin.

Lupulin is official both in the British Pharmacopoeia and the United States Pharmacopoeia.

Medicinal Action and Uses

Hops have tonic, nervine, diuretic and anodyne properties. Their volatile oil produces sedative and soporific effects, and the Lupamaric acid or bitter principle is stomachic and tonic. For this reason Hops improve the appetite and promote sleep.

The official preparations are an infusion and a tincture. The infusion is employed as a vehicle, especially for bitters and tonics: the tincture is stomachic and is used to improve the appetite and digestion. Both preparations have been considered to be sedative, were formerly much given in nervousness and hysteria and at bedtime to induce sleep; in cases of nervousness, delirium and inflammation being considered to produce a most soothing effect, frequently procuring for the patient sleep after long periods of sleeplessness in overwrought conditions of the brain.

The bitter principle in the Hop proves one of the most efficacious vegetable bitters obtainable. An infusion of 1/2 oz. Hops to 1 pint of water will be found the proper quantity for ordinary use. It has proved of great service also in heart disease, fits, neuralgia and nervous disorders, besides being a useful tonic in indigestion, jaundice, and stomach and liver affections generally. It gives prompt ease to an irritable bladder, and is said to be an excellent drink in cases of delirium tremens. Sherry in which some Hops have been steeped makes a capital stomachic cordial.

A pillow of warm Hops will often relieve toothache and earache and allay nervous irritation.

An infusion of the leaves, strobiles and stalks, as Hop Tea, taken by the wine glassful two or three times daily in the early spring, is good for sluggish livers. Hop Tea in the leaf, as frequently sold by grocers, consists of Kentish Hop leaves, dried, crushed under rollers and then mixed with ordinary Ceylon or Indian Tea. The infusion combines the refreshment of the one herb with the sleepinducing virtues of the other.

Hop juice cleanses the blood, and for calculus trouble nothing better can be found than the bitter principle of the Hop. A decoction of the root has been esteemed as of equal benefit with Sarsaparilla.

As an external remedy, an infusion of Hops is much in demand in combination with chamomile flowers or poppy heads as a fomentation for swelling of a painful nature, inflammation, neuralgic and rheumatic pains, bruises, boils and gatherings. It removes pain and allays inflammation in a very short time. The Hops may also be applied as a poultice.

The drug Lupulin is an aromatic bitter and is reputed to be midly sedative, inducing sleep without causing headache.

It is occasionally administered as a hypnotic, either in pills with alcohol, or enclosed in a cachet.

Preparations of Lupulin are not much used in this country, although official, but in the United States they are considered preferable for internal use.

Recipes for Herb Beers

Formerly every farmhouse inn had a brewing plant and brewhouse attached to the buildings, and all brewed their own beer till the large breweries were established and supplanted home-brewed beers. Many of these farmhouses then began to brew their own 'stingo' from wayside herbs, employing old rustic recipes that had been carried down from generation to generation. The true value of vegetable bitters and of herb beers have yet to be recognized by all sections of the community. Workmen in puddling furnaces and potteries in the Midland and Northern counties find, however, that a tea made of tonic herbs is cheaper and less intoxicating than ordinary beer and patronize the herb beers freely, Dandelion Stout ranking as one of the favorites. It is also made in Canada.

Dandelion is a good ingredient in many digestive or diet drinks. A dinner drink may be made as follows: Take 2 OZ. each of dried Dandelion and Nettle herbs and 1 OZ. of Yellow Dock. Boil in 1 gallon of water for 15 minutes and then strain the liquor while hot on to 2 Lb. of sugar, on the top of which is sprinkled 2 tablespoonsful of powdered Ginger. Leave till milk-warm, then add boiled water gone cold to bring the quantity up to 2 gallons. The temperature must then not be above 75 degrees F. Now dissolve 1/2 oz. solid yeast in a little of the liquid and stir into the bulk. Allow to ferment 24 hours, skim and bottle, and it will be ready for use in a day or two.

A good, pleasant-tasting botanic beer is also made of the Nettle alone. Quantities of the young fresh tops are boiled in a gallon of water, with the juice of two lemons, a teaspoonful of crushed ginger and 1 Lb. of brown sugar. Fresh yeast is floated on toast in the liquor, when cold, to ferment it, and when it is bottled the result is a specially wholesome sort of ginger beer.

Meadow Sweet was also formerly much in favour. The mash when worked with barm made a pleasant drink, either in the harvest field or at the table. It required little sugar, some even made it without any sugar at all.

Another favorite brew was that of armsful of Meadowsweet, Yarrow, Dandelion and Nettles, and the mash when 'sweetened with old honey' and well worked with barm, and then bottled in big stoneware bottles, made a drink strong enough to turn even an old toper's head.

Old honeycomb from the thatch of an ancient cottage, filled with rich and nearly black honey, when boiled into syrup and then strained, was used in the making of herb beer, while the wax was put at the mouths of the hives for the bees.

Dandelion, Meadowsweet and Agrimony, equal quantities of each, would also be boiled together for 20 minutes (about 2 OZ. each of the dried herbs to 2 gallons of water), then strained and 2 lb. of sugar and 1/2 pint of barm or yeast added. This was bottled after standing in a warm place for 12 hours. This recipe is still in use.

A Herb Beer that needs no yeast is made from equal quantities of Meadowsweet, Betony, Agrimony and Raspberry leaves (2 OZ. of each) boiled in 2 gallons of water for 15 minutes, strained, then 2 lb. of white sugar added and bottled when nearly cool.

In some outlying islands of the Hebrides there is still brewed a drinkable beer by making two-thirds Heath tops with one-third of malt.

HOP BITTERS, as an appetiser, to be taken in tablespoonful doses three times in the day before eating, may be made as follows: Take 2 OZ. of Buchu leaves and 1/2 lb. of Hops. Boil these in 5 quarts of water in an iron vessel for an hour. When lukewarm add essence of Winter green (Pyrola) 2 OZ. and 1 pint alcohol.

Another way of making Hop Bitters is to take 1/2 oz. Hops, 1 OZ. Angelica Herb and 1 OZ. Holy Thistle. Pour 3 pints of boiling water on them and strain when cold. A wine glassful may be taken four times a day.

To make a good HOP BEER, put 2 OZ. Hops in 2 quarts of water for 15 minutes. Then strain and dissolve 1 lb. of sugar in the liquor. To this add 4 quarts of cold water and 2 tablespoonsful of fresh barm. Allow to stand for 12 hours in a warm place and it will then be ready for bottling.

HOREHOUND, WHITE

Botanical: Marrubium vulgare (LINN.)
Family: N.O. Labiatae
Synonym: Hoarhound.
Part Used: Herb.

Habitat

White Horehound is a perennial herbaceous plant, found all over Europe and indigenous to Britain. Like many other plants of the Labiate tribe, it flourishes in waste places and by roadsides, particularly in the counties of Norfolk and Suffolk, where it is also cultivated in the corners of cottage gardens for making tea and candy for use in coughs and colds. It is also brewed and made into Horehound Ale, an appetizing and healthful beverage, much drunk in Norfolk and other country districts.

DESCRIPTION

The plant is bushy, producing numerous annual, quadrangular and branching stems, a foot or more in height, on which the whitish flowers are borne in crowded, axillary, woolly whorls. The leaves are much wrinkled, opposite, petiolate, about 1 inch long, covered with white, felted hairs, which give them a woolly appearance. They have a curious, musky smell, which is diminished by drying and lost on keeping. Horehound flowers from June to September.

The Romans esteemed Horehound for its medicinal properties, and its Latin name of Marrubium is said to be derived from Maria urbs, an ancient town of Italy. Other authors derive its name from the Hebrew marrob (a bitter juice), and state that it was one of the bitter herbs which the Jews were ordered to take for the Feast of Passover.

The Egyptian Priests called this plant the 'Seed of Horus,' or the 'Bull's Blood,' and the 'Eye of the Star.' It was a principal ingredient in the negro Caesar's antidote for vegetable poisons.

Gerard recommends it, in addition to its uses in coughs and colds, to 'those that have drunk poyson or have been bitten of serpents,' and it was also administered for 'mad dogge's biting.'

It was once regarded as an anti-magical herb.

According to Columella, Horehound is a serviceable remedy against Cankerworm in trees, and it is stated that if it be put into new milk and set in a place pestered with flies, it will speedily kill them all.

CULTIVATION

White Horehound is a hardy plant, easily grown, and flourishes best in a dry, poor soil. It can be propagated from seeds sown in spring, cuttings, or by dividing the roots (the most usual method). If raised from seed, the seedlings should be planted out in the spring, in rows, with a space of about 9 inches or more between each plant. No further culture will be needed than weeding. It does not blossom until it is two years old.

Until recently, it was chiefly collected in Southern France, where it is much cultivated. It is in steady demand, and it would probably pay to cultivate it more in this country.

White Horehound is distinguished from other species by its woolly stem, the densely felted hairs on the leaves, and the tentoothed teeth of the calyx.

CONSTITUENTS

The chief constituent is a bitter principle known as Marrubium, with a little volatile oil, resin, tannin, wax, fat, sugar, etc.

MEDICINAL ACTION AND USES

White Horehound has long been noted for its efficacy in lung troubles and coughs. Gerard says of this plant:

'Syrup made of the greene fresh leaves and sugar is a most singular remedie against the cough and wheezing of the lungs . . . and doth wonderfully and above credit ease such as have been long sicke of any consumption of the lungs, as hath beene often proved by the learned physitions of our London College.'

And Culpepper says:

'It helpeth to expectorate tough phlegm from the chest, being taken with the roots of Irris or Orris.... There is a syrup made of this plant which I would recommend as an excellent help to evacuate tough phlegm and cold rheum from the lungs of aged persons, especially those who are asthmatic and short winded.'

Preparations of Horehound are still largely used as expectorants and tonics. It may, indeed, be considered one of the most popular pectoral remedies, being given with benefit for chronic cough, asthma, and some cases of consumption.

Horehound is sometimes combined with Hyssop, Rue, Liquorice root and Marshmallow root, 1/2 oz. of each boiled in 2 pints of water, to 1 1/2 pint, strained and given in 1/2 teacupful doses, every two to three hours.

For children's coughs and croup, it is given to advantage in the form of syrup, and is a most useful medicine for children, not only for the complaints mentioned, but as a tonic and a corrective of the stomach. It has quite a pleasant taste.

Taken in large doses, it acts as a gentle purgative.

The powdered leaves have also been employed as a vermifuge and the green leaves, bruised and boiled in lard, are made into an ointment which is good for wounds.

For ordinary cold, a simple infusion of Horehound (Horehound Tea) is generally sufficient in itself. The tea may be made by pouring boiling water on the fresh or dried leaves, 1 OZ. of the herb to the pint. A wine glassful may be taken three or four times a day.

Candied Horehound is best made from the fresh plant by boiling it down until the juice is extracted, then adding sugar before boiling this again, until it has become thick enough in consistence to pour into a paper case and be cut into squares when cool.

Two or three teaspoonsful of the expressed juice of the herb may also be given as a dose in severe colds.

Preparations and Dosages

Fluid extract, 1/2 to 1 drachm. Syrup, 2 to 4 drachms. Solid extract, 5 to 15 grains.

HOREHOUND, BLACK

Botanical: Ballota nigra (LINN.)
Family: N.O. Labiatae
Synonyms: Marrubium nigrum. Black Stinking Horehound.
Part Used: Herb.

Description

Black Horehound is distinguished by its disagreeable odor. It also belongs to the Labiatae order, among which it is distinguished by the strongly ten-ribbed salver-shaped calyx. The Ballota are natives of the temperate regions of the Eastern Hemisphere, and are remarkable for their strong offensive odor, on account of which they are for the most part rejected by cattle; hence the name from the Greek ballo (to reject). This plant (Ballota nigra) is sometimes given the opprobrious name of 'Black Stinking Horehound.' It is a common wayside perennial, has stout-branched stems, eggshaped wrinkled leaves, and whorls of numerous dull purple flowers.

The whole plant is as offensive in odor as it is unattractive in appearance. It is mostly found growing near towns and villages, and has accompanied our colonists to many remote countries.

It has a perennial root of a woody and fibrous nature. The leaves are arranged in pairs on the stem, each pair being at right angles to the pair it succeeds. They are stalked, with margins coarsely serrate, dull green in color, their surfaces clothed with soft grey hairs, and with rather conspicuous veining.

The flowers are arranged in more or less dense whorls at the axils of the leaves; their color occasionally varies to white.

The corolla of the Horehound has its upper lip erect and slightly concave, and the lower lip cleft into three, the lateral lobes being considerably smaller than the central ones. The calyx is tubular, its mouth having five short spreading teeth terminating in a stiff bristly point. The body of the calyx is sharply ridged and furrowed.

It is found in flower from June to October. The name ballote was given to this plant as early as the time of Dioscorides.

It has been suggested that the name Horehound came from two Anglo-Saxon words signifying the hoary honey-yielding plant; but other authorities find other derivations.

Dioscorides (like Gerard) declared that the Ballota was an antidote for the bite of a mad dog.

Beaumont and Fletcher's Faithful Shepherdess has a reference to this property of the plant:

'This is the clote bearing a yellow flower,
And this black horehound: both are very good

For sheep or shepherd bitten by a wood-Dog's venom'd tooth.'

Medicinal Action and Uses

Antispasmodic, stimulant and vermifuge.

Preparation

Liquid extract.

HORSENETTLE

Botanical: Solanum carolinense (LINN.)
Family: N.O. Solanaceae
Synonyms: Bull Nettle. Treadfoot. Sand Brier. Apple of Sodom. Poisonous Potato.
Parts Used: Air-dried ripe berries, root.

Habitat

United States of America. This weed is a hardy, coarse perennial, found growing in waste sandy ground as far west as Iowa and south to Florida.

Description

Bears orange yellow berries which is the most active part of the plant, they are glabrous and fleshy, with an odor like pepper, taste, bitter and acrid.

Constituents

Probably Solanine and Solanidine and an organic acid.

Medicinal Action and Uses

Sedative, antispasmodic; has long been used by the Southern negroes in the treatment ofepilepsy; is a useful remedy in infantile convulsions and menstrual hysteria, has no unpleasant effects, but its usefulness is said to be limited, unless given with bromides.

Preparations and Dosages

Fluid drachm three times a day. Berries are given in doses of 5 to 60 grains. Root, 10 grains.

HORSERADIS

Botanical:Cochlearia Armoracia (LINN.)
Family: N.O. Cruciferae
Synonyms: Mountain Radish. Great Raifort. Red Cole.
Part Used: Root.

Habitat

This plant has been in cultivation from the earliest times, but its exact place of origin seems to be obscure. Hooker considers that it is possibly a cultivated form of Cochlearia macrocarpa, a native of Hungary; other authorities consider it indigenous to the eastern parts of Europe, from the Caspian and through Russia and Poland to Finland. In Britain and other parts of Europe from Sicily northwards, it occurs cultivated, or semi-wild as a garden escape. It is probably the plant mentioned by Pliny under the name of Amoracia, and recommended by him for its medicinal qualities, being then apparently employed exclusively in physic, not as food or condiment It is possible that the Wild Radish, or Raphanos agrios of the Greeks was this plant It is said to be one of the five bitter herbs, with Coriander, Horehound, Lettuce and Nettle. which the Jews were made to eat during the Feast of Passover.

Both the root and leaves of Horseradish were universally used as a medicine during the Middle Ages, and as a condiment in Denmark and Germany. It was known in England as 'Red Cole' in the time of Turner (1548), but is not mentioned by him as a condiment. Gerard (1597), who describes it under the name of Raphanus rusticanus, states that it occurs wild in several parts of England, and after referring to its medicinal uses, goes on to say:

'the Horse Radish stamped with a little vinegar put thereto, is commonly used among the Germans for sauce to eate fish with and such like meates as we do mustarde,'

showing that the custom was unfamiliar to his countrymen, with whom the root had not yet passed from a drug to a condiment. He mentions this plant as an illustration of the old idea of 'Antipathies,' saying:

'Divers thinke that this Horse Radish is an enimie to Vines, and that the hatred between them is so great, that if the rootes heerof be planted neere to the vine, it bendeth backward from it as not willing to have fellowship with it.'

Nearly half a century later, the taste for Horseradish as a condiment had spread to England, for Parkinson, writing in 1640, describes its use as a sauce 'with country people and strong labouring men in some countries of Germany,' and adds 'and in our owne land also, but, as I said, it is too strong for tender and gentle stomaches,' and a few years later, in 1657, Coles states as a commonly-known fact, 'that the root, sliced thin and mixed with vinegar is eaten as a sauce with meat, as among the Germans.' That the use of Horseradish in France was in like manner a custom adopted from their neighbours, is proved by its old French name, Moutarde des Allemands.

The root was included in the Materia Medica of the London Pharmacopoeias of the eighteenth century, under the name of R. rusticanus, the same name Gerard gave it. Its present botanical name, Cochlearia Armoracia, was given it by Linnaeus, Cochleare being the name of an old-fashioned spoon to which its long leaves are supposed to bear a resemblance. The popular English name, Horseradish, means a coarse radish, to distinguish it from the edible radish (R. sativus), the prefix 'Horse' being often used thus, comp. Horse-Mint, Horse Chestnut. It was formerly also known as the Mountain Radish and Great Raifort.

The common Scurvy-grass (C. officinalis) is of the same genus, as are also the English Scurvy-grass (C. Anglica) and the Danish Scurvy-grass (C. Danica).

Cultivation

To grow fine Horseradish roots a plot of tilled ground must be chosen, manure being placed 18 to 24 inches deep; the ground in which they are planted ought to be very rich, or they will not thrive.

In order to obtain good sticks for winter an early start must be made, and some time in January the ground should be deeply dug. Planting is carried out in February by means of root cuttings, straight, young roots, 8 or 9 inches long, and about 1/2 inch wide being chosen, each having a crown or growing point. Make deep holes with the dibber, 12 to 15 inches deep and 12 to 18 inches apart each way; carefully divest the sets of all side roots and drop each in a hole, trickling a little fine soil round them before filling up the holes firmly. Beyond hoeing to keep the soil clear of weeds, no further care is needed.

During winter, the crop may either be lifted or stored like Beetroot, or the roots be lifted as required. In the latter case, the ground must be protected in frosty weather. The roots may be preserved for some time in their juicy state by putting them in dry sand.

It is necessary every few years to replant the bed, otherwise the crop deteriorates. The plants will stand through two seasons without deterioration. They may either be replanted elsewhere or another bed made on the same site, just as may be expedient. When it is desired to destroy plantations of Horseradish, it is absolutely necessary to rid the soil of even the smallest particle of root: if this is not done, much annoyance will be caused the following summer.

Part Used

The root is the only part now used, and in the fresh state only. It is nearly cylindrical, except at the crown, where it is somewhat enlarged.

Constituents

When unbroken, it is inodorous, but exhales a characteristic pungent odor when scraped or bruised, and has a hot, biting taste, combined with a certain sweetness. It has properties very similar to Black Mustard seeds, containing Sinigrin, a crystalline glucoside, which is decomposed in the presence of water by Myrosin, an enzyme found also in the root, the chief produce being the volatile oil Allyl, isothiocyanate, which is identical with that of Black Mustard seed. This volatile oil, which is easily developed by scraping the root when in a fresh state, does not preexist in the root, the reaction not taking place in the root under normal conditions, because the Sinigrin and Myrosin exist in separate cells, and it is only the bruising of the cells that brings their contents together.

The oil is highly diffusible and pungent on account of the Myrosin contained, 1 drop being sufficient to odorize the atmosphere of a whole room. On exposure to the air, the root quickly turns color and loses its volatile strength. It likewise becomes vapid and inert by being boiled. It contains also a bitter resin, sugar, starch, gum, albumin and acetates.

Medicinal Action and Uses

Stimulant, aperient, rubefacient, diuretic and antiseptic. It is a powerful stimulant, whether applied internally or externally as a rubefacient, and has aperient and antiseptic properties. Taken with oily fish or rich meat, either by itself or steeped in vinegar, or in a plain sauce, it acts as an excellent stimulant to the digestive organs, and as a spur to complete digestion.

It is a very strong diuretic, and was employed by old herbalists in calculus and like affections. It is useful in the treatment of dropsy. Boerhaave recommended it to be given in scurvy when there was not much fever, and administered it for various other complaints.

An infusion for dropsy is prepared by pouring 1 pint of boiling water on 1 OZ. of Horseradish and 1/2 oz. of Mustard seed, crushed. The dose is 2 to 3 tablespoonsful three times a day.

The chief official preparation of Horseradish in the British Pharmacopoeia is Comp. Sp. Horseradish; a fluid extract is also prepared. A compound spirit of Horseradish may be prepared with slices of the fresh root, orange peel, nutmeg and spirit of wine, which proves effective in languid digestion, as well as for chronic rheumatism, 1 or 2 teaspoonsful being taken two or three times daily after meals with half a wine glassful of water.

The root is expectorant, antiscorbutic, and if taken too freely, emetic. It contains so much sulphur that it is serviceable used externally as a rubefacient in chronic rheumatism and in paralytic complaints. Culpepper says.: 'If bruised and laid to a part grieved with the sciatica, gout, joint-ache or hard swellings of the spleen and liver, it doth wonderfully help them all.' A poultice of the scraped root serves instead of a mustard plaister. Scraped horseradish if applied to chilblains, secured with a light bandage, will help to cure them. For facial neuralgia, some of the fresh scrapings, if held in the hand of the affected side, will give relief - the hand in some cases within a short time becoming bloodlessly white and benumbed.

When infused in wine, Horseradish root will stimulate the whole nervous system and promote perspiration.

An infusion of sliced Horseradish in milk, by its stimulating pungency and the sulphur it contains, makes an excellent cosmetic for the skin when lacking clearness and freshness of color. Horseradish juice mixed with white vinegar will also, applied externally, help to remove freckles. The same mixture, well diluted with water and sweetened with glycerine, gives marked relief to children in whooping-cough, 1 or 2 desertspoonsful being taken at a time. Horseradish syrup is very effectual in hoarseness: 1 drachm of the root, fresh scraped, with 4 oz. of water, is infused two hours in a close vessel and made into a syrup with double its weight in sugar. The dose is a teaspoonful or two, occasionally repeated.

If eaten at frequent intervals during the day and at meals, Horseradish is said to be most efficacious in getting rid of the persistent cough following influenza.

Horseradish was formerly much employed as a remedy for worms in children. Coles says: 'Of all things given to children for worms, horseradish is not the least, for it soon killeth and expelleth them.'

Preparations and Dosages

Fluid extract, 1/2 to 1 drachm. Comp. Spirit of Horseradish, B.P., 1 to 2 drachms.

HORSETAILS

Botanical: Equisetum arvense, Equisetum hyemale, Equisetum maximum, Equisetum sylvaticum
Family: N.O. Equisetaceae
Synonyms: Shave-grass. Bottle-brush. Paddock-pipes. Dutch Rushes. Pewterwort.
Part Used: Herb.

Habitat

They are chiefly distributed in the temperate northern regions: seven of the twenty-five known species are British, the most frequent being Equisetum arvense, E. sylvaticum, E. maximum and E. hyemale. E. arvense, the CORN HORSETAIL, is a very troublesome weed, most difficult to extirpate from cultivated land. Many of the species are very variable.

The Horsetails belong to a class of plants, the Equisetaceae, that has no direct affinity with any other group of British plants. They are nearest allied to the Ferns. The class includes only a single genus, Equisetum, the name derived from the Latin words equus (a horse) and seta (a bristle), from the peculiar bristly appearance of the jointed stems of the plants, which have also earned them their popular names of Horsetail, Bottle-brush and Paddock-pipes.

Large plants of this order probably formed a great proportion of the vegetation during the carboniferous period, the well-known fossils Calamites being the stems of gigantic fossil Equisetaceae, which in this period attained their maximum development - those now existing being mere dwarfish representatives.

The Equisetaceae have an external resemblance in habit to Casuarina or Ephedra, and as regards the heads of fructification to Zamia (a genus of Cycadaceae). The Casuarina have very much the appearance of gigantic Horsetails, being trees with threadlike, jointed, furrowed, pendent branches without leaves, but with small toothed sheaths at the joints. They are met with most abundantly in tropical Australia, less frequently in the Indian Islands, New Caledonia, etc. In Australia they are said by Dr. Bennett to be called Oaks. The wood is used for fires, as it burns readily and the ashes retain the heat for a long time. The wood is much valued for steam-engines, ovens, etc., and the timber furnished by these trees is appreciated for its extreme hardness. From its color it is called in the Colonies 'Beefwood.'

Though mostly inhabitants of watery places, flourishing where they can lodge their perennial roots in water or string clay which holds the wet, the Equisetums will grow in a garden near water, under a wall, or in the shade and will spread rapidly.

Description

The stems spring from a creeping rhizome, or root-stock, which produces at its joints a number of roots. Two kinds of stems are produced fertile and barren: they are erect, jointed, brittle and grooved, hollow except at the joints and with air-cells in their walls under the grooves. There are no leaves, the joints terminating in toothed sheathes, the teeth corresponding with the ridges and representing leaves. Branches, if present, arise from the sheathbases and are solid. In most cases, the fertile or fruiting stem is unbranched and withers in spring, almost before the barren fronds appear. It bears a terminal cone-like catkin, consisting of numerous closely-packed peltae, upon the under margins of which are the sporanges, containing microscopic spores, attached to elastic threads, which are coiled round the spore when moist and uncoil when dry.

The development of young Horsetails from the spores is similar to that of Ferns, germination and impregnation being effected in the same manner. The Equisitaceae are also propagated in a vegetative nonsexual manner by means of subterranean stolons and by tubers.

The barren summer fronds give off numerous, slender, jointed branches in whorls of about a dozen; in some British species, the fruiting and barren stems are often both unbranched.

A quantity of silica is deposited in the stems, especially in the epidermis or outer skin. In one species, E. hyemale (Linn.), the epidermis contains so much silica that bunches of the stem have been sold for polishing metal and used to be imported from Holland for the purpose, hence the popular name of Dutch Rushes. It is also called Scouring Rush, and by old writers Shavegrass, and was formerly much used by white smiths and cabinet-makers. Gerard tells us that in his time it was employed for scouring pewter and wooden kitchen utensils, and thence called Pewterwort, and that fletchers and combmakers rubbed and polished their work with it, and long after his day, the dairymaids of the northern counties of England used it for scouring their milk-pails. Linnaeus tells us that this species, among others, forms excellent food for horses in some parts of Sweden, but that cows are apt to lose their teeth by feeding on it and to be afflicted with diarrhrea. As a matter of fact, cattle, in this country, usually instinctively avoid these plants and would probably only eat them in the absence of better fodder.

The young shoots of the larger species of Horsetail, especially E. maximum (Lamk.) the E. fluviatile of Linnaeus - were formerly said to be eaten, dressed like asparagus, or fried with flour and butter. It is recorded that the poorer classes among the Romans occasionally ate them as a vegetable, but they are neither palatable nor very nutritious. Linnaeus stated that the reindeer, who refuses ordinary hay, will eat this kind of Horsetail, which is about 3 feet high and juicy, and that it is cut as fodder in the north of Sweden for cows, with a view to increasing their milk, but that horses will not touch it.

Several of the species have been used medicinally, and the older herbalists considered them useful vulneraries, and recommended them for consumption and dysentery. The FIELD HORSETAIL (E. arvense), the species of British Horsetail most commonly met with, is the one now generally collected and sold for medicinal purposes . It is common in cornfields and wet meadows, its presence being supposed to indicate subterranean, flowing waters or springs. In this species, the fruiting stems are simple, very rarely branched, appearing early in spring and soon decaying. The barren stems which appear later are branched, six to nineteen grooved, the angles rough and sharp, and terminate generally in a long, naked point; the joints are about 1 inch long and 1/24 to 1/16 inch in diameter, the teeth of the sheaths long and acute. The shoots have neither color nor taste. The fertile stems are yellowish, shorter and stouter, somewhat succulent, with only two to five joints.

In warmer climates, and even in Lisbon, as E. debile and elongatum, they require the support of bushes to which they cling. They sometimes attain a great size as does E. giganteum, though they never reach the dimensions of the fossil Equisetaceae.

The rhizomes contain a considerable quantity of starch-cells.

E. sylvaticum, the WOOD HORSETAIL, which grows in copses and on hedgebanks, has slender, angular stems, 1 to 2 feet high, nearly smooth, ten to eighteen grooved. It is readily recognized by the elegant appearance of the whorls of recurved branches, generally twelve or more branches to a whorl, which are very slender, about 5 inches long, quadrangular and beset by several secondary whorls so that the plant resembles a miniature pine tree. The cones of the fertile stems are 3/4 to 1 inch long.

It is this species that Linnaeus informs us is a principal food for horses in some parts of Sweden. It is used medicinally in the same manner as the preceding species.

E. maximum, the GREAT or RIVER HORSETAIL, already mentioned, is found in bogs, ditches, and on the banks of rivers and ponds. It is the largest of the European species, the barren stems attaining a height of from 3 to 6 feet, sometimes nearly an inch in diameter. They are twenty to forty grooved, with numerous joints, pale in color and smooth, the branchlets quadrangular. The fertile stems are quite short, only 8 to 10 inches high, but thicker; their cones, 2 to 3 inches long.

Part Used Medicinally

The barren stems only are used medicinally, appearing after the fruiting stems have died down, and are used in their entirety, cut off just above the root. The herb is used either fresh or dried, but is said to be most efficacious when fresh. A fluid extract is prepared from it. The ashes of the plant are also employed.

Medicinal Action and Uses

Diuretic and astringent. Horsetail has been found beneficial in dropsy, gravel and kidney affections generally, and a drachm of the dried herb, powdered, taken three or four times a day, has proved very effectual in spitting of blood.

The ashes of the plant are considered very valuable in acidity of the stomach, dyspepsia, etc., administered in doses of 3 to 10 grains.

Besides being useful in kidney and bladder trouble, a strong decoction acts as an emmenagogue; being cooling and astringent, it is of efficacy for hemorrhage, cystic ulceration and ulcers in the urinary passages.

The decoction applied externally will stop the bleeding of wounds and quickly heal them, and will also reduce the swelling of eyelids.

Preparation and Dosage

Fluid extract, 10 to 60 drops.

Horsetail was formerly official under the name of Cauda equina and was much esteemed as an astringent. Culpepper quotes Galen in saying that it will heal sinews, 'though they be cut in sunder,' and speaks of it highly for bleeding of the nose, a use to which it is still put by country people.

Culpepper says:

'It is very powerful to stop bleeding, either inward or outward, the juice or the decoction being drunk, or the juice, decoction or distilled water applied outwardly... It also heals inward ulcers.... It solders together the tops of green wounds and cures all ruptures in children. The decoction taken in wine helps stone and strangury; the distilled water drunk two or three times a day eases and strengthens the intestines and is effectual in a cough that comes by distillation from the head. The juice or distilled water used as a warm fomentation is of service in inflammations and breakings-out in the skin.'

HOUND'S TONGUE

Botanical: Cynoglossum officinale (LINN.)
Family: N.O. Boraginaceae
Synonyms: Lindefolia spectabilis. Dog's Tongue.
Part Used: Herb.

Hound's Tongue is a rough, bristly perennial, belonging to the Borage tribe. Its scientific name of Cynoglossum is derived from the Greek, and signifies ' Dog's Tongue,' from the shape and texture of the leaves, under which name, and still more frequently as Hound's Tongue, it is properly known.

It is a stout, herbaceous plant, found occasionally in this country on waste ground, though more frequently on the Continent, especially in Switzerland and Germany.

The stem, hairy and leafy, 1 to 2 feet high, branched above, arises from amidst large, narrow, radical, stalked leaves.

In Culpepper's days, the root was also used in decoction and as pills for coughs, colds in the head and shortness of breath, and the leaves were boiled in wine as a cure for dysentery. He also tells us:

'Bruising the leaves or the juice of them boiled in hog's lard and applied helpeth to preserve the hair from falling and easeth the pain of a scald or burn. A bruised leaf laid to a green wound speedily heals the same. The baked roots are good for piles, also the distilled water of the herb and root is used with good effect for all the aforesaid purposes, taken inwardly or applied outwardly, especially as a wash for wounds or punctures.'

Gerard says of this plant: 'It will tye the tongues of Houndes so that they shall not bark at you, if it be laid under the bottom of your feet,' and in his days the ointment and decoction were very generally reputed to be a cure for the bites of mad dogs.

In modern medicine it is often used internally and externally to relieve piles. It is soothing to the digestive organs.

HOUSELEEK

Botanical: Sempervivum tectorum (LINN.)
Family: N.O. Crassulaceae
Synonyms: Jupiter's Eye. Thor's Beard. Jupiter's Beard. Bullock's Eye. Sengreen. Ayron. Ayegreen.

Part Used: Fresh leaves.

The Houseleek was dedicated of old to Jupiter or Thor, and bore also the names of Jupiter's Eye, Thor's Beard, Jupiter's Beard, Barba Jovis (in France, Joubarbe des toits), from its massive clusters of flowers, which were supposed to resemble the beard of Jupiter. The German name of Donnersoart and the English Thunderbeard have the same meaning, being derived from Jupiter the Thunderer.

It was in high esteem among the Romans, who grew it in vases before their houses.

It is not really indigenous to this country, being a native of the mountain ranges of Central and Southern Europe and of the Greek islands, but it was introduced into Great Britain many centuries ago and is now found abundantly throughout the country, its large rosettes of fleshy leaves being a familiar sight on many an old cottage roof.

The word Leek is from the Anglo-Saxon leac, a plant, so that Houseleek means literally the House Plant. It was also called, in the fourteenth century, Ayron, Ayegreen and Sengreen, i.e. Evergreen.

The generic name Sempervivum, from the Latin semper (always) and vivo (I live), refers to its retention of vitality under almost all conditions, and the specific name tectorum bears witness to its usual place of growth - a roof.

It was supposed to guard what it grows upon against fire and lightning, and we read that Charlemagne ordered it to be planted upon the roof of every house, probably with this view. Whatever the origin of the custom, it prevails in many other parts of Europe, as well as in England and France. Welsh peasants believe it protects their houses from storms, and ensures the prosperity of their inmates. Superstitious country-folk in Wiltshire are often found to have a strong objection to the removal of a plant of Houseleek from their roof, or even to the plucking of the flowers by a stranger, believing it will bring death to the dwellers; it was formerly believed to be an efficient guard against sorcery as well as against lightning.

The root is perennial and is fibrous. The thick succulent leaves enable the plant to retain vitality even in the driest weather, acting as reservoirs of moisture. The leaves, arising directly from the root, grow in compact, rose-like tufts, 2 to 4 inches in diameter. They are extremely fleshy and juicy, flat, 1 to 2 inches long, sessile, oblong, though broader towards the middle of the rosette, sharply pointed, and the edges fringed with hairs and of a purple color.

The flowers are produced in July, but generally very sparingly. The flower-stems do not arise from the rosettes of leaves, but are on separate, upright shoots, which are from 9 inches to a foot or more in height, round, fleshy and stout, slightly downy, with the leaves scattered thickly on them. The flowers are clustered together on only one side of the stem and are numerous, 2/3 to 1 inch in diameter, of a dull, pale red-purple. Like other flowers in this genus they are absolutely regular and symmetrical throughout, the sepals, petals and pistils being all of the same number - twelve in this species - and the stamens just twice as many, twentyfour in this case, twelve of which are arranged alternately with the petals and are imperfect, frequently bearing in their anthers instead of pollen dust, embryo seeds, which never attain maturity. The flowers are quite scentless.

This is a most useful as well as effective plant for an old wall, or to cover the high part of a rock-garden; it can be absolutely relied upon to withstand drought.

Cultivation

This species will grow on rock-work, as well as on a roof, flourishing better than on ordinary ground. When once fixed, it will spread fast by means of its offsets. It may easily be made to cover the whole roof of a building, whether of tiles, thatch or wood, by sticking the offsets on with a little earth. Linnaeus stated that the plant was used in this manner as a preservative to the coverings of houses in certain parts of Sweden, and it is certain that it tends to preserve thatched roofs.

The flowering-heads die soon after they have blossomed, but the offsets soon supply their places.

Part Used Medicinally

The fresh leaves and the expressed juice from them. The leaves have a saline, astringent and acid taste, but no odor.

Constituents

The leaves contain malic acid in combination with lime.

Medicinal Action and Uses

Refrigerant, astringent, diuretic. In rural districts, the bruised leaves of the fresh plant, or its juice, are often applied as a poultice to burns, scalds, contusions, scrofulous ulcers, and in inflammatory conditions of the skin generally, giving immediate relief. If the juice be mixed with clarified lard and applied to an inflamed surface, the inflammation is quickly reduced.

It can be used in many skin diseases. Some old authorities recommend mixing the juice with cream.

With honey, the juice has been used to assuage the soreness and ulcerated condition of the mouth in thrush, the mixture being used with a hair pencil.

Boerhaave, the famous Dutch physician, found 10 oz. of the juice beneficial in dysentery, but it is not admitted into modern practice.

In large doses, Houseleek juice is emetic and purgative.

Dose, 2 to 10 drops.

It is said to remove warts and corns. Parkinson tells us:

'The juice takes away corns from the toes and feet if they be bathed therewith every day, and at night emplastered as it were with the skin of the same House Leek.'

The leaves sliced in two and the inner surface applied to warts, act as a positive cure for them.

Culpepper informs us that:

'Our ordinary Houseleek is good for all inward heats, as well as outward, and in the eyes or other parts of the body: a posset made of the juice is singularly good in all hot agues, for it cooleth and tempereth the blood and spirits and quencheth the thirst; and is also good to stay all defluction or sharp and salt rheums in the eyes, the juice being dropped into them. If the juice be dropped into the ears, it easeth pain.... It cooleth and restraineth all hot inflammations St. Anthony's fire (Erysipelas), scaldings and burnings, the shingles, fretting ulcers, ringworms and the like; and much easeth the pain and the gout.'

After describing the use of the leaves in the cure of corns, he goes on to say:

'it easeth also the headache, and the distempered heat of the brain in frenzies, or through want of sleep, being applied to the temples and forehead. The leaves bruised and laid upon the crown or seam of the head, stayeth bleeding at the nose very quickly. The distilled water of the herb is profitable for all the purposes aforesaid. The leaves being gently rubbed on any place stung with nettles or bees, doth quickly take away the pain.'

Gerard tells us the:

'iuice of Houseleeke, Garden Nightshade and the buds of Poplar, boiled in hog's grease, maketh the most singular Populeon that ever was used in Chirugerie.'

Galen recommends Houseleek for erysipelas and shingles, and Dioscorides as a remedy for weak and inflamed eyes. Pliny says it never fails to produce sleep.

In the fourteenth century it was used as an ingredient of a preparation for neuralgia, called hemygreyne, i.e. megrim, and an ointment used at that time for scalds and burns.

Culpepper speaks of the Small Houseleek, the Stonecrop Houseleek, the Common Stonecrop or Wallpepper, the Orpine, the Kidneywort and the Water Houseleek, some of which are known now under different names, the name Houseleek nowadays being reserved exclusively for the above-described species, Sempervivum tectorum.

HYACINTH, GRAPE

Botanical: Muscari racemosum (MILL.)
Family: N.O. Liliaceae
Synonym: Starch Hyacinth.

The Grape Hyacinth, very much cultivated in England as a garden plant and occasionally met with in sandy soils in the eastern and southern counties, has, like the Wild Hyacinth, a poisonous bulb. The leaves are narrow and rather thick, 6 inches to a foot long, the flower-stem usually shorter, with a close, terminal raceme, or head of small, dark blue flowers, looking almost like little berries and having a sweet scent. A few of the uppermost are of a pale blue, erect, much narrower and without stamens or pistils. As the flowers of the various species of Muscari secrete much nectar, they are like the garden Scillas - to be reckoned among the useful bee plants of the spring.

The Grape Hyacinth has sometimes been called Starch Hyacinth, as the flowers have been supposed to smell of wet starch. The name of the genus, Muscari, comes from the Greek word for musk, a smell yielded by some species.

Medicinal Action and Uses

The American species Muscari comosum (Mill.) (Feather Hyacinth), or Purse Tassel, has been used, as well as other species of Muscari, for its diuretic and stimulant properties. Comisic acid has been extracted from the bulb, and apparently acts like Saponin.

The innumerable varieties of Garden Hyacinth are derived from an Eastern plant, Hyacinthus orientalis.

HYACINTH, WILD

Botanical: Hyacinthus nonscriptus
Family: N.O. Rosaceae
Synonyms---Bluebell. Scilla nutans. Nodding Squill. Scilla nonscriptus. Agraphis nutans.
Part Used: Roots.
Habitat: Woods of Britain.

History The Wild Hyacinth is in flower from early in April till the end of May, and being a perennial, and spreading rapidly, is found year after year in the same spot, forming a mass of rich color in the woods where it grows. The long leaves remain above ground until late in the autumn. From the midst of very long, narrow leaves, rising from the small bulb and overtopping them, rises the flower-stem, bearing the pendulous 'bluebells' arranged in a long, curving line. Each flower has two small bracts at the base of the short flower-stalk of pedicel. The perianth (the term applied when the parts of the calyx and corolla are so similar in form and color that no difference is perceptible) is bluish-purple and composed of six leaflets. The flowers have a slight, starch-like scent.

This is the 'fair-hair'd hyacinth' of Ben Jonson, a name alluding to the old myth, for tradition associates the flower with the Hyacinth of the Ancients, the flower of grief and mourning, so Linnaeus first called it Hyacinthus. Hyacinthus was a charming and handsome Spartan youth, loved by both Apollo and Zephyrus. Hyacinthus preferred the Sun-God to the God of the West, who sought to be revenged. One day, when Apollo was playing quoits with the youth, a quoit that he threw was blown by Zephyrus out of its proper course and it struck and killed Hyacinthus. Apollo, stricken with grief, raised from his blood a purple flower on which the letters 'ai, ai,' were traced, so that the cry of woe might for evermore have existence on the earth. As our English variety of Hyacinth had no trace of these mystic letters, our older botanists called it Hyacinthus nonscriptus, or 'not written on.' A later generic name, Agraphis, is of similar meaning, being a compound of two Greek words, meaning 'not to mark.'

The bulbs are poisonous in the fresh state. The viscid juice so abundantly contained in them and existing in every part of the plant has been used as a substitute for starch and in the days when stiff ruffs were worn was much in request, being thought second only to Wake-robin roots. It was also used for fixing feathers on arrows, instead of glue and as bookbinders' gum for the covers of books.

The roots, dried and powdered, are balsamic, having some styptic properties which have not been fully investigated.

It has been found to be one of the best remedies for leucorrhoea. The decoction of the juice of the root operates by urine.

Dosage

From 1 to 3 grains.

HYDRANGEA

Botanical: Hydrangea arborescens (LINN.)
Family: N.O. Saxifragaceae
Synonyms: Wild Hydrangea. Seven Barks. Hydrangea vulgaris. Common Hydrangea.
Parts Used: Dried rhizome, roots.
Habitat: The United States.

History

The Hydrangeas are marsh or aquatic plants, and hence the name is derived from a Greek compound signifying water-vessel. Four of the known species are natives of America; one, the garden Hydrangea (Hydrangea hortensis), is widely cultivated in the gardens of China and Japan. Many methods are employed in this country for imparting the blue tinge to its petals. The oak-leaved Hydrangea (H. quercifolia), a native of Florida, is also cultivated for its beauty.

The bark of H. arborescens is rough, with a tendency to peel, each layer being of a different color, from which it has probably derived its name 'Seven Barks.' The roots are of variable length and thickness, having numerous radicles, reaching a diameter of more than half an inch. They are externally pale grey, tough, with splintery fracture; white inside, without odor, having a sweetish, rather pungent taste. When fresh, the root and stalks are very succulent, containing much water, and can easily be cut. When dry, they are tough and resistant, so that they should be bruised or cut into short, transverse sections while fresh. The taste of the bark of the dried root resembles that of cascarilla. The stalks contain a pith which is easily removed, and they are used in some parts of the country for pipe-stems.

Constituents

The root has been found to contain two resins, gum, sugar, starch, albumen, soda, lime potassa, magnesia, sulphuric and phosphoric acids, a protosalt of iron, and a glucoside, Hydrangin. No tannin has been found, but a fixed oil and a volatile oil have been obtained. From the alcoholic extract of the flowers of H. hortensia, two crystalline substances were isolated, Hydragenol and Hydrangeaic acid.

Medicinal Action and Uses

Diuretic, cathartic, tonic. The decoction is said to have been used with great advantage by the Cherokee Indians, and later, by the settlers, for calculous diseases. It does not cure stone in the bladder, but, as demonstrated to the medical profession by Dr. S. W. Butler, of Burlington, N.J., it removes gravelly deposits and relieves the pain consequent on their emission. As many as 120 calculi have been known to come from one person under its use.

The fluid extract is principally used for earthy deposits, alkaline urine, chronic gleet, and mucous irritations of the bladder in aged persons. A concentrated syrup with sugar or honey, or a simple decoction of the root, may also be used. In overdoses, it will cause vertigo, oppressions of the chest, etc. The leaves are said by Dr. Eoff to be tonic, silagogue, cathartic and diuretic.

Dosage

30 grains. Of fluid extract, 30 to 100 minims. Of syrup, 1 teaspoonful, three times a day.

HYDROCOTYLE

Botanical: Hydrocotyle Asiatica (LINN.)
Family: N.O. Umbelliferae
Synonyms: Indian Pennywort. Marsh Penny. White Rot. Thick-leaved Pennywort.
Part Used: Leaves.
Habitat: Asia and Africa.

Description

A small umbelliferous plant growing in Southern Africa and India, indigenous to the Southern United States. The special characteristics of the leaflets are petiolate, reniform, crenate, seven nerved and nearly glabrous.

Constituents

An oily volatile liquid called vellarin (which has a strong smell reminiscent of the plant, and a bitter, pungent, persistent taste) and tannic acid.

Medicinal Action and Uses

A valuable medicine for its diuretic properties; has long been used in India as an aperient or alterative tonic, useful in fever and bowel complaints and a noted remedy for leprosy, rheumatism and ichthyosis; employed as a poultice for syphilitic ulcers. In small doses it acts as a stimulant, in large doses as a narcotic, causing stupor and headache and with some people vertigo and coma.

Other Species

The native species is not unlike the Indian variety, but there is a slight difference in the leaves.

European hydrocotyle vulgaris (syn. Common Pennywort). Leaves orbicular and peltate. The plant appears to have no noxious qualities; it grows freely in boggy places on the edges of lakes and rivers.

The plant has come into disfavour because it is said to cause footrot in sheep.

HYDROPHILIA

Botanical: Hydrophilia spinosa
Family: N.O. Acanthaceae
Synonym: Asteracantha Longifolia.
Parts Used: Root, seeds, dried herb.
Habitat: India, widely distributed in the sub-tropical regions of the world.

Description

The name is derived from the Greek, and refers to the medical doctrine of fluids in the body. It has tapering roots, a number of rootlets, and upright square stems; leaves and branches opposite, nodes swollen near them; the stem and leaves have three- to five-celled stiff hairs. Flowers, four pairs awl-shaped and like leaves in shape. Corolla glabrous on lower lip. Fruit has four to eight flattened brownish seeds, which contain a quantity of strong mucilage. The drug has no special odor or taste.

Constituents

Chiefly mucilage, fixed oil, phytosterol, and a trace of an alkaloidal substance, properties similar to Couchgrass.

Medicinal Action and Uses

Demulcent and a diuretic for catarrh of the urinary organs; the dried herb and root, or rhizome, has long been used in India for dropsy, especially when accompanied by hepatic obstruction. It is a popular aphrodisiac. In Southern India the root is the commercial part, but in Bombay the seeds are mostly used.

Preparation

Decoction, 2 oz. of root to 3 pints of water boiled down to 1 pint. Dose, 1/2 to 2 fluid ounces. Official in India and the Eastern Colonies.

HYSSOP

Botanical: Hyssopus officinalis (LINN.)
Family: N.O. Labiatae
Part Used: Herb.

Hyssop is a name of Greek origin. The Hyssopos of Dioscorides was named from azob (a holy herb), because it was used for cleaning sacred places. It is alluded to in the Scriptures: 'Purge me with Hyssop, and I shall be clean.'

Cultivation

It is an evergreen, bushy herb, growing 1 to 2 feet high, with square stem, linear leaves and flowers in whorls, six- to fifteen-flowered. Is a native of Southern Europe not indigenous to Britain, though stated to be naturalized on the ruins of Beaulieu Abbey in the New Forest.

Hyssop is cultivated for the use of its flower-tops, which are steeped in water to make an infusion, which is sometimes employed as an expectorant. There are three varieties, known respectively by their blue, red and white flowers, which are in bloom from

June to October, and are sometimes employed as edging plants. Grown with catmint, it makes a lovely border, backed with Lavender and Rosemary. As a kitchen herb, it is mostly used for broths and decoctions, occasionally for salad. For medicinal use the flower-tops should be cut in August.

It may be propagated by seeds, sown in April, or by dividing the plants in spring and autumn, or by cuttings, made in spring and inserted in a shady situation. Plants raised from seeds or cuttings, should, when large enough, be planted out about 1 foot apart each way, and kept watered till established. They succeed best in a warm aspect and in a light, rather dry soil. The plants require cutting in, occasionally, but do not need much further attention.

Medicinal Action and Uses

Expectorant, diaphoretic, stimulant, pectoral, carminative. The healing virtues of the plant are due to a particular volatile oil, which is stimulative, carminative and sudorific. It admirably promotes expectoration, and in chronic catarrh its diaphoretic and stimulant properties combine to render it of especial value. It is usually given as a warm infusion, taken frequently and mixed with Horehound. Hyssop Tea is also a grateful drink, well adapted to improve the tone of a feeble stomach, being brewed with the green tops of the herb, which are sometimes boiled in soup to be given for asthma. In America, an infusion of the leaves is used externally for the relief of muscular rheumatism, and also for bruises and discoloured contusions, and the green herb, bruised and applied, will heal cuts promptly.

The infusion has an agreeable flavor and is used by herbalists in pulmonary diseases.

It was once much employed as a carminative in flatulence and hysterical complaints, but is now seldom employed.

A tea made with the fresh green tops, and drunk several times daily, is one of the oldfashioned country remedies for rheumatism that is still employed. Hyssop baths have also been recommended as part of the cure, but the quantity used would need to be considerable.

Preparation

Fluid extract, 30 to 60 drops. The Hyssop of commerce (Hyssopus officinalis) occurs in Palestine, but is not conspicuous among the numerous Labiatae of the Syrian hillsides, which include thyme and marjoram, mint, rosemary and lavender. Tradition identifies the Hyssop of Scripture with the familiar herb, Marjoram (origanum), of which six species are found in the Holy Land. The common kind, so well known in cottage gardens (O. vulgare), grows only in the north, but an allied species (O. maru) abounds through the central hills, and a variety is common in the southern desert.

Dr. J. F. Royle disagrees, and identifies the Hyssop of the Bible with the Caper-plant (Capparis spinosa) which grows in the Jordan Valley, in Egypt, and the Desert, in the gorges of Lebanon, and in the Kedron Valley. It 'springs out of the walls' of the old Temple area. This view is supported by Canon Tristram and others. The Arabs call it azaf.

The leaves, stems and flowers of H. officinalis possess a highly aromatic odor and yield by distillation an essential oil of exceedingly fine odor, much appreciated by perfumers, its value being even greater than Oil of Lavender. It is also much employed in the manufacture of liqueurs, forming an important constituent in Chartreuse. Bees feed freely on the plant and the odor of the honey obtained from this source is remarkably good. The leaves are used locally as a medicinal tea. As a kitchen herb it has gone out of use because of its strong flavor, but on account of its aroma it was formerly employed as a strewing herb.

RECIPE FOR HYSSOP TEA

'Infuse a quarter of an ounce of dried hyssop flowers in a pint of boiling water for ten minutes; sweeten with honey, and take a wine glassful three times a day, for debility of the chest. It is also considered a powerful vermifuge.' (Old Cookery Book.)

HYSSOP, HEDGE

Botanical: Gratiola officinalis (LINN.)
Family: N.O. Scrophulariaceae
Parts Used: Root, herb.

Description

Hedge-Hyssop was formerly an official drug. The root and herb are still used in herbal medicine.

The plant, a perennial, is a native of the south of Europe, growing in meadows and moist grounds. The square stem rises from a creeping, scaly rhizome to the height of 6 to 12 inches, and has opposite stalkless, lanceshaped, finely serrate, smooth, pale-green leaves, and whitish, or reddish flowers, placed singly in the axils of the upper pairs of leaves, the corollas two-lipped, with yellow hairs in the tube.

The plant is inodorous, but has a bitter, nauseous, somewhat acrid taste, which earns it the name of Hedge Hyssop.

Constituents

Its active constituent is the bitter crystalline glucoside Gratiolin and a reddish, amorphous, bitter principle, Gratiosolin, likewise a glucoside.

Medicinal Action and Uses

A drastic cathartic and emetic, possessing also diuretic properties. Has been used for the relief of dropsy, and is recommended in scrofula, chronic affections of the liver, jaundice, and enlargement of the spleen, and as a worm dispeller.

Preparations

The infusion of 1/2 oz. of powdered root is taken in tablespoonful doses. Powdered root, 15 to 30 grains.

Gratiola officinalis was in former times called Gratia Dei, on account of its active medicinal properties. In large doses it is said to be poisonous. Haller says that the abundance of this plant in some of the Swiss meadows renders it dangerous to allow cattle to feed in them. G. peruviane has similar properties.' (Treasury of Botany.)

The tropical American herb Vandellia diffusa (Linn.) is used like Gratiola. The dried plant has a strong odor of tobacco.

A decoction of V. diffusa is employed medicinally in Guiana in fevers and disorders of the liver. The species are natives of the East Indies, China, Burma, and South America. Some of them are grown in this country. The generic name commemorates a Professor of Botany at Lisbon.

Curanga amara (Juss.), known as Herpestis amara (Benth.) and Gratiola amara (Roxb.), yields the important East Indian tonic and febrifuge Curanja or Koen-tao-tjao. It contains the bitter alcohol-soluble glucoside curanjiin.

Bonnaya rotundifolia (Benth.) is the East Indian Tsjanga-puspam used as an antispasmodic.

Scoparia dulcis (Linn.), a common weed of tropical America, is used as an astringent and antispasmodic under the name Vacourinha.

Many other species, native to different parts of the world, belonging to this family, are in medicinal use in a lesser degree. Nearly all of them contain bitter substances, and many possess anthelmintic properties.

HYSTERONICA

Botanical: Hysteronica Baylahuen
Family: N.O. Compositae
Synonym: Haplopappus Baylahuen.
Habitat: Western United States of America, Chile.

Description

Belongs to the same group as Solidago (Golden Rod) and is closely allied to Grindelia botanically and as a drug.

Constituents

Volatile oil, fatty oil which has the same odor as the plant, acid resin which is a mixture of four other resines, and tannin.

Medicinal Action and Uses

Stimulant, expectorant. The medicinal properties lie principally in its resin and volatile oil, the resin acting chiefly on the bowels and urinary passages, and the volatile oil on the lungs. It does not cause disorder to the stomach and bowels, it is a valuable remedy in dysentery, chronic diarrhea specially of tuberculous nature and in chronic cystitis.

The tincture, by its stimulating and protective action (like tinc. benzoin), has served as a dressing for wounds and ulcers.

Preparations

Infusion (1 : 150) has been advised, also a tincture (100 : 500) in a dose of 15 to 25 drops.

Index

A

B

C

D

E

F

G

H

I

N

O

P

Q

R

S

T

U

www.ingramcontent.com/pod-product-compliance
Lightning Source LLC
Chambersburg PA
CBHW080810280326
41926CB00091B/4120